NINTH EDITION

Burton's

MICROBIOLOGY FOR THE HEALTH SCIENCES

Paul G. Engelkirk, PhD, MT(ASCP), SM(AAM)

Biomedical Educational Services (Biomed Ed)
Belton, Texas
Adjunct Faculty, Biology Department
Temple College, Temple, TX

Janet Duben-Engelkirk, EdD, MT(ASCP)

Biomedical Educational Services (Biomed Ed)
Belton, Texas
Adjunct Faculty, Biotechnology Department
Temple College, Temple, TX

Wolters Kluwer | Lippincott Williams & Wilkins
Health

Philadelphia · Baltimore · New York · London
Buenos Aires · Hong Kong · Sydney · Tokyo

Acquisitions Editor: David B. Troy
Product Manager: John Larkin
Managing Editor: Laura S. Horowitz, Hearthside Publishing Services
Marketing Manager: Allison Powell
Designer: Steve Druding
Compositor: Maryland Composition/Absolute Service Inc.

Ninth Edition

351 West Camden Street   530 Walnut Street
Baltimore, MD 21201   Philadelphia, PA 19106

Printed in the People's Republic of China

9 8 7 6 5 4 3 2

Library of Congress Cataloging-in-Publication Data

Engelkirk, Paul G.
  Burton's microbiology for the health sciences / Paul G. Engelkirk, Janet Duben-Engelkirk. — 9th ed.
     p. ; cm.
  Includes bibliographical references and index.
  ISBN 978-1-60547-673-5
  1. Microbiology. 2. Medical microbiology. 3. Allied health personnel. I. Burton, Gwendolyn R. W.
(Gwendolyn R. Wilson) II. Duben-Engelkirk, Janet L. III. Title. IV. Title: Microbiology for the health sciences.
  [DNLM: 1. Microbiological Processes. 2. Communicable Diseases—microbiology. QW 4 E575b 2011]
  QR41.2.B88 2010
  616.9'041—dc22

                                                                                    2009036495

DISCLAIMER

Care has been taken to confirm the accuracy of the information present and to describe generally accepted practices. However, the authors, editors, and publisher are not responsible for errors or omissions or for any consequences from application of the information in this book and make no warranty, expressed or implied, with respect to the currency, completeness, or accuracy of the contents of the publication. Application of this information in a particular situation remains the professional responsibility of the practitioner; the clinical treatments described and recommended may not be considered absolute and universal recommendations.

The authors, editors, and publisher have exerted every effort to ensure that drug selection and dosage set forth in this text are in accordance with the current recommendations and practice at the time of publication. However, in view of ongoing research, changes in government regulations, and the constant flow of information relating to drug therapy and drug reactions, the reader is urged to check the package insert for each drug for any change in indications and dosage and for added warnings and precautions. This is particularly important when the recommended agent is a new or infrequently employed drug.

Some drugs and medical devices presented in this publication have Food and Drug Administration (FDA) clearance for limited use in restricted research settings. It is the responsibility of the healthcare provider to ascertain the FDA status of each drug or device planned for use in their clinical practice.

To purchase additional copies of this book, call our customer service department at **(800) 638-3030** or fax orders to **(301) 223-2320**. International customers should call **(301) 223-2300**.

Visit Lippincott Williams & Wilkins on the Internet: **http://www.lww.com**. Lippincott Williams & Wilkins customer service representatives are available from 8:30 AM to 6:00 PM, EST.

Dedicated to the original author of this book,
Dr. Gwendolyn R.W. Burton,
whose spirit lives on within its pages.

Gwen,
we will remember you,
think of you,
pray for you.
And when another day is through,
we'll still be friends with you.

(paraphrased lyrics of a song by the late and much loved John Denver)

AND

To our parents,
without whose love and support,
we could have never
fulfilled our dreams.

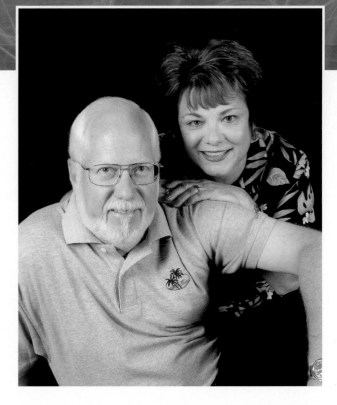

Paul G. Engelkirk, PhD, MT(ASCP), SM(AAM), is a retired professor of biological sciences in the Science Department at Central Texas College in Killeen, Texas, where he taught introductory microbiology for 12 years. Before joining Central Texas College, he was an associate professor at the University of Texas Health Science Center in Houston, Texas, where he taught diagnostic microbiology to medical technology students for 8 years. Prior to his teaching career, Dr. Engelkirk served 22 years as an officer in the U.S. Army Medical Department, supervising various immunology, clinical pathology, and microbiology laboratories in Germany, Vietnam, and the United States. He retired from the Army with the rank of Lieutenant Colonel.

Dr. Engelkirk received his bachelor's degree in biology from New York University and his master's and doctorate degree (both in microbiology and public health) from Michigan State University. He received additional medical technology and tropical medicine training at Walter Reed Army Hospital in Washington, D.C., and specialized training in anaerobic bacteriology, mycobacteriology, and virology at the Centers for Disease Control and Prevention in Atlanta, Georgia.

Dr. Engelkirk is the author or coauthor of four microbiology textbooks, 10 additional book chapters, five medical laboratory-oriented self-study courses, and many scientific articles. He also served for 14 years as coeditor of four separate newsletters for clinical microbiology laboratory personnel. Dr. Engelkirk has been engaged in various aspects of clinical microbiology for more than 45 years and is a past president of the Rocky Mountain Branch of the American Society for Microbiology. He and his wife, Janet, currently provide biomedical educational services through their consulting business (Biomed Ed), located in Belton, Texas. Dr. Engelkirk's hobbies include RVing, hiking, kayaking, nature photography, writing, and working in his yard.

Janet Duben-Engelkirk, EdD, MT(ASCP), has over 30 years of experience in clinical laboratory science and higher education. She received her bachelor's degrees in biology and medical technology and her master's degree in technical education from the University of Akron, and her doctorate in allied health education and administration from a combined program through the University of Houston and Baylor College of Medicine in Houston, Texas.

Dr. Duben-Engelkirk began her career in clinical laboratory science education teaching students "on the bench" in a community hospital in Akron, Ohio. She then became Education Coordinator for the Clinical Laboratory Science Program at the University of Texas Health Science Center at Houston, where she taught clinical chemistry and related subjects for 12 years. In 1992, Dr. Duben-Engelkirk assumed the position of Director of Allied Health and Clinical Laboratory Science Education at Scott and White Hospital in Temple, Texas, wherein her responsibilities included teaching microbiology and clinical chemistry. She also served as Interim Program Director for the Medical Laboratory Technician program at Temple College. In 2006, Dr. Duben-Engelkirk assumed the position of chair of the biotechnology department at the Texas Bioscience Institute and Temple College, where she was responsible for curriculum development and administration of the biotechnology degree programs. She is now semiretired and teaching online biotechnology courses for the Temple College Biotechnology Department. She and her husband, Paul, are also co-owners of a biomedical education consulting business.

Dr. Duben-Engelkirk was coeditor of a widely used clinical chemistry textbook and coauthored a clinical anaerobic bacteriology textbook with Paul. She has authored or coauthored numerous book chapters, journal articles, self-study courses, newsletters, and other educational materials over the course of her career.

Dr. Duben-Engelkirk has received many awards during her career, including Outstanding Young Leader in Allied Health, the American Society for Clinical Laboratory Science's Omicron Sigma Award for outstanding service, and Teaching Excellence Awards. Her professional interests include instructional technology, computer-based instruction, and distance education. Outside of the office and classroom, Dr. Duben-Engelkirk enjoys taking cruises, reading, music, yoga, movies, hiking, and camping.

Microbiology—the study of microbes—is a fascinating subject that impacts our daily lives in numerous ways. Microbes live on us and in us. They are vital in many industries. Microbes are essential for the cycling and recycling of elements such as carbon, oxygen, and nitrogen, and provide most of the oxygen in our atmosphere. They are used to clean up toxic wastes. Microbes are used in genetic engineering and gene therapy. And, of course, many microbes cause disease. In recent years, the public has been bombarded with news reports about microbe-associated medical problems such as swine flu, bird flu, severe acute respiratory syndrome (SARS), flesh-eating bacteria, mad cow disease, superbugs, black mould in buildings, West Nile virus, bioterrorism, anthrax, smallpox, food recalls as a result of *Escherichia coli* and *Salmonella* contamination, and epidemics of meningitis, hepatitis, influenza, tuberculosis, and diarrheal diseases.

WRITTEN FOR HEALTHCARE PROFESSIONALS

Burton's Microbiology for the Health Sciences has been written primarily for nurses and other healthcare professionals. This book provides students of these professions with vital microbiology information that will enable them to carry out their duties in an informed, safe, and efficient manner. It is appropriate for use in any one-semester introductory microbiology course, whether for students of the healthcare professions or for science or biology majors. Unlike many of the other introductory microbiology texts on the market, *all* of the material in this book can be covered in a single semester.

Chapters of special importance to students of the healthcare professions include those dealing with antibiotics and other antimicrobial agents, epidemiology and public health, healthcare-associated infections, infection control, how microbes cause disease, how our bodies protect us from pathogens and infectious diseases, and the major viral, bacterial, fungal, and parasitic diseases of humans.

NEW TO THE NINTH EDITION

The most obvious changes in the ninth edition are an increased number of color illustrations and the redistribution of information about infectious diseases. The eighth edition's lengthy and somewhat cumbersome chapter on infectious diseases (Chapter 17) has been divided into five chapters (Chapters 17 through 21 in the ninth edition). The artwork has been expanded and updated to make it more useful and more appealing. Color illustrations appear throughout the book, rather than being grouped together in one location. The book is divided into eight major sections, containing a total of 21 chapters. Each chapter contains a Chapter Outline, Learning Objectives, Self-Assessment Exercises, and information about the contents of the Student CD-ROM. Interesting historical information, in the form of "Historical Notes," is spread throughout the book and is presented in appropriate chapters.

STUDENT-FRIENDLY FEATURES

The authors have made every attempt to create a student-friendly book. The book can be used by all types of students, including those with little or no science background and mature students returning to school after an absence of several years. It is written in a clear and concise manner. It contains more than 30 Study Aid boxes, which summarize important information and explain difficult concepts and similar-sounding terms. New terms are highlighted and defined in the text, and are included in a Glossary at the back of the book.

Answers to Self-Assessment Exercises contained in the book can be found in Appendix A. Appendix B contains a summary of key points about the most important bacterial pathogens discussed in the book. In the past, students have found this appendix to be especially helpful. Appendix C contains useful formulas for conversion of one type of unit to another (e.g., Fahrenheit to Celsius and vice versa). Because Greek letters are commonly used in microbiology, the Greek alphabet can be found in Appendix D.

STUDENT CD-ROM

The Student CD-ROM included with the book provides a vast amount of supplemental information.

Each section of the CD-ROM includes the primary objectives of the chapter, a list of new terms introduced in the chapter, a review of key points, and sections entitled "Insight," "Increase Your Knowledge," and "Critical Thinking." Case Studies are provided for the chapters on infectious diseases. The Student CD-ROM also contains answers to the Self-Assessment Exercises found in the book, and additional Self-Assessment Exercises with answers. Instructor information on "thePoint" includes suggested laboratory exercises, suggested audiovisual aids, an image bank, a test generator, and answers to the various Case Studies and Self-Assessment Exercises in the book and on the Student CD-ROM.

TO OUR READERS

As you will discover, the concise nature of this book makes each sentence significant. Thus, you will be intellectually challenged to learn each new concept as it is presented. It is our hope that you will enjoy your study of microbiology and be motivated to further explore this exciting field, especially as it relates to your occupation. Many students who have used this textbook in their introductory microbiology course have gone on to become infection control nurses, epidemiologists, clinical laboratory scientists (medical technologists), and microbiologists.

OUR THANKS

We are deeply indebted to all of the people who helped with the editing and publication of this book. Special thanks to our extremely efficient Managing Editor, Ms. Laura Horowitz, who was an absolute delight to work with; to Gregory Bond, MSN, for his thorough review of the previous edition; to the authors of other Lippincott Williams & Wilkins textbooks, whose illustrations appear throughout the book; to Dr. Patrick Hidy, RN, and Christine Vernon, for providing many of the drawings; and to David B. Troy, Acquisitions Editor; Allison Powell, Marketing Manager; and Meredith Brittain and John Larkin, Product Managers from Lippincott Williams & Wilkins.

Paul G. Engelkirk, PhD, MT(ASCP), SM(AAM)
Janet Duben-Engelkirk, EdD, MT(ASCP)

In today's health careers, a thorough understanding of microbiology is more important than ever. *Burton's Microbiology for the Health Sciences, Ninth Edition*, not only provides the conceptual knowledge you will need but also teaches you how to apply it. This User's Guide introduces you to the features and tools of this innovative textbook. Each feature is specifically designed to enhance your learning experience, preparing you for a successful career as a health professional.

CHAPTER OPENER FEATURES

The features that open each chapter are an introduction to guide you through the remainder of the lesson.

Chapter Outline

Serves as a "roadmap" to the material ahead.

Learning Objectives

Highlight important concepts—helping you to organize and prioritize learning.

Introduction

Familiarizes you with the material covered in the chapter.

CHAPTER FEATURES

The following features appear throughout the body of the chapter. They are designed to hone critical thinking skills and judgment, build clinical proficiency, and promote comprehension and retention of the material.

Historical Note Boxes

Provide insight into the history and development of microbiology and healthcare.

Spotlighting Boxes

A new feature spotlighting healthcare careers.

Study Aid Boxes

Summarize key information, explain difficult concepts, and differentiate similar-sounding terms.

Clinical Procedure Boxes

Set forth step-by-step instructions for common procedures.

Something To Think About

These boxes contain information that will stimulate students to ponder interesting possibilities.

Test Preparation Features

These features help you review chapter content and test yourself before exams.

Highlighted Key Points

Help you pinpoint the main ideas of the text.

Self-Assessment Exercises

Help you gauge your understanding of what you have learned.

On the CD-ROM Box

Directs you to additional content and exercises for review on the companion CD-ROM.

BONUS CD-ROM

Packaged with this textbook, the CD-ROM is a powerful learning tool. It includes the following features that help reinforce and review the material covered in the book:

Chapter Learning Tools

- Primary Objectives of Each Chapter
- Lists of New Terms Introduced in Each Chapter
- Review of Key Points
- Answers to Text-Based Exercises
- Additional Self-Assessment Exercises with Answers

Also included are special "Insight," "Increase Your Knowledge," "Critical Thinking," and "Case Study" sections that provide additional information and exercises as well as fun facts on selected topics from the text.

Additional Appendices

1. Microbial Intoxications
2. Phyla and Medically Significant Genera within the Domain *Bacteria*
3. Basic Chemistry Concepts
4. Responsibilities of the Clinical Microbiology Laboratory
5. Clinical Microbiology Laboratory Procedures
6. Preparing Solutions and Dilutions

CONTENTS

APPENDICES

MICROBIOLOGY—THE SCIENCE

1

LEARNING OBJECTIVES

AFTER STUDYING THIS CHAPTER, YOU SHOULD BE ABLE TO:

- Define microbiology, pathogen, nonpathogen, and opportunistic pathogen
- Differentiate between acellular microbes and microorganisms and list several examples of each
- List several reasons why microbes are important (e.g., as a source of antibiotics)
- Explain the relationship between microbes and infectious diseases
- Differentiate between infectious diseases and microbial intoxications
- Outline some of the contributions of Leeuwenhoek, Pasteur, and Koch to microbiology
- Differentiate between biogenesis and abiogenesis
- Explain the germ theory of disease
- Outline Koch's Postulates and cite some circumstances in which they may not apply
- Discuss two medically related fields of microbiology

INTRODUCTION

Welcome to the fascinating world of microbiology, where you will learn about creatures so small that they cannot be seen with the naked eye. In this chapter, you will discover the effects that these tiny creatures have on our daily lives and the environment around us, and why knowledge of them is of great importance to healthcare professionals. You will learn that some of them are our friends, whereas others are our enemies. You are about to embark on an exciting journey. Enjoy the adventure!

WHAT IS MICROBIOLOGY?

The study of microbiology is essentially an advanced biology course. Ideally, students taking microbiology will have some background in biology. Although **biology** is the study of *living* organisms (from *bios*, referring to living organisms, and *logy*, meaning "the study of"), microbiology includes the study of certain nonliving entities as well as certain living organisms. Collectively, these nonliving entities and living organisms are called **microbes**. *Micro* means very small—anything so small that it must be viewed with a **microscope** (an optical instrument used to observe very small objects). Therefore, **microbiology** can be defined as the *study of microbes*. Individual microbes can be observed only with the use of various types of microscopes. Microbes are said to be *ubiquitous*, meaning they are virtually everywhere.

> Microbiology is the study of microbes. Individual microbes can be observed only with the use of various types of microscopes.

The various categories of microbes include viruses, bacteria, archaea, protozoa, and certain types of algae and fungi (Fig. 1-1). These categories of microbes are discussed in detail in Chapters 4 and 5. Because most scientists do not consider viruses to be living organisms, they are often referred to as "acellular microbes" or "infectious particles" rather than microorganisms.

> The two major categories of microbes are called acellular microbes (also called infectious particles) and cellular microbes (also called microorganisms). Acellular microbes include viruses and prions. Cellular microbes include all bacteria, all archaea, some algae, all protozoa, and some fungi.

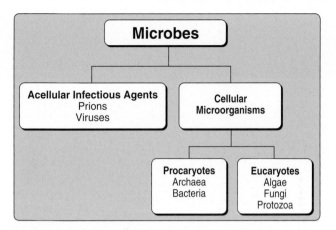

FIGURE 1-1. Acellular and cellular microbes.
Acellular microbes (also known as infectious particles) include prions and viruses. Cellular microbes include the less complex procaryotes (organisms composed of cells that lack a true nucleus, such as archaea and bacteria) and the more complex eucaryotes (organisms composed of cells that contain a true nucleus, such as algae, protozoa, and fungi). Procaryotes and eucaryotes are discussed more fully in Chapter 3.

Your first introduction to microbes may have been when your mother warned you about "germs" (Fig. 1-2). Although not a scientific term, germs are the microbes that cause disease.
Your mother worried that you might become infected with these types of microbes. Disease-causing microorganisms are technically known as **pathogens** (also referred to as infectious agents) (Table 1-1). Actually, only about 3% of known microbes are capable of causing disease (i.e., only about 3% are pathogenic). Thus, the vast majority of known microbes are **nonpathogens**—microbes that do not cause disease. Some nonpathogens are beneficial to us, whereas others have no effect on us at all. In newspapers and on television, we read and hear more about pathogens than we do about nonpathogens, but in this book you will learn about both categories—the microbes that help us ("microbial allies") and those that harm us ("microbial enemies").

> Microbes that cause disease are known as pathogens. Those that do not cause disease are called nonpathogens.

WHY STUDY MICROBIOLOGY?

Although they are very small, microbes play significant roles in our lives. Listed below are a few of the many reasons to take a microbiology course and to learn about microbes:

- We have, living on and in our bodies (e.g., on our skin and in our mouths and intestinal tract), approximately 10 times as many microbes

> The microbes that live on and in the human body are referred to as our indigenous microflora.

as the total number of cells (i.e., epithelial cells, nerve cells, muscle cells, etc.) that make up our bodies (10 trillion cells × 10 = 100 trillion microbes). It has been estimated that perhaps as many as 500 to 1,000 different species of microbes live on and in us. Collectively, these microbes are known as our **indigenous microflora** (or indigenous microbiota) and, for the most part, they are of benefit to us. For example, the indigenous microflora inhibit the growth of pathogens in those areas of the body where they live by occupying space, depleting the food supply, and secreting materials (waste products, toxins, antibiotics, etc.) that may prevent or reduce the growth of pathogens. Indigenous microflora are discussed more fully in Chapter 10.

- Some of the microbes that colonize (inhabit) our bodies are known as **opportunistic pathogens** (or *opportunists*). Although these microbes usually do not cause us any problems, they have the potential to cause infections if they gain access to a part of our anatomy where they do not belong. For example,

> Opportunistic pathogens do not cause disease under ordinary conditions, but have the potential to cause disease should the opportunity present itself.

Don't touch that filthy thing. It's covered with germs.

FIGURE 1-2. "Germs." In all likelihood, your mother was your first microbiology instructor. Not only did she alert you to the fact that there were "invisible" critters in the world that could harm you, she also taught you the fundamentals of hygiene—like handwashing.

TABLE 1-1	Pathogens
CATEGORY	**EXAMPLES OF DISEASES THEY CAUSE**
Algae	A very rare cause of infections; intoxications (which result from ingestion of toxins)
Bacteria	Anthrax, botulism, cholera, diarrhea, diphtheria, ear and eye infections, food poisoning, gas gangrene, gonorrhea, hemolytic uremic syndrome (HUS), intoxications, Legionnaires' disease, leprosy, Lyme disease, meningitis, plague, pneumonia, Rocky Mountain spotted fever, scarlet fever, staph infections, strep throat, syphilis, tetanus, tuberculosis, tularemia, typhoid fever, typhus, urethritis, urinary tract infections, whooping cough
Fungi	Allergies, cryptococcosis, histoplasmosis, intoxications, meningitis, pneumonia, thrush, tinea (ringworm) infections, yeast vaginitis
Protozoa	African sleeping sickness, amebic dysentery, babesiosis, Chagas' disease, cryptosporidiosis, diarrhea, giardiasis, malaria, meningoencephalitis, pneumonia, toxoplasmosis, trichomoniasis
Viruses	Acquired immunodeficiency syndrome (AIDS), "bird flu," certain types of cancer, chickenpox, cold sores (fever blisters), common cold, dengue, diarrhea, encephalitis, genital herpes infections, German measles, hantavirus pulmonary syndrome (HPS), hemorrhagic fevers, hepatitis, infectious mononucleosis, influenza, measles, meningitis, monkeypox, mumps, pneumonia, polio, rabies, severe acute respiratory syndrome (SARS), shingles, smallpox, warts, yellow fever

a bacterium called *Escherichia coli* (*E. coli*) lives in our intestinal tracts. This organism does not cause us any harm as long as it remains in our intestinal tract but can cause disease if it gains access to our urinary bladder, bloodstream, or a wound. Other opportunistic pathogens strike when a person becomes run-down, stressed-out, or debilitated (weakened) as a result of some disease or condition. Thus, opportunistic pathogens can be thought of as microbes awaiting the opportunity to cause disease.

• Microbes are essential for life on this planet as we know it. For example, some microbes produce oxygen by the process known as **photosynthesis** (discussed in Chapter 7). Actually, microbes contribute more oxygen to our atmosphere than do plants. Thus, organisms that require oxygen—humans, for example—owe a debt of gratitude to the algae and cyanobacteria (a group of photosynthetic bacteria) that produce oxygen.

• Many microbes are involved in the decomposition of dead organisms and the waste products of living organisms. Collectively, they are referred to as **decomposers** or **saprophytes**. By definition, a saprophyte is an organism that lives on dead or decaying organic matter. Imagine living in a world with no decomposers. Not a pleasant thought! Saprophytes aid in fertilization by returning inorganic nutrients to the soil. They break down dead and dying organic materials (plants and animals) into nitrates, phosphates, and other chemicals necessary for the growth of plants (Fig. 1-3).

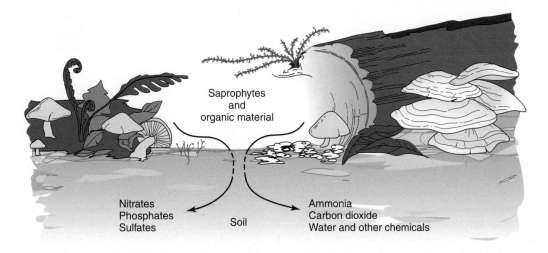

Saprophytes and organic material

Nitrates
Phosphates
Sulfates

Soil

Ammonia
Carbon dioxide
Water and other chemicals

FIGURE 1-3. Saprophytes. Saprophytes break down dead and decaying organic material into inorganic nutrients in the soil.

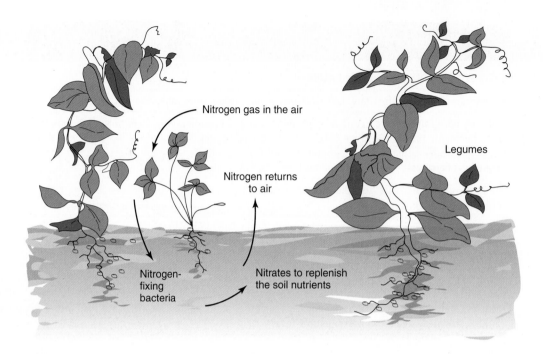

FIGURE 1-4. Nitrogen fixation. Nitrogen-fixing bacteria that live on or near the roots of legumes convert free nitrogen from the air into ammonia in the soil. Nitrifying bacteria then convert the ammonia into nitrites and nitrates, which are nutrients used by plants.

- Some microbes are capable of decomposing industrial wastes (oil spills, for example). Thus, we can use microbes—genetically engineered microbes, in some cases—to clean up after ourselves. The use of microbes in this manner is called **bioremediation**, a topic discussed in more detail in Chapter 10. **Genetic engineering** is discussed briefly in a following section and more fully in Chapter 7.
- Many microbes are involved in elemental cycles, such as the carbon, nitrogen, oxygen, sulfur, and phosphorous cycles. In the nitrogen cycle, certain bacteria convert nitrogen gas in the air to ammonia in the soil. Other soil bacteria then convert the ammonia to nitrites and nitrates. Still other bacteria convert the nitrogen in nitrates to nitrogen gas, thus completing the cycle (Fig. 1-4). Knowledge of these microbes is important to farmers who practice crop rotation to replenish nutrients in their fields and to gardeners who keep compost pits as a source of natural fertilizer. In both cases, dead organic material is broken down into inorganic nutrients (e.g., nitrates and phosphates) by microbes. The study of the relationships between microbes and the environment is called **microbial ecology**. Microbial ecology and the nitrogen cycle are discussed more fully in Chapter 10.
- Algae and bacteria serve as food for tiny animals. Then, larger animals eat the smaller creatures, and so on. Thus, microbes serve as important links in food chains (Fig. 1-5). Microscopic organisms in the ocean, collectively referred to as **plankton**, serve as the starting point of many food chains. Tiny marine plants and algae are called **phytoplankton**, whereas tiny marine animals are called **zooplankton**.
- Some microbes live in the intestinal tracts of animals, where they aid in the digestion of food and, in some cases, produce substances that are of value to the host animal. For example, the *E. coli* bacteria that live in the human intestinal tract produce vitamins K and B_1, which are absorbed and used by the human body. Although termites eat wood, they cannot digest wood. Fortunately for them, termites have cellulose-eating protozoa in their intestinal tracts that break down the wood that the termites consume into smaller molecules that the termites can use as nutrients.

FIGURE 1-5. Food chain. Tiny living organisms such as bacteria, algae, microscopic aquatic plants (e.g., phytoplankton), and microscopic aquatic animals (e.g., zooplankton) are eaten by larger animals, which in turn are eaten by still larger animals, etc., until an animal in the chain is consumed by a human. Humans are at the top of the food chain.

TABLE 1-2	Products Requiring Microbial Participation in the Manufacturing Process
CATEGORY	**EXAMPLES**
Foods	Acidophilus milk, bread, butter, buttermilk, chocolate, coffee, cottage cheese, cream cheese, fish sauces, green olives, kimchi (from cabbage), meat products (e.g., country-cured hams, sausage, salami), pickles, poi (fermented taro root), sauerkraut, sour cream, sourdough bread, soy sauce, various cheeses (e.g., cheddar, Swiss, Limburger, Camembert, Roquefort and other blue cheeses), vinegar, yogurt
Alcoholic beverages	Ale, beer, brandy, sake (rice wine), rum, sherry, vodka, whiskey, wine
Chemicals	Acetic acid, acetone, butanol, citric acid, ethanol, formic acid, glycerol, isopropanol, lactic acid
Antibiotics	Amphotericin B, bacitracin, cephalosporins, chloramphenicol, cycloheximide, cycloserine, erythromycin, griseofulvin, kanamycin, lincomycin, neomycin, novobiocin, nystatin, penicillin, polymyxin B, streptomycin, tetracycline

- Many microbes are essential in various food and beverage industries, whereas others are used to produce certain enzymes and chemicals (Table 1-2). The use of living organisms or their derivatives to make or modify useful products or processes is called **biotechnology**, an exciting and timely topic that is discussed more fully in Chapter 10.

- Some bacteria and fungi produce antibiotics that are used to treat patients with infectious diseases. By definition, an **antibiotic** is a substance produced by a microbe that is effective in killing or inhibiting the growth of other microbes. The use of microbes in the antibiotic industry is an example of biotechnology. Production of antibiotics by microbes is discussed in Chapter 9.

- Microbes are essential in the field of genetic engineering. In genetic engineering, a gene or genes from one organism (e.g., from a bacterium, a human, an animal, or a plant) is/are inserted into a bacterial or yeast cell. Because a gene contains the instructions for the production of a gene product (usually a protein), the cell that receives a new gene can now produce whatever product is coded for by that gene; so too can all of the cells that arise from the original cell. Microbiologists have engineered bacteria and yeasts to produce a variety of useful substances, such as insulin, various types of growth hormones, interferons, and materials for use as vaccines. Genetic engineering is discussed more fully in Chapter 7.

- For many years, microbes have been used as "cell models." The more that scientists learned about the structure and functions of microbial cells, the more they learned about cells in general. The intestinal bacterium *E. coli* is one of the most studied of all microbes. By studying *E. coli*, scientists have learned a great deal about the composition and inner workings of cells, including human cells.

- Finally, we come to diseases. Microbes cause two categories of diseases: infectious diseases and microbial intoxications (Fig. 1-6). An **infectious disease** results when a pathogen colonizes the body and subsequently causes disease. A **microbial intoxication** results when a person ingests a *toxin* (poisonous substance) that has been produced by a microbe. Of the two categories, infectious diseases cause far more illnesses and deaths. Infectious diseases are the

> Pathogens cause two major types of diseases: infectious diseases and microbial intoxications.

FIGURE 1-6. The two categories of diseases caused by pathogens. Infectious diseases result when a pathogen colonizes (inhabits) the body and subsequently causes disease. Microbial intoxications result when a person ingests a toxin (poisonous substance) that has been produced by a pathogen in vitro (outside the body).

leading cause of death in the world and the third leading cause of death in the United States (after heart disease and cancer). Worldwide, infectious diseases cause about 50,000 deaths per day, with the majority of deaths occuring in developing countries. Anyone pursuing a career in a healthcare profession must be aware of infectious diseases, the pathogens that cause them, the sources of the pathogens, how these diseases are transmitted, and how to protect yourself and your patients from these diseases. Physicians' assistants, nurses, surgical technologists, dental assistants, laboratory technologists, respiratory therapists, orderlies, nurses' aides, and all others who are associated with patients and patient care must take precautions to prevent the spread of pathogens. Harmful microbes may be transferred from health workers to patients; from patient to patient; from contaminated mechanical devices, instruments, and syringes to patients; from contaminated bedding, clothes, dishes, and food to patients; and from patients to healthcare workers, hospital visitors, and other susceptible persons. To limit the spread of pathogens, sterile, aseptic, and antiseptic techniques (discussed in Chapter 12) are used everywhere in hospitals, nursing homes, operating rooms, and laboratories. In addition, the bioterrorist activities of recent years serve to remind us that everyone should have an understanding of the agents (pathogens) that are involved and how to protect ourselves from becoming infected. Bioterrorist and biological warfare agents are discussed in Chapter 11. Additional information about microbial intoxications can be found in CD-ROM Appendix 1 ("Microbial Intoxications").

FIRST MICROORGANISMS ON EARTH

Perhaps you have wondered how long microbes have existed on Earth. Scientists tell us that the Earth was formed about 4.5 billion years ago and, for the first 800 million to 1 billion years of Earth's existence, there was no life on this planet. Fossils of primitive microbes (as many as 11 different types) found in ancient rock formations in northwestern Australia date back to about 3.5 billion years ago. By comparison, animals and humans are relative newcomers. Animals made their appearance on Earth between 900 and 650 million years ago (there is some disagreement in the scientific community about the exact date), and, in their present form, humans (*Homo sapiens*) have existed for only the past 100,000 years or so. Candidates for the first microbes on Earth are archaea and cyanobacteria; these types of microbes are discussed in Chapter 4.

EARLIEST KNOWN INFECTIOUS DISEASES

In all likelihood, infectious diseases of humans and animals have existed for as long as humans and animals have

inhabited the planet. We know that human pathogens have existed for thousands of years because damage caused by them has been observed in the bones and internal organs of mummies and early human fossils. By studying mummies, scientists have learned that bacterial diseases, such as tuberculosis and syphilis, and parasitic worm infections, such as schistosomiasis, dracunculiasis (guinea worm infection), and tapeworm infections, have been around for a very long time.

The earliest known account of a "pestilence" occurred in Egypt about 3180 BC. This may represent the first recorded epidemic, although words like *pestilence* and *plague* were used without definition in early writings. Around 1900 BC, near the end of the Trojan War, the Greek army was decimated by an epidemic of what is thought to have been bubonic plague. The Ebers papyrus, describing epidemic fevers, was discovered in a tomb in Thebes, Egypt; it was written around 1500 BC. A disease thought to be smallpox occurred in China around 1122 BC. Epidemics of plague occurred in Rome in 790, 710, and 640 BC and in Greece around 430 BC.

In addition to the diseases already mentioned, there are early accounts of rabies, anthrax, dysentery, smallpox, ergotism, botulism, measles, typhoid fever, typhus fever, diphtheria, and syphilis. The syphilis story is quite interesting. It made its first appearance in Europe in 1493. Many people believe that syphilis was carried to Europe by Native Americans who were brought to Portugal by Christopher Columbus. The French called syphilis the *Neapolitan disease*; the Italians called it the *French or Spanish disease*; and the English called it the *French pox*. Other names for syphilis were Spanish, German, Polish, and Turkish pocks. The name "syphilis" was not given to the disease until 1530.

PIONEERS IN THE SCIENCE OF MICROBIOLOGY

Bacteria and protozoa were the first microbes to be observed by humans. It then took about 200 years before a connection was established between microbes and infectious diseases. Among the most significant events in the early history of microbiology were the development of microscopes, bacterial staining procedures, techniques that enabled microorganisms to be cultured (grown) in the laboratory, and steps that could be taken to prove that specific microbes were responsible for causing specific infectious diseases. During the past 400 years, many individuals contributed to our present understanding of microbes. Three early microbiologists are discussed in this chapter; others are discussed at appropriate points throughout the book.

Anton van Leeuwenhoek (1632–1723)

Because Anton van Leeuwenhoek was the first person to see live bacteria and protozoa, he is sometimes referred to as the "Father of Microbiology," the "Father of

FIGURE 1-7. Portrait of Anton van Leeuwenhoek by Jan Verkolje. (Courtesy of en.wikipedia.org)

ined scrapings from his teeth, water from ditches and ponds, water in which he had soaked peppercorns, blood, sperm, and even his own diarrheal stools. In many of these specimens, he observed various tiny living creatures, which he called "animalcules." Leeuwenhoek recorded his observations in the form of letters, which he sent to the Royal Society of London. The following passage is an excerpt from one of those letters (*Milestones in Microbiology*, edited by Thomas Brock. American Society for Microbiology, Washington, DC, 1961):

> Tho my teeth are kept usually very clean, nevertheless when I view them in a Magnifying Glass, I find growing between them a little white matter as thick as wetted flower . . . I therefore took some of this flower and mixt it . . . with pure rain water wherein were no Animals . . . and then to my great surprize perceived that the aforesaid matter contained very many small living Animals, which moved themselves very extravagantly . . . The number of these Animals in the scurf of a mans Teeth, are so many that I believe they exceed the number of Men in a kingdom. For upon the examination of a small parcel of it, no thicker than a Horse-hair, I found too many living Animals therein, that I guess there might have been 1000 in a quantity of matter no bigger than the 1/100 part of a sand.

Bacteriology," and the "Father of Protozoology".[a] Interestingly, Leeuwenhoek was not a trained scientist. At various times in his life, he was a fabric merchant, a surveyor, a wine assayer, and a minor city official in Delft, Holland. As a hobby, he ground tiny glass lenses, which he mounted in small metal frames, thus creating what today are known as **single-lens microscopes** or **simple microscopes**. During his lifetime, he made more than 500 of these microscopes. Leeuwenhoek's fine art of grinding lenses that would magnify an object to 200 to 300 times its size was lost at his death because he had not taught this skill to anyone during his lifetime. In one of the hundreds of letters that he sent to the Royal Society of London, he wrote:

> My method for seeing the very smallest animalcules I do not impart to others; nor how to see very many animalcules at one time. This I keep for myself alone.

Apparently, Leeuwenhoek had an unquenchable curiosity, as he used his microscopes to examine almost anything he could get his hands on (Fig. 1-7). He exam-

Leeuwenhoek's letters finally convinced scientists of the late 17th century of the existence of microbes. Leeuwenhoek never speculated on their origin, nor did he associate them with the cause of disease. Such relationships were not established until the work of Louis Pasteur and Robert Koch in the late 19th century.

The following quote is from Paul de Kruif's book, *Microbe Hunters*, Harcourt Brace, 1926:

> [Leeuwenhoek] had stolen and peeped into a fantastic sub-visible world of little things, creatures that had lived, had bred, had battled, had died, completely hidden from and unknown to all men from the beginning of time. Beasts these were of a kind that ravaged and annihilated whole races of men ten million times larger than they were themselves. Beings these were, more terrible than fire-spitting dragons or hydra-headed monsters. They were silent assassins that murdered babes in warm cradles and kings in sheltered places. It was this invisible, insignificant, but implacable—and sometimes friendly—world that Leeuwenhoek had looked into for the first time of all men of all countries.

Once scientists became convinced of the existence of tiny creatures that could not be observed with the naked eye, they began to speculate on their origin. On the basis of observation, many of the scientists of that time believed that life could develop spontaneously from inanimate

---

[a] Although Leeuwenhoek was probably the first person to see *live* protozoa, he may not have been the first person to observe protozoa. Many scholars believe that Robert Hooke (1635-1703), an English physician, was the first person to observe and describe microbes, including a fossilized protozoan and two species of live microfungi.

substances, such as decaying corpses, soil, and swamp gases. The idea that life can arise spontaneously from nonliving material is called the theory of spontaneous generation or **abiogenesis**. For more than 2 centuries, from 1650 to 1850, this theory was debated and tested. Following the work of others, Louis Pasteur (discussed later) and John Tyndall (discussed in Chapter 3) finally disproved the theory of spontaneous generation and proved that life can only arise from preexisting life. This is called the theory of **biogenesis**, first proposed by a German scientist named Rudolf Virchow in 1858. Note that the theory of biogenesis does not speculate on the *origin* of life, a subject that has been discussed and debated for hundreds of years.

Louis Pasteur (1822–1895)

Louis Pasteur (Fig. 1-8), a French chemist, made numerous contributions to the newly emerging field of microbiology and, in fact, his contributions are considered by many people to be the foundation of the science of microbiology and a cornerstone of modern medicine. Listed below are some of his most significant contributions:

- While attempting to discover why wine becomes contaminated with undesirable substances, Pasteur

FIGURE 1-8. Pasteur in his laboratory. A 1925 wood engraving by Timothy Cole. (From Zigrosser C. Medicine and the Artist [Ars Medica]. New York: Dover Publications, Inc., 1970. By permission of the Philadelphia Museum of Art.)

discovered what occurs during alcoholic fermentation (discussed in Chapter 7). He also demonstrated that different types of microbes produce different fermentation products. For example, yeasts convert the glucose in grapes to ethyl alcohol (ethanol) by fermentation, but certain contaminating bacteria, such as *Acetobacter*, convert glucose to acetic acid (vinegar) by fermentation, thus, ruining the taste of the wine.

- Through his experiments, Pasteur dealt the fatal blow to the theory of spontaneous generation.
- Pasteur discovered forms of life that could exist in the absence of oxygen. He introduced the terms "aerobes" (organisms that require oxygen) and "anaerobes" (organisms that do not require oxygen).
- Pasteur developed a process (today known as pasteurization) to kill microbes that were causing wine to spoil—an economic concern to France's wine industry. **Pasteurization** can be used to kill pathogens in many types of liquids. Pasteur's process involved heating wine to 55°C[b] and holding it at that temperature for several minutes. Today, pasteurization is accomplished by heating liquids to 63° to 65°C for 30 minutes or to 73° to 75°C for 15 seconds. It should be noted that pasteurization does not kill *all* of the microbes in liquids—just the pathogens.
- Pasteur discovered the infectious agents that caused the silkworm diseases that were crippling the silk industry in France. He also discovered how to prevent such diseases.
- Pasteur made significant contributions to the germ theory of disease—the theory that specific microbes cause specific infectious diseases. For example, anthrax is caused by a specific bacterium (*Bacillus anthracis*), whereas tuberculosis is caused by a different bacterium (*Mycobacterium tuberculosis*).
- Pasteur championed changes in hospital practices to minimize the spread of disease by pathogens.
- Pasteur developed vaccines to prevent chicken cholera, anthrax, and swine erysipelas (a skin disease). It was the development of these vaccines that made him famous in France. Before the vaccines, these diseases were decimating chickens, sheep, cattle, and pigs in that country—a serious economic problem.
- Pasteur developed a vaccine to prevent rabies in dogs and successfully used the vaccine to treat human rabies.

To honor Pasteur and continue his work, especially in the development of a rabies vaccine, the Pasteur Institute was created in Paris in 1888. It became a clinic for rabies treatment, a research center for infectious diseases, and a teaching center. Many scientists who studied under Pasteur went on to make important discoveries of

---

[b] "C" is an abbreviation for Celsius. Although Celsius is also referred to as centigrade, Celsius is preferred. Formulas for converting Celsius to Fahrenheit and vice versa can be found in Appendix C ("Useful Conversions").

An Ethical Dilemma for Louis Pasteur

In July 1885, while he was developing a vaccine that would prevent rabies in dogs, Louis Pasteur faced an ethical decision. A 9-year-old boy, named Joseph Meister, had been bitten 14 times on the legs and hands by a rabid dog. At the time, it was assumed that virtually anyone who was bitten by a rabid animal would die. Meister's mother begged Pasteur to use his vaccine to save her son. Pasteur was a chemist, not a physician, and thus was not authorized to treat humans. Also, his experimental vaccine had never been administered to a human being. Nonetheless, 2 days after the boy had been bitten, Pasteur injected Meister with the vaccine in an attempt to save the boy's life. The boy survived, and Pasteur realized that he had developed a rabies vaccine that could be administered to a person after they had been infected with rabies virus.

their own and create a vast international network of Pasteur Institutes. The first of the foreign institutes was founded in Saigon, Vietnam, which today is known as Ho Chi Minh City. One of the directors of that institute was Alexandre Emile Jean Yersin—a former student of Robert Koch and Louis Pasteur—who, in 1894, discovered the bacterium that causes plague.

Robert Koch (1843–1910)

Robert Koch (Fig. 1-9), a German physician, made numerous contributions to the science of microbiology. Some of them are listed here:

- Koch made many significant contributions to the germ theory of disease. For example, he proved that the anthrax bacillus (*B. anthracis*), which had been discovered earlier by other scientists, was truly the cause of anthrax. He accomplished this using a series of scientific steps that he and his colleagues had developed; these steps later became known as Koch's Postulates (described later in this chapter).
- Koch discovered that *B. anthracis* produces spores, capable of resisting adverse conditions.
- Koch developed methods of fixing, staining, and photographing bacteria.
- Koch developed methods of cultivating bacteria on solid media. One of Koch's colleagues, R.J. Petri, invented a flat glass dish (now known as a **Petri dish**) in which to culture bacteria on solid media. It was Frau Hesse—the wife of another of Koch's colleagues—who suggested the use of agar (a polysaccharide obtained from seaweed) as a solidifying agent. These methods enabled Koch to obtain pure cultures of bacteria. The term **pure culture** refers to a condition in which only

FIGURE 1-9. Robert Koch. (Courtesy of www.wpclipart.com).

one type of organism is growing on a solid culture medium or in a liquid culture medium in the laboratory; no other types of organisms are present.
- Koch discovered the bacterium (*M. tuberculosis*) that causes tuberculosis and the bacterium (*Vibrio cholerae*) that causes cholera.
- Koch's work on tuberculin (a protein derived from *M. tuberculosis*) ultimately led to the development of a skin test valuable in diagnosing tuberculosis.

Koch's Postulates

During the mid- to late-1800s, Robert Koch and his colleagues established an experimental procedure to prove that a specific microbe is the cause of a specific infectious disease. This scientific procedure, published in 1884, became known as **Koch's Postulates** (Fig. 1-10).

Koch's Postulates (paraphrased):

1. A particular microbe must be found in all cases of the disease and must not be present in healthy animals or humans.
2. The microbe must be isolated from the diseased animal or human and grown in pure culture in the laboratory.

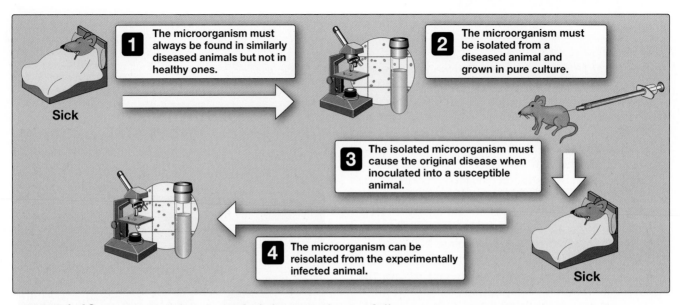

FIGURE 1-10. Koch's Postulates: proof of the germ theory of disease. (From Harvey RA et al. Lippincott's Illustrated Reviews, Microbiology, 2nd ed. Philadelphia: Lippincott Williams & Wilkins, 2007.)

3. The same disease must be produced when microbes from the pure culture are inoculated into healthy susceptible laboratory animals.
4. The same microbe must be recovered from the experimentally infected animals and grown again in pure culture.

After completing these steps, the microbe is said to have fulfilled Koch's Postulates and has been proven to be the cause of that particular infectious disease. Koch's Postulates not only helped to prove the germ theory of disease, but also gave a tremendous boost to the development of microbiology by stressing laboratory culture and identification of microbes.

Exceptions to Koch's Postulates

Circumstances do exist in which Koch's Postulates cannot be fulfilled. Examples of such circumstances are as follows:

• To fulfill Koch's Postulates, it is necessary to grow (culture) the pathogen in the laboratory (in vitro[c]) in or on artificial culture media. However, certain pathogens will not grow on artificial media. Such pathogens include viruses, rickettsias (a category of bacteria), chlamydias (another category of bacteria), and the bacteria that cause leprosy and syphilis. Viruses, rickettsias, and chlamydias are called *obligate intracellular pathogens* (or *obligate intracellular parasites*) because they can only survive and multiply within living host cells. Such

organisms can be grown in cell cultures (cultures of living human or animal cells of various types), embryonated chicken eggs, or certain animals (referred to as laboratory animals). In the laboratory, the leprosy bacterium (*Mycobacterium leprae*) is propagated in armadillos, and the spirochetes of syphilis (*Treponema pallidum*) grow well in the testes of rabbits and chimpanzees. Microbes having complex and demanding nutritional requirements are said to be **fastidious** (meaning fussy). Although certain fastidious organisms can be grown in the laboratory by adding special mixtures of vitamins, amino acids, and other nutrients to the culture media, others cannot be grown in the laboratory because no one has discovered what ingredient(s) to add to the medium to enable them to grow.

• To fulfill Koch's Postulates, it is necessary to infect laboratory animals with the pathogen being studied. However, many pathogens are species-specific, meaning that they infect only one species of animal. For example, some pathogens that infect humans will *only* infect humans. Thus, it is not always possible to find a laboratory animal that can be infected with a pathogen that causes human disease. Because human volunteers are difficult to obtain and ethical reasons limit their use, the researcher may only be able to observe the changes caused by the pathogen in human cells that can be grown in the laboratory (called cell cultures).

• Some diseases, called **synergistic infections**, are caused not by one particular microbe, but by the combined effects of two or more different microbes. Examples of such infections include acute necrotizing ulcerative gingivitis (ANUG; also known as "trench mouth") and bacterial vaginosis. It is very difficult to reproduce such synergistic infections in the laboratory.

---

[c] As used in this book, the term **in vitro** refers to something that occurs *outside* the living body, whereas the term **in vivo** refers to something that occurs *within* the living body. In vitro often refers to something that occurs in the laboratory.

• Another difficulty that is sometimes encountered while attempting to fulfill Koch's Postulates is that certain pathogens become altered when grown in vitro. Some become less pathogenic, whereas others become non-pathogenic. Thus, they will no longer infect animals after being cultured on artificial media.

It is also important to keep in mind that not all diseases are caused by microbes. Many diseases, such as rickets and scurvy, result from dietary deficiencies. Some diseases are inherited because of an abnormality in the chromosomes, as in sickle cell anemia. Others, such as diabetes, result from malfunction of a body organ or system. Still others, such as cancer of the lungs and skin, are influenced by environmental factors. However, all infectious diseases are caused by microbes, as are all microbial intoxications.

> All infectious diseases and microbial intoxications are caused by microbes.

CAREERS IN MICROBIOLOGY

A **microbiologist** is a scientist who studies microbes. He or she might have a bachelor's, master's, or doctoral degree in microbiology.

There are many career fields within the science of microbiology. For example, a person may specialize in the study of just one particular category of microbes. A **bacteriologist** is a scientist who specializes in **bacteriology**—the study of the structure, functions, and activities of bacteria. Scientists specializing in the field of **phycology** (or algology) study the various types of algae and are called **phycologists** (or algologists). **Protozoologists** explore the area of **protozoology**—the study of protozoa and their activities. Those who specialize in the study of fungi, or **mycology**, are called **mycologists**. **Virology** encompasses the study of viruses and their effects on living cells of all types. **Virologists** and cell biologists may become genetic engineers who transfer genetic material (deoxyribonucleic acid or DNA) from one cell type to another. Virologists may also study prions and viroids, acellular infectious agents that are even smaller than viruses (discussed in Chapter 4).

Other career fields in microbiology pertain more to applied microbiology—that is, how a knowledge of microbiology can be applied to different aspects of society, medicine, and industry. Two medically related career fields are discussed here; other microbiology career fields are discussed on the CD-ROM that accompanies this book. The scope of microbiology has broad, far-reaching effects on humans and their environment.

Medical and Clinical Microbiology

Medical microbiology is an excellent career field for individuals having interests in medicine and microbiology. The field of medical microbiology involves the study of pathogens, the diseases they cause, and the body's defenses against disease. This field is concerned with epidemiology, transmission of pathogens, disease-prevention measures, aseptic techniques, treatment of infectious diseases, immunology, and the production of vaccines to protect people and animals against infectious diseases. The complete or almost complete eradication of diseases like smallpox and polio, the safety of modern surgery, and the successful treatment of victims of infectious diseases are attributable to the many technological advances in this field. A branch of medical microbiology, called **clinical microbiology** or **diagnostic microbiology**, is concerned with the laboratory diagnosis of infectious diseases of humans. This is an excellent career field for individuals with interests in laboratory sciences and microbiology. Diagnostic microbiology and the clinical microbiology laboratory are discussed in Chapter 13.

> **ON THE CD-ROM**
> • Terms Introduced in This Chapter
> • Review of Key Points
> • Insight: Additional Careers in Microbiology
> • Increase Your Knowledge
> • Critical Thinking
> • Additional Self-Assessment Exercises

SELF-ASSESSMENT EXERCISES

After studying this chapter, answer the following multiple-choice questions.

1. Which of the following individuals is considered to be the "Father of Microbiology?"
   a. Anton von Leeuwenhoek ✓
   b. Louis Pasteur
   c. Robert Koch
   d. Rudolf Virchow
2. The microbes that usually live on or in a person are collectively referred to as:
   a. germs.
   b. indigenous microflora. ✓
   c. nonpathogens.
   d. opportunistic pathogens.
3. Microbes that live on dead and decaying organic material are known as:
   a. indigenous microflora.
   b. parasites.
   c. pathogens.
   d. saprophytes. ✓
4. The study of algae is called:
   a. algaeology.
   b. botany.
   c. mycology.
   d. phycology. ✓

5. The field of parasitology involves the study of which of the following types of organisms?
   a. arthropods, bacteria, fungi, protozoa, and viruses
   b. arthropods, helminths, and certain protozoa
   c. bacteria, fungi, and protozoa
   d. bacteria, fungi, and viruses
6. Rudolf Virchow is given credit for proposing which of the following theories?
   a. abiogenesis
   b. biogenesis
   c. germ theory of disease
   d. spontaneous generation
7. Which of the following microbes are considered obligate intracellular pathogens?
   a. chlamydias, rickettsias, *M. leprae*, and *T. pallidum*
   b. *M. leprae* and *T. pallidum*
   c. *M. tuberculosis* and viruses
   d. rickettsias, chlamydias, and viruses

8. Which of the following statements is true?
   a. Koch developed a rabies vaccine.
   b. Microbes are ubiquitous.
   c. Most microbes are harmful to humans.
   d. Pasteur conducted experiments that proved the theory of abiogenesis.
9. Which of the following are even smaller than viruses?
   a. chlamydias
   b. prions and viroids
   c. rickettsias
   d. cyanobacteria
10. Which of the following individuals introduced the terms "aerobes" and "anaerobes"?
   a. Anton von Leeuwenhoek
   b. Louis Pasteur
   c. Robert Koch
   d. Rudolf Virchow

VIEWING THE MICROBIAL WORLD

2

LEARNING OBJECTIVES

AFTER STUDYING THIS CHAPTER, YOU SHOULD BE ABLE TO:

- Explain the interrelationships among the following metric system units of length: centimeters, millimeters, micrometers, and nanometers
- State the metric units used to express the sizes of bacteria, protozoa, and viruses
- Compare and contrast the various types of microscopes, to include simple microscopes, compound light microscopes, electron microscopes, and atomic force microscopes

INTRODUCTION

Microbes are very tiny. But how tiny are they? Generally, some type of microscope is required to see them; thus, microbes are said to be *microscopic*. Various types of microscopes are discussed in this chapter. The metric system will be discussed first, however, because metric system units of length are used to express the sizes of microbes and the resolving power of optical instruments.

USING THE METRIC SYSTEM TO EXPRESS THE SIZES OF MICROBES

In microbiology, metric units (primarily micrometers and nanometers) are used to express the sizes of mi-crobes. The basic unit of length in the metric system, the meter (m), is equivalent to approximately 39.4 inches and is, therefore, about 3.4 inches longer than a yard. A meter may be divided into 10 (10^1) equally spaced units called **decimeters**; or 100 (10^2) equally spaced units called **centimeters**; or 1,000 (10^3) equally spaced units called **millimeters**; or 1 million (10^6) equally spaced units called **micrometers**; or 1 billion (10^9) equally spaced units called **nanometers**. Interrelationships among these units are shown in Figure 2-1. Formulas that can be used to convert inches into centimeters, millimeters, etc., can be found in Appendix C ("Useful Conversions") at the back of the book.

It should be noted that the old terms *micron* (μ)[a] and *millimicron* (mμ) have been replaced by the terms *micrometer* (μm) and *nanometer* (nm), respectively. An *angstrom* (Å) is 0.1 nanometer (0.1 nm). Using this scale, human red blood cells are about 7 μm in diameter.

The sizes of bacteria and protozoa are usually expressed in terms of micrometers. For example, a typical spherical bacterium (**coccus**; pl., **cocci**) is approximately 1 μm in diameter. About seven cocci could fit side by side across a human red blood cell. If the head of a pin was 1 mm (1,000 μm) in diameter, then

> The sizes of bacteria are expressed in micrometers, whereas the sizes of viruses are expressed in nanometers.

---

[a] The Greek letter μ is pronounced "mew." Greek letters are frequently used in science, including the science of microbiology. To aid students who are unfamiliar with the Greek alphabet, Appendix D contains the complete Greek alphabet.

FIGURE 2-1. Representations of metric units of measure and numbers.

1 meter

	Centimeters	Millimeters	Micrometers	Nanometers
One meter contains	100	1,000	1,000,000	1,000,000,000
One centimeter contains	1	10	10,000	10,000,000
One millimeter contains		1	1,000	1,000,000
One micrometer contains			1	1,000
One nanometer contains				1

$$10 = 1 \times 10^1$$
$$100 = 1 \times 10^2$$
$$1,000 = 1 \times 10^3$$
$$1,000,000 = 1 \times 10^6$$
$$1,000,000,000 = 1 \times 10^9$$

1,000 cocci could be placed side by side on the pinhead. A typical rod-shaped bacterium (**bacillus**; pl., **bacilli**) is about 1 μm wide × 3 μm long, although some bacilli are shorter and some form very long filaments. The sizes of viruses are expressed in terms of nanometers. Most of the viruses that cause human disease range in size from about 10 to 300 nm, although some (e.g., Ebola virus, a cause of hemorrhagic fever) can be as long as 1,000 nm (1 μm). Some very large protozoa reach a length of 2,000 μm (2 mm).

In the microbiology laboratory, the sizes of cellular microbes are measured using an ocular micrometer, a tiny ruler within the eyepiece (ocular) of the compound light microscope (described later). Before it can be used to measure objects, however, the ocular micrometer must first be calibrated, using a measuring device called a **stage micrometer**. Calibration must be performed for each of the objective lenses to determine the distance between the marks on the ocular micrometer. The ocular micrometer can then be used to measure lengths and widths of microbes and other objects on the specimen slide. The sizes of some microbes are shown in Figure 2-2 and Table 2-1.

> An ocular micrometer is used to measure the dimensions of objects being viewed with a compound light microscope.

MICROSCOPES

The human eye, a telescope, a pair of binoculars, a magnifying glass, and a microscope can all be thought of as various types of optical instruments. A **microscope** is an optical instrument that is used to observe tiny objects, often objects that cannot be seen at all with the unaided human eye (the "naked eye"). Each optical instrument has a limit as to what can be seen using that instrument. This limit is referred to as the **resolving power** or **resolution** of the instrument. Resolving power is discussed in more detail later in the chapter. Table 2-2 contains the resolving powers for various optical instruments.

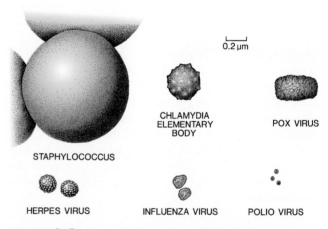

0.2 μm

STAPHYLOCOCCUS

CHLAMYDIA ELEMENTARY BODY

POX VIRUS

HERPES VIRUS

INFLUENZA VIRUS

POLIO VIRUS

FIGURE 2-2. The relative sizes of *Staphylococcus* and *Chlamydia* bacteria and several viruses.
Poliovirus is one of the smallest viruses that infect humans. (From Winn WC Jr, et al. Koneman's Color Atlas and Textbook of Diagnostic Microbiology, 6th ed. Philadelphia: Lippincott Williams & Wilkins, 2006.)

TABLE 2-1   Relative Sizes of Microbes

MICROBE OR MICROBIAL STRUCTURE	DIMENSION(S)	APPROXIMATE SIZE (μm)
Viruses (most)	Diameter	0.01–0.3
Bacteria		
Cocci (spherical bacteria)	Diameter	average = 1
Bacilli (rod-shaped bacteria)	Width × length	average = 1 × 3
	Filaments (width)	1
Fungi		
Yeasts	Diameter	3–5
Septate hyphae (hyphae containing cross-walls)	Width	2–15
Aseptate hyphae (hyphae without cross-walls)	Width	10–30
Pond water protozoa		
Chlamydomonas	Length	5–12
Euglena	Length	35–55
Vorticella	Length	50–145
Paramecium	Length	180–300
Volvox[a]	Diameter	350–500
Stentor[a]	Length (when extended)	1,000–2,000

[a]These organisms are visible with the unaided human eye.

TABLE 2-2   Characteristics of Various Types of Microscopes

TYPE	RESOLVING POWER	USEFUL MAGNIFICATION	CHARACTERISTICS
Brightfield	0.2000 μm	×1,000	Used to observe morphology of microorganisms such as bacteria, protozoa, fungi, and algae in living (unstained) and nonliving (stained) state Cannot observe microbes less than 0.2 μm in diameter or thickness, such as spirochetes and viruses
Darkfield	0.2000 μm	×1,000	Unstained organisms are observed against a dark background Useful for examining thin spirochetes Slightly more difficult to operate than brightfield
Phase-contrast	0.2000 μm	×1,000	Can be used to observe unstained living microorganisms
Fluorescence	0.2000 μm	×1,000	Fluorescent dye attached to organism Primarily an immunodiagnostic technique (immunofluorescence) Used to detect microbes in cells, tissues, and clinical specimens
Transmission electron microscope (TEM)	0.0002 mm (0.2 nm)	×200,000	Specimen is viewed on a screen Excellent resolution Allows examination of cellular and viral ultrastructure Specimen is nonliving Reveals internal features of thin specimens
Scanning electron microscope (SEM)	0.0200 mm (20 nm)	×10,000	Specimen is viewed on a screen Gives the illusion of depth (three-dimensions) Useful for examining surface features of cells and viruses Specimen is nonliving Resolution is less than that of TEM

FIGURE 2-3. Leeuwenhoek's microscopes. (A) Leeuwenhoek's microscopes were very simple devices. Each had a tiny glass lens, mounted in a brass plate. The specimen was placed on the sharp point of a brass pin, and two screws were used to adjust the position of the specimen. The entire instrument was about 3 to 4 inches long. It was held very close to the eye.
(B) Although his microscopes had a magnifying capability of only around ×200 to ×300, Leeuwenhoek was able to create remarkable drawings of different types of bacteria that he observed. (From Volk WA, et al. Essentials of Medical Microbiology, 5th ed. Philadelphia: Lippincott-Raven, 1996.)

Simple Microscopes

A **simple microscope** is defined as a microscope containing only one magnifying lens. Actually, a magnifying glass could be considered a simple microscope. Images seen when using a magnifying glass usually appear about 3 to 20 times larger than the object's actual size. During the late 1600s, Anton van Leeuwenhoek, who was discussed in Chapter 1, used simple microscopes to observe many tiny objects, including bacteria and protozoa (Fig. 2-3). Because of his unique ability to grind glass lenses, scientists believe that Leeuwenhoek's simple microscopes had a maximum magnifying power of about ×300 (300 times).

Compound Microscopes

A **compound microscope** is a microscope that contains more than one magnifying lens. Although the first person to construct and use a compound microscope is not known with certainty, Hans Jansen and his son Zacharias are often given credit for being the first (see the following "Historical Note"). Compound light microscopes usually magnify objects about 1,000 times. Photographs taken through the lens system of compound microscopes are called **photomicrographs**.

> A simple microscope contains only one magnifying lens, whereas a compound microscope contains more than one magnifying lens.

Because visible light (from a built-in light bulb) is used as the source of illumination, the compound microscope is also referred to as a **compound light microscope**. It is the wavelength of visible light (approximately 0.45 μm) that limits the size of objects that can be seen using the compound light microscope. When using the compound light microscope, objects cannot be seen if they are smaller than half of the wavelength of

HISTORICAL NOTE

Early Compound Microscopes

Hans Jansen, an optician in Middleburg, Holland, is often given credit for developing the first compound microscope, sometime between 1590 and 1595. Although his son, Zacharias, was only a young boy at the time, Zacharias apparently later took over production of the Jansen microscopes. The Jansen microscopes contained two lenses and achieved magnifications of only ×3 to ×9. Compound microscopes having a three-lens system were later used by Marcello Malpighi in Italy and Robert Hooke in England, both of whom published papers between 1660 and 1665 describing their microscopic findings. In his 1665 book entitled *Micrographia*, Hooke described a fossilized shell of a foraminiferan—a type of protozoan—and two species of microscopic fungi. Some scientists consider these to be the first written descriptions of microorganisms and feel that Hooke (rather than Leeuwenhoek) should be given credit for discovering microbes. Some early compound microscopes are shown in Figure 2-4.

FIGURE 2-4. **A Leeuwenhoek microscope (center), surrounded by examples of early compound light microscopes.** (Not to scale.)

visible light. A compound light microscope is shown in Figure 2-5, and the functions of its various components are described in Table 2-3.

The compound light microscopes used in today's laboratories contain two magnifying lens systems. Within the eyepiece or ocular is a lens called the **ocular lens**; it usually has a magnifying power of ×10. The second magnifying

Total magnification of the compound light microscope is calculated by multiplying the magnifying power of the ocular lens by the magnifying power of the objective being used.

lens system is in the objective, which is positioned immediately above the object to be viewed. The four objectives used in most laboratory compound light microscopes are ×4, ×10, ×40, and ×100 objectives. As shown in Table 2-4, total magnification is calculated by multiplying the magnifying power of the ocular (×10) by the magnifying power of the objective that you are using.

The ×4 objective is rarely used in microbiology laboratories. Usually, specimens are first observed using the ×10 objective. Once the specimen is in focus, the high-power or "high-dry" objective is then swung into position.

FIGURE 2-5. A modern compound light microscope.

This lens can be used to study algae, protozoa, and other large microorganisms. However, the oil-immersion objective (total magnification = ×1,000) must be used to study bacteria, because they are so tiny. To use the oil-immersion objective, a drop of immersion oil must first be placed between the specimen and the objective; the immersion oil reduces the scattering of light and ensures that the light will enter the oil-immersion lens. The oil-immersion objective cannot be used without immersion oil. The oil is not required when using the other objectives.

For optimal observation of the specimen, the light must be properly adjusted and focused. The condenser, located beneath the stage, focuses light onto the specimen, adjusts the amount of light, and shapes the cone of light entering the objective. Generally, the higher the magnification, the more light that is needed.

As magnification is increased, the amount of light striking the object being examined must also be increased. There are three correct ways to accomplish this: (a) by opening the iris diaphragm in the condenser, (b) by opening the field diaphragm, and (c) by increasing the intensity of light being emitted from the microscope's light bulb, by turning the rheostat knob clockwise. Turning the knob that raises and lowers the condenser is an *incorrect* way to adjust lighting.

Magnification alone is of little value unless the enlarged image possesses increased detail and clarity. Image clarity depends on the microscope's resolving power (or resolution), which is the ability of the lens system to distinguish between two adjacent objects. If two objects are moved closer and closer together, there comes a point when the objects are so close together that the lens system can no longer resolve them as two separate objects (i.e., they are so close together that they appear to be one object). That distance between them, at which they cease to be seen as separate objects, is referred to as the resolving power of the optical instrument. Knowing the resolving power of an optical instrument also defines the smallest object that can be seen with that instrument. For example, the resolving power of the unaided human eye is approximately 0.2 mm. Thus, the unaided human eye is unable to see objects smaller than 0.2 mm in diameter.

> The resolving power or resolution of an optical instrument is its ability to distinguish between two adjacent objects. The resolving power of the unaided human eye is 0.2 mm.

TABLE 2-3   Components of the Compound Light Microscope

COMPONENT	LOCATION	FUNCTION
(A) Ocular lens (also known as an eyepiece); a monocular microscope has one; a binocular microscope (such as shown in Fig. 2-5) has two	At the top of the microscope	The ocular lens is an ×10 magnifying lens
(B) Revolving nosepiece	Above the stage	Holds the objective lenses
(C) Objective lenses	Held in place above the stage stage by the revolving nosepiece	Used to magnify objects placed on the stage
(D) Stage	Directly beneath the nosepiece and objective lenses	Flat surface on which the specimen is placed
Stage adjustment knobs (not shown in Fig. 2-5)	Beneath the stage	Used to move the stage and microscope slide
(E) Iris diaphragm control arm	On the condenser	Used to adjust the amount of light passing through the condenser
(F) Condenser	Beneath the stage	Contains a lens system that focuses light onto the specimen
(G) Collector lens with field diaphragm	Beneath the condenser	Controls the amount of light entering the condenser
(H) Rheostat control knob	Front side of the base	Controls the amount of light emitted from the light source
(I) Field diaphragm lever	Attached to the field diaphragm	Used to adjust the amount of light passing through the collector lens
(J) On/off switch	On the side of the base	Turns the light source on and off
(K) Base		Contains the light source
(L) Condenser control knob	Beneath and behind the condenser	Used to adjust the height of the condenser
(M & N) Fine and coarse adjustment knobs	On the arm of the microscope near the base	Used to focus the objective lenses
(O) Arm		Supports the binocular body and the revolving nosepiece; held with one hand when carrying the microscope, with the other hand beneath the base to support the weight of the microscope
(P) Binocular body		Holds the ocular lenses in their proper locations

NOTE: Letters in parentheses refer to parenthesized letters in Figure 2-5.

TABLE 2-4   Magnifications Achieved Using the Compound Light Microscope

OBJECTIVE	TOTAL MAGNIFICATION ACHIEVED WHEN THE OBJECTIVE IS USED IN CONJUNCTION WITH AN ×10 OBJECTIVE OCULAR LENS
×4 (scanning objective)	×40
×10 (low-power objective)	×100
×40 (high-dry objective)	×400
×100 (oil-immersion objective)	×1,000

The resolving power of the compound light microscope is approximately 1,000 times better than the resolving power of the unaided human eye. In practical terms, this means that objects can be examined with the compound microscope that are as much as 1,000 times smaller than the smallest objects that can be seen with the unaided human eye. Using a compound light microscope, we can see objects down to about 0.2 μm in diameter.

> The resolving power of the compound light microscope is approximately 0.2 μm, which is approximately one half the wavelength of visible light.

Additional magnifying lenses could be added to the compound light microscope, but this would not increase the resolving power. As stated earlier, as long as visible light is used as the source of illumination, objects smaller than half of the wavelength of visible light cannot be seen. Increasing magnification without increasing the resolving power is called **empty magnification**. It does no good to increase magnification without increasing resolving power.

Because objects are observed against a bright background (or "bright field") when using a compound light microscope, that microscope is sometimes referred to as a **brightfield microscope**. If the regularly used condenser is replaced with what is known as a darkfield condenser, illuminated objects are seen against

> When using a brightfield microscope, a person observes objects against a bright background. When using a darkfield microscope, a person observes illuminated objects against a dark background.

a dark background (or "dark field"), and the microscope has been converted into a **darkfield microscope**. In the clinical microbiology laboratory, darkfield microscopy is routinely used to diagnose primary syphilis (the initial stage of syphilis). The etiologic (causative) agent of syphilis—a spiral-shaped bacterium, named *Treponema pallidum*—cannot be seen with a brightfield microscope because it is thinner than 0.2 μm and, therefore, is beneath the resolving power of the compound light microscope. *T. pallidum* can be seen using a darkfield microscope, however, much in the same way that you can "see" dust particles in a beam of sunlight. Dust particles are actually beneath the resolving power of the unaided eye and, therefore, cannot really be seen. What you see in the beam is sunlight being reflected off the dust particles. With the darkfield microscope, laboratory technologists do not really see the treponemes—they see the light being reflected off the bacteria, and that light is easily seen against the dark background (Fig. 2-6).

Other types of compound microscopes include phase-contrast microscopes and fluorescence microscopes. **Phase-contrast microscopes** can be used to observe unstained living microorganisms. Because the light refracted by living cells is different from the light refracted by the

FIGURE 2-6. Spiral-shaped *T. pallidum* bacterium. The etiologic agent of syphilis, as seen by darkfield microscopy. (Courtesy of the Centers for Disease Control and Prevention.)

surrounding medium, contrast is increased, and the organisms are more easily seen. **Fluorescence microscopes** contain a built-in ultraviolet (UV) light source. When UV light strikes certain dyes and pigments, these substances emit a longer wavelength light, causing them to glow against a dark background. Fluorescence microscopy is often used in immunology laboratories to demonstrate that antibodies stained with a fluorescent dye have combined with specific antigens; this is a type of immunodiagnostic procedure. (Immunodiagnostic procedures are described in Chapter 16.)

Electron Microscopes

Although extremely small infectious agents, such as rabies and smallpox viruses, were known to exist, they could not be seen until the electron microscope was developed. It should be noted that electron microscopes cannot be used to observe living organisms. Organisms are killed during the specimen-processing procedures. Even if they were not, they would be unable to survive in the vacuum created within the electron microscope.

Electron microscopes use an electron beam as a source of illumination and magnets to focus the beam. Because the wavelength of electrons traveling in a vacuum is much shorter than the wavelength of visible light—about 100,000 times shorter—electron microscopes have a much greater resolving power than compound light microscopes. There are two types of electron microscopes: transmission electron microscopes and scanning electron microscopes.

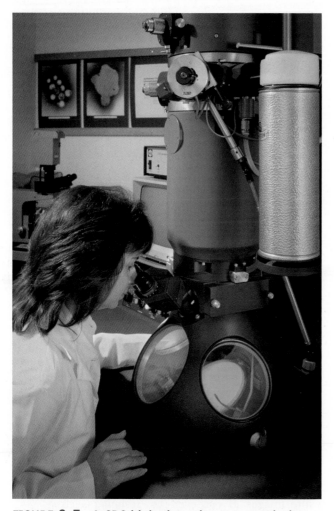

FIGURE 2-7. A CDC biologist using a transmission electron microscope. (Courtesy of James Gathany and the Centers for Disease Control and Prevention.)

FIGURE 2-8. Transmission electron micrograph of influenza virus A. (From Winn WC Jr, et al. Koneman's Color Atlas and Textbook of Diagnostic Microbiology, 6th ed. Philadelphia: Lippincott Williams & Wilkins, 2006.)

are examined, transmission electron microscopy enables scientists to study the internal structure of cells. Special staining procedures are used to increase contrast between different parts of the cell. The first transmission electron microscopes were developed during the late 1920s and early 1930s, but it was not until the early 1950s that electron microscopes began to be used routinely to study cells.

A **scanning electron microscope** (Fig. 2-9) has a shorter column and instead of being placed into the electron beam, the specimen is placed at the bottom of the column. Electrons that bounce off the surface of the specimen are captured by detectors, and an image of the specimen appears on a monitor. Scanning electron microscopes are used to observe the outer

Scanning electron microscopes have a resolving power of about 20 nm—about 100 times less than the resolving power of transmission electron microscopes.

A **transmission electron microscope** (Fig. 2-7) has a very tall column, at the top of which an electron gun fires a beam of electrons downward. When an extremely thin specimen (less than 1 μm thick) is placed into the electron beam, some of the electrons are transmitted through the specimen, and some are blocked. An image of the specimen is produced on a phosphor-coated screen at the bottom of the microscope's column. The object can be magnified up to approximately 1 million times. Thus, using a transmission electron microscope, a magnification is achieved that is about 1,000 times greater than the maximum magnification achieved using a compound light microscope. Even very tiny microbes (e.g., viruses) can be observed using a transmission electron microscope (Fig. 2-8). Because thin sections of cells

The resolving power of a transmission electron microscope is approximately 0.2 nm, which is about one million times better than the resolving power of the unaided human eye and 1,000 times better than the resolving power of the compound light microscope.

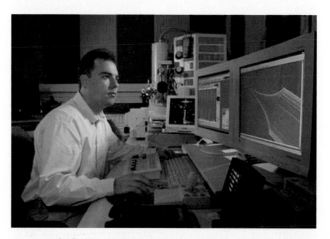

FIGURE 2-9. Scanning electron microscope. (Courtesy of the National Institute of Standards and Technology, U.S. Commerce Department.)

FIGURE 2-10. *Staphylococcus aureus* **and red blood cells, as seen by light microscopy.** (From Marler LM, et al. Direct Smear Atlas. Philadelphia: Lippincott Williams & Wilkins, 2001.)

FIGURE 2-12. Scanning electron micrograph of *S. aureus.* (Courtesy of Janice Carr, Matthew J. Arduino, and the Centers for Disease Control and Prevention.)

surfaces of specimens (i.e., surface detail). Although the resolving power of scanning electron microscopes (about 20 nm) is not quite as good as the resolving power of transmission electron microscopes (about 0.2 nm), it is still possible to observe extremely tiny objects using a scanning electron microscope. Scanning electron microscopes became available during the late 1960s.

FIGURE 2-11. Transmission electron micrograph of *S. aureus.* *S. aureus* cells in various stages of binary fission. (From Volk WA, et al. Essentials of Medical Microbiology, 5th ed. Philadelphia: Lippincott-Raven, 1996.)

Both types of electron microscopes have built-in camera systems. The photographs taken using transmission and scanning electron microscopes are called **transmission electron micrographs** (TEMs) and **scanning electron micrographs** (SEMs), respectively. They are black and white images. If you ever see *electron micrographs* in color, they have been artificially colorized. Figures 2-10, 2-11, and 2-12 show the differences in magnification and detail between photomicrographs and electron micrographs. Note that Figures 2-10, 2-11, and 2-12 all depict the same organism, but each of these illustrations was made using a different type of microscope. Refer to Table 2-2 for the characteristics of various types of microscopes.

Photographs taken using compound light microscopes are called photomicrographs. Those taken using transmission and scanning electron microscopes are called transmission electron micrographs and scanning electron micrographs, respectively.

Atomic Force Microscopes

Neither transmission nor scanning electron microscopes enable scientists to observe live microbes because of the required specimen processing procedures and subjection of the specimens to a vacuum. Atomic force microscopy (AFM) enables scientists to observe living cells at extremely high magnification and resolution under physiological conditions. Using AFM, it is possible to observe single live cells in aqueous solutions where dynamic physiological processes can be observed in real time. Unlike the scanning electron microscope, which provides a two-dimensional image of a sample, the AFM provides a true three-dimensional surface profile.

Figure 2-13 is a diagrammatic representation of an AFM. A silicon or silicon nitride cantilever having a sharp tip (probe) at its end is used to scan the specimen surface.

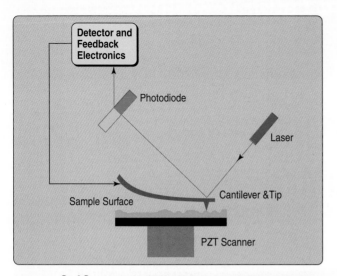

FIGURE 2-13. Atomic force microscope. See text for details. PZT, lead zirconate titanate. (Courtesy of Askewmind at en.wikipedia.)

When the tip is brought into proximity of a sample surface, forces between the tip and the sample lead to a deflection of the cantilever. Typically, the deflection is measured using a laser spot reflected from the top surface of the cantilever into an array of photodiodes, creating an image on a monitor screen. Additional information regarding AFM can be found by using an Internet search engine.

ON THE CD-ROM
- Terms Introduced in This Chapter
- Review of Key Points
- Increase Your Knowledge
- Critical Thinking
- Additional Self-Assessment Exercises

SELF-ASSESSMENT EXERCISES

After studying this chapter, answer the following multiple-choice questions.

1. A millimeter is equivalent to how many nanometers?
   a. 1,000
   b. 10,000
   c. 100,000
   d. 1,000,000
2. Assume that a pinhead is 1 mm in diameter. How many spherical bacteria (cocci), lined up side by side, would fit across the pinhead? (Hint: Use information from Table 2-1.)
   a. 100
   b. 1,000

   c. 10,000
   d. 100,000
3. What is the length of an average rod-shaped bacterium (bacillus)?
   a. 3 μm
   b. 3 nm
   c. 0.3 mm
   d. 0.03 mm
4. What is the total magnification when using the high-power (high-dry) objective of a compound light microscope equipped with a ×10 ocular lens?
   a. 40
   b. 50
   c. 100
   d. 400
5. How many times better is the resolution of the transmission electron microscope than the resolution of the unaided human eye?
   a. 1,000
   b. 10,000
   c. 100,000
   d. 1,000,000
6. How many times better is the resolution of the transmission electron microscope than the resolution of the compound light microscope?
   a. 100
   b. 1,000
   c. 10,000
   d. 100,000
7. How many times better is the resolution of the transmission electron microscope than the resolution of the scanning electron microscope?
   a. 100
   b. 1,000
   c. 10,000
   d. 100,000
8. The limiting factor of any compound light microscope (i.e., the thing that limits its resolution to 0.2 μm) is the:
   a. number of condenser lenses it has.
   b. number of magnifying lenses it has.
   c. number of ocular lenses it has.
   d. wavelength of visible light.
9. Which of the following individuals is given credit for developing the first compound microscope?
   a. Anton van Leeuwenhoek
   b. Hans Jansen
   c. Louis Pasteur
   d. Robert Hooke
10. A compound light microscope differs from a simple microscope in that the compound light microscope contains more than one:
    a. condenser lens.
    b. magnifying lens.
    c. objective lens.
    d. ocular lens.

3 CELL STRUCTURE AND TAXONOMY

LEARNING OBJECTIVES

AFTER STUDYING THIS CHAPTER, YOU SHOULD BE ABLE TO:

- Explain what is meant by the cell theory (see Historical Note: Cells)
- State the contributions of Hooke, Schleiden and Schwann, and Virchow to the study of cells
- Cite one function for each of the following parts of a eucaryotic cell: cell membrane, nucleus, ribosomes, Golgi complex, lysosomes, mitochondria, plastids, cytoskeleton, cell wall, flagella, and cilia
- Cite a function for each of the following parts of a bacterial cell: cell membrane, chromosome, cell wall, capsule, flagella, pili, and endospores
- Compare and contrast plant, animal, and bacterial cells
- Define the terms genus, specific epithet, and species
- Describe the Five-Kingdom and Three-Domain Systems of classification

INTRODUCTION

Recall from Chapter 1 that there are two major categories of microbes: **acellular microbes** (also called **in-** fectious particles) and **cellular microbes** (also called **microorganisms**). In this chapter, you will learn about the structure of microorganisms. Because they are so small, very little detail concerning their structure can be determined using the compound light microscope. Our knowledge of the ultrastucture of microbes has been gained through the use of electron microscopes. Ultrastructure refers to the very detailed views of cells that are beyond the resolving power of the compound light microscope. Also discussed in this chapter are the ways in which microbes and their cells reproduce and how microorganisms are classified.

In biology, a **cell** is defined as the fundamental unit of any living organism because, like the total organism, the cell exhibits the basic characteristics of life. A cell obtains food (nutrients) from the environment to produce energy for metabolism and other activities. **Metabolism** refers to all of the chemical reactions that occur within a cell (see Chapter 7 for a detailed discussion of metabolism and metabolic reactions). Because of its metabolism, a cell can grow and reproduce. It can respond to stimuli in its environment such as light, heat, cold, and the presence of chemicals. A cell can mutate (change genetically) as a result of accidental changes in its genetic material—

Cells

In 1665, an English physicist named Robert Hooke published a book, entitled *Micrographia*, containing descriptions of objects he had observed using a compound light microscope that he had made. These objects included molds, rusts, fleas, lice, fossilized plants and animals, and sections of cork. Hooke referred to the small empty chambers in the structure of cork as "cells," probably because they reminded him of the bare rooms (called cells) in a monastery. Hooke was the first person to use the term *cells* in this manner. Around 1838 to 1839, a German botanist named Matthias Schleiden and a German zoologist named Theodor Schwann concluded that all plant and animal tissues were composed of cells; this later became known as the **cell theory**. Then, in 1858, the German pathologist Rudolf Virchow proposed the theory of *biogenesis*—that life can only arise from preexisting life and, therefore, that cells can only arise from preexisting cells. Biogenesis does not address the issue of the origin of life on Earth, a complex topic about which much has been written.

Microorganisms

- **Acellular**
  Viroids
  Prions
  Viruses
- **Cellular**
  - **Procaryotes**
    Archaea
    Bacteria
    Cyanobacteria
  - **Eucaryotes**
    Algae
    Protozoa
    Fungi

FIGURE 3-1. Acellular and cellular microbes. Acellular microbes include viroids, prions, and viruses. Cellular microbes include the less complex procaryotes (archaea and bacteria) and the more complex eucaryotes (some algae, all protozoa, and some fungi).

the **deoxyribonucleic acid** (DNA) that makes up the genes of its chromosomes—and, thus, can become better or less suited to its environment. As a result of these genetic changes, the mutant organism may be better adapted for survival and development into a new **species** (pl., **species**) of organism.

Bacterial cells exhibit all the characteristics of life, although they do not have the complex system of membranes and *organelles* (tiny organlike structures) found in the more advanced single-celled organisms. These less complex cells, which include *Bacteria* and *Archaea*, are called **procaryotes** or **procaryotic cells**.[a] The more complex cells, containing a true nucleus and many membrane-bound organelles, are called **eucaryotes** or **eucaryotic cells**.[a] Eucaryotes include such organisms as algae, protozoa, fungi, plants, animals, and humans. Some microorganisms are procaryotic, some are eucaryotic, and some are not cells at all (Fig. 3-1).

Viruses appear to be the result of regressive or reverse evolution. They are composed of only a few genes protected by a protein coat, and sometimes may contain one or a few enzymes. Viruses depend on the energy and metabolic machinery of a host cell to reproduce. Because viruses are acellular (not composed of cells), they are placed in a completely separate category. They are discussed in detail in Chapter 4.

> Eucaryotic cells possess a true nucleus, whereas procaryotic cells do not.

For those in the health professions, it is important to learn differences in the structure of various cells, not only for identification purposes, but also to understand differences in their metabolism. These factors must be known before one can determine or explain why antimicrobial agents (drugs) attack and destroy pathogens, but do not harm human cells.

Cytology, the study of the structure and function of cells, has developed during the past 75 years with the aid of the electron microscope and sophisticated biochemical research. Many books have been written about the details of these tiny functional factories—cells—but only a brief discussion of their structure and activities is presented here.

EUCARYOTIC CELL STRUCTURE

Eucaryotes (*eu* = true; *caryo* refers to a nut or nucleus) are so named because they have a true nucleus, in that their DNA is enclosed by a nuclear membrane. Most animal and plant cells are 10 to 30 μm in diameter, about 10 times larger than most procaryotic cells. Figure 3-2 illustrates a typical eucaryotic animal cell. This illustration is a composite of most of the structures that might be found in the various types of human body cells. Figure 3-3 is a transmission electron micrograph (TEM) of an actual yeast cell. A discussion of the functional parts of eucaryotic cells can be better understood by keeping the illustrated structures in mind.

Cell Membrane

The cell is enclosed and held intact by the *cell membrane*, which is also referred to as the plasma, cytoplasmic, or cellular membrane. Structurally, it is a mosaic composed of large

> Cell membranes have selective permeability, allowing only certain substances to pass through them.

---

[a] Alternate spellings of procaryote and eucaryote are prokaryote and eukaryote.

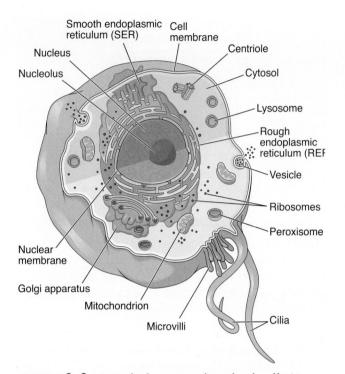

FIGURE 3-2. A typical eucaryotic animal cell. (From Cohen BJ. Memmler's The Human Body in Health and Disease, 11th ed. Philadelphia: Lippincott Williams & Wilkins, 2009.)

Eucaryotic chromosomes consist of linear DNA molecules and proteins (histones and nonhistone proteins). **Genes** are located along the DNA molecules. Although genes are sometimes described as "beads on a string," each bead (gene) is actually a particular segment of the DNA molecule. Each gene contains the genetic information that enables the cell to produce one or more **gene products**. Most gene products are proteins, but some genes code for the production of two types of **ribonucleic acid** (RNA): ribosomal ribonucleic acid (rRNA) and transfer ribonucleic acid (tRNA) molecules (discussed in Chapter 6). The organism's complete collection of genes is referred to as that organism's **genotype** (or **genome**). To understand more about how genes control the activities of the entire organism, refer to Chapters 6 and 7.

An organism's complete collection of genes is referred to as its genotype or genome.

The number and composition of chromosomes and the number of genes on each chromosome are characteristic of the particular species of organism. Different species have different numbers and sizes of chromosomes. Human diploid cells, for example, have 46 chromosomes (23 pairs), each consisting of thousands of

molecules of proteins and phospholipids (certain types of fats). The cell membrane is like a "skin" around the cell, separating the contents of the cell from the outside world. The cell membrane regulates the passage of nutrients, waste products, and secretions into and out of the cell. Because the cell membrane has the property of *selective permeability*, only certain substances may enter and leave the cell. The cell membrane is similar in structure and function to all of the other membranes that are found in eucaryotic cells.

Nucleus

As previously mentioned, the primary difference between procaryotic and eucaryotic cells is that eucaryotic cells possess a "true nucleus," whereas procaryotic cells do not. The

A "true nucleus" consists of nucleoplasm, chromosomes, and a nuclear membrane.

nucleus (pl., **nuclei**) controls the functions of the entire cell and can be thought of as the "command center" of the cell. The nucleus has three components: nucleoplasm, chromosomes, and a nuclear membrane. **Nucleoplasm** (a type of **protoplasm**) is the gelatinous matrix or base material of the nucleus. The **chromosomes** are embedded or suspended in the nucleoplasm. The membrane that serves as a "skin" around the nucleus is called the **nuclear membrane**; it contains holes (nuclear pores) through which large molecules can enter and exit the nucleus.

FIGURE 3-3. Cross section through a yeast cell. The cross section shows the nucleus (N) with nuclear pores (P), mitochondrion (M), and vacuole (V). The cytoplasm is surrounded by the cell membrane. The thick outer portion is the cell wall. (From Lechavalier HA, Pramer D. The Microbes. Philadelphia: JB Lippincott, 1970.)

genes. It has been estimated that the human genome consists of between 20,000 and 30,000 genes.[b]

When observed using a transmission electron microscope, a dark (electron dense) area can be seen in the nucleus. This area is called the **nucleolus**; it is here that rRNA molecules are manufactured. The rRNA molecules then exit the nucleus and become part of the structure of ribosomes (discussed later in this chapter).

Cytoplasm

Cytoplasm (a type of protoplasm) is a semifluid, gelatinous, nutrient matrix. Within the cytoplasm are found insoluble storage granules and various cytoplasmic organelles, including endoplasmic reticulum, ribosomes, Golgi complexes, mitochondria, centrioles, microtubules, lysosomes, and other membrane-bound vacuoles. Each of these organelles has a highly specific function, and all of the functions are interrelated to maintain the cell and allow it to properly perform its activities. The cytoplasm is where most of the cell's metabolic reactions occur. The semifluid portion of the cytoplasm, excluding the granules and organelles, is sometimes referred to as the *cytosol*.

Endoplasmic Reticulum

The **endoplasmic reticulum** (ER) is a highly convoluted system of membranes that are interconnected and arranged to form a transport network of tubules and flattened sacs within the cytoplasm. Much of the ER has a rough, granular appearance when observed by transmission electron microscopy and is designated as **rough endoplasmic reticulum** (RER). This rough appearance is caused by the many *ribosomes* attached to the outer surface of the membranes. ER to which ribosomes are not attached is called **smooth endoplasmic reticulum** (SER).

Ribosomes

Eucaryotic ribosomes are 18 to 22 nm in diameter. They consist mainly of rRNA and protein and play an important part in the synthesis (manufacture) of proteins. Clusters of ribosomes (called **polyribosomes** or **polysomes**), held together by a molecule of messenger RNA (mRNA), are sometimes observed by electron microscopy.

> Ribosomes are the sites of protein synthesis.

---

[b] Although the Human Genome Project was completed in 2003, the exact number of genes encoded by the human genome is still unknown. The reason for the uncertainty is that the various predictions are derived from different computational methods and gene-finding programs. Defining a gene is problematic for a number of reasons, including (1) small genes can be difficult to detect, (2) one gene can code for several protein products, (3) some genes code only for RNA, and (4) two genes can overlap. Even with improved genome analysis, computation alone is insufficient to generate an accurate gene number. Gene predictions must be verified by labor-intensive work in the laboratory before the scientific community can reach any real consensus. (From http://www.ornl.gov/hgmis.)

Each eucaryotic ribosome is composed of two subunits—a large subunit (the 60S subunit) and a small subunit (the 40S subunit)—that are produced in the nucleolus. The subunits are then transported to the cytoplasm where they remain separate until such time as they join together with an mRNA molecule to initiate protein synthesis (Chapter 6). When united, the 40S and 60S subunits form an 80S ribosome. (The "S" refers to Svedberg units, and 40S, 60S, and 80S are sedimentation coefficients. A sedimentation coefficient expresses the rate at which a particle or molecule moves in a centrifugal field; it is determined by the size and shape of the particle or molecule.)

Most of the proteins released from the ER are not mature. They must undergo further processing in an organelle known as a Golgi complex before they are able to perform their functions within or outside of the cell.

Golgi Complex

A **Golgi complex**, also known as a Golgi apparatus or Golgi body, connects or communicates with the ER. This stack of flattened, membranous sacs completes the transformation of newly synthesized proteins into mature, functional ones and packages them into small, membrane-enclosed vesicles for storage within the cell or export outside the cell (exocytosis or secretion). Golgi complexes are sometimes referred to as "packaging plants."

> Golgi complexes can be considered "packaging plants."

Lysosomes and Peroxisomes

Lysosomes are small (about 1 μm diameter) vesicles that originate at the Golgi complex. They contain lysozyme and other digestive enzymes that break down foreign material taken into the cell by *phagocytosis* (the engulfing of large particles by amebas and certain types of white blood cells called **phagocytes**). These enzymes also aid in breaking down worn out parts of the cell and may destroy the entire cell by a process called **autolysis** if the cell is damaged or deteriorating. Lysosomes are found in all eucaryotic cells.

Peroxisomes are membrane-bound vesicles in which hydrogen peroxide is both generated and broken down. Peroxisomes contain the enzyme catalase, which catalyzes (speeds up) the breakdown of hydrogen peroxide into water and oxygen. Peroxisomes are found in most eucaryotic cells, but are especially prominent in mammalian liver cells.

Mitochondria

The energy necessary for cellular function is provided by the formation of high-energy phosphate molecules such as adenosine triphosphate (ATP). ATP molecules are the major energy-carrying or energy-storing molecules within cells. **Mitochondria** (sing., **mitochondrion**) are referred to as the "power

> Mitochondria can be considered "power plants" or "energy factories."

plants," "powerhouses," or "energy factories" of the eucaryotic cell, because this is where most of the ATP molecules are formed by cellular respiration. During this process, energy is released from glucose molecules and other nutrients to drive other cellular functions (see Chapter 7). The number of mitochondria in a cell varies greatly depending on the activities required of that cell. Mitochondria are about 0.5 to 1 μm in diameter and up to 7 μm in length. Many scientists believe that mitochondria and chloroplasts arose from bacteria living within eucaryotic cells (see "Insight: The Origin of Mitochondria and Chloroplasts" on the CD-ROM).

Plastids

Plant cells contain both mito-chondria and another type of energy-producing organelle, called a plastid. **Plastids** are membrane-bound structures containing various photosynthetic pigments; they are the sites of photosynthesis. **Chloroplasts**, one type of plastid, contain a green, photosynthetic pigment called chlorophyll. Chloroplasts are found in plant cells and algae. **Photosynthesis** is the process by which light energy is used to convert carbon dioxide and water into carbohydrates and oxygen (Chapter 7). The chemical bonds in the carbohydrate molecules represent stored energy. Thus, photosynthesis is the conversion of light energy into chemical energy.

> Plastids are the sites of photosynthesis.

Cytoskeleton

Present throughout the cytoplasm is a system of fibers, collectively known as the **cytoskeleton**. The three types of cytoskeletal fibers are microtubules, microfilaments (actin filaments), and intermediate filaments. All three types serve to strengthen, support, and stiffen the cell, and give the cell its shape. In addition to their structural roles, microtubules and microfilaments are essential for various activities, such as cell division, contraction, motility (see the section on flagella and cilia), and the movement of chromosomes within the cell. **Microtubules** are slender, hollow tubules composed of spherical protein subunits called *tubulins*.

Cell Wall

Some eucaryotic cells contain *cell walls*—external structures that provide rigidity, shape, and protection (Fig. 3-4). Eucaryotic cell walls, which are much simpler in structure than procaryotic cell walls, may contain cellulose, pectin, lignin, chitin, and some mineral salts (usually found in algae). The cell walls of algae contain a polysaccharide—*cellulose*—that is not found in the cell walls of any other microorganisms. Cellulose is also found in the cell walls of plants. The cell walls of fungi contain a polysaccharide—*chitin*—that is not found in the cell walls of any other microorganisms. Chitin, which is similar in structure to cellulose, is also found in the exoskeletons of beetles and crabs.

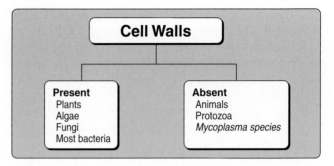

FIGURE 3-4. Presence or absence of cell wall in various types of cells. *Mycoplasma* is a genus of bacteria.

Flagella and Cilia

Some eucaryotic cells (e.g., spermatozoa and certain types of protozoa and algae) possess relatively long, thin structures called **flagella** (sing., **flagellum**). Such cells are said to be flagellated or motile; flagellated protozoa are called flagellates. The whipping motion of the flagella enables flagellated cells to "swim" through liquid environments; flagella are said to be whiplike. Flagella are referred to as organelles of locomotion (cell movement). Flagellated cells may possess one flagellum or two or more flagella. **Cilia** (sing., **cilium**) are also organelles of locomotion, but they tend to be shorter (more hairlike), thinner, and more numerous than flagella. Cilia can be found on some species of protozoa (called ciliates) and on certain types of cells in our bodies (e.g., the ciliated epithelial cells that line the respiratory tract). Unlike flagella, cilia tend to beat with a coordinated, rhythmic movement. Eucaryotic flagella and cilia, which contain an internal "9 + 2" arrangement of microtubules (Fig. 3-5), are structurally more complex than bacterial flagella.

> Motile eucaryotic cells possess either flagella or cilia.

PROCARYOTIC CELL STRUCTURE

Procaryotic cells are about 10 times smaller than eucaryotic cells. A typical *Escherichia coli* cell is about 1 μm wide and 2 to 3 μm long. Structurally, *procaryotes* are very simple cells when compared with eucaryotic cells, and yet they are able to perform the necessary processes of life. Reproduction of procaryotic cells is by *binary fission*—the simple division of one cell into two cells, after DNA replication (Chapter 6) and the formation of a separating membrane and cell wall. All bacteria are procaryotes, as are the archaea.

Embedded within the cytoplasm of procaryotic cells are a chromosome, ribosomes, and other cytoplasmic particles (Fig. 3-6). Unlike eucaryotic cells, the cytoplasm of procaryotic cells is not filled with internal membranes. The cytoplasm is surrounded by a cell membrane, a cell wall (usually), and sometimes a capsule or slime layer.

FIGURE 3-5. Cilia. TEM showing cross sections of mouse respiratory cilia. Note the 9 + 2 arrangement of microtubules within each cilium: two single microtubules in the center, surrounded by nine doublet microtubules. (Courtesy of Louisa Howard and Michael Binder.)

These latter three structures make up the bacterial cell envelope. Depending on the particular species of bacterium, flagella, pili (description follows), or both may be observed outside the cell envelope, and a spore may sometimes be seen within the cell.

Cell Membrane

Enclosing the cytoplasm of a procaryotic cell is the cell membrane (or plasma, cytoplasmic, or cellular membrane). This membrane is similar in structure and function to the eucaryotic cell membrane. Chemically, the cell membrane consists of proteins and phospholipids, which are discussed further in Chapter 6. Being selectively permeable, the membrane controls which substances may enter or leave the cell. It is flexible and so thin that it cannot be seen with a compound light microscope. However, it is frequently observed in TEMs of bacteria.

Many enzymes are attached to the cell membrane, and various metabolic reactions take place there. Some scientists believe that inward foldings of the cell membranes—called **mesosomes**—are where cellular respiration takes place in bacteria. This process is similar to that which occurs in the mitochondria of eucaryotic cells, in which nutrients are broken down to produce energy in the form of ATP molecules. On the other hand, some scientists think that mesosomes are nothing more than artifacts created during the processing of bacterial cells for electron microscopy.

In cyanobacteria and other photosynthetic bacteria (bacteria that convert light energy into chemical energy), infoldings of the cell membrane contain chlorophyll and other pigments that serve to trap light energy for photosynthesis. However, procaryotic cells do not have complex internal membrane systems similar to the ER and Golgi complex of eucaryotic cells. Procaryotic cells do not contain any membrane-bound organelles or vesicles.

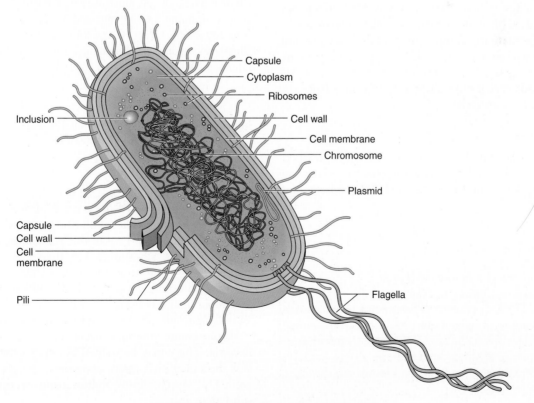

FIGURE 3-6. A typical procaryotic cell.

Chromosome

The procaryotic chromosome usually consists of a single, long, supercoiled, circular DNA molecule, which serves as the control center of the bacterial cell. <mark>Bacterial cells possess only one chromosome, whereas eucaryotic cells may possess many.</mark>
It is capable of duplicating itself, guiding cell division, and directing cellular activities. A procaryotic cell contains neither nucleoplasm nor a nuclear membrane. The chromosome is suspended or embedded in the cytoplasm. The DNA-occupied space within a bacterial cell is sometimes referred to as the bacterial nucleoid.

The thin and tightly folded chromosome of *E. coli* is about 1.5 mm (1,500 μm) long and only 2 nm wide. Because a typical *E. coli* cell is about 2 to 3 μm long, its chromosome is approximately 500 to 750 times longer than the cell itself—quite a packaging feat! Bacterial chromosomes contain between 450 and 8,000 genes, depending on the species. Each gene codes for one or more gene products (enzymes, other proteins, and rRNA and tRNA molecules). In comparison, the chromosomes within a human cell contain between 20,000 and 30,000 genes.

Small, circular molecules of double-stranded DNA that are not part of the chromosome (referred to as **extrachromosomal DNA** or **plasmids**) may also be present in the cytoplasm of procaryotic cells (Fig. 3-7). A plasmid may contain anywhere from fewer than 10 genes to several hundred genes. A bacterial cell may not contain any plasmids, or it may contain one plasmid, multiple copies of the same plasmid, or more than one type of plasmid (i.e., plasmids containing different genes). (Additional information about bacterial plasmids is found in Chapter 7.) Plasmids have also been found in yeast cells. <mark>A bacterial cell may not contain any plasmids, or it may contain one plasmid, multiple copies of the same plasmid, or more than one type of plasmid.</mark>

Cytoplasm

The semiliquid cytoplasm of procaryotic cells consists of water, enzymes, dissolved oxygen (in some bacteria), waste products, essential nutrients, proteins, carbohydrates, and

STUDY AID
Beware of Similar Sounding Words

A **plasmid** is a small, circular molecule of double-stranded DNA. It is referred to as extrachromosomal DNA because it is not part of the chromosome. Plasmids are found in most bacteria. A **plastid** is a cytoplasmic organelle, found only in certain eucaryotic cells (e.g., algae and plants). Plastids are the sites of photosynthesis.

CHROMOSOME
- Circular, double-stranded DNA
- 3000 genes (3000 kilobases)
- Single copy per cell
- Highly folded in cell

Cell wall

BACTERIUM

PLASMID
- Circular, double-stranded DNA
- 5-100 genes (5-100 kilobases)
- 1-20 copies per cell

FIGURE 3-7. A typical bacterial genome. The hypothetical bacterial cell illustrated here possesses a chromosome containing 3,000 genes and a plasmid containing 5 to 100 genes. (From Harvey RA et al. Lippincott's Illustrated Reviews, Microbiology, 2nd ed. Philadelphia: Lippincott Williams & Wilkins, 2007.)

lipids—a complex mixture of all the materials required by the cell for its metabolic functions.

Cytoplasmic Particles

Within the bacterial cytoplasm, many tiny particles have been observed. Most of these are ribosomes, often occurring in clusters called polyribosomes or polysomes (*poly* meaning many). Procaryotic ribosomes are smaller than eucaryotic ribosomes, but their function is the same—they are the sites of protein synthesis. A 70S procaryotic ribosome is composed of a 30S subunit and a 50S subunit. It has been estimated that there are about 15,000 ribosomes in the cytoplasm of an *E. coli* cell.

Cytoplasmic granules occur in certain species of bacteria. These may be stained by using a suitable stain, and then identified microscopically. The granules may consist of starch, lipids, sulfur, iron, or other stored substances.

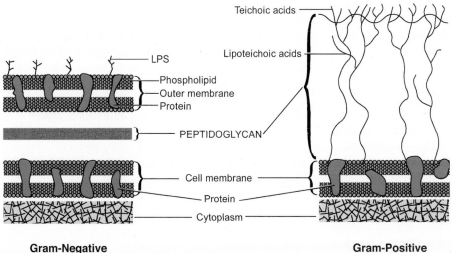

Teichoic acids

Lipoteichoic acids

LPS

Phospholipid
Outer membrane
Protein

PEPTIDOGLYCAN

Cell membrane

Protein

Cytoplasm

**Gram-Negative
Cell Wall**

**Gram-Positive
Cell Wall**

FIGURE 3-8. Differences between Gram-negative and Gram-positive cell walls. The relatively thin Gram-negative cell wall contains a thin layer of peptidoglycan, an outer membrane, and lipopolysaccharide (LPS). The thicker Gram-positive cell wall contains a thick layer of peptidoglycan and teichoic and lipoteichoic acids.

Bacterial Cell Wall

The rigid exterior cell wall that defines the shape of bacterial cells is chemically complex. Thus, the structure of bacterial cell walls is quite different from the relatively simple structure of eucaryotic cell walls, although they serve the same functions—providing rigidity, strength, and protection. The main constituent of most bacterial cell walls is a complex macromolecular polymer known as peptidoglycan (murein), consisting of many polysaccharide chains linked together by small peptide (protein) chains. Peptidoglycan is only found in bacteria. The thickness of the cell wall and its exact composition vary with the species of bacteria. The cell walls of certain bacteria, called **Gram-positive bacteria** (to be explained in Chapter 4), have a thick layer of peptidoglycan combined with teichoic acid and lipoteichoic acid molecules. The cell walls of **Gram-negative bacteria** (also explained in Chapter 4) have a much thinner layer of peptidoglycan, but this layer is covered with a complex layer of lipid macromolecules, usually referred to as the outer membrane, as shown in Figures 3-8 and 3-9. These macromolecules are discussed in Chapter 6. Although most bacteria have cell walls, bacteria in the genus *Mycoplasma* do not. Archaea (described in Chapter 4) have cell walls, but their cell walls do not contain peptidoglycan.

Some bacteria lose their ability to produce cell walls, transforming into tiny variants of the same species, referred to as **L-form** or **cell wall–deficient** (CWD) bacteria. Over 50 different species of bacteria are capable of transforming into CWD bacteria, some of which are responsible for chronic diseases such as chronic fatigue syndrome, Lyme disease, rheumatoid arthritis, and sarcoidosis. Clinicians are often unaware that CWD bacteria are present in their patients because they will not grow under standard laboratory conditions;

> Most bacteria possess cell walls. Exceptions include cell wall–deficient bacteria and bacteria in the genus *Mycoplasma*.

they must be cultured in a different medium and at a different temperature than classical bacteria.

Glycocalyx (Slime Layers and Capsules)

Some bacteria have a thick layer of material (known as glycocalyx) located outside their cell wall. **Glycocalyx** is a slimy, gelatinous material produced by the cell membrane and secreted outside of the cell wall. There are two types of glycocalyx. One type, called a **slime layer**, is not highly organized and is not firmly attached to the cell wall. It easily detaches from the cell wall and

> Depending on the species, bacterial cells may or may not be surrounded by glycocalyx. The two types of glycocalyx are slime layers and capsules.

FIGURE 3-9. Bacterial cell walls. (A) A portion of the Gram-positive bacterium, *Bacillus fastidious*; note the cell wall's thick peptidoglycan layer, beneath which can be seen the cell membrane. **(B)** The Gram-negative bacterium, *Enterobacter aerogenes*; both the cell membrane and the outer membrane are visible along some sections of the cell wall. (From Volk WA, et al. Essentials of Medical Microbiology, 5th ed. Philadelphia: Lippincott-Raven, 1996.)

drifts away. Bacteria in the genus *Pseudomonas* produce a slime layer, which sometimes plays a role in diseases caused by *Pseudomonas* species. Slime layers enable certain bacteria to glide or slide along solid surfaces.

The other type of glycocalyx, called a **capsule**, is highly organized and firmly attached to the cell wall. Capsules usually consist of polysaccharides, which may be combined with lipids and proteins, depending on the bacterial species. Knowledge of the chemical composition of capsules is useful in differentiating among different types of bacteria within a particular species; for example, different strains of *Haemophilus influenzae*, a cause of meningitis and ear infections in children, are identified by their capsular types. A vaccine, called Hib vaccine, is available for protection against disease caused by *H. influenzae* capsular type b. Other examples of encapsulated bacteria are *Klebsiella pneumoniae*, *Neisseria meningitidis*, and *Streptococcus pneumoniae*.

Capsules can be detected using a capsule staining procedure, which is a type of *negative stain*. The bacterial cell

FIGURE 3-10. Capsule stain. (A) Drawing illustrating the results of the capsule staining technique.
(B) Photomicrograph of encapsulated bacteria that have been stained using the capsule staining technique.
The capsule stain is an example of a negative staining technique. Note that the bacterial cells and the background stain, but the capsules do not. The capsules are seen as unstained "halos" around the bacterial cells.
([B] From Winn WC Jr, et al. Koneman's Color Atlas and Textbook of Diagnostic Microbiology, 6th ed. Philadelphia: Lippincott Williams & Wilkins, 2006.)

and background become stained, but the capsule remains unstained (Fig. 3-10). Thus, the capsule appears as an unstained halo around the bacterial cell. Antigen–antibody tests (described in Chapter 16) may be used to identify specific strains of bacteria possessing unique capsular molecules (antigens).

Encapsulated bacteria usually produce colonies on nutrient agar that are smooth, mucoid, and glistening; they are referred to as **S-colonies**. Nonencapsulated bacteria tend to grow as dry, rough colonies, called **R-colonies**. Capsules serve an antiphagocytic func-

> Bacterial capsules serve an antiphagocytic function, meaning that they protect encapsulated bacteria from being phagocytized by white blood cells.

tion, protecting the encapsulated bacteria from being phagocytized (ingested) by phagocytic white blood cells. Thus, encapsulated bacteria are able to survive longer in the human body than nonencapsulated bacteria.

Flagella

Flagella (sing., **flagellum**) are threadlike, protein appendages that enable bacteria to move. Flagellated bacteria are said to be motile, whereas nonflagel-

> Motile bacteria usually possess flagella. Bacteria never possess cilia.

lated bacteria are usually nonmotile. Bacterial flagella are about 10 to 20 nm thick; too thin to be seen with the compound light microscope.

The number and arrangement of flagella possessed by a certain species of bacterium are characteristic of that species and can, thus, be used for classification and identification purposes (Fig. 3-11). Bacteria possessing flagella over their entire surface (perimeter) are called **peritrichous bacteria** (Fig. 3-12). Bacteria with a tuft of flagella at one end are described as being **lophotrichous bacteria,** whereas those having one or more flagella at each end are said to be **amphitrichous bacteria.** Bacteria possessing a single polar flagellum are described as **monotrichous bacteria.** In the laboratory, the number of flagella that a cell possesses and their locations on the cell can be determined using what is known as a flagella stain. The stain adheres to the flagella, making them thick enough to be seen under the microscope.

Bacterial flagella consist of three, four, or more threads of protein (called **flagellin**) twisted like a rope. Thus, the structures of bacterial flagella and eucaryotic flagella are quite different. You will recall that eucaryotic flagella (and cilia) contain a complex arrangement of internal microtubules, which run the length of the membrane-bound flagellum. Bacterial flagella do not contain microtubules, and their flagella are not membrane-bound. Bacterial flagella arise from a basal body in the cell membrane and project outward through the cell wall and capsule (if present), as shown in Figure 3-6.

Some **spirochetes** (spiral-shaped bacteria) have two flagella-like fibrils called **axial filaments**, one attached to each end of the bacterium. These axial filaments extend

FIGURE 3-11. Flagellar arrangement. The four basic types of flagellar arrangement on bacteria: peritrichous, flagella all over the surface; lophotrichous, a tuft of flagella at one end; amphitrichous, one or more flagella at each end; monotrichous, one flagellum.

toward each other, wrap around the organism between the layers of the cell wall, and overlap in the midsection of the cell. As a result of its axial filaments, spirochetes can move in a spiral, helical, or inchworm manner.

Pili (Fimbriae)

Pili (sing., **pilus**) or **fimbriae** (sing., **fimbria**) are hair-like structures, most often observed on Gram-negative bacteria. They are composed of polymerized protein molecules called pilin. Pili are much thinner than fla-gella, have a rigid structure, and are not associated with motility. These tiny appendages arise from the cyto-plasm and extend through the plasma membrane, cell wall, and capsule (if present). There are two types of pili: one type merely enables bacteria to adhere or at-tach to surfaces; the other type (called a **sex pilus**) enables transfer of genetic material from one bacterial

cell to another following attachment of the cells to each other.

The pili that merely enable bacteria to anchor themselves to surfaces (e.g., tissues within the human body) are usually quite numerous (Fig. 3-13). In some species of bacteria, piliated strains (those possess-ing pili) are able to cause diseases like urethritis and cystitis, whereas nonpiliated strains (those not possess-ing pili) of the same organisms are unable to cause these diseases.

> Pili are organelles of attachment. That is, they enable bacteria to adhere to surfaces.

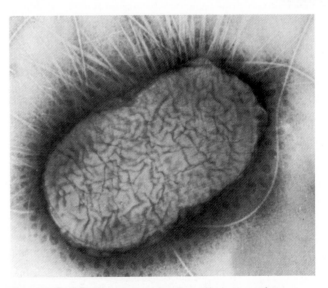

FIGURE 3-13. *Proteus vulgaris* cell, possessing numerous short, straight pili and several longer, curved flagella; the cell is undergoing binary fission. *P. vulgaris* is a bacterial species. (From Volk WA, et al. Essentials of Medical Microbiology, 5th ed. Philadelphia: Lippincott-Raven, 1996.)

FIGURE 3-12. A *Salmonella* cell, showing peritri-chous flagella. *Salmonella* is a bacterial genus. (From Volk WA, et al. Essentials of Medical Microbiology, 5th ed. Philadelphia: Lippincott-Raven, 1996.)

A bacterial cell possessing a sex pilus (called a **donor cell**)—and the cell only possesses one sex pilus—is able to attach to another bacterial cell (called a recipient cell) by means of the sex pilus. Genetic material (usually in the form of a plasmid) is then transferred through the hollow sex pilus from the donor cell to the recipient cell—a process known as **conjugation** (described more fully in Chapter 7).

> A sex pilus enables the transfer of genetic material from one bacterial cell (the donor cell) to another (the recipient cell).

Spores (Endospores)

A few genera of bacteria (e.g., *Bacillus* and *Clostridium*) are capable of forming thick-walled spores as a means of survival when their moisture or nutrient supply is low. Bacterial spores are referred to as **endospores**,

> Endospores enable bacteria to survive adverse conditions, such as temperature extremes, desiccation, and lack of nutrients.

and the process by which they are formed is called **sporulation.** During sporulation, a copy of the chromosome and some of the surrounding cytoplasm becomes enclosed in several thick protein coats. Spores are resistant to heat, cold, drying, and most chemicals. Spores have been shown to survive for many years in soil or dust, and some are quite resistant to disinfectants and boiling. When the dried spore lands on a moist, nutrient-rich surface, it germinates, and a new vegetative bacterial cell (a cell capable of growing and dividing) emerges. Germination of a spore may be compared with germination of a seed. However, in bacteria, spore formation is related to the survival of the bacterial cell, not to reproduction. Usually, only one spore is produced in a bacterial cell and it germinates into only one vegetative bacterium (Fig. 3-14). In the laboratory, endospores can be stained using what is known as a spore stain. Once a particular bacterium's endospores are stained, the laboratory technologist can determine whether the organism is producing terminal or subterminal spores. A terminal spore is produced at the very end of the bacterial cell, whereas a subterminal spore is produced elsewhere in the cell. Where a spore is being produced within the cell and whether or not it causes a swelling of the cell serve as clues to the identity of the organism.

FIGURE 3-14. A bacillus with a well-defined endospore (arrow). A bacillus is a rod-shaped bacterium. (From Lechavalier HA, Pramer D. The Microbes. Philadelphia: JB Lippincott, 1970.)

SUMMARY OF STRUCTURAL DIFFERENCES BETWEEN PROCARYOTIC AND EUCARYOTIC CELLS

Eucaryotic cells contain a true nucleus, whereas procaryotic cells do not. Eucaryotic cells are divided into plant and animal types. Animal cells do not have a cell wall, whereas plant cells have a simple cell wall, usually containing cellulose.

> Eucaryotic cells contain numerous membranes and membrane-bound structures. The only membrane possessed by a procaryotic cell is its cell membrane.

Cellulose, a type of polysaccharide, is a rigid polymer of glucose (polymers and polysaccharides are described in Chapter 6). Procaryotic cells have complex cell walls consisting of proteins, lipids, and polysaccharides. Eucaryotic cells contain membranous structures (such as ER and Golgi complexes) and many membrane-bound organelles (such as mitochondria and plastids). Procaryotic cells possess no membranes other than the cell membrane that encloses the cytoplasm. Eucaryotic ribosomes (referred to as 80S ribosomes) are larger and denser than those found in procaryotes (70S ribosomes). The fact that

TABLE 3-1	Comparison between Eucaryotic and Procaryotic Cells		
	EUCARYOTIC CELLS		PROCARYOTIC CELLS
	Plant Type	Animal Type	
Biologic distribution	All plants, fungi, and algae	All animals and protozoa	All bacteria
Nuclear membrane	Present	Present	Absent
Membranous structures other than cell membranes	Present	Present	Generally absent except for mesosomes and photosynthetic membranes
Microtubules	Present	Present	Absent
Cytoplasmic ribosomes (density)	80S	80S	70S
Chromosomes	Composed of DNA and proteins	Composed of DNA and proteins	Composed of DNA alone
Flagella or cilia	When present, have a complex structure	When present, have a complex structure	When present, flagella have a simple twisted protein structure; procaryotic cells do not possess cilia
Cell wall	When present, of simple chemical constitution; usually contains cellulose	Absent	Of complex chemical constitution, containing peptidoglycan
Photosynthesis (chlorophyll)	Present	Absent	Present in cyanobacteria and some other bacteria

70S ribosomes are found in the mitochondria and chloroplasts of eucaryotes may indicate that these structures were derived from parasitic procaryotes during their evolutionary development. Other differences between procaryotic and eucaryotic cells are listed in Table 3-1.

REPRODUCTION OF ORGANISMS AND THEIR CELLS

Reproduction (referring to the manner in which organisms reproduce) and cell reproduction (referring to the process by which individual cells reproduce) are complex topics, which can only be briefly discussed in a book of this size. The following topics are discussed briefly on the CD-ROM:

- asexual versus sexual reproduction
- life cycles
- eucaryotic cell reproduction (mitosis and meiosis)

Procaryotic Cell Reproduction

Procaryotic cell reproduction is quite simple when compared with eucaryotic cell division. Procaryotic cells reproduce by a process known as *binary fission*, **Bacterial cells reproduce by binary fission—one cell splits in half to become two cells.**

in which one cell (the parent cell) splits in half to become two daughter cells. Before a procaryotic cell can divide in half, its chromosome must be duplicated (a process known as DNA replication; discussed in Chapter 6), so that each daughter cell will possess the same genetic information as the parent cell (Fig. 3-15).

The time it takes for binary fission to occur (i.e., the time it takes for one procaryotic cell to become two cells) is called the **generation time**. The generation time varies from one bacterial species to another and **The length of time it takes for one bacterial cell to split into two cells is referred to as the organism's generation time.** also depends on the growth conditions (e.g., pH, temperature, availability of nutrients). In the laboratory (in vitro), under ideal conditions, *E. coli* has a generation time of about 20 minutes—the number of cells will double every 20 minutes. Bacterial generation times range from as short as 10 minutes to as long as 24 hours, or even longer in some cases.

TAXONOMY

According to *Bergey's Manual of Systematic Bacteriology* (described in Chapter 4 and on the CD-ROM), **taxonomy** (the science of classification of living organisms) consists

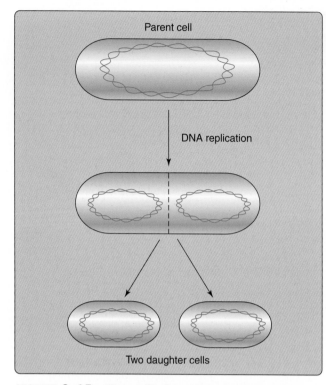

FIGURE 3-15. Binary fission. Note that DNA replication must occur prior to the actual splitting (fission) of the parent cell.

of three separate but interrelated areas: classification, nomenclature, and identification. *Classification* is the arrangement of organisms into taxonomic groups (known as **taxa** [sing., **taxon**]) on the basis of similarities or relationships. Taxa include kingdoms or domains, divisions or phyla, classes, orders, families, genera, and species. Closely related organisms (i.e., organisms having similar characteristics) are placed into the same taxon. *Nomenclature* is the assignment of names to the various taxa according to international rules. *Identification* is the process of determining whether an isolate belongs to one of the established, named taxa or represents a previously unidentified species.

STUDY AID

A Way to Remember the Sequence of Taxa From Kingdom to Species

Abbreviations and phrases are often helpful when trying to learn new material. A former student used the phrase "King David Came Over For Good Spaghetti" (KDCOFGS) to help her remember the sequence of taxa from kingdom to species (K for Kingdom, D for Division, C for Class, O for Order, F for Family, G for Genus, and S for Species). Or, if phylum is preferred, rather than division, King Philip can be substituted for King David (KPCOFGS).

When attempting to identify an organism that has been isolated from a clinical specimen, laboratory technologists are very much like detectives. They gather "clues" (characteristics, attributes, properties, traits) about the organism until they have sufficient clues to identify (speciate) the organism. In most cases, the clues that have been gathered will match the characteristics of an established species. (Note: throughout this book, the term "to identify an organism" means to learn the organism's species name—i.e., to speciate it.) An organism's complete collection of physical characteristics is known as the organism's phenotype.

> An organism's complete collection of genes is referred to as the organism's genotype or genome. An organism's complete collection of physical characteristics is known as the organism's phenotype.

Microbial Classification

Since Aristotle's time, scientists have attempted to name and classify living organisms in a meaningful way, based on their appearance and behavior. Thus, the science of taxonomy was established, based on the binomial system of nomenclature developed in the 18th century by the Swedish scientist, Carolus Linnaeus. In the binomial system, each organism is given two names (e.g., *Homo sapiens* for humans). The first name is the **genus** (pl., **genera**), and the second name is the **specific epithet**. The first and second names together are referred to as the *species*.

> In the binomial system of nomenclature, the first name (e.g., *Escherichia*) is the genus, and the second name (e.g., *coli*) is the specific epithet. When used together, the first and second names (e.g., *Escherichia coli*) are referred to as a species.

Because written reference is often made to genera and species, biologists throughout the world have adopted a standard method of expressing these names. To express the genus, capitalize the first letter of the word and underline or italicize the whole word—for example, *Escherichia*. To express the species, capitalize the first letter of the genus name (the specific epithet is not capitalized) and then underline or italicize the entire species name—for example, *Escherichia coli*. Frequently, the genus is designated by a single-letter abbreviation; in the example just given, *E. coli* indicates the species. In an essay or article about *Escherichia coli*, *Escherichia* would be spelled out the first time the organism is mentioned; thereafter, the abbreviated form, *E. coli*, could be used. The abbreviation "sp." is used to designate a single species, whereas the abbreviation "spp." is used to designate more than one species.

In addition to the proper scientific names for bacteria, acceptable terms like staphylococci (for *Staphylococcus* spp.), streptococci (for *Streptococcus* spp.), clostridia (for *Clostridium* spp.), pseudomonads (for *Pseudomonas* spp.), mycoplasmas (for *Mycoplasma* spp.), rickettsias (for

BACTERIUM	DISEASE

TABLE 3-2 — Examples of Bacteria Named for the Diseases That They Cause[a]

BACTERIUM	DISEASE
Bacillus anthracis	Anthrax
Chlamydophila pneumoniae	Pneumonia
Chlamydophila psittaci	Psittacosis ("parrot fever")
Chlamydia trachomatis	Trachoma
Clostridium botulinum	Botulism
Clostridium tetani	Tetanus
Corynebacterium diphtheriae	Diphtheria
Francisella tularensis	Tularemia ("rabbit fever")
Klebsiella pneumoniae	Pneumonia
Mycobacterium leprae	Leprosy (Hansen's disease)
Mycobacterium tuberculosis	Tuberculosis
Mycoplasma pneumoniae	Pneumonia
Neisseria gonorrhoeae	Gonorrhea
Neisseria meningitidis	Meningitis
Streptococcus pneumoniae	Pneumonia
Vibrio cholerae	Cholera

[a]In some cases, these bacteria cause more than one disease.

HISTORICAL NOTE

What's in a Name?

Sometimes, bacteria and other microorganisms are named for the person who discovered the organism. An interesting example is the name of the plague bacillus. The bacterium that causes plague was discovered in 1894 by Alexandre Emile Jean Yersin (1863-1943), a French bacteriologist of Swiss descent, who worked for many years at various Pasteur Institutes in Vietnam. Yersin originally named the organism *Bacillus pestis*, but in 1896 the name was changed to *Pasteurella pestis*, to honor Louis Pasteur, with whom Yersin had studied. Then, many years later, taxonomists changed the name to *Yersinia pestis* to honor Yersin—the person who discovered the organism. Other genera named for bacteriologists include *Bordetella* (Jules Bordet), *Escherichia* (Theodore Escherich), *Neisseria* (Albert Ludwig Neisser), and *Salmonella* (Daniel Elmer Salmon).

- Plants are in the Kingdom Plantae
- Animals are in the Kingdom Animalia (Although humans are in the Kingdom Animalia, in this book, the word "animals" refers to animals other than humans.)

Viruses are not included in the Five-Kingdom System of Classification because they are not living cells; they are acellular. Note that four of the five kingdoms consist of eucaryotic organisms. Each kingdom consists of divisions or phyla, which, in turn, are divided into classes, orders, families, genera, and species (Table 3-3). In some cases, species are subdivided into subspecies, their names consisting of a genus, a specific epithet, and a subspecific epithet (abbreviated "ssp."); an example would be *H. influenzae* ssp. *aegyptius*, the most common cause of "pinkeye." Although Whittaker's Five-Kingdom System of Classification has been the most popular classification system for the past 30 or so years, not all scientists agree with it; other taxonomic classification schemes exist. For example, some scientists do not agree that algae and protozoa should be placed into the same kingdom, and in some classification schemes, protozoa are placed into a subkingdom of the Animal Kingdom.

In the late 1970s, Carl R. Woese (see "Historical Note") devised a Three-Domain System of Classification, which is gaining in popularity among scientists. In this Three-Domain System, there are two domains of procaryotes (*Archaea* and *Bacteria*) and one domain (*Eucarya* or *Eukarya*), which includes all eucaryotic organisms. *Archaea* comes from *archae*, meaning "ancient." Although members of the Domain *Archaea*

> The three domains in the Three-Domain System are *Archaea*, *Bacteria*, and *Eucarya*. Note that the domain names are italicized.

Rickettsia spp.), and chlamydias (for *Chlamydia* spp.) are commonly used. Nicknames and slang terms frequently used within hospitals are GC and gonococci (for *Neisseria gonorrhoeae*), meningococci (for *N. meningitidis*), pneumococci (for *S. pneumoniae*), staph (for *Staphylococcus* or staphylococcal), and strep (for *Streptococcus* or streptococcal). It is common to hear healthcare workers using terms like meningococcal meningitis, pneumococcal pneumonia, staph infection, and strep throat.

Quite often, bacteria are named for the disease that they cause (see Table 3-2 for examples). In a few cases, bacteria are misnamed. For example, *H. influenzae* does not cause influenza, which is a respiratory disease caused by influenza viruses.

Organisms are categorized into larger groups based on their similarities and differences. In 1969, Robert H. Whittaker proposed a Five-Kingdom System of Classification, in which all organisms are placed into five kingdoms:

- Bacteria and archaea are in the Kingdom Procaryotae (or Monera)
- Algae and protozoa are in the Kingdom Protista (organisms in this kingdom are referred to as **protists**)
- Fungi are in the Kingdom Fungi

TABLE 3-3	Comparison of Human and Bacterial Classification		
	HUMAN BEING	ESCHERICHIA COLI (A MEDICALLY IMPORTANT GRAM-NEGATIVE BACILLUS)[a]	STAPHYLOCOCCUS AUREUS (A MEDICALLY IMPORTANT GRAM-POSITIVE COCCUS)[a]
Kingdom (Domain)	Animalia (Eucarya)	Procaryotae (Bacteria)	Procaryotae (Bacteria)
Phylum	Chordata	Proteobacteria	Firmicutes
Class	Mammalia	Gammaproteobacteria	Bacilli
Order	Primates	Enterobacteriales	Bacillales
Family	Hominidae	Enterobacteriaceae	Staphylococcaceae
Genus	Homo	Escherichia	Staphylococcus
Species (a species has two names; the first name is the genus, and the second name is the specific epithet)	Homo sapiens	Escherichia coli	Staphylococcus aureus

[a]Based on Bergey's Manual of Systematic Bacteriology, vol. 1, 2nd ed. New York: Springer-Verlag, 2001. A bacillus is a rod-shaped bacterium. A coccus is a spherical-shaped bacterium.

have been referred to in the past as archaebacteria and archaeobacteria (meaning ancient bacteria), these names have fallen out of favor because the **archaea** are so different from bacteria. Similarly, organisms in the Domain *Bacteria* have, at times, been referred to as eubacteria, meaning "true" bacteria, but are now usually referred to simply as **bacteria.** Note that the domain names are italicized. Domain *Archaea* contains 2 phyla and Domain *Bacteria* contains 23. The Three-Domain System of Classification is based on differences in the structure of certain rRNA molecules among organisms in the three domains.

HISTORICAL NOTE

Carl R. Woese

During the 1970s, a molecular biologist named Carl Woese and his colleagues at the University of Illinois shook up the scientific community by developing a system of classifying organisms that was based on the sequences of nucleotide bases in their ribosomal RNA molecules. They demonstrated that procaryotic organisms can be divided into two major groups (referred to as domains), based on differences in their rRNA sequences, and that the rRNA from these two groups differed from the rRNA of eucaryotic organisms. Although this system of classification was not widely accepted at first, Woese's Three-Domain System of Classification has become the classification system most favored by microbiologists.

DETERMINING RELATEDNESS AMONG ORGANISMS

How do scientists determine how closely related one organism is to another? The most widely used technique for gauging diversity or relatedness is called rRNA sequencing. Ribosomes are made up of
two subunits: a small subunit and a large subunit. The small subunit contains only one RNA molecule, which is referred to as the "small subunit rRNA" or SSUrRNA. The SSUrRNA in procaryotic ribosomes is a 16S rRNA molecule, whereas the SSUrRNA in eucaryotes is an 18S rRNA molecule. (The "S" in 16S and 18S refers to Svedberg units, which were discussed earlier.) The gene that codes for the 16S rRNA molecule contains about 1,500 DNA nucleotides, whereas the gene that codes for the 18S rRNA molecule contains about 2,000 nucleotides. The sequence of nucleotides in the gene that codes for the 16S rRNA molecule is called the 16s rDNA sequence. To determine "relatedness," researchers compare the sequence of nucleotide base pairs in the gene, rather than comparing the actual SSUrRNA molecules. If the 16S rDNA sequence of one procaryotic organism is quite similar to the 16S rDNA sequence of another procaryotic organism, then the organisms are closely related. The less similar the 16S rDNA sequences in procaryotes (or the 18S rDNA sequences in eucaryotes), the less related are the organisms. For example, the 18S rDNA sequence of a human is much more similar to

> Relatedness among organisms is determined by analysis of genes that code for small subunit ribosomal RNA (SSUrRNA).

the 18S rDNA sequence of a chimpanzee than to the 18S rDNA sequence of a fungus.

Not only can rRNA be used for taxonomic purposes, it can also be used in the clinical microbiology laboratory to identify pathogens. Microorganisms are identified by comparing the rRNA gene sequences that are recovered from clinical specimens to sequences contained in high-quality reference databanks.

Perhaps taxonomists will some day combine the Three-Domain System and the Five-Kingdom System, producing either a Six-Kingdom System (Bacteria, Archaea, Protista, Fungi, Plantae, and Animalia) or a Seven-Kingdom System (Bacteria, Archaea, Algae, Protozoa, Fungi, Plantae, and Animalia).

ON THE CD-ROM
- Terms Introduced in This Chapter
- Review of Key Points
- Insight
  - Asexual versus Sexual Reproduction; Life Cycles; Eucaryotic Cell Reproduction (Mitosis and Meiosis)
  - The Origin of Mitochondria and Chloroplasts
- Increase Your Knowledge
- Critical Thinking
- Additional Self-Assessment Exercises

SELF-ASSESSMENT EXERCISES

After studying this chapter, answer the following multiple-choice questions.

1. Molecules of extrachromosomal DNA are also known as:
   a. Golgi bodies.
   b. lysosomes.
   c. plasmids.
   d. plastids.
2. A bacterium possessing a tuft of flagella at one end of its cell would be called what kind of bacterium?
   a. amphitrichous
   b. lophotrichous
   c. monotrichous
   d. peritrichous
3. One way in which an archaean would differ from a bacterium is that the archaean would possess no:
   a. DNA in its chromosome.
   b. peptidoglycan in its cell walls.
   c. ribosomes in its cytoplasm.
   d. RNA in its ribosomes.
4. Some bacteria stain Gram-positive and others stain Gram-negative as a result of differences in the structure of their:
   a. capsule.
   b. cell membrane.
   c. cell wall.
   d. ribosomes.
5. Of the following, which one is *not* found in procaryotic cells?
   a. cell membrane
   b. chromosome
   c. mitochondria
   d. plasmids
6. The Three-Domain System of Classification is based on differences in which of the following molecules?
   a. mRNA
   b. peptidoglycan
   c. rRNA
   d. tRNA
7. Which of the following is in the correct sequence?
   a. Kingdom, Class, Division, Order, Family, Genus
   b. Kingdom, Division, Class, Order, Family, Genus
   c. Kingdom, Division, Order, Class, Family, Genus
   d. Kingdom, Order, Division, Class, Family, Genus
8. Which one of the following is *never* found in procaryotic cells?
   a. flagella
   b. capsule
   c. cilia
   d. ribosomes
9. The semipermeable structure controlling the transport of materials between the cell and its external environment is the:
   a. cell membrane.
   b. cell wall.
   c. cytoplasm.
   d. nuclear membrane.
10. In eucaryotic cells, what are the sites of photosynthesis?
    a. mitochondria
    b. plasmids
    c. plastids
    d. ribosomes

4 MICROBIAL DIVERSITY

PART 1 | Acellular and Procaryotic Microbes

LEARNING OBJECTIVES

AFTER STUDYING THIS CHAPTER, YOU SHOULD BE ABLE TO:

- Describe the characteristics used to classify viruses (e.g., DNA vs. RNA)
- List five specific properties of viruses that distinguish them from bacteria
- List at least three important viral diseases of humans
- Discuss differences between viroids and virions, and the diseases they cause
- List various ways in which bacteria can be classified
- State the three purposes of fixation
- Define the terms diplococci, streptococci, staphylococci, tetrad, octad, coccobacilli, diplobacilli, streptobacilli, and pleomorphism
- Define the terms obligate aerobe, microaerophile, facultative anaerobe, aerotolerant anaerobe, obligate anaerobe, and capnophile
- State key differences among rickettsias, chlamydias, and mycoplasmas
- Identify several important bacterial diseases of humans
- State several ways in which archaea differ from bacteria

INTRODUCTION

Imagine the excitement that Anton van Leeuwenhoek experienced as he gazed through his tiny glass lenses and became the first person to see live microbes. In the years that have followed his eloquently written late 17th to early 18th century accounts of the bacteria and protozoa that he observed, tens of thousands of microbes have been discovered, described, and classified. In this chapter and the next, you will be introduced to the diversity of form and function that exists in the microbial world.

As you will recall, microbiology is the study of microbes, which are too small to be seen by the naked eye. Microbes can be divided into those that are truly cellular (bacteria, archaea, algae, protozoa, and fungi) and those that are acellular (viruses, viroids, and prions). The cellular microorganisms can be subdivided into those that are procaryotic (bacteria and archaea) and those that are eucaryotic (algae, protozoa, and fungi). For a variety of reasons, acellular microorganisms are not considered by most scientists to be living organisms. Thus, rather than using the term microorganisms to describe them, viruses, viroids, and prions are more correctly referred to as acellular microbes or infectious particles.

ACELLULAR MICROBES

Viruses

Complete virus particles, called *virions*, are very small and simple in structure. Most viruses range in size from 10 to 300 nm in diameter, although some—like Ebola virus—can be up to 1 μm in length. The smallest virus is about the size of the large hemoglobin molecule of a red blood cell. Scientists were unable to see viruses until electron microscopes were invented in the 1930s. The first photographs of viruses were obtained in 1940. A negative staining procedure, developed in 1959, revolutionized the study of viruses, making it possible to observe unstained viruses against an electron-dense, dark background.

> Viruses are extremely small. They are observed using electron microscopes.

No type of organism is safe from viral infections; viruses infect humans, animals, plants, fungi, protozoa, algae, and bacterial cells (Table 4-1). Many human diseases are caused by viruses (refer back to Table 1-1). Many of the viruses that infect humans are shown in Figure 4-1. Some viruses—called oncogenic viruses or

> Viruses are not alive. To replicate, viruses must invade live host cells.

oncoviruses—cause specific types of cancer, including human cancers such as lymphomas, carcinomas, and some types of leukemia.

Viruses are said to have five specific properties that distinguish them from living cells:

- The vast majority of viruses possess *either* DNA or RNA, unlike living cells, which possess both.
- They are unable to replicate (multiply) on their own; their replication is directed by the viral nucleic acid once it has been introduced into a host cell.
- Unlike cells, they do not divide by binary fission, mitosis, or meiosis.
- They lack the genes and enzymes necessary for energy production.
- They depend on the ribosomes, enzymes, and metabolites ("building blocks") of the host cell for protein and nucleic acid production.

> Except in very rare cases, a particular virus contains either DNA or RNA—not both.

A typical virion consists of a genome of either DNA or RNA, surrounded by a *capsid* (protein coat), which is composed of many small protein units called *capsomeres*. Together, the nucleic acid and the capsid are referred to as the nucleocapsid (Fig. 4-2). Some viruses (called enveloped viruses) have an outer envelope composed of lipids and polysaccharides (Fig. 4-3). Bacterial viruses may also have a tail, sheath, and tail fibers. There are no ribosomes for protein synthesis or sites of energy production; hence, the virus must invade and take over a functioning cell to produce new virions.

> The simplest of human viruses consists of nothing more than nucleic acid surrounded by a protein coat (the capsid). The capsid plus the enclosed nucleic acid are referred to as the nucleocapsid.

Viruses are classified by the following characteristics: (a) type of genetic material (either DNA or RNA), (b) shape of the capsid, (c) number of capsomeres, (d) size of the capsid, (e) presence or absence of an envelope, (f) type of host that it infects, (g) type of disease it produces, (h) target cell, and (i) immunologic or antigenic properties.

There are four categories of viruses, based on the type of genome they possess. The genome of most viruses is either double-stranded DNA or single-stranded RNA, but a few viruses possess single-stranded DNA or double-stranded RNA. Viral genomes are usually circular molecules, but some are linear (having two ends). Capsids of viruses have various shapes and symmetry. They may be polyhedral (many sided), helical (coiled tubes), bullet shaped, spherical, or a complex combination of these shapes. Polyhedral capsids have 20 sides or facets; geometrically, they are referred to as icosahedrons. Each facet consists of several capsomeres; thus, the size of the virus is determined by the size of each facet and the number of capsomeres in each.

TABLE 4-1	Relative Sizes and Shapes of Some Viruses		
VIRUSES	NUCLEIC ACID TYPE	SHAPE	SIZE RANGE (nm)
Animal Viruses			
Vaccinia	DNA	Complex	200 × 300
Mumps	RNA	Helical	150–250
Herpes simplex	DNA	Polyhedral	100–150
Influenza	RNA	Helical	80–120
Retroviruses	RNA	Helical	100–120
Adenoviruses	DNA	Polyhedral	60–90
Retroviruses	RNA	Polyhedral	60–80
Papovaviruses	DNA	Polyhedral	40–60
Polioviruses	RNA	Polyhedral	28
Plant Viruses			
Turnip yellow mosaic	RNA	Polyhedral	28
Wound tumor	RNA	Polyhedral	55–60
Alfalfa mosaic	RNA	Polyhedral	18 × 36–40
Tobacco mosaic	RNA	Helical	18 × 300
Bacteriophages			
T2	DNA	Complex	65 × 210
L	DNA	Complex	54 × 194
F_x-174	DNA	Complex	25

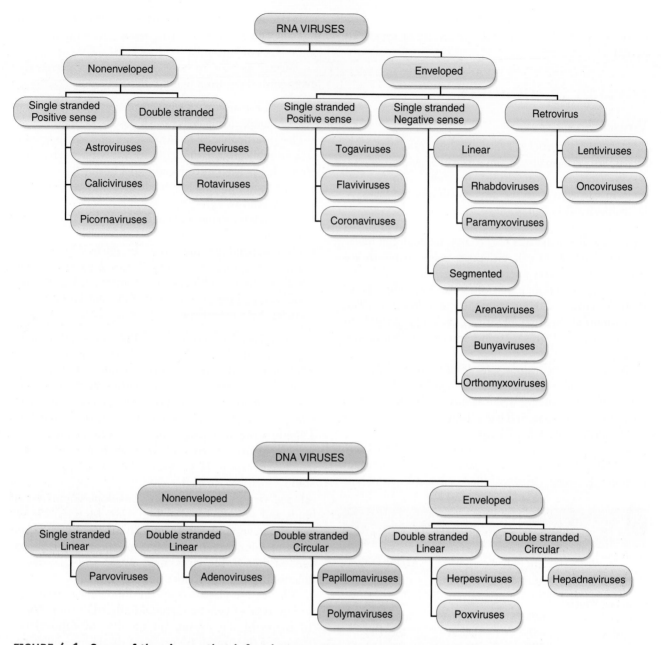

FIGURE 4-1. Some of the viruses that infect humans. Note that some viruses contain RNA, whereas others contain DNA, and that the nucleic acid that they possess may either be single or double stranded. Within the host cell, single-stranded positive sense RNA functions as messenger RNA (mRNA), whereas single-stranded negative sense RNA serves as a template for the production of mRNA. Some of the viruses possess an envelope, whereas others do not. (From Engleberg NC et al. Schaechter's Mechanisms of Microbial Diseases, 4th ed. Philadelphia: Lippincott Williams & Wilkins, 2007.)

Frequently, the envelope around the capsid makes the virus appear spherical or irregular in shape in electron micrographs. The envelope is acquired by certain animal viruses as they escape from the nucleus or cytoplasm of the host cell by budding (Figs. 4-4 and 4-5). In other words, the envelope is derived from either the host cell's nuclear membrane or cell membrane. Apparently, viruses are then able to alter these membranes by adding protein fibers, spikes, and knobs that enable the virus to recognize the next host cell to be in-

vaded. A list of some viruses, their characteristics, and diseases they cause is presented in Table 4-2. Sizes of some viruses are depicted in Figure 4-6.

Origin of Viruses

Where did viruses come from? Two main theories have been proposed to explain the origin of viruses. One theory states that viruses existed before cells, but this seems unlikely in view of the fact that viruses require cells for their replication. The other theory states that cells came first and

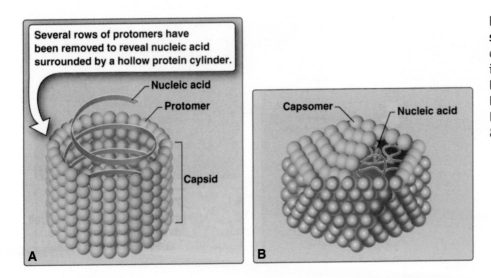

FIGURE 4-2. Viral nucleocapsids. (A) Nucleocapsid of a helical virus. **(B)** Nucleocapsid of an icosahedral virus. (From Harvey RA et al. Lippincott's Illustrated Reviews: Microbiology, 2nd ed. Philadelphia: Lippincott Williams & Wilkins, 2007.)

that viruses represent ancient derivatives of degenerate cells or cell fragments. The question of whether viruses are alive depends on one's definition of life and, thus, is not an easy question to answer. However, most scientists agree that viruses lack most of the basic features of cells; thus, they consider viruses to be nonliving entities.

Because they are not composed of cells, viruses are not considered to be living organisms. They are referred to as acellular microbes or infectious particles.

Bacteriophages

The viruses that infect bacteria are known as *bacteriophages* (or simply, *phages*). Like all viruses, they are obligate intracellular pathogens, in that they must enter a bacterial cell to replicate. There are three categories of bacteriophages, based on their shape:

- Icosahedron bacteriophages: an almost spherical shape, with 20 triangular facets; the smallest icosahedron phages are about 25 nm in diameter.
- Filamentous bacteriophages: long tubes formed by capsid proteins assembled into a helical structure; they can be up to about 900 nm long.

- Complex bacteriophages: icosahedral heads attached to helical tails; may also possess base plates and tail fibers.

In addition to shape, bacteriophages can be categorized by the type of nucleic acid that they possess; there are single-stranded DNA phages, double-stranded DNA phages, single-stranded RNA phages, and double-stranded RNA phages. From this point, only DNA phages will be discussed.

Bacteriophages can be categorized by the events that occur after invasion of the bacterial cell: some are virulent phages, whereas others are temperate phages. Phages in either category do not actually enter the bacterial cell—rather, they inject their nucleic acid into the cell. It is what happens next that distinguishes virulent phages from temperate phages.

Virulent bacteriophages always cause what is known as the *lytic cycle*, which ends with the destruction (lysis) of the bacterial cell. For most phages, the whole process (from attachment to lysis) takes less than 1 hour.

Once it enters a host cell, a virulent bacteriophage always initiates the lytic cycle, which results in the destruction of the cell.

The steps in the lytic cycle are shown in Table 4-3.

FIGURE 4-3. Enveloped viruses. (A) Enveloped helical virus. **(B)** Enveloped icosahedral virus. (From Harvey RA et al. Lippincott's Illustrated Reviews: Microbiology, 2nd ed. Philadelphia: Lippincott Williams & Wilkins, 2007.)

1 Virus-specific glycoproteins are synthesized and transported to the host cell membrane.

Host cell membrane

Viral protein

2 The cytoplasmic domains of membrane proteins bind nucleocapsids.

Nucleocapsid

3 A nucleocapsid is enveloped by the host cell membrane.

4 The host cell membrane provides the viral envelope by a process of "budding".

5 The enveloped virion is released from the host cell.

FIGURE 4-4. Virus particle becoming enveloped in the process of budding from a host cell.
(From Harvey RA et al. Lippincott's Illustrated Reviews: Microbiology, 2nd ed. Philadelphia: Lippincott Williams & Wilkins, 2007.)

FIGURE 4-5. Herpesviruses acquiring their envelopes as they leave a host cell's nucleus by budding. (1–3) Viruses within the nucleus. **(4)** Virus in the process of leaving the nucleus by budding. **(5, 6)** Viruses that have already acquired their envelopes. (From Volk WA, et al. Essentials of Medical Microbiology, 5th ed. Philadelphia: Lippincott-Raven, 1996.)

The first step in the lytic cycle is *attachment* (adsorption) of the phage to the surface of the bacterial cell. The phage can only attach to bacterial cells that possess the appropriate receptor—a protein or polysaccharide molecule on the surface of the cell that is recognized by a molecule on the surface of the phage. Most bacteriophages are species- and strain-specific, meaning that they only infect a particular species or strain of bacteria. Those that infect *Escherichia coli* are called coliphages. Some bacteriophages can attach to more than one species of bacterium. Figure 4-7 shows numerous bacteriophages attached to the surface of a *Vibrio cholerae* cell.

> Bacteriophages can only attach to bacteria that possess surface molecules (receptors) that can be recognized by molecules on the phage surface.

The second step in the lytic cycle is called *penetration*. In this step, the phage injects its DNA into the bacterial cell, acting much like a hypodermic needle (Fig. 4-8). From this point on, the phage DNA "dictates" what occurs within the bacterial cell. This is sometimes described as the phage DNA taking over the host cell's "machinery."

The third step in the lytic cycle is called *biosynthesis*. It is during this step that the phage genes are expressed, resulting in the production (biosynthesis) of viral pieces. It is also during this step that the host cell's enzymes (e.g., DNA polymerase and RNA polymerase), nucleotides, amino acids, and ribosomes are used to make viral DNA and viral proteins. In the fourth step of the lytic cycle, called *assembly*, the viral pieces are assembled to produce complete viral particles (virions). It is during this step that viral DNA is packaged up into capsids.

The final step in the lytic cycle, called *release*, is when the host cell bursts open and all of the new virions

TABLE 4-2	Selected Important Groups of Viruses and Viral Diseases		
VIRUS TYPE	**VIRAL CHARACTERISTICS**	**VIRUS**	**DISEASE**
Poxviruses	Large, brick shape with envelope, dsDNA	Variola Vaccinia	Smallpox Cowpox
Polyoma-papilloma	dsDNA, polyhedral	Papillomavirus Polyomavirus	Warts Some tumors, some cancer
Herpesvirus	Polyhedral with envelope, dsDNA	Herpes simplex I Herpes simplex II Herpes zoster Varicella	Cold sores or fever blisters Genital herpes Shingles Chickenpox
Adenovirus	dsDNA, icosahedral, with envelope		Respiratory infections, pneumonia, conjunctivitis, some tumors
Picornaviruses (the name means small RNA viruses)	ssRNA, tiny icosahedral, with envelope	Rhinovirus Poliovirus Hepatitis types A and B Coxsackievirus	Colds Poliomyelitis Hepatitis Respiratory infections, meningitis
Reoviruses	dsRNA, icosahedral with envelope	Enterovirus	Intestinal infections
Myxoviruses	RNA, helical with envelope	Orthomyxoviruses types A and B Myxovirus parotidis Paramyxovirus Rhabdovirus	Influenza Mumps Measles (rubeola) Rabies
Arbovirus	Arthropodborne RNA, cubic	Mosquitoborne type B Mosquitoborne types A and B Tickborne, coronavirus	Yellow fever Encephalitis (many types) Colorado tick fever
Retrovirus	dsRNA, helical with envelope	RNA tumor virus HTLV virus HIV	Tumors Leukemia AIDS

ds, double-stranded; ss, single-stranded.

(about 50–1,000) escape from the cell. Thus, the lytic cycle ends with lysis of the host cell. Lysis is caused by an enzyme that is coded for by a phage gene. At the appropriate time—after assembly—the appropriate viral gene is expressed, the enzyme is produced, and the bacterial cell wall is destroyed. With certain bacteriophages, a phage gene codes for an enzyme that interferes with cell wall synthesis, leading to weakness and, finally, collapse of the cell wall. The lytic cycle is summarized in Figure 4-9.

The other category of bacteriophages—*temperate phages* (also known as *lysogenic phages*)—do not immediately initiate the lytic cycle, but rather, their DNA remains integrated into the bacterial cell chromosome, generation after generation. Temperate bacteriophages are discussed further in Chapter 7.

Bacteriophages are involved in two of the four major ways in which bacteria acquire new genetic information. These processes—called lysogenic conversion and transduction—are discussed in Chapter 7.

Because bacteriophages destroy bacteria, there has been much speculation and experimentation through the years regarding their use to destroy bacterial pathogens and treat bacterial infections. The earliest research of this nature was conducted in the 1930s, but ended when antibiotics were discovered in the 1940s. However, since

Unlike virulent bacteriophages, temperate bacteriophages do not immediately initiate the lytic cycle. Their DNA can remain integrated into the host cell's chromosome for generation after generation.

FIGURE 4-6. Comparative sizes of virions, their nucleic acids, and bacteria. (From Davis BD, et al. Microbiology, 4th ed. Philadelphia: JB Lippincott, 1990.)

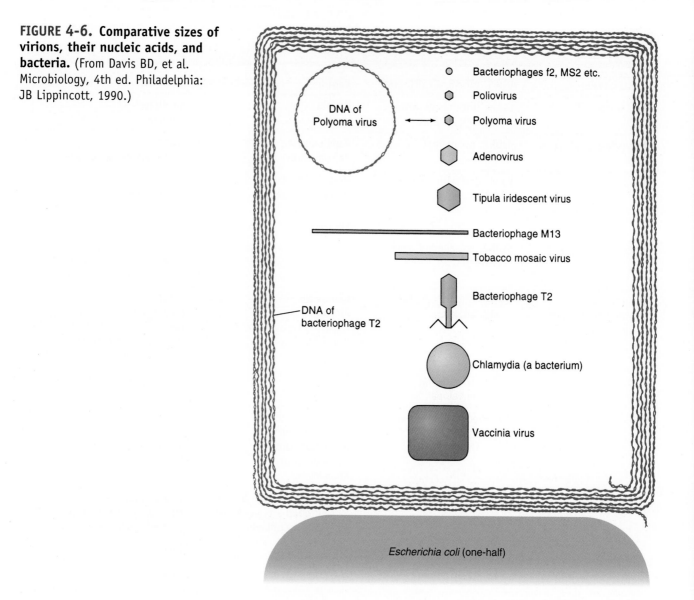

Bacteriophages f2, MS2 etc.

Poliovirus

Polyoma virus

DNA of Polyoma virus

Adenovirus

Tipula iridescent virus

Bacteriophage M13

Tobacco mosaic virus

Bacteriophage T2

DNA of bacteriophage T2

Chlamydia (a bacterium)

Vaccinia virus

Escherichia coli (one-half)

TABLE 4-3	Steps in the Multiplication of Bacteriophages (Lytic Cycle)	
STEP	**NAME OF STEP**	**WHAT OCCURS DURING THIS STEP**
1	Attachment (adsorption)	The phage attaches to a protein or polysaccharide molecule (receptor) on the surface of the bacterial cell
2	Penetration	The phage injects its DNA into the bacterial cell; the capsid remains on the outer surface of the cell
3	Biosynthesis	Phage genes are expressed, resulting in the production of phage pieces or parts (i.e., phage DNA and phage proteins)
4	Assembly	The phage pieces or parts are assembled to create complete phages
5	Release	The complete phages escape from the bacterial cell by lysis of the cell

FIGURE 4-7. A partially lysed cell of a *Vibrio cholerae* bacterium, with many attached virions of phage CP-T1. (Courtesy of R.W. Taylor and J.E. Ogg, Colorado State University, Fort Collins, CO.)

the emergence of multidrug-resistant bacteria ("superbugs"), research into the use of bacteriophages to treat bacterial diseases has been renewed. Additionally, bacteriophage enzymes that destroy cell walls or prevent their synthesis are currently being studied for use as therapeutic agents. It is possible that, in the future, certain bacterial diseases will be treated using orally administered or injected pathogen-specific bacteriophages or bacteriophage enzymes.

Animal Viruses

Viruses that infect humans and animals are collectively referred to as *animal viruses*. Some animal viruses are DNA viruses; others are RNA viruses. Animal viruses may consist solely of nucleic acid surrounded by a protein coat (capsid), or they may be more complex. For example, they may be enveloped or they may contain enzymes that play a role in viral multiplication within host cells. The steps in the multiplication of animal viruses are shown in Table 4-4.

The first step in the multiplication of animal viruses is *attachment* (or adsorption) of the virus to the cell. Like bacteriophages, animal viruses can only attach to cells bearing **Like bacteriophages, animal viruses can only attach to and invade cells bearing appropriate surface receptors.**

the appropriate protein or polysaccharide receptors on their surface. Did you ever wonder why certain viruses cause infections in dogs, but not in humans, or vice versa? Did you ever wonder why certain viruses cause respiratory infections, whereas others cause gastrointestinal infections? It all boils down to receptors. Viruses can only attach to and invade cells that bear a receptor that they can recognize.

The second step in the multiplication of animal viruses is *penetration*, but, unlike bacteriophages, the entire virion usually enters the host cell, sometimes because the cell phagocytizes the virus (Figs. 4-10, 4-11, and 4-12). This necessitates a third step that was not required for bacteriophages—*uncoating*—whereby the viral nucleic acid escapes from the capsid.

As with bacteriophages, from this point on, the viral nucleic acid "dictates" what occurs within the host cell. The fourth step is *biosynthesis*, whereby many viral pieces (viral nucleic acid and viral proteins) are produced. This step can be quite complicated, depending on what type of virus infected the cell (i.e., whether it was a single-stranded DNA virus, a double-stranded DNA virus, a single-stranded RNA virus, or a double-stranded RNA virus). Some animal viruses do not initiate biosynthesis right away, but rather, remain latent within the host cell for variable periods. Latent viral infections are discussed in more detail in a subsequent section.

The fifth step—*assembly*—involves fitting the virus pieces together to produce complete virions. After the virus particles are assembled, they must escape from the cell—a sixth step called *release*. How they escape from the cell depends **Animal viruses escape from their host cells either by lysis of the cell or budding. Viruses that escape by budding become enveloped viruses.**

on the type of virus that it is. Some animal viruses escape by destroying the host cell, leading to cell destruction and some of the symptoms associated with infection with that particular virus. Other viruses escape the cell by a process known as budding. Viruses that escape from the host cell cytoplasm by budding become surrounded with

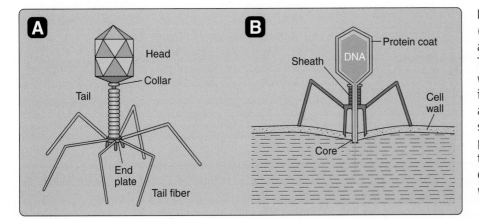

FIGURE 4-8. Bacteriophages. (A) The bacteriophage T4 is an assembly of protein components. The head is a protein membrane with 20 facets, filled with DNA. It is attached to a tail consisting of a hollow core surrounded by a sheath and based on a spiked end plate to which six fibers are attached. **(B)** The sheath contracts, driving the core through the cell wall, and viral DNA enters the cell.

1 Attachment of phage to cell surface receptor

← Bacteriophage

Cell wall of bacterium

0 MINUTES

2 Injection of phage DNA into cell

DNA

1 MINUTE

3 Synthesis of new phage DNA and phage proteins

10 MINUTES

Phage proteins

4 Assembly of new phage particles

25 MINUTES

Complete phage particle

5 Lysis of cell and release of progeny phage

30 MINUTES

FIGURE 4-9. Summary of the lytic process.
(From Harvey RA et al. Lippincott's Illustrated Reviews: Microbiology, 2nd ed. Philadelphia: Lippincott Williams & Wilkins, 2007.)

diagnostic tool to identify certain viral diseases. Inclusion bodies may be found in the cytoplasm (cytoplasmic inclusion bodies) or within the nucleus (intranuclear inclusion bodies), depending on the particular disease. In rabies, the cytoplasmic inclusion bodies in nerve cells are called Negri bodies. The inclusion bodies of AIDS and the Guarnieri bodies of smallpox are also cytoplasmic. Herpes and poliomyelitis viruses cause intranuclear inclusion bodies. In each case, inclusion bodies may represent aggregates or collections of viruses. Some important human viral diseases include AIDS, chickenpox, cold sores, the common cold, Ebola virus infections, genital herpes infections, German measles, Hantavirus pulmonary syndrome, infectious mononucleosis, influenza, measles, mumps, poliomyelitis, rabies, severe acute respiratory syndrome (SARS), and viral encephalitis. In addition, all human warts are caused by viruses.

Latent Virus Infections

Herpes virus infections, such as cold sores (fever blisters), are good examples of latent virus infections. Although the infected person is always harboring the virus in nerve cells, the cold sores come and go. A fever, stress, or excessive sunlight can trigger the viral genes to take over the cells and produce more viruses; in the process, cells are destroyed and a cold sore develops. Latent viral infections are usually limited by the defense systems of the human body—phagocytes and antiviral proteins called interferons that are produced by virus-infected cells (discussed in Chapter 15). Shingles, a painful nerve disease that is also caused by a herpesvirus, is another example of a latent viral infection. After a chickenpox infection, the virus can remain latent in the human body for many years. Then, when the body's immune defenses become weakened by old age or disease, the latent chickenpox virus resurfaces to cause shingles.

Antiviral Agents

Antibiotics function by inhibiting certain metabolic activities within cellular pathogens, and viruses are not cells. However, for certain patients with colds and influenza, antibiotics may be prescribed in an attempt to prevent secondary bacterial infections that might follow the virus infection. In recent years, a relatively small number of chemicals—called antiviral agents—have been developed to interfere with virus-specific enzymes and virus production by either disrupting critical phases in viral cycles or inhibiting the synthesis of viral DNA, RNA, or proteins. Antiviral agents are discussed further in Chapter 9.

It is very important for healthcare professionals to understand that antibiotics are not effective against viral infections.

Drugs used to treat viral infections are called antiviral agents.

pieces of the cell membrane, thus becoming enveloped viruses. If it is an enveloped virus, you know that it escaped from its host cell by budding.

Remnants or collections of viruses, called *inclusion bodies*, are often seen in infected cells and are used as a

TABLE 4-4	Steps in the Multiplication of Animal Viruses	
STEP	**NAME OF STEP**	**WHAT OCCURS DURING THIS STEP**
1	Attachment (adsorption)	The virus attaches to a protein or polysaccharide molecule (receptor) on the surface of a host cell
2	Penetration	The entire virus enters the host cell, in some cases because it was phagocytized by the cell
3	Uncoating	The viral nucleic acid escapes from the capsid
4	Biosynthesis	Viral genes are expressed, resulting in the production of pieces or parts of viruses (i.e., viral DNA and viral proteins)
5	Assembly	The viral pieces or parts are assembled to create complete virions
6	Release	The complete virions escape from the host cell by lysis or budding

Oncogenic Viruses

Viruses that cause cancer are called *oncogenic viruses* or *on-coviruses*. The first evidence that viruses cause cancers came from experiments with chickens. Subsequently, viruses were shown to be the cause of various types of cancers in rodents, frogs, and cats.

> Viruses that cause cancer are known as oncogenic viruses or oncoviruses.

Although the causes of many (perhaps most) types of human cancers remain unknown, it is known that *some* human cancers are caused by viruses. Epstein-Barr virus (a type of herpesvirus) causes infectious mononucleosis (not a type of cancer), but also causes three types of human cancers: nasopharyngeal carcinoma, Burkitt lymphoma, and B-cell lymphoma. Kaposi sarcoma, a type of cancer common in AIDS patients, is caused by human

FIGURE 4-10. Penetration of a host cell by a nonenveloped virus via endocytosis. (From Harvey RA et al. Lippincott's Illustrated Reviews: Microbiology, 2nd ed. Philadelphia: Lippincott Williams & Wilkins, 2007.)

FIGURE 4-11. Penetration of a host cell by an enveloped virus. (From Harvey RA et al. Lippincott's Illustrated Reviews: Microbiology, 2nd ed. Philadelphia: Lippincott Williams & Wilkins, 2007.)

FIGURE 4-12. Infection of host cells by Herpes simplex virus. Adsorption **(A)**, penetration **(B–D)**, and uncoating and digestion of the capsid **(E–G)** of herpes simplex on HeLa cells, as deduced from electron micrographs of infected cell sections. Penetration involves local digestion of the viral and cellular membranes **(B, C)**, resulting in fusion of the two membranes and release of the nucleocapsid into the cytoplasmic matrix **(D)**. The naked nucleocapsid is intact in **E**, is partially digested in **F**, and has disappeared in **G**, leaving a core containing DNA and protein. (From Morgan C, et al. *J Virol* 1968;2:507.)

herpesvirus 8. Associations between hepatitis B and C viruses and hepatocellular (liver) carcinoma have been established. Human papillomaviruses (HPV; wart viruses) can cause different types of cancer, including cancers of the cervix and other parts of the genital tract. A retrovirus that is closely related to human immunodeficiency virus (HIV; the cause of acquired immunodeficiency syndrome [AIDS]), called human T-lymphotrophic virus type 1 (HTLV-1), causes a rare type of adult T-cell leukemia. All of the mentioned oncogenic viruses, except HTLV-1, are DNA viruses. HTLV-1 is an RNA virus.

Human Immunodeficiency Virus

Human immunodeficiency virus, the cause of AIDS, is an enveloped, single-stranded RNA virus[a] (Fig. 4-13). It is a member of a genus of viruses called lentiviruses, in a family of

AIDS is caused by a single-stranded RNA virus known as human immunodeficiency virus (HIV).

viruses called Retroviridae (retroviruses). HIV is able to attach to and invade cells bearing receptors that the virus recognizes. The most important of these receptors is designated CD4, and cells possessing that receptor are called CD4[+] cells. The most important of the CD4[+] cells is the helper T cell (discussed in Chapter 16); HIV infections destroy these important cells of the immune system. Macrophages also possess CD4 receptors and can, thus,

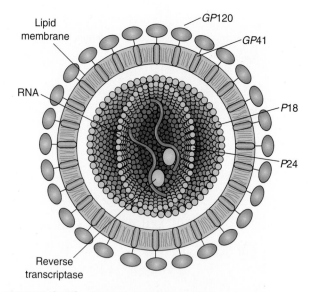

FIGURE 4-13. Human immunodeficiency virus (HIV). HIV is an enveloped virus, containing two identical single-stranded RNA molecules. Each of its 72 surface knobs contains a glycoprotein (designated *gp*120) capable of binding to a CD4 receptor on the surface of certain host cells (e.g., T-helper cells). The "stalk" that supports the knob is a transmembrane glycoprotein (designated *gp*41), which may also play a role in attachment to host cells. Reverse transcriptase is an RNA-dependent DNA polymerase. (From Porth CM. Pathophysiology: Concepts of Altered Health States, 5th ed. Philadelphia: Lippincott Williams & Wilkins, 1998.)

[a] The HIV virion contains two single-stranded RNA molecules.

be invaded by HIV. In addition, HIV is able to invade certain cells that do not possess CD4 receptors, but do possess other receptors that HIV is able to recognize.

Mimivirus

An extremely large double-stranded DNA virus, called Mimivirus, has been recovered from amebas. The virus was given the name Mimivirus because it "mimics" bacteria. It is so large that it can be observed using a standard compound light microscope. The Mimivirus particle has a 7 nm thick capsid with a diameter of 750 nm. An array of 80- to 125-nm long closely packed fibers project outward from the capsid surface (Fig. 4-14). Within the capsid, its DNA is surrounded by two 4-nm thick lipid membranes. Its genome is at least 10 times larger than that of the large viruses in the smallpox family and larger than the genome of some of the smallest bacteria. Some of its genes code for functions which were previously thought to be the exclusive province of cellular organisms, such as the translation of proteins and DNA repair

enzymes. Mimivirus contains several genes for sugar, lipid, and amino acid metabolism. And, unlike most DNA viruses, Mimivirus contains some RNA molecules. A limited number of reports suggest that Mimivirus may be the cause of some cases of human pneumonia.

Plant Viruses

More than 1,000 different viruses cause plant diseases, including diseases of citrus trees, cocoa trees, rice, barley, tobacco, turnips, cauliflower, potatoes, tomatoes, and many other fruits, vegetables, trees, and grains. These diseases result in huge economic losses, estimated to be in excess of $70 billion per year worldwide. Plant viruses are usually transmitted via insects (e.g., aphids, leaf hoppers, whiteflies); mites; nematodes (round worms); infected seeds, cuttings, and tubers; and contaminated tools (e.g., hoes, clippers, and saws).

Viroids and Prions

Although viruses are extremely small nonliving infectious agents, viroids and prions are even smaller and less complex infectious agents. *Viroids* con-

> Viroids are infectious RNA molecules that cause a variety of plant diseases.

sist of short, naked fragments of single-stranded RNA (about 300–400 nucleotides in length) that can interfere with the metabolism of plant cells and stunt the growth of plants, sometimes killing the plants in the process. They are transmitted between plants in the same manner as viruses. Plant diseases thought or known to be caused by viroids include potato spindle tuber (producing small, cracked, spindle-shaped potatoes), citrus exocortis (stunting of citrus trees), and diseases of chrysanthemums, coconut palms, and tomatoes. Thus far, no animal diseases have been discovered that are caused by viroids.

Prions (pronounced "pree-ons") are small infectious proteins that apparently cause fatal neurological diseases in animals, such as scrapie (pronounced "scrape-ee") in sheep and goats;

> Prions are infectious protein molecules that cause a variety of animal and human diseases.

bovine spongiform encephalopathy (BSE; "mad cow disease"; see "Insight: Microbes in the News: 'Mad Cow Disease'" on the CD-ROM); and kuru, Creutzfeldt-Jakob (C-J) disease, Gerstmann-Sträussler-Scheinker (GSS) disease, and fatal familial insomnia in humans. Similar diseases in mink, mule deer, Western white-tailed deer, elk,

FIGURE 4-14. Mimivirus structure. The Mimivirus virion consists of a double-stranded DNA core, surrounded by two lipid membranes and a protein capsid. Numerous fibrils extend outward from the capsid surface. (Courtesy of Xanthine at http://en.wikipedia.org.)

Labels on figure: Capsid · Inner Membranes · Fibrils · Core · 400nm

STUDY AID
Beware of Similar Sounding Terms
A **virion** is a complete viral particle (i.e., one that has all its parts, including nucleic acid and a capsid). A **viroid** is an infectious RNA molecule.

and cats may also be caused by prions. The name "scrapie" comes from the observation that infected animals scrape themselves against fence posts and other objects in an effort to relieve the intense pruritus (itching) associated with the disease. The disease in deer and elk is called "chronic wasting disease," in reference to the irreversible weight loss that the animals experience.

Kuru is a disease that was once common among natives in Papua, New Guinea, where women and children ate human brains as part of a traditional burial custom (ritualistic cannibalism). If the brain of the deceased person contained prions, then persons who ate that brain developed kuru. Kuru, C-J disease, and GSS disease involve loss of coordination and dementia. Dementia, a general mental deterioration, is characterized by disorientation and impaired memory, judgment, and intellect. In fatal familial insomnia, insomnia and dementia follow difficulty sleeping. All these diseases are fatal spongiform encephalopathies, in which the brain becomes riddled with holes (spongelike).

Scientists have been investigating the link between "mad cow disease" and a form of C-J disease (called variant CJD or vCJD) in humans. As of December 2008, 207 cases of vCJD had been diagnosed worldwide, including 164 in the United Kingdom; these cases probably resulted from eating prion-infected beef. The cattle may have acquired the disease through ingestion of cattle feed that contained ground-up parts of prion-infected sheep.

The 1997 Nobel Prize for Physiology or Medicine was awarded to Stanley B. Prusiner, the scientist who coined the term prion and studied the role of these proteinaceous infectious particles in disease. Of all pathogens, prions are believed to be the most resistant to disinfectants. The mechanism by which prions cause disease remains a mystery, although it is thought that prions convert normal protein molecules into nonfunctional ones by causing the normal molecules to change their shape. Many scientists remain unconvinced that proteins alone can cause disease.

THE DOMAIN *BACTERIA*

Characteristics

Recall from Chapter 3 that there are two domains of procaryotic organisms: Domain *Bacteria* and Domain *Archaea*. The bacteriologist's most important reference (sometimes referred to as the bacteriologist's "bible") is a five-volume set of books entitled *Bergey's Manual of Systematic Bacteriology* (*Bergey's Manual* for short), which is currently being rewritten. (An outline of these volumes can be found on CD-ROM Appendix 2: "Phyla and Medically Significant Genera Within the Domain *Bacteria*.") When all five volumes have been completed, they will contain descriptions of more than 5,000 validly named species of bacteria. Some authorities believe that this number represents only from less than 1% to a few percent of the total number of bacteria that exist in nature.

According to *Bergey's Manual*, the Domain *Bacteria* contains 23 phyla, 32 classes, 5 subclasses, 77 orders, 14 suborders, 182 families, 871 genera, and 5,007 species. Organisms in this domain are broadly divided into three phenotypic categories (i.e., categories based on their physical characteristics): (a) those that are Gram-negative and have a cell wall, (b) those that are Gram-positive and have a cell wall, and (c) those that lack a cell wall. (The terms Gram-positive and Gram-negative are explained in a subsequent section of this chapter.) Using computers, microbiologists have established numerical taxonomy systems that not only help to identify bacteria by their physical characteristics, but also can help establish how closely related these organisms are by comparing the composition of their genetic material and other cellular characteristics. (Note: as previously mentioned, throughout this book, the term "to identify an organism" means to learn the organism's species name [i.e., to speciate it].)

Many characteristics of bacteria are examined to provide data for identification and classification. These characteristics include cell shape and morphological arrangement, staining reactions, motility, colony morphology, atmospheric requirements, nutritional requirements, biochemical and metabolic activities, specific enzymes that the organism produces, pathogenicity (the ability to cause disease), and genetic composition.

> A bacterium's Gram reaction (Gram-positive or Gram-negative), basic cell shape, and morphological arrangement of the cells are very important clues to the organism's identification.

Cell Morphology

With the compound light microscope, the size, shape, and morphologic arrangement of various bacteria are easily observed. Bacteria vary greatly in size, usually ranging from spheres measuring about 0.2 μm in diameter to 10.0-μm–long spiral-shaped bacteria, to even longer filamentous bacteria. As previously mentioned, the average coccus is about 1 μm in diameter, and the average bacillus is about 1 μm wide × 3 μm long. Some unusually large bacteria and unusually small bacteria have also been discovered (discussed later).

There are three basic shapes of bacteria (Fig. 4-15): (a) round or spherical bacteria—the *cocci* (sing., *coccus*); (b) rectangular or rod-shaped bacteria—the *bacilli* (sing., *bacillus*); and (c) curved and spiral-shaped bacteria (sometimes referred to as spirilla).

> The three general shapes of bacteria are round (cocci), rod-shaped (bacilli), and spiral-shaped.

Recall from Chapter 3 that bacteria divide by binary fission—one cell splits in half to become two daughter cells. The time it takes for one cell to

> Bacteria reproduce by binary fission. The time it takes for one bacterial cell to split into two cells is referred to as that organism's generation time.

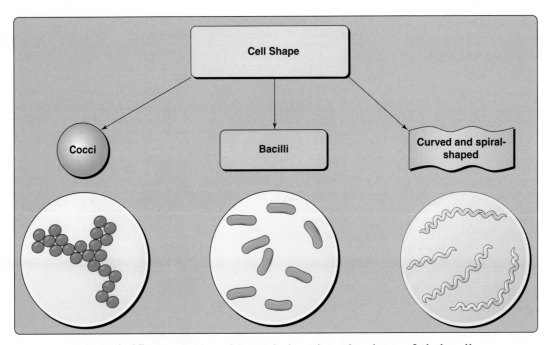

FIGURE 4-15. Categories of bacteria based on the shape of their cells.

split into two cells is referred to that organism's generation time. After binary fission, the daughter cells may separate completely from each other or may remain connected, forming various morphologic arrangements.

Cocci may be seen singly or in pairs (*diplococci*), chains (*streptococci*), clusters (*staphylococci*), packets of four (*tetrads*), or packets of eight (*octads*), depending on the particular species and the manner in which the cells divide (Figs. 4-16 and 4-17). Examples of medically important cocci include *Enterococcus* spp., *Neisseria* spp., *Staphylococcus* spp., and *Streptococcus* spp.

> Pairs of cocci are known as diplococci. Chains of cocci are known as streptococci. Clusters of cocci are known as staphylococci.

STUDY AID

Bacterial Names Sometimes Provide a Clue to Their Shape

If "coccus" appears in the name of a bacterium, you automatically know the shape of the organism—spherical. Examples include genera such as *Enterococcus*, *Peptococcus*, *Peptostreptococcus*, *Staphylococcus*, and *Streptococcus*. However, not all cocci have "coccus" in their names (e.g., *Neisseria* spp.). If "bacillus" appears in the name of a bacterium, you automatically know the shape of the organism—rod-shaped or rectangular. Examples include genera such as *Actinobacillus*, *Bacillus*, *Lactobacillus*, and *Streptobacillus*. However, not all bacilli have "bacillus" in their names (e.g., *E. coli*).

Bacilli (often referred to as rods) may be short or long, thick or thin, and pointed or with curved or blunt ends. They may occur singly, in pairs (*diplobacilli*), in chains (*streptobacilli*), in long filaments, or branched. Some rods are quite short, resembling elongated cocci; they are called *coccobacilli*. *Listeria monocytogenes* and *Haemophilus influenzae* are examples of coccobacilli. Some bacilli stack up next to each other, side by side in a palisade arrangement, which is characteristic of *Corynebacterium diphtheriae* (the cause of diphtheria) and organisms that resemble it in appearance (called *diphtheroids*). Examples of medically important bacilli include members of the family *Enterobacteriaceae* (e.g., *Enterobacter*, *Escherichia*, *Klebsiella*, *Proteus*, *Salmonella*, and *Shigella* spp.), *Pseudomonas aeruginosa*, *Bacillus* spp., and *Clostridium* spp.

Curved and spiral-shaped bacilli are placed into a third morphologic grouping. For example, *Vibrio* spp., such as *V. cholerae* (the cause of cholera) and *V. parahaemolyticus* (a cause of diarrhea), are curved (comma-shaped) bacilli. Curved bacteria usually occur singly, but some species may form pairs. A pair of curved bacilli

STUDY AID

Beware the Word "Bacillus"

Whenever you see the word *Bacillus*, capitalized and underlined or italicized, it is a particular genus of rod-shaped bacteria. However, if you see the word bacillus, and it is not capitalized, underlined, or italicized, it refers to any rod-shaped bacterium.

FIGURE 4-16. Morphologic arrangements of cocci and examples of bacteria having these arrangements.

Arrangement	Description	Appearance	Example	Disease
Diplococci	Cocci in pairs		*Neisseria gonorrhoeae*	Gonorrhea
Streptococci	Cocci in chains		*Streptococcus pyogenes*	Strep throat
Staphylococci	Cocci in clusters		*Staphylococcus aureus*	Boils
Tetrad	A packet of 4 cocci		*Micrococcus luteus*	Rarely pathogenic
Octad	A packet of 8 cocci		*Sarcina ventriculi*	Rarely pathogenic

FIGURE 4-17. Morphologic arrangements of cocci. (A) Photomicrograph of Gram-stained *Staphylococcus aureus* cells illustrating Gram-positive (blue) cocci in grapelike clusters. A pink-stained white blood cell can also be seen in the lower portion of the photomicrograph. **(B)** Scanning electron micrograph of *Streptococcus mutans* illustrating cocci in chains. **([A]** From Winn WC Jr, et al. Koneman's Color Atlas and Textbook of Diagnostic Microbiology, 6th ed. Philadelphia: Lippincott Williams & Wilkins, 2006. **[B]** From Volk WA, et al. Essentials of Medical Microbiology, 5th ed. Philadelphia: Lippincott-Raven, 1996.)

resembles a bird and is described as having a gull-wing morphology. *Campylobacter* spp. (a common cause of diarrhea) have a gull-wing morphology. Spiral-shaped bacteria are referred to as spirochetes. Different species of spirochetes vary in size, length, rigidity, and the number and amplitude of their coils. Some are tightly coiled, such as *Treponema pallidum*, the cause of syphilis, with a flexible cell wall that enables them to move readily through tissues (Fig. 4-18). Its morphology and characteristic motility—spinning around its long axis— make *T. pallidum* easy to recognize in wet preparations of clinical specimens obtained from patients with primary syphilis. *Borrelia* spp., the causative agents of Lyme disease and relapsing fever, are examples of less tightly coiled spirochetes (Fig. 4-19).

Some bacteria may lose their characteristic shape because adverse growth conditions (e.g., the presence of certain antibiotics) prevent the production of normal cell walls. They are referred to as cell wall–deficient (CWD) bacteria. Some CWD bacteria revert to their original shape when placed in favorable growth conditions, whereas others do not. Bacteria in the genus *Mycoplasma* do not have cell walls; thus, when examined microscopically, they appear in various shapes. Bacteria that exist in a variety of shapes are described as being *pleomorphic*; the ability to exist in a variety of shapes is known as *pleomorphism*. Because they have no cell walls, mycoplasmas are resistant to antibiotics that inhibit cell wall synthesis.

> A bacterial species having cells of different shapes is said to be pleomorphic.

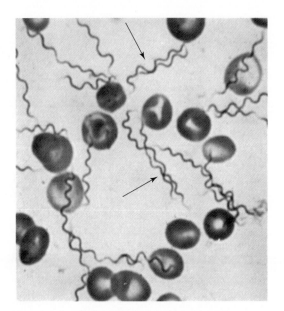

FIGURE 4-19. Spiral-shaped *Borrelia hermsii* (arrows), a cause of relapsing fever, in a stained blood smear. (From Volk WA, et al. Essentials of Medical Microbiology, 5th ed. Philadelphia: Lippincott-Raven, 1996.)

Staining Procedures

As they exist in nature, most bacteria are colorless, transparent, and difficult to see. Therefore, various staining methods have been devised to enable scientists to examine bacteria. In preparation for staining, the bacteria are smeared onto a glass microscope slide (resulting in what is known as a "smear"), air-dried, and then "fixed." (Methods for preparing and fixing smears are further described in CD-ROM Appendix 5: "Clinical Microbiology Laboratory Procedures.") The two most common methods of fixation are heat fixation and methanol fixation. Heat fixation is usually accomplished by passing the smear through a Bunsen burner flame. If not performed properly, excess heat can distort the morphology of the cells. Methanol fixation, which is accomplished by flooding the smear with absolute methanol for 30 seconds, is a more satisfactory fixation technique. In general, fixation serves three purposes:

1. It kills the organisms.
2. It preserves their morphology (shape).
3. It anchors the smear to the slide.

Specific stains and staining techniques are used to observe bacterial cell morphology (e.g., size, shape, morphologic arrangement, composition of cell wall, capsules, flagella, endospores).

A *simple stain* is sufficient to determine bacterial shape and morphologic arrangement (e.g., pairs, chains, clusters). For this method, shown in Figure 4-20, a dye (such

FIGURE 4-18. Scanning electron micrograph of *Treponema pallidum*, the bacterium that causes syphilis. (Courtesy of Dr. David Cox and the Centers for Disease Control and Prevention.)

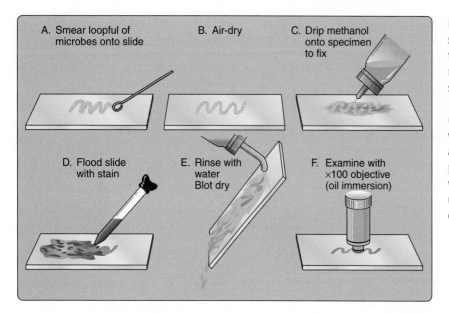

A. Smear loopful of microbes onto slide
B. Air-dry
C. Drip methanol onto specimen to fix
D. Flood slide with stain
E. Rinse with water Blot dry
F. Examine with ×100 objective (oil immersion)

FIGURE 4-20. Simple bacterial staining technique. (A) With a flamed loop, smear a loopful of bacteria suspended in broth or water onto a slide. **(B)** Allow slide to air-dry. **(C)** Fix the smear with absolute (100%) methanol. **(D)** Flood the slide with the stain. **(E)** Rinse with water and blot dry with bibulous paper or paper towel. **(F)** Examine the slide with the ×100 microscope objective, using a drop of immersion oil directly on the smear.

as methylene blue) is applied to the fixed smear, rinsed, dried, and examined using the oil immersion lens of the microscope. The procedures used to observe bacterial capsules, spores, and flagella are collectively referred to as *structural staining procedures.*

In 1883, Dr. Hans Christian Gram developed a staining technique that bears his name—the Gram stain or Gram staining procedure. The Gram stain has become the most important staining procedure in the bacteriology laboratory, because it differentiates between "Gram-positive" and "Gram-negative" bacteria (these terms will be explained shortly). The organism's Gram reaction serves as an extremely important "clue" when

HISTORICAL NOTE
The Origin of the Gram Stain

While working in a laboratory in the morgue of a Berlin hospital in the 1880s, a Danish physician named **Hans Christian Gram** developed what was to become the most important of all bacterial staining procedures. He was developing a staining technique that would enable him to see bacteria in the lung tissues of patients who had died of pneumonia. The procedure he developed—now called the *Gram stain*—demonstrated that two general categories of bacteria cause pneumonia: some of them stained blue and some of them stained red. The blue ones came to be known as Gram-positive bacteria, and the red ones came to be known as Gram-negative bacteria. It was not until 1963 that the mechanism of Gram differentiation was explained by M.R.J. Salton.

attempting to learn the identity (species) of a particular bacterium. The steps in the Gram staining procedure are described in CD-ROM Appendix 5: "Clinical Microbiology Laboratory Procedures" and illustrated in Fig. 4-21.

The color of the bacteria at the end of the Gram staining procedure depends on the chemical composition of their cell wall (Table 4-5). If the bacteria were not decolorized during the decolorization step, they will be blue to purple at the conclusion of the Gram staining procedure; such bacteria are said to be "Gram-positive." The thick layer of peptidoglycan in the cell walls of Gram-positive bacteria makes it difficult to remove the crystal violet–iodine complex during the decolorization step. Figures 4-22 through 4-26 depict various Gram-positive bacteria.

If, on the other hand, the crystal violet was removed from the cells during the decolorization step, and the cells were subsequently stained by the safranin (a red dye), they will be pink to red at the conclusion of the Gram staining procedure; such bacteria are said to be "Gram-negative." The thin layer of peptidoglycan in the cell walls of Gram-negative bacteria makes it easier to remove the crystal violet–iodine complex during decolorization. In addition, the decolorizer dissolves the lipid in the cell walls of Gram-negative bacteria; this destroys the integrity of the cell wall and makes it much easier to remove the crystal violet–iodine complex. Figures 4-27 and 4-28 depict various Gram-negative bacteria.

> If a bacterium is blue to purple at the end of the Gram staining procedure, it is said to be Gram-positive. If, on the other hand, it ends up being pink to red, it is said to be Gram-negative.

FIGURE 4-21. Steps in the Gram staining technique. (From Harvey RA et al. Lippincott's Illustrated Reviews: Microbiology, 2nd ed. Philadelphia: Lippincott Williams & Wilkins, 2007.)

1. Heat-fix specimen to slide. Flood slide with crystal violet solution; allow to act for 1 minute.

Crystal violet solution

2. Rinse the slide, then flood with iodine solution; allow iodine to act for 1 minute. Before acetone decolorization (next step), all organisms appear purple, that is, gram-positive.

Iodine solution

3. Rinse off excess iodine. Decolorize with acetone, approximately 5 seconds (time depends on density of specimen).

Acetone

4. Wash slide immediately in water. After acetone decolorization, those organisms that are gram-negative are no longer visible.

5. Apply safranin counterstain for 30 seconds.

Safranin

6. Wash in water, blot, and dry in air. Gram-negative organisms are visualized after application of the counterstain.

Key: ● = Gram-positive violet. ▬ = Gram-negative red. ⬭ = Colorless.

TABLE 4-5	Differences between Gram-Positive and Gram-Negative Bacteria	
	GRAM-POSITIVE BACTERIA	**GRAM-NEGATIVE BACTERIA**
Color at the end of the Gram staining procedure	Blue-to-purple	Pink-to-red
Peptidoglycan in cell walls	Thick layer	Thin layer
Teichoic acids and lipoteichoic acids in cell walls	Present	Absent
Lipopolysaccharide in cell walls	Absent	Present

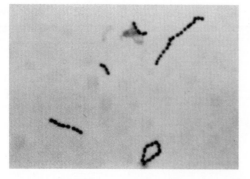

FIGURE 4-22. Chains of Gram-positive streptococci in a Gram-stained smear from a broth culture. (From Winn WC Jr, et al. Koneman's Color Atlas and Textbook of Diagnostic Microbiology, 6th ed. Philadelphia: Lippincott Williams & Wilkins, 2006.)

FIGURE 4-23. Gram-positive *Streptococcus pneumoniae* in a Gram-stained smear of a blood culture. Note the pairs of cocci, known as diplococci (arrows). (From Winn WC Jr, et al. Koneman's Color Atlas and Textbook of Diagnostic Microbiology, 6th ed. Philadelphia: Lippincott Williams & Wilkins, 2006.)

FIGURE 4-24. Gram-positive bacilli (*Clostridium perfringens*) in a Gram-stained smear prepared from a broth culture. Individual bacilli and chains of bacilli (streptobacilli) can be seen. (From Winn WC Jr, et al. Koneman's Color Atlas and Textbook of Diagnostic Microbiology, 6th ed. Philadelphia: Lippincott Williams & Wilkins, 2006.)

FIGURE 4-25. Gram-positive bacilli (*Clostridium tetani*) in a Gram-stained smear from a broth culture. Terminal spores can be seen on some of the cells (arrows). (From Winn WC Jr, et al. Koneman's Color Atlas and Textbook of Diagnostic Microbiology, 6th ed. Philadelphia: Lippincott Williams & Wilkins, 2006.)

FIGURE 4-26. Many Gram-positive bacteria can be seen on the surface of a pink-stained epithelial cell in this Gram-stained sputum specimen. Several smaller pink-staining polymorphonuclear leukocytes can also be seen. (From Winn WC Jr, et al. Koneman's Color Atlas and Textbook of Diagnostic Microbiology, 6th ed. Philadelphia: Lippincott Williams & Wilkins, 2006.)

FIGURE 4-27. Gram-negative bacilli in a Gram-stained smear prepared from a bacterial colony. Individual bacilli and a few short chains of bacilli can be seen. (From Koneman E, et al. Color Atlas and Textbook of Diagnostic Microbiology, 5th ed. Philadelphia: Lippincott Williams & Wilkins, 1997.)

FIGURE 4-28. Loosely coiled Gram-negative spirochetes. *Borrelia burgdorferi* is the etiologic agent (cause) of Lyme disease. (From Winn WC Jr, et al. Koneman's Color Atlas and Textbook of Diagnostic Microbiology, 6th ed. Philadelphia: Lippincott Williams & Wilkins, 2006.)

Figure 4-29 illustrates the various shapes of bacteria that may be observed in a Gram-stained clinical specimen. Some strains of bacteria are neither consistently blue to purple nor pink to red after Gram staining; they are referred to as Gram-variable bacteria. Examples of Gram-variable bacteria are members of the genus *Mycobacterium*, such as *M. tuberculosis* and *M. leprae*. Refer to Table 4-6 and Figures 4-22 through 4-28 for the staining characteristics of certain pathogens.

Mycobacterium species are more often identified using a staining procedure called the *acid-fast stain*. In this procedure, carbol fuchsin (a bright red dye) is first driven into the bacterial cell using heat (usually by flooding the smear with carbol fuchsin, and then holding a Bunsen burner flame under the slide until steaming of the carbol fuchsin occurs). The heat is necessary because the cell walls of mycobacteria contain waxes, which prevent the stain from penetrating the cells. The heat softens the waxes, enabling the stain to penetrate. A decolorizing agent (a mixture of acid and alcohol) is then used in an attempt to remove the red color from the cells. Because mycobacteria are not decolorized by the acid–alcohol mixture (again owing to the waxes in their cell walls), they are said to be acid-fast. Most other bacteria are decolorized by the acid–alcohol treatment; they are said to be non–acid-fast. The acid-fast stain is especially useful in the tuberculosis laboratory ("TB lab") where the acid-fast mycobacteria are readily seen as red bacilli (referred to as acid-fast bacilli or AFB) against a blue or green background in a sputum specimen from a tuberculosis patient. Figures 4-30 and 4-31 depict the appearance of mycobacteria after the acid-fast staining procedure. The acid-fast staining procedure was developed in 1882 by Paul Ehrlich—a German chemist.

The Gram and acid-fast staining procedures are referred to as *differential staining procedures* because they enable microbiologists to differentiate one group of bacteria from another (i.e., Gram-positive bacteria from Gram-negative bacteria, and acid-fast bacteria from non–acid-fast bacteria). Table 4-7 summarizes the various types of bacterial staining procedures.

> The acid-fast stain is of value in the diagnosis of tuberculosis. Acid-fast bacteria are red at the end of the acid-fast staining procedure.

FIGURE 4-29. Various forms of bacteria that might be observed in Gram-stained smears. Shown here are single cocci, diplococci, tetrads, octads, streptococci, staphylococci, single bacilli, diplobacilli, streptobacilli, branching bacilli, loosely coiled spirochetes, and tightly coiled spirochetes. (See text for explanation of terms.)

STUDY AID

A Method of Remembering a Particular Bacterium's Gram Reaction

A former student used this method to remember the Gram reaction of a particular bacterium. In her notebook, she drew two large circles. She lightly shaded in one circle, using a blue colored pencil. The other circle was lightly shaded red. Within the blue circle, she wrote the names of bacteria studied in the course that were Gram-positive. Within the red circle, she wrote the names of bacteria that were Gram-negative. She then studied the two circles. Later, whenever she encountered the name of a particular bacterium, she would remember which circle it was in. If it was in the blue circle, then the bacterium was Gram-positive. If it was in the red circle, the bacterium was Gram-negative. Clever!

TABLE 4-6	Characteristics of Some Important Pathogenic Bacteria		
STAINING REACTION	**MORPHOLOGY**	**BACTERIUM**	**DISEASE(S)**
Gram-positive	Cocci in clusters	*Staphylococcus aureus*	Wound infections, boils, pneumonia, septicemia, food poisoning
	Cocci in chains	*Streptococcus pyogenes*	Strep throat, scarlet fever, necrotizing fasciitis, septicemia
	Diplococci	*Streptococcus pneumoniae*	Pneumonia, meningitis, ear and sinus infections
	Bacillus	*Corynebacterium diphtheriae*	Diphtheria
	Spore-forming bacillus	*Bacillus anthracis*	Anthrax
		Clostridium botulinum	Botulism
		Clostridium perfringens	Wound infections, gas gangrene, food poisoning
		Clostridium tetani	tetanus
Gram-negative	Diplococci	*Neisseria gonorrhoeae*	gonorrhea
		Neisseria meningitidis	Meningitis, respiratory infections
	Bacillus	*Bordetella pertussis*	Whooping cough (pertussis)
		Brucella abortus	Brucellosis
		Chlamydia trachomatis	Genital infections, trachoma
		Escherichia coli	Urinary tract infections, septicemia
		Francisella tularensis	Tularemia
		Haemophilus ducreyi	Chancroid
		Haemophilus influenzae	Meningitis; respiratory, ear and sinus infections
		Klebsiella pneumoniae	Urinary tract and respiratory infections
		Proteus vulgaris	Urinary tract infections
		Pseudomonas aeruginosa	Respiratory, urinary, and wound infections
		Rickettsia rickettsii	Rocky Mountain spotted fever
		Salmonella typhi	Typhoid fever
		Salmonella spp.	Gastroenteritis
		Shigella spp.	Gastroenteritis
		Yersinia pestis	Plague
	Curved bacillus	*Vibrio cholerae*	Cholera
	Spirochete	*Treponema pallidum*	Syphillis
Acid-fast, Gram-variable	Branching bacilli	*Mycobacterium leprae*	Leprosy (Hansen disease)
		Mycobacterium tuberculosis	Tuberculosis

FIGURE 4-30. Many red acid-fast mycobacteria can be seen in this acid-fast stained liver biopsy specimen. (From Winn WC Jr, et al. Koneman's Color Atlas and Textbook of Diagnostic Microbiology, 6th ed. Philadelphia: Lippincott Williams & Wilkins, 2006.)

FIGURE 4-31. Many red acid-fast bacilli (*Mycobacterium tuberculosis*) can be seen in this acid-fast stained concentrate from a digested sputum specimen. (From Koneman, E, et al. Color Atlas and Textbook of Diagnostic Microbiology, 5th ed. Philadelphia: Lippincott Williams & Wilkins, 1997.)

TABLE 4-7   Types of Bacterial Staining Procedures

CATEGORY	EXAMPLE(S)	PURPOSE
Simple staining procedure	Staining with methylene blue	Merely to stain the cells so that their size, shape, and morphologic arrangement can be determined
Structural staining procedures	Capsule stains	To determine whether the organism is encapsulated
	Flagella stains	To determine whether the organism possesses flagella and, if so, their number and location on the cell
	Endospore stains	To determine whether the organism is a spore-former and, if so, to determine whether the spores are terminal or subterminal spores
Differential staining procedures	Gram stain	To differentiate between Gram-positive and Gram-negative bacteria
	Acid-fast stain	To differentiate between acid-fast and non–acid-fast bacteria

Motility

If a bacterium is able to "swim," it is said to be motile. Bacteria unable to swim are said to be nonmotile. Bacterial motility is most often associated with the presence of flagella or axial filaments, although some bacteria exhibit a type of gliding motility on secreted slime. Bacteria never possess cilia. Most spiral-shaped bacteria and about one half of the bacilli are motile by means of flagella, but cocci are generally nonmotile. A flagella stain can be used to demonstrate the presence, number, and location of flagella on bacterial cells. Various terms (e.g., monotrichous, amphitrichous, lophotrichous, peritrichous) are used to describe the number and location of flagella on bacterial cells (see Chapter 3).

Motility can be demonstrated by stabbing the bacteria into a tube of semisolid agar or by using the hanging-drop technique. Growth (multiplication) of bacteria in semisolid agar produces turbidity (cloudiness). Nonmotile organisms will grow only along the stab line (thus, turbidity will be seen only along the stab line), but motile organisms will spread away from the stab line (thus, producing turbidity throughout the medium; see Fig. 4-32). In the hanging-drop method (Fig. 4-33), a drop of a bacterial suspension is placed onto a glass coverslip. The coverslip is then inverted over a depression slide. When the preparation is examined microscopically, motile bacteria within the "hanging drop" will be seen darting around in every direction.

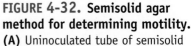

FIGURE 4-32. Semisolid agar method for determining motility. **(A)** Uninoculated tube of semisolid agar. **(B)** Same tube being inoculated by stabbing the inoculating wire into the medium. **(C)** Pattern of growth of a nonmotile organism, after incubation. **(D)** Pattern of growth of a motile organism, after incubation.

A.   B.   C.   D.

FIGURE 4-33. Hanging-drop preparation for study of living bacteria.
(A) Depression slide. **(B)** Depression slide with coverglass over the depression area. **(C)** Side view of hanging-drop preparation showing the drop of liquid culture medium hanging from the center of the coverglass above the depression.

Colony Morphology

A single bacterial cell that lands on the surface of a solid culture medium cannot be seen, but after it divides over and over again, it produces a mound or pile of bacteria, known as a bacterial colony (Fig. 4-34). A colony contains millions of organisms. The colony morphology (appearance of the colonies) of bacteria varies from one species to another. Colony morphology includes the size, color, overall shape, elevation, and the appearance of the edge or margin of the colony. As is true for cell morphology and staining characteristics, colony features serve as important "clues" in the identification of bacteria. Size of colonies is determined by the organism's rate of growth (generation time), and is an important characteristic of a particular bacterial species. Colony morphology also includes the results of enzymatic

> A mound or pile of bacteria on a solid culture medium is known as a bacterial colony.

activity on various types of culture media, such as those shown in Figures 8-3 through 8-5 in Chapter 8.

Atmospheric Requirements

In the microbiology laboratory, it is useful to classify bacteria on the basis of their relationship to oxygen (O_2) and carbon dioxide (CO_2). With respect to oxygen, a bacterial isolate can be classified into one of five major groups: obligate aerobes, microaerophilic aerobes (microaerophiles), facultative anaerobes, aerotolerant anaerobes, and obligate anaerobes (Fig. 4-35). In a liquid medium such as thioglycollate broth, the region of the medium in which the organism grows depends on the oxygen needs of that particular species.

To grow and multiply, *obligate aerobes* require an atmosphere containing molecular oxygen in concentrations comparable to that found in room air (i.e., 20%–21% O_2). Mycobacteria and certain fungi are examples of microorganisms that are obligate aerobes. *Microaerophiles* (microaerophilic aerobes) also require oxygen for

> Obligate aerobes and microaerophiles require oxygen. Obligate aerobes require an atmosphere containing about 20% to 21% oxygen, whereas microaerophiles require reduced oxygen concentrations (usually around 5% oxygen).

FIGURE 4-34. Formation of a bacterial colony on solid growth medium. In this illustration, the generation time is assumed to be 30 minutes. (From Harvey RA, et al. Lippincott's Illustrated Reviews: Microbiology, 2nd ed. Philadelphia: Lippincott Williams & Wilkins, 2007.)

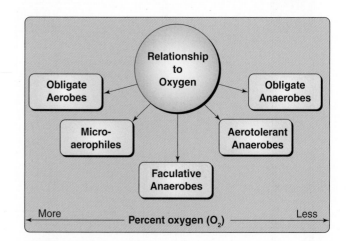

FIGURE 4-35. Categories of bacteria based on their relationship to oxygen.

multiplication, but in concentrations lower than that found in room air. *Neisseria gonorrhoeae* (the causative agent of gonorrhea) and *Campylobacter* spp. (which are major causes of bacterial diarrhea) are examples of microaerophilic bacteria that prefer an atmosphere containing about 5% oxygen.

Anaerobes can be defined as organisms that do not require oxygen for life and reproduction. However, they vary in their sensitivity to oxygen. The terms obligate anaerobe, aerotolerant anaerobe, and facultative anaerobe are used to describe the organism's relationship to molecular oxygen. An *obligate anaerobe* is an anaerobe that can only grow in an anaerobic environment (i.e., an environment containing no oxygen) (see "Insight: Life in the Absence of Oxygen" on the CD-ROM).

An *aerotolerant anaerobe* does not require oxygen, grows better in the absence of oxygen, but can survive in atmospheres containing molecular oxygen (such as air and a CO_2 incubator). The concentration of oxygen that an aerotolerant anaerobe can tolerate varies from one species to another. *Facultative anaerobes* are capable of surviving in either the presence or absence of oxygen; anywhere from 0% O_2 to 20% to 21% O_2. Many of the bacteria routinely isolated from clinical specimens are facultative anaerobes (e.g., members of the family *Enterobacteriaceae*, most streptococci, most staphylococci).

> Obligate anaerobes, aerotolerant anaerobes, and facultative anaerobes can thrive in an atmosphere devoid of oxygen.

Room air contains less than 1% CO_2. Some bacteria, referred to as *capnophiles* (capnophilic organisms), grow better in the laboratory in the presence of increased concentrations of CO_2. Some anaerobes (e.g., *Bacteroides* and *Fusobacterium* species) are capnophiles, as are some aerobes (e.g., certain *Neisseria*, *Campylobacter*, and *Haemophilus* species). In the clinical microbiology laboratory, CO_2 incubators are routinely calibrated to contain between 5% and 10% CO_2.

> For optimum growth in the laboratory, capnophiles require an atmosphere containing 5% to 10% carbon dioxide.

Nutritional Requirements

All bacteria need some form of the elements carbon, hydrogen, oxygen, sulfur, phosphorus, and nitrogen for growth. Special elements, such as potassium, calcium, iron, manganese, magnesium, cobalt, copper, zinc, and uranium, are required by some bacteria. Certain microbes have specific vitamin requirements and some need organic substances secreted by other living microorganisms during their growth. Organisms with especially demanding nutritional requirements are said to be fastidious; think of them as being "fussy." Special enriched media must be used to grow fastidious organisms in the laboratory. The nutritional needs of a particular organism are usually characteristic for that species of bacteria and sometimes serve as important clues when attempting to identify the organism. Nutritional requirements are discussed further in Chapters 7 and 8.

Biochemical and Metabolic Activities

As bacteria grow, they produce many waste products and secretions, some of which are enzymes that enable them to invade their host and cause disease. The pathogenic strains of many bacteria, such as staphylococci and streptococci, can be tentatively identified by the enzymes they secrete. Also, in particular environments, some bacteria are characterized by the production of certain gases, such as carbon dioxide, hydrogen sulfide, oxygen, or methane. To aid in the identification of certain types of bacteria in the laboratory, they are inoculated into various substrates (e.g., carbohydrates and amino acids) to determine whether they possess the enzymes necessary to break down those substrates. Learning whether a particular organism is able to break down a certain substrate serves as a clue to the identity of that organism. Different types of culture media are also used in the laboratory to learn information about an organism's metabolic activities (to be discussed in Chapter 8).

Pathogenicity

The characteristics that enable bacteria to cause disease are discussed in Chapter 14. Many pathogens are able to cause disease because they possess capsules, pili, or endotoxins (biochemical components of the cell walls of Gram-negative bacteria), or because they secrete exotoxins and exoenzymes that damage cells and tissues. Frequently, pathogenicity (the ability to cause disease) is tested by injecting the organism into mice or cell cultures. Some common pathogenic bacteria are listed in Table 4-6.

Genetic Composition

Most modern laboratories are moving toward the identification of bacteria using some type of test procedure that analyzes the organism's deoxyribonucleic acid (DNA) or ribonucleic acid (RNA). These test procedures are collectively referred to as molecular diagnostic procedures. The composition of the genetic material (DNA) of an organism is unique to each species. DNA probes make it possible to identify an isolate without relying on phenotypic characteristics. A DNA probe is a single-stranded DNA sequence that can be used to identify an organism by hybridizing with a unique complimentary sequence on the DNA or rRNA of that organism. Also, through the use of 16S rRNA sequencing (see Chapter 3), a researcher can determine the degree of relatedness between two different bacteria.

Unique Bacteria

Rickettsias, chlamydias, and mycoplasmas are bacteria, but they do not possess all the attributes of typical bacterial cells. Thus, they are often referred to as "unique" or "rudimentary" bacteria. Because they are so small and difficult to isolate, they were formerly thought to be viruses.

Rickettsias, Chlamydias, and Closely Related Bacteria

Rickettsias and chlamydias are bacteria with a Gram-negative–type cell wall. They are obligate intracellular pathogens that cause diseases in humans and other animals. As the name implies, an obligate intracellular pathogen is a pathogen that must live within a host cell. To grow such organisms in the laboratory, they must be inoculated into embryonated chicken eggs, laboratory animals, or cell cultures. They will not grow on artificial (synthetic) culture media.

The genus *Rickettsia* was named for Howard T. Ricketts, a U.S. pathologist; these organisms have no connection to the disease called rickets, which is the result of vitamin D deficiency. Because they appear to have leaky cell membranes, most rickettsias must live inside another cell to retain all necessary cellular substances (Fig. 4-36). All diseases caused by *Rickettsia* species are arthropod-borne, meaning that they are transmitted by arthropod *vectors* (carriers); see Table 4-8.

Arthropods such as lice, fleas, and ticks transmit the rickettsias from one host to another by their bites or waste products. Diseases caused by *Rickettsia* spp. include typhus and typhuslike diseases (e.g., Rocky Mountain spotted fever). All these diseases involve production of a rash. Medically important bacteria that are closely related to rickettsias include *Coxiella burnetii*, *Bartonella quintana* (formerly *Rochalimaea quintana*), *Ehrlichia* spp., and *Anaplasma* spp. *C. burnetii* (the cause of Q fever) is

FIGURE 4-36. *Rickettsia prowazekii* (arrows), the cause of epidemic louseborne typhus, in experimentally infected tick tissue. (From Volk WA, et al. Essentials of Medical Microbiology, 5th ed. Philadelphia: Lippincott-Raven, 1996.)

transmitted primarily by aerosols, but can be transmitted to animals by ticks. *B. quintana* is associated with trench fever (a louseborne disease), cat scratch disease, bacteremia, and endocarditis. *Ehrlichia* and *Anaplasma* spp. cause human tickborne diseases such as human monocytic ehrlichiosis (HME) and human granulocytic

TABLE 4-8	Human Diseases Caused by Unique Bacteria	
GENUS	**SPECIES**	**HUMAN DISEASE(S)**
Rickettsia	*R. akari*	Rickettsialpox (a miteborne disease)
	R. prowazekii	Epidemic typhus (a louseborne disease)
	R. rickettsii	Rocky Mountain spotted fever (a tickborne disease)
	R. typhi	Endemic or murine typhus (a fleaborne disease)
Ehrlichia spp.	*E. chaffeensis*	Human monocytic ehrlichiosis
Anaplasma spp.	*Anaplasma phagocytophilum*	Human granulocytic ehrlichiosis
Chlamydia (and *Chlamydia*-like bacteria)	*Chlamydophila pneumoniae*	Pneumonia
	Chlamydophila psittaci	Psittacosis (a respiratory disease; a zoonosis; sometimes called "parrot fever")
	Chlamydia trachomatis	Different serotypes cause different diseases, including trachoma (an eye disease) inclusion conjunctivitis (an eye disease), nongonococcal urethritis (NGU; a sexually transmitted disease), lymphogranuloma venereum (LGV; a sexually transmitted disease)
Mycoplasma	*M. pneumoniae*	Atypical pneumonia
	M. genitalium	Nongonococcal urethritis (NGU)
Orientia	*O. tsutsugamushi*	Scrub typhus (a miteborne disease)
Ureaplasma	*U. urealyticum*	Nongonococcal urethritis (NGU)

ehrlichiosis (HGE). *Ehrlichia* and *Anaplasma* spp. are intraleukocytic pathogens, meaning that they live within certain types of white blood cells.

The term "chlamydias" refers to *Chlamydia* spp. and closely related organisms (such as *Chlamydophila* spp.). Chlamydias are referred to as "energy parasites." Although they can produce adenosine

> Rickettsias and chlamydias are examples of obligate intracellular organisms—organisms that can only exist *within* host cells.

triphosphate (ATP) molecules, they preferentially use ATP molecules produced by their host cells. ATP molecules are the major energy-storing or energy-carrying molecules of cells (see Chapter 7). Chlamydias are obligate intracellular pathogens that are transferred by inhalation of aerosols or by direct contact between hosts—*not* by arthropods. Medically important chlamydias include *Chlamydia trachomatis*, *Chlamydophila pneumoniae*, and *Chlamydophila psittaci*. Different serotypes of *C. trachomatis* cause different diseases, including trachoma (the leading cause of blindness in the world), inclusion conjunctivitis (another type of eye disease), and nongonococcal urethritis (NGU; a term given to urethritis that is not caused by *Neisseria gonorrhoeae*). *C. pneumoniae* causes a type of pneumonia, and *C. psittaci* causes a respiratory disease called psittacosis. Chlamydial diseases are listed in Table 4-8.

Mycoplasmas

Mycoplasmas are the smallest of the cellular microbes (Fig. 4-37). Because they lack cell walls, they assume many shapes, from coccoid to fila-

> Because they do not possess cell walls, *Mycoplasma* spp. are pleomorphic.

mentous; thus, they appear pleomorphic when examined microscopically. Sometimes they are confused with cell wall–deficient (CWD) forms of bacteria, described earlier; however, even in the most favorable growth media, mycoplasmas are not able to produce cell walls,

FIGURE 4-37. Scanning electron micrograph of *Mycoplasma pneumoniae*. (From Strohl WA, et al. Lippincott's Illustrated Reviews: Microbiology. Philadelphia: Lippincott Williams & Wilkins, 2001.)

"Strains" versus "Serotypes"
Within a given species, there are usually different *strains*. For example, there are many different strains of *E. coli*. If the *E. coli* that has been isolated from Patient X is producing an enzyme that is not being produced by the *E. coli* from Patient Z, the two *E. coli* isolates are considered to be different strains. Or, if one isolate of *E. coli* is resistant to ampicillin (an antibiotic), and the other *E. coli* isolate is susceptible to ampicillin, then these isolates are considered to be different strains of *E. coli*. Also, there are usually different *serotypes* (sometimes called serovars) within a given species. Serotypes of an organism differ from each other as a result of differences in their surface molecules (surface antigens). Sometimes, as is true for *C. trachomatis* and *E. coli*, different serotypes of a given species cause different diseases.

which is not true for CWD. Mycoplasmas were formerly called pleuropneumonia-like organisms (PPLO), first isolated from cattle with lung infections. They may be free-living or parasitic and are pathogenic to many animals and some plants. In humans, pathogenic mycoplasmas cause primary atypical pneumonia and genitourinary infections; some species can grow intracellularly. Because they have no cell wall, they are resistant to treatment with penicillin and other antibiotics that work by inhibiting cell wall synthesis. Mycoplasmas can be cultured on artificial media in the laboratory, where they produce tiny colonies (called "fried egg colonies") that resemble sunny-side-up fried eggs in appearance. The absence of a cell wall prevents mycoplasmas from staining with the Gram stain procedure. Diseases caused by mycoplasmas and a closely related organism (*Ureaplasma urealyticum*) are shown in Table 4-8.

Especially Large and Especially Small Bacteria

The size of a typical coccus (e.g., a *Staphylococcus aureus* cell) is 1 μm in diameter. A typical bacillus (e.g., an *E. coli* cell) is about 1.0 μm wide × 3.0 μm long, although some bacilli are long thin filaments—up to about 12 μm in length or even longer—but still only about 1 μm wide. Thus, most bacteria are microscopic, requiring the use of a microscope to be seen.

Perhaps the largest of all bacteria—large enough to be seen with the unaided human eye—is *Thiomargarita namibiensis*, a colorless, marine, sulfide-oxidizing bacterium. Single spherical cells of *T. namibiensis* are 100 to 300 μm, but may be as large as 750 μm (0.75 mm). In terms of size, comparing a *T. namibiensis* cell to an *E. coli* cell would be like comparing a blue whale to a newly born mouse. Other marine sulfide-oxidizing bacteria in the genera *Beggiatoa* and *Thioploca* are also especially large, having diameters from 10 μm to more than 100 μm. Although *Beggiatoa* and *Thioploca* form filaments, *Thiomargarita* cells do not.

Another enormous bacterium, named *Epulopiscium fishelsonii*, has been isolated from the intestines of the reef surgeonfish; this bacillus is about 80 μm wide × 600 μm (0.6 mm) long. *Epulopiscium* cells are about five times longer than eucaryotic *Paramecium* cells.[b] The volume of an *Epulopiscium* cell is about a million times greater than the volume of a typical bacterial cell. Spore-forming bacteria called metabacteria, found in the intestines of herbivorous rodents, are closely related to *Epulopiscium*, but they reach lengths of only 20 to 30 μm. Although shorter than *Epulopiscium*, metabacteria are much longer than most bacteria.

At the other end of the spectrum, there are especially tiny bacteria called *nanobacteria*. Their sizes are expressed in nanometers because these bacteria are less than 1 μm in diameter; hence the name, nanobacteria. In some cases, they are as small as 20 nm in diameter. Nanobacteria have been found in soil, minerals, ocean water, human and animal blood, human dental calculus (plaque), arterial plaque, and even rocks (meteorites) of extraterrestrial origin. The existence of nanobacteria is controversial, however. Some scientists believe that these tiny structures were formed by geological, rather than biological, processes. They feel that nanobacteria are smaller than the minimum possible size for a living cell.

Photosynthetic Bacteria

Photosynthetic bacteria include purple bacteria, green bacteria, and cyanobacteria (erroneously referred to in the past as blue-green algae). Although all three groups use light as an energy source, they do not all carry out photosynthesis in the same way. For example, purple and green bacteria (which, in some cases, are not actually those colors) do not produce oxygen, whereas cyanobacteria do. Photosynthesis that produces oxygen is called *oxygenic photosynthesis*, whereas photosynthesis that does not produce oxygen is called *anoxygenic photosynthesis*.

> Photosynthetic bacteria are bacteria capable of converting light energy into chemical energy. Cyanobacteria are examples of photosynthetic bacteria.

In photosynthetic eucaryotes (algae and plants), photosynthesis takes place in plastids, which were discussed in Chapter 3. In cyanobacteria, photosynthesis takes place on intracellular membranes known as thylakoids. Thylakoids are attached to the cell membrane at various points and are thought to represent invaginations of the cell membrane. Attached to the thylakoids, in orderly rows, are numerous phycobilisomes—complex protein pigment aggregates where light harvesting occurs.

Many scientists believe that cyanobacteria were the first organisms capable of carrying out oxygenic photosynthesis and, thus, played a major part in the oxygenation of the atmosphere. Fossil records reveal that cyanobacteria were already in existence 3.3 to 3.5 billion years ago. Photosynthesis is discussed further in Chapter 7. Cyanobacteria vary widely in shape; some are cocci, some are bacilli, and others form long filaments.

When appropriate conditions exist, cyanobacteria in pond or lake water will overgrow, creating a water bloom—a "pond scum" that resembles a thick layer of bluish green (turquoise) oil paint. The conditions include a mild or no wind, a balmy water temperature (15°–30°C), a water pH of 6 to 9, and an abundance of the nutrients nitrogen and phosphorous in the water. Many cyanobacteria are able to convert nitrogen gas (N_2) from the air into ammonium ions (NH_4^+) in the soil or water; this process is known as *nitrogen fixation* (Chapter 10).

Some cyanobacteria produce toxins (poisons), such as neurotoxins (which affect the central nervous system), hepatotoxins (which affect the liver), and cytotoxins (which affect other types of cells). These cyanotoxins can cause disease and even death in wildlife species and humans that consume contaminated water. Additional information about these toxins can be found in the CD-ROM Appendix 1, entitled "Microbial Intoxications."

> Some cyanobacteria produce toxins (called cyanotoxins) that can cause disease and even death in animals and humans.

THE DOMAIN *ARCHAEA*

Procaryotic organisms thus far described in this chapter are all members of the Domain *Bacteria*. Procaryotic organisms in the Domain *Archaea* were discovered in 1977. Although they were once referred to as archaebacteria (or archaeobacteria), most scientists now feel that there are sufficient differences between archaea and bacteria to stop referring to archaea as bacteria. *Archae* means "ancient," and the name *archaea* was originally assigned when it was thought that these procaryotes evolved earlier than bacteria. Now, there is considerable debate as to whether bacteria or archaea came first. Genetically, even though they are procaryotes, archaea are more closely related to eucaryotes than they are to bacteria; some possess genes otherwise found only in eucaryotes. Many scientists believe that bacteria and archaea diverged from a

---

[b] *Paramecium* is a genus of freshwater protozoa.

TABLE 4-9	Examples of Extremophiles
TYPE OF EXTREME ENVIRONMENT	**NAME GIVEN TO THESE TYPES OF EXTREMOPHILES**
Extremely acidic	Acidophiles
Extremely alkaline	Alkaliphiles
Extremely hot	Thermophiles
Extremely cold	Psychrophiles
Extremely salty	Halophiles
Extremely high pressure	Piezophiles (formerly barophiles)

common ancestor relatively soon after life began on this planet. Later, the eucaryotes split off from the archaea.

According to *Bergey's Manual of Systematic Bacteriology*, the Domain *Archaea* contains 2 phyla, 8 classes, 12 orders, 21 families, 69 genera, and 217 species. Archaea vary widely in shape; some are cocci, some are bacilli, and others form long filaments. Many, but not all, archaea are "extremophiles," in the sense that they live in extreme environments, such as extremely acidic, alkaline, hot, cold, or salty environments, or environments where there is extremely high pressure (Table 4-9).

Some live at the bottom of the ocean in and near thermal vents, where, in addition to heat and salinity, there is extreme pressure. Other archaea, called methanogens, produce methane, which is a flammable gas. Although virtually all archaea possess cell walls, their cell walls contain no peptidoglycan. In contrast, all bacterial cell walls contain peptidoglycan. The 16S rRNA sequences of archaea are quite different from the 16S rRNA sequences of bacteria. The 16S rRNA sequence data suggest that archaea are more closely related to eucaryotes than they are to bacteria. You will recall from Chapter 3 that differences in rRNA structure form the basis of the Three-Domain System of Classification.

> Many archaea are extremophiles, meaning that they live in extreme environments; e.g., environments that are extremely hot, dry, or salty.

ON THE CD-ROM
* Terms Introduced in This Chapter
* Review of Key Points
* Insight
  * Microbes in the News: "Mad Cow Disease"
  * Life in the Absence of Oxygen
* Increase Your Knowledge
* Critical Thinking
* Additional Self-Assessment Exercises

SELF-ASSESSMENT EXERCISES

After studying this chapter, answer the following multiple-choice questions.

1. Which one of the following steps occurs during the multiplication of animal viruses, but not during the multiplication of bacteriophages?
   a. assembly
   b. biosynthesis
   c. penetration
   d. uncoating
2. Which one of the following diseases or groups of diseases is not caused by prions?
   a. certain plant diseases
   b. chronic wasting disease of deer and elk
   c. Creutzfeldt-Jacob disease of humans
   d. "mad cow disease"
3. Most procaryotic cells reproduce by:
   a. binary fission.
   b. budding.
   c. gamete production.
   d. spore formation.
4. The group of bacteria that lack rigid cell walls and take on irregular shapes is:
   a. chlamydias.
   b. mycobacteria.
   c. mycoplasmas.
   d. rickettsias.
5. At the end of the Gram staining procedure, Gram-positive bacteria will be:
   a. blue to purple.
   b. green.
   c. orange.
   d. pink to red.
6. Which one of the following statements about rickettsias is false?
   a. Diseases caused by rickettsias are arthropod-borne.
   b. Rickets is caused by a *Rickettsia* species.
   c. *Rickettsia* species cause typhus and typhuslike diseases.
   d. Rickettsias have leaky membranes.
7. Which one of the following statements about *Chlamydia* and *Chlamydophila* spp. is false?
   a. They are obligate intracellular pathogens.
   b. They are considered to be "energy parasites."
   c. The diseases they cause are all arthropod-borne.
   d. They are considered to be Gram-negative bacteria.
8. Which one of the following statements about cyanobacteria is false?
   a. Although cyanobacteria are photosynthetic, they do not produce oxygen as a result of photosynthesis.
   b. At one time, cyanobacteria were called blue-green algae.
   c. Some cyanobacteria are capable of nitrogen fixation.
   d. Some cyanobacteria are important medically because they produce toxins.

9. Which one of the following statements about archaea is false?
   a. Archaea are more closely related to eucaryotes than they are to bacteria.
   b. Both archaea and bacteria are procaryotic organisms.
   c. Some archaea live in extremely hot environments.
   d. The cell walls of archaea contain a thicker layer of peptidoglycan than the cell walls of bacteria.

10. An organism that does not require oxygen, grows better in the absence of oxygen, but can survive in atmospheres containing some molecular oxygen is known as a(n):
   a. aerotolerant anaerobe.
   b. capnophile.
   c. facultative anaerobe.
   d. microaerophile.

MICROBIAL DIVERSITY

PART 2 | Eucaryotic Microbes

5

LEARNING OBJECTIVES

AFTER STUDYING THIS CHAPTER, YOU SHOULD BE ABLE TO:

- Compare and contrast the differences among algae, protozoa, and fungi (e.g., photosynthetic ability, chitin in cell walls, etc.)
- Explain what is meant by a "red tide" (i.e., what causes it) and its medical significance
- List the four major categories of protozoa and their most important differentiating characteristics (e.g., their mode of locomotion)
- Define the terms pellicle, cytostome, and stigma
- List five major infectious diseases of humans that are caused by protozoa and five that are caused by fungi
- Define and state the importance of phycotoxins and mycotoxins
- Explain the differences between aerial and vegetative hyphae, septate and aseptate hyphae, sexual and asexual spores
- Explain the major difference between a lichen and a slime mould

INTRODUCTION

Acellular and procaryotic microbes were described in Chapter 4. This chapter describes the eucaryotic microbes, which include some species of algae, all protozoa, some species of fungi, all lichens, and all slime moulds. Scientists have not yet determined when the first eucaryotic organisms appeared on Earth. The best guesses are between 2 and 3.5 billion years ago.

> Eucaryotic microbes include some species of algae and fungi, and all protozoa, lichens, and slime moulds.

ALGAE

Characteristics and Classification

Algae (sing., *alga*) are photosynthetic, eucaryotic organisms that, together with protozoa, are classified in the second kingdom (Protista) of the Five-Kingdom System of Classification. Collectively, they are referred to as protists. Not all taxonomists agree, however, that algae and protozoa should be combined in the same kingdom. The study of algae is called phycology (or algology), and a person who studies algae is called a phycologist (or algologist).

> Algae and protozoa are referred to as protists because they are in the kingdom Protista.

All algal cells consist of cytoplasm, a cell wall (usually), a cell membrane, a nucleus, plastids, ribosomes, mitochondria, and Golgi bodies. In addition, some algal cells have a *pellicle* (a thickened cell membrane), a *stigma* (a light-sensing organelle, also known as an eyespot), and flagella. Although they are not plants, algae are more

TABLE 5-1	Similarities and Differences between Algae and Plants	
	ALGAE	**PLANTS**
Eucaryotic	Yes	Yes
Photosynthetic	Yes	Yes
Cells contain chlorophyll	Yes	Yes
Use carbon dioxide as an energy source	Yes	Yes
Store energy in the form of starch	Yes	Yes
Composed of roots, stems, and leaves	No	Most (bryophytes, such as mosses, are the exception)
Cell walls contain cellulose	Most (exceptions include diatoms and dinoflagellates; *Euglena* and *Volvox* do not have cell walls)	Yes
Method of reproduction	Both asexual and sexual	Sexual
Contain a vascular system to transport internal fluids	No	Most (mosses and other bryophytes are avascular)

plantlike than protozoa (see Table 5-1 for similarities and differences between algae and plants). Algae lack true roots, stems, and leaves.

Algae range in size from tiny, unicellular, microscopic organisms (e.g., diatoms, dinoflagellates, desmids) to large, multicellular, plantlike seaweeds (e.g., kelp; Table 5-2). Thus, not all algae are microorganisms. Algae may be arranged in colonies or strands and are found in freshwater and salt water, in wet soil, and on wet rocks. Algae produce their energy by photosynthesis, using energy from the sun, carbon dioxide, water, and inorganic nutrients from the soil to build cellular material. However, a few species use organic nutrients, and others survive with very little sunlight. Most algal cell walls contain cellulose, a polysaccharide not found in the cell walls of any other microorganisms. Depending on the types of photosynthetic pigments they possess, algae are classified as green, golden (or golden brown), brown, or red.

Diatoms are tiny, usually unicellular algae that live in both freshwater and seawater. They are important members of the phytoplankton. Diatoms have silicon dioxide in their cell walls; thus, they have cell walls made of glass. Deposits of diatoms are used to make diatomaceous earth, which is used in filtration systems, insulation, and abrasives. Because of their attractive, geometric, and varied appearance, diatoms are quite interesting to observe microscopically.

Dinoflagellates are microscopic, unicellular, flagellated, often photosynthetic algae. Like diatoms, they are important members of the phytoplankton, producing much of the oxygen in our atmosphere and serving as important links in food chains. Some dinoflagellates produce light and, for this reason, are sometimes referred to as fire algae. Dinoflagellates are responsible for what are known as "red tides" (discussed in CD-ROM Appendix 1: "Microbial Intoxications").

Green algae include desmids, *Spirogyra*, *Chlamydomonas*, *Volvox*, and *Euglena*, all of which can be found in pond water (Fig. 5-1). Desmids are unicellular algae, some of which resemble a microscopic banana. *Spirogyra* is an example of a filamentous alga, often producing long green strands in pond water. *Chlamydomonas* is a unicellular, biflagellated alga, containing one chloroplast and a stigma.

> Algae considered to be microorganisms include diatoms, dinoflagellates, desmids, and species of *Chlamydomonas*, *Euglena, Spirogyra, and Volvox.*

Volvox is a multicellular alga (sometimes referred to as a colonial alga or colony), consisting of as many as 60,000 interconnected, biflagellated cells, arranged to form a hollow sphere. The flagella beat in a coordinated manner, causing the *Volvox* colony to move through the water in a rolling motion. Sometimes, daughter colonies can be seen within a *Volvox* colony.

Euglena is a rather interesting alga, in that it possesses features possessed by both algae and protozoa. Like algae, *Euglena* contains chloroplasts, is photosynthetic, and stores energy in the form of starch. Protozoan features include the presence of a primitive mouth (called a *cytostome*) and the absence of a cell wall (hence, no cellulose). *Euglena* possesses a photosensing organelle called a stigma and a single flagellum. With its stigma, it can sense light; with its flagellum, it can swim into the light. When there is no light, *Euglena* can continue to obtain nutrients by ingesting food through its cytostome. Although it has no cell wall, *Euglena* does possess a pellicle, which serves the same function as a cell wall—protection.

TABLE 5-2	Characteristics of Algae			
PHYLUM (AND COMMON NAME)	**STRUCTURAL ARRANGEMENT**	**PREDOMINANT COLOR**	**PHOTOSYNTHETIC PIGMENTS**[a]	**HABITAT**
Bacillariophyta (diatoms)	Unicellular	Olive brown	Chlorophyll c, carotenoids, xanthophylls	Freshwater and seawater
Chlorophyta (green algae)	Unicellular and multicellular	Green	Chlorophyll b, carotenoids	Freshwater (predominantly) and seawater
Chrysophyta (golden algae)	Unicellular	Golden olive	Chlorophyll c, carotenoids, xanthophylls	Freshwater
Dinoflagellata (dinoflagellates)	Unicellular	Brown	Chlorophyll c, carotenoids, xanthophylls	Freshwater and seawater
Euglenophyta (*Euglena* spp. and closely related organisms)	Unicellular	Green	Chlorophyll b, carotenoids, xanthophylls	Freshwater
Phaeophyta (brown algae)	Multicellular seaweeds	Olive brown	Chlorophyll c, carotenoids, xanthophylls	Seawater; most commonly, cold environments
Rhodophyta (red algae)	Multicellular seaweeds	Red to black	Chlorophyll d (in some), carotenoids, phycobilins	Seawater (predominantly) and freshwater; most commonly, tropical environments

[a]In addition to chlorophyll a, which is possessed by all algae. Carotenoids are yellow-orange; chlorophylls are greenish; phycobilins are red and blue; and xanthophylls are brownish.

FIGURE 5-1. Common pond water algae and protozoa. (A) *Amoeba* sp., **(B)** *Euglena* sp., **(C)** *Stentor* sp., **(D)** *Vorticella* sp., in extended and contracted positions. **(E)** *Volvox* sp., **(F)** *Paramecium* sp., **(B)**, and **(E)** are algae. **(A)**, **(C)**, **(D)**, and **(F)** are protozoa.

FIGURE 5-2. Green algae growing on shoreline rocks. (Courtesy of http://www.imageafter.com)

Algae are easy to find. They include large seaweeds of various colors, brown kelp (up to 10 m in length) found along ocean shores, the green scum floating on ponds, and the slippery green material on wet rock (Fig. 5-2). There are also many microscopic forms in pond water that differ from the colorless, nonphotosynthetic protozoa in that they are pigmented and photosynthetic. Some algae (e.g., *Chlamydomonas*, *Euglena*, and *Volvox*) have characteristics (e.g., cytostome, pellicle, flagella) that cause them to be classified as protozoa by some taxonomists. (Although there is some disagreement among taxonomists as to where *Chlamydomonas*, *Volvox*, and *Euglena* should be classified, they are referred to as algae in this book, primarily because they are photosynthetic. In this book, photosynthetic protists are considered to be algae, and nonphotosynthetic protists are considered to be protozoa.)

> In this book, photosynthetic protists are considered to be algae, and nonphotosynthetic protists are considered to be protozoa.

Algae are an important source of food, iodine and other minerals, fertilizers, emulsifiers for pudding, and stabilizers for ice cream and salad dressings; they are also used as a gelling agent for jams and nutrient media for bacterial growth. Because algae are nearly 50% oil, scientists are studying them as a source of biofuels. The agar used as a solidifying agent in laboratory culture media is a complex polysaccharide derived from a red marine alga. On the down side, damage to water systems is frequently caused by algae clogging filters and pipes if many nutrients are present.

Medical Significance

One genus of algae (*Prototheca*) is a very rare cause of human infections (causing a disease known as protothecosis). *Prototheca* lives in soil and can enter wounds,

> Algae are only a very rare cause of human infections. Protothecosis is an example of a human algal infection.

especially those located on the feet. It produces a small subcutaneous lesion that can progress to a crusty, wartylooking lesion. If the organism enters the lymphatic system, it may cause a debilitating, sometimes fatal infection, especially in immunosuppressed individuals. Algae in several other genera secrete substances (*phycotoxins*) that are poisonous to humans, fish, and other animals. For additional information on these toxins, see CD-ROM Appendix 1: "Microbial Intoxications."

PROTOZOA

Characteristics

Protozoa (sing., *protozoan*) are eucaryotic organisms that, together with algae, are classified in the second kingdom (Protista) of the Five-Kingdom System of Classification. As previously stated, not all taxonomists agree that algae and protozoa should be combined in the same kingdom. The study of protozoa is called protozoology, and a person who studies protozoa is called a protozoologist.

Most protozoa are unicellular (single-celled), ranging in length from 3 to 2,000 μm. Most of them are free-living organisms, found in soil and water (Fig. 5-1). Protozoal cells are more animallike than plantlike. All protozoal cells possess a variety of eucaryotic structures and organelles, including cell membranes, nuclei, endoplasmic reticulum, mitochondria, Golgi bodies, lysosomes, centrioles, and food vacuoles. In addition, some protozoa possess pellicles, cytostomes, contractile vacuoles, pseudopodia, cilia, and flagella. Protozoa have no chlorophyll and, therefore, cannot make their own food by photosynthesis. Some ingest whole algae, yeasts, bacteria, and smaller protozoans as their source of nutrients; others live on dead and decaying organic matter.

> Most protozoa are single-celled free-living microorganisms.

Protozoa do not have cell walls, but some, including some flagellates and some ciliates, possess a pellicle, which serves the same purpose as a cell wall—protection. Some flagellates and some ciliates ingest food through a primitive mouth or opening, called a cytostome. *Paramecium* spp. (common pond water ciliates) possess both a pellicle and a cytostome. Some pond water protozoa (such as amebae and *Paramecium*) contain an organelle called a *contractile vacuole*, which pumps water out of the cell. *Vorticella* spp. (pond water ciliates) have a contractile stalk (Fig. 5-1). Within the stalk is a primitive muscle fiber called a myoneme.

> *Paramecium* and *Vorticella* spp. are examples of free-living pond protozoa.

A typical protozoan life cycle consists of two stages: the trophozoite stage and the cyst stage. The **trophozoite** is the motile, feeding, dividing stage in a protozoan's life cycle, whereas the *cyst* is the nonmotile, dormant, survival stage.

> A typical protozoan life cycle consists of two stages: a motile trophozoite stage and a nonmotile cyst stage.

In some ways (e.g., a thick outer wall), cysts are like bacterial spores.

Some protozoa are parasites. Parasitic protozoa break down and absorb nutrients from the body of the host in which they live. Many parasitic protozoa are pathogens, such as those that cause malaria, giardiasis, African sleeping sickness, and amebic dysentery (see Chapter 21). Other protozoa coexist with the host animal in a type of mutualistic symbiotic relationship—a relationship in which both organisms benefit. A typical example of such a symbiotic relationship is the termite and its intestinal protozoa. The protozoa digest the wood eaten by the termite, enabling both organisms to absorb the nutrients necessary for life. Without the intestinal protozoa, the termite would be unable to digest the wood that it eats and would starve to death. Symbiotic relationships are discussed in greater detail in Chapter 10.

> Malaria, giardiasis, African sleeping sickness, and amebic dysentery are examples of human diseases caused by parasitic protozoa.

Classification and Medical Significance

Protozoa are divided into groups (referred to in various classification schemes as phyla, subphyla, or classes) according to their method of locomotion (Table 5-3).

Amebae (amebas) move by means of cytoplasmic extensions called **pseudopodia** (sing., *pseudopodium*; false feet). An **ameba** (pl., *amebae*) first extends a pseudopodium in the direction the ameba intends to move, and then the rest of the cell slowly flows into it; this process is called ameboid movement. An ameba ingests

> Protozoa are classified taxonomically by their mode of locomotion. Some move by pseudopodia, others by flagella, others by cilia, and some are nonmotile.

a food particle (e.g., a yeast or bacterial cell) by surrounding the particle with pseudopodia, which then fuse together; this process is known as phagocytosis. The ingested particle, surrounded by a membrane, is referred to as a food vacuole (or phagosome). Digestive enzymes, released from lysosomes, then digest or break down the food into nutrients. Some of the white blood cells in our bodies ingest and digest materials in the same manner as amebae. (Phagocytosis by white blood cells is discussed further in Chapter 15). When fluids are ingested in a similar manner, the process is known as *pinocytosis*. One medically important ameba is *Entamoeba histolytica*, which causes amebic dysentery (amebiasis) and extraintestinal (meaning away from the intestine) amebic abscesses. Other amebae of medical significance, described in Chapter 21, include *Naegleria fowleri* (the cause of primary amebic meningoencephalitis) and *Acanthamoeba* spp. (which cause eye infections).

> Amebae (amebas), such as *Acanthamoeba*, *Entamoeba*, and *Naegleria* spp. move by means of cytoplasmic extensions called pseudopodia (false feet).

Ciliates (sing., *ciliate*) move about by means of large numbers of hairlike cilia on their surfaces. Cilia exhibit an oarlike motion. Ciliates are the most complex of all protozoa. A pathogenic ciliate, *Balantidium coli*, causes dysentery in underdeveloped countries (Fig. 5-3). It is usually transmitted to humans from drinking water that has been contaminated by swine feces. *B. coli* is the only ciliated protozoan that causes disease in humans. Examples of pond water ciliates are *Blepharisma, Didinium, Euplotes,*

> Ciliates, such as *Balantidium*, *Paramecium, Stentor,* and *Vorticella* spp., move about by means of large numbers of hairlike cilia on their surfaces.

TABLE 5-3	Characteristics of Major Protozoa			
CATEGORY	MEANS OF MOVEMENT	METHOD OF ASEXUAL REPRODUCTION	METHOD OF SEXUAL REPRODUCTION	REPRESENTATIVES
Ciliates	Cilia	Transverse fission	Conjugation	*Balantidium coli, Paramecium, Stentor, Tetrahymena, Vorticella*
Amebae (amebas)	Pseudopodia (false feet)	Binary fission	When present, involves flagellated sex cells	*Amoeba, Naegleria, Entamoeba histolytica*
Flagellates	Flagella	Binary fission	None	*Chlamydomonas, Giardia lamblia, Trichomonas, Trypanosoma*
Sporozoa	Generally nonmotile except for certain sex cells	Multiple fission	Involves flagellated sex cells	*Plasmodium, Toxoplasma gondii, Cryptosporidium*

FIGURE 5-3. Photomicrograph of *B. coli*, the only ciliated protozoan that causes human disease. *B. coli* causes a diarrheal disease called balantidiasis. Note the numerous short cilia (arrows) around the periphery of the cell. (Courtesy of the Oregon Public Health Laboratory and the Division of Parasitic Diseases, CDC.)

Paramecium, Stentor, and *Vorticella* spp., some of which are shown in Figure 5-1.

Flagellated protozoa or **flagellates** (sing., *flagellate*) move by means of whiplike flagella. A basal body (also called a kinetosome or kinetoplast) anchors each flagellum within the cytoplasm. Flagella exhibit a wavelike motion. Some flagellates are pathogenic. For example, *Trypanosoma brucei* subspecies *gambiense*, transmitted by the tsetse fly, causes African sleeping sickness in humans; *Trypanosoma cruzi* causes American trypanosomiasis (Chagas' disease); *Trichomonas vaginalis* causes persistent sexually transmitted infections (trichomoniasis) of the male and female genital tracts; and *Giardia lamblia* (also known as *Giardia intestinalis*) causes a persistent diarrheal disease (giardiasis; Fig. 5-4).

Nonmotile protozoa—protozoa lacking pseudopodia, flagella, or cilia—are classified together in a category called sporozoa. The most important sporozoan pathogens are the *Plasmodium* spp. that cause malaria in many areas of the world. One of these species, *Plasmodium vivax*, causes a few cases of malaria annually in the United States. Malarial parasites are transmitted by female *Anopheles* mosquitoes, which become infected when they take a blood meal from a person with malaria. Another sporozoan, *Cryptosporidium parvum*, causes severe diarrheal disease (cryptosporidiosis) in immunosuppressed patients, especially those with acquired immunodeficiency syndrome

> Flagellated protozoa (flagellates), such as *Trypanosoma, Trichomonas,* and *Giardia* spp., move by means of whiplike flagella.

> *Babesia, Cryptosporidium, Cyclospora, Plasmodium,* and *Toxoplasma* spp. are examples of sporozoan protozoa that cause human infections. Sporozoan protozoa are nonmotile.

FIGURE 5-4. Scanning electron micrograph of *G. lamblia*, a flagellated protozoan that causes human disease. *G. lamblia* causes a diarrheal disease called giardiasis. (Courtesy of Janice Carr and the Centers for Disease Control and Prevention.)

(AIDS). A 1993 epidemic in Milwaukee, Wisconsin, caused by *Cryptosporidium* oocysts in drinking water, resulted in more than 400,000 cases of cryptosporidiosis, including some fatal cases. Other pathogenic sporozoans include *Babesia* spp. (the cause of babesiosis), *Cyclospora cayetanensis* (the cause of a diarrheal disease called cyclosporiasis), and *Toxoplasma gondii* (the cause of toxoplasmosis). Pathogenic protozoa are described in Chapter 21.

FUNGI

Characteristics

In the Five-Kingdom System of Classification, **fungi** (sing., *fungus*) are in a kingdom all by themselves—the Kingdom Fungi. The study of fungi is called mycology, and a person who studies fungi is called a mycologist.

> The study of fungi is called mycology.

Fungi are found almost everywhere on earth; some (the saprophytic fungi) living on organic matter in water and soil, and others (the parasitic fungi) living on and within animals and plants. Some are harmful, whereas others are beneficial. Fungi also live on many unlikely materials, causing deterioration of leather and plastics and spoilage of jams, pickles, and many other foods. Beneficial fungi are important in the production of cheeses, beer, wine, and other foods, as well as certain drugs (e.g., the immunosuppressant drug cyclosporine) and antibiotics (e.g., penicillin).

Fungi are a diverse group of eucaryotic organisms that include yeasts, moulds, and mushrooms. As saprophytes, their main source of food is dead and decaying organic matter. Fungi are the "garbage disposers" of nature—the "vultures" of the microbial world. By secreting digestive enzymes into dead plant and animal matter, they decompose this material into absorbable nutrients for themselves and other living organisms; thus, they are the original "recyclers." Imagine living in a world without saprophytes, stumbling through endless piles of dead plants and animals and animal waste products. Not a pleasant thought!

Fungi are sometimes incorrectly referred to as plants. They are not plants. One way that fungi differ from plants and algae is that they are not photosynthetic; they have no chlorophyll or other photosynthetic pigments. The cell walls of algal and plant cells contain cellulose (a polysaccharide), but fungal cell walls do not. Fungal cell walls do contain a polysaccharide called chitin, which is not found in the cell walls of any other microorganisms. Chitin is also found in the exoskeletons of arthropods.

> Neither algae nor fungi are plants. Algae are photosynthetic, but fungi are not.

Although many fungi are unicellular (e.g., yeasts), others grow as filaments called **hyphae** (sing., *hypha*), which intertwine to form a mass called a **mycelium** (pl., *mycelia*) or thallus; thus, they are quite different from bacteria, which are always unicellular. Also remember that bacteria are procaryotic, whereas fungi are eucaryotic. Some fungi have *septate hyphae* (meaning that the cytoplasm within the hypha is divided into cells by cross-walls or septa), whereas others have *aseptate hyphae* (the cytoplasm within the hypha is not divided into cells; no septa). Aseptate hyphae contain multinucleated cytoplasm (described as being coenocytic). Learning whether the fun-

> Yeasts are unicellular, whereas moulds are multicellular.

STUDY AID
Decomposer versus Saprophyte
The term **decomposer** relates to what an organism "does for a living," so to speak—decomposers break materials down. The term **saprophyte** (or saprobe) relates to how an organism obtains nutrients; saprophytes absorb nutrients from dead and decaying organic matter. Sometimes the terms decomposer and saprophyte are used to describe the same organism. For example, all saprophytes are decomposers—they decompose organic materials, such as corpses, dead plants, and feces. However, not all decomposers are saprophytes. Some decomposers decompose materials such as minerals, rocks, inorganic industrial wastes, rubber, plastic, and textiles. Also note the difference between a saprophyte and a parasite. A parasite obtains nutrients from living organisms, whereas a saprophyte obtains nutrients from dead ones.

gus possesses septate or aseptate hyphae is an important "clue" when attempting to identify a fungus that has been isolated from a clinical specimen (Fig. 5-5).

Reproduction

Depending on the particular species, fungal cells can reproduce by budding, hyphal extension, or the formation of spores. There are two general categories of fungal spores: sexual spores and asexual spores.

> One of the ways in which fungi reproduce is by spore production. The two general types of fungal spores are sexual and asexual spores.

Sexual spores are produced by the fusion of two gametes (thus, by the fusion of two nuclei). Sexual spores have a variety of names (e.g., ascospores, basidiospores, zygospores), depending on

> Asexual fungal spores are known as conidia.

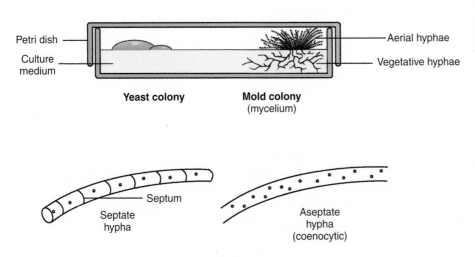

FIGURE 5-5. Fungal colonies and terms relating to hyphae.

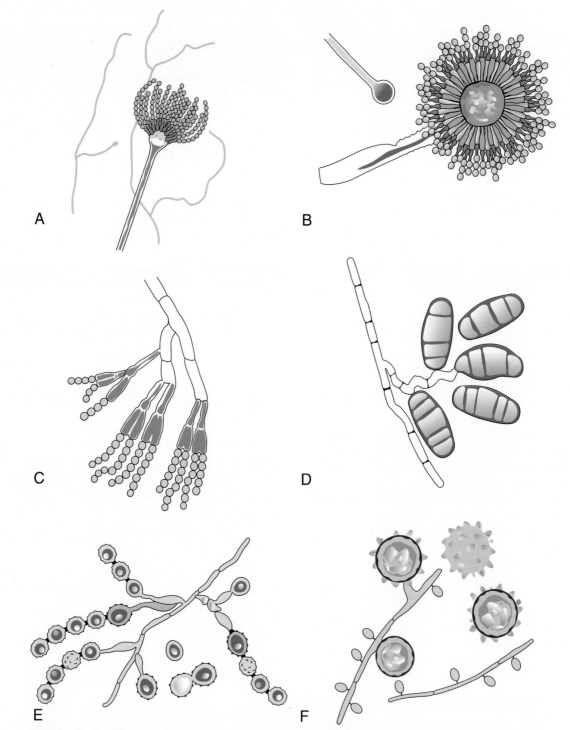

FIGURE 5-6. Microscopic appearance of various fungi. (A) *Aspergillus fumigatus.* **(B)** *Aspergillus flavus.* **(C)** *Penicillium* sp. **(D)** *Curvularia* sp. **(E)** *Scopulariopsis* sp. **(F)** *Histoplasma capsulatum.* (From Winn WC Jr, et al. Koneman's Color Atlas and Textbook of Diagnostic Microbiology, 6th ed. Philadelphia: Lippincott Williams & Wilkins, 2006.)

the exact manner in which they are formed. Fungi are classified taxonomically in accordance with the type of sexual spore that they produce or the type of structure on which the spores are produced (Fig. 5-6). Asexual spores are formed in many different ways, but not by the fusion of gametes (Fig. 5-7). Asexual spores are also called **conidia** (sing., *conidium*). Some species of fungi produce both asexual and sexual spores. Fungal spores are very resistant structures that are carried great distances by wind. They are resistant to heat, cold, acids, bases, and other chemicals. Many people are allergic to fungal spores.

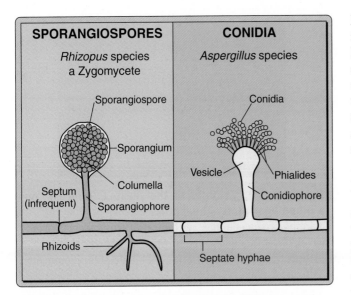

FIGURE 5-7. Asexual reproduction in *Rhizopus* and *Aspergillus* moulds. Illustrating the types of structures within and upon which asexual spores are produced. (From Winn WC Jr, et al. Koneman's Color Atlas and Textbook of Diagnostic Microbiology, 6th ed. Philadelphia: Lippincott Williams & Wilkins, 2006.)

Classification

The taxonomic classification of fungi changes periodically. One current classification divides the Kingdom Fungi into five phyla. Classification of fungi into these phyla is based primarily on their mode of sexual reproduction. The two phyla known as "lower fungi" are the Zygomycotina (or Zygomycota) and the Chytridiomycotina (or Chytridiomycota). Zygomycotina include the common bread moulds and other fungi that cause food spoilage. Chytridiomycotina, which are not considered to be true fungi by some taxonomists, live in water ("water moulds") and soil. The two phyla known as "higher fungi" are the Ascomycotina (or Ascomycota) and the Basidiomycotina (or Basidiomycota). Ascomycotina include certain yeasts and some fungi that cause plant diseases (e.g., Dutch Elm disease). Basidiomycotina include some yeasts, some fungi that cause plant diseases, and the large "fleshy fungi" that live in the woods (e.g., mushrooms, toadstools, bracket fungi, puffballs). The fifth phylum—Deuteromycotina (or Deuteromycota)—contains fungi having no mode of sexual reproduction, or in which the mode of sexual reproduction is not known. This phylum is sometimes referred to as Fungi Imperfecti. Deuteromycetes include certain medically important moulds such as *Aspergillus* and *Penicillium*. Characteristics of each of these phyla are shown in Table 5-4.

Yeasts

Yeasts are eucaryotic single-celled (unicellular) organisms that lack mycelia. Individual yeast cells, sometimes referred to as blastospores or blasto-conidia, can only be observed using a microscope. They usually reproduce by budding (Fig. 5-8), but occasionally do so by a type of spore formation. Sometimes a string of elongated buds is formed; this string of elongated buds is called a **pseudohypha** (pl., *pseudohyphae*). It resembles a hypha, but it is *not* a hypha (Fig. 5-9). Some yeasts produce thick-walled, sporelike structures called chlamydospores (or chlamydoconidia; Fig. 5-9).

> Yeasts are microscopic, single-celled organisms that usually reproduce by budding.

Yeasts are found in soil and water and on the skins of many fruits and vegetables. Wine, beer, and alcoholic beverages had been produced for centuries before Louis Pasteur discovered that naturally occurring yeasts on the skin of grapes and other fruits and grains were responsible for these fermentation processes. The common yeast *Saccharomyces cerevisiae* ("baker's yeast") ferments sugar to alcohol under anaerobic conditions. Under aerobic conditions, this yeast breaks down simple sugars to carbon dioxide and water; for this reason, it has long been used to leaven light bread. Yeasts are also a good source of nutrients for humans because they produce many vitamins and proteins. Some yeasts (e.g., *Candida albicans* and *Cryptococcus neoformans*) are human pathogens. *C. albicans* is the yeast most frequently isolated from human clinical specimens, and is also the fungus most frequently isolated from human clinical specimens.

> *C. albicans* and *C. neoformans* are examples of yeasts that cause human infections.

PHYLUM	TYPE OF HYPHAE	TYPE OF SEXUAL SPORE	TYPE OF ASEXUAL SPORE
Zygomycotina (Zygomycota)	Aseptate	Zygospore	Nonmotile sporangiospores
Chytridiomycotina (Chytridiomycota)	Aseptate	Oospore	Motile zoospores
Ascomycotina (Ascomycota)	Septate	Ascospore	Conidiospores
Basidiomycotina (Basidiomycota)	Septate	Basidiospore	Rare
Deuteromycotina (Deuteromycota)	Septate	None observed	Conidiospores

TABLE 5-4   Selected Characteristics of the Phyla of Fungi

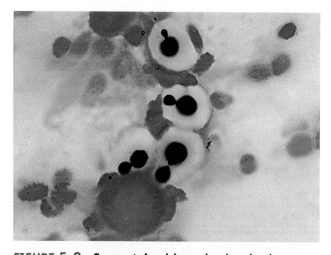

FIGURE 5-8. Gram-stained bronchoalveolar lavage specimen containing four darkly stained, narrow-necked, budding yeasts, suggestive of a *Cryptococcus* species. The negatively stained halos surrounding the yeast cells are dense polysaccharide capsules. (From Marler LM, Siders JA, Allen SD. Direct Smear Atlas. Philadelphia: Lippincott Williams & Wilkins, 2001.)

In the laboratory, yeasts produce colonies that are quite similar in appearance to bacterial colonies (Figs. 5-5 and 5-10). To distinguish between a yeast colony and a bacterial colony, a wet mount can be performed. A small portion of the colony is mixed with a drop of water or saline on a microscope slide, a coverslip is added, and the preparation is examined under the microscope.

FIGURE 5-10. Colonies of the yeast, *C. albicans*, on a blood agar plate. The footlike extensions from the margins of the colonies are typical of this species. (Winn WC Jr, et al. Koneman's Color Atlas and Textbook of Diagnostic Microbiology, 6th ed. Philadelphia: Lippincott Williams & Wilkins, 2006.)

Alternatively, the preparation can be stained using the Gram staining procedure. Yeasts are usually larger than bacteria (ranging from 3 to 8 μm in diameter) and are usually oval-shaped; some may be observed in the process of budding (Fig. 5-11). Bacteria do not produce buds.

Moulds

Although this category of fungi is frequently spelled "molds," mycologists prefer to use "moulds." Moulds are the fungi often seen in water and soil and on food. They grow in the form of cytoplasmic filaments or hyphae that make up the mycelium of the mould. Some of

FIGURE 5-9. Microscopic examination of a culture of *Candida albicans*. Seen here are **(A)** chlamydospores, **(B)** pseudohyphae (elongated yeast cells, linked end to end), and **(C)** budding yeast cells (blastospores). (From Davis BD, et al. Microbiology, 4th ed. Philadelphia: Harper & Row, 1987.)

FIGURE 5-11. Gram-stained wound aspirate, illustrating the size differences among yeasts, bacteria, and white blood cells. Included in this photomicrograph are numerous white blood cells (red objects), two blue-stained budding yeast cells (top, center), and several Gram-positive cocci (small blue spheres near the bottom). The yeast and bacterial cells have been phagocytized by white blood cells. (From Marler LM, Siders JA, Allen SD. Direct Smear Atlas. Philadelphia: Lippincott Williams & Wilkins, 2001.)

the hyphae (called *aerial hyphae*) extend above the surface of whatever the mould is growing on, and some (called *vegetative hyphae*) are beneath the surface (Fig. 5-5). Reproduction is by spore formation, either sexually or asexually, on the aerial hyphae; for this reason, aerial hyphae are sometimes referred to as reproductive hyphae. Various species of moulds are found in each of the classes of fungi except Basidiomycotina. An interesting mould in class Chytridiomycotina is *Phytophthora infestans*, the potato blight mould that caused a famine in Ireland in the mid-19th century (see the following Historical Note).

Moulds have great commercial importance. For example, within the Ascomycotina and the Basidiomycotina classes are found many antibiotic-producing moulds, such as *Penicillium* and *Cephalosporium*. Penicillin, the first antibiotic to be discovered by a scientist, was actually discovered by accident (discussed in Chapter 9). Many additional antibiotics were later developed by culturing soil samples in laboratories and isolating any moulds that inhibited growth of bacteria. Today, to increase their spectrum of activity, antibiotics can be chemically altered in pharmaceutical company laboratories, as has been done with the various semisynthetic penicillins (e.g., ampicillin, amoxicillin, and carbenicillin).

> Many of the commonly used antibiotics are produced by moulds.

Some moulds are also used to produce large quantities of enzymes (such as amylase, which converts starch to glucose), citric acid, and other organic acids that are used commercially. The flavor of cheeses such as bleu cheese, Roquefort, camembert, and limburger are the result of moulds that grow in them.

HISTORICAL NOTE
The Great Potato Famine
Although St. Patrick may have driven the snakes out of Ireland, it was a mould named *Phytophthora infestans* that drove away many of the Irish people. The mould killed off Ireland's potato crops in 1845, 1846, and 1848, causing more than 1 million people to die of starvation and illnesses resulting from malnutrition. When their crops failed, many people could not pay their rent; about 800,000 were forced out of their homes. Nearly 2 million Irish abandoned their homeland to start new lives in America and other countries; many died aboard ship while en route. Ireland lost about one third of its population between 1847 and 1860. Some blamed the "little people" for the potato disease; others blamed the devil. It was not until 1861 that Antoine De Bary proved that it was a fungus that had caused the blight. Late blight of potato was the first disease known with certainty to be caused by a microorganism.

FIGURE 5-12. Fleshy fungi growing on the forest floor. The toxins produced by some fleshy fungi can cause human disease. (Photograph by PG Engelkirk.)

Fleshy Fungi

The large fungi that are encountered in forests, such as mushrooms, toadstools, puffballs, and bracket fungi, are collectively referred to as fleshy fungi (Fig. 5-12). Obviously, they are not microorganisms. Mushrooms are a class of true fungi that consist of a network of filaments or strands (the mycelium) that grow in the soil or in a rotting log, and a fruiting body (the mushroom that rises above the ground) that forms and releases spores. Each spore, much like the seed of a plant, germinates into a new organism. Many mushrooms are delicious to eat, but others, including some that resemble edible fungi, are extremely toxic and may cause permanent liver and brain damage or death if ingested.

> Mushrooms, toadstools, puffballs, and bracket fungi (collectively referred to as fleshy fungi) are examples of fungi that are not microorganisms.

Medical Significance

A variety of fungi (including yeasts, moulds, and some fleshy fungi) are of medical, veterinary, and agricultural importance because of the diseases they cause in humans, animals, and plants. Many diseases of crop plants, grains, corn, and potatoes, are caused by moulds. Some of these plant diseases are referred to as blights and rusts. Not only do these fungi destroy crops, but some produce toxins (*mycotoxins*) that cause disease in humans and animals (discussed in CD-ROM Appendix 1: "Microbial Intoxications"). Moulds and yeasts also cause a variety of infectious diseases of humans and animals—collectively referred to as *mycoses* (discussed later and in Chapter 20). Considering the large number of fungal species, very few are pathogenic for humans.

> A variety of yeasts and moulds cause human infections (known as mycoses). Some moulds and fleshy fungi produce mycotoxins, which can cause human diseases called microbial intoxications.

TABLE 5-5	Selected Fungal Diseases of Humans	
CATEGORY	**GENUS/SPECIES**	**DISEASES**
Yeasts	*Candida albicans*	Thrush; yeast vaginitis; nail infections; systemic infection
	Cryptococcus neoformans	Cryptococcosis (lung infection; meningitis, etc.)
Moulds	*Aspergillus* spp.	Aspergillosis (lung infection; systemic infection)
	Mucor and *Rhizopus* spp. and other species of bread moulds	Mucormycosis or zygomycosis (lung infection; systemic infection)
	Various dermatophytes	Tinea ("ringworm") infections
Dimorphic fungi	*Blastomyces dermatitidis*	Blastomycosis (primarily a disease of lungs and skin)
	Coccidioides immitis	Coccidioidomycosis (lung infection; systemic infection)
	Histoplasma capsulatum	Histoplasmosis (lung infection; systemic infection)
	Sporothrix schenckii	Sporotrichosis (a skin disease)
Other	*Pneumocystis jiroveci*	*Pneumocystis* pneumonia (PCP)

Fungal Infections of Humans

Fungal infections are known as **mycoses** (sing., *mycosis*), and are categorized as superficial, cutaneous, subcutaneous, or systemic mycoses. In some cases the infection may progress through all these stages. Representative mycoses are listed in Table 5-5.

Superficial and Cutaneous Mycoses. Superficial mycoses are fungal infections of the outermost areas of the human body: hair, fingernails, toenails, and the dead, outermost layers of the skin (the epidermis). Cutaneous mycoses are fungal infections of the living layers of skin (the dermis). A group of moulds, collectively referred to as dermatophytes, cause tinea infections, which are often referred to as "ringworm" infections. (Please note that ringworm infections have absolutely nothing to do with worms.) Tinea infections are named in accordance with the part of the anatomy that is infected; examples include tinea pedis (athlete's foot), tinea unguium (fingernails and toenails), tinea capitis (scalp), tinea barbae (face and neck), tinea corporis (trunk of the body), and tinea cruris (groin area).

C. albicans is an opportunistic yeast that lives harmlessly on the skin and mucous membranes of the mouth, gastrointestinal tract, and genitourinary tract. However, when conditions cause a reduction in the number of indigenous bacteria at these anatomic locations, *C. albicans* flourishes, leading to yeast infections of the mouth (thrush), skin, and vagina (yeast vaginitis). This type of local infection may become a focal site from which the organisms invade the bloodstream to become a generalized or systemic infection in many internal areas of the body.

Subcutaneous and Systemic Mycoses. Subcutaneous and systemic mycoses are more severe types of mycoses. Subcutaneous mycoses are fungal infections of the dermis and underlying tissues. These conditions can be quite grotesque in appearance. An example is Madura foot (a type of eucaryotic mycetoma), in which the patient's foot becomes covered with large, unsightly, fungus-containing bumps.

Systemic or generalized mycoses are fungal infections of internal organs of the body, sometimes affecting two or more different organ systems simultaneously (e.g., simultaneous infection of the respiratory system and the bloodstream, or simultaneous infection of the respiratory tract and the central nervous system).

Spores of some pathogenic fungi may be inhaled with dust from contaminated soil or dried bird and bat feces (guano), or they may enter through wounds of the hands and feet. If the spores are inhaled into the lungs, they may germinate there to cause a respiratory infection similar to tuberculosis. Examples of deep-seated pulmonary infections are blastomycosis, coccidioidomycosis, cryptococcosis, and histoplasmosis. In each case, the pathogens may invade further to cause widespread systemic infections, especially in immunosuppressed individuals (see Insight: Microbes in the News: "Sick Building Syndrome" [Black Mould in Buildings] on the CD-ROM).

Did you know that common bread moulds can cause human disease—even death? Inhalation of spores of bread moulds like *Rhizopus* and *Mucor* spp. by an immunosuppressed patient can lead to a respiratory disease called zygomycosis or mucormycosis. The mould can then become disseminated throughout the patient's body and can lead to death. *Rhizopus, Mucor,* and other bread moulds are primitive moulds with aseptate hyphae. As previously mentioned, the cytoplasm of aseptate hyphae is not divided into individual cells by cross-walls (septa).

To diagnose mycoses, clinical specimens are submitted to the mycology section of the clinical microbiology laboratory (discussed in Chapter 13). When isolated from clin-

ical specimens, yeasts are identified (speciated) by inoculating
them into a series of biochemical tests. In this way, the laboratory technologist can determine
which substrates (usually carbohydrates) the yeast is able to use
as nutrients; this depends on what enzymes the yeast possesses. Minisystems (miniaturized biochemical test systems) are commercially available for the identification of
clinically important yeasts.

> In the mycology laboratory, yeasts are identified (speciated) by determining which substrates they are able to use as nutrients.

Biochemical tests are rarely
used, however, for identification of moulds isolated from
clinical specimens. Rather,
moulds are identified by a
combination of macroscopic
and microscopic observations
and the speed at which they
grow. Macroscopic observa-
tions include the color, texture, and topography of the
mould colony (mycelium). Microscopic examination of
the mould reveals the types of structures on which or
within which spores are produced (Fig. 5-6); the method
of spore production varies from one species of mould to
another. Immunodiagnostic procedures, including skin

> In the mycology laboratory, moulds are identified by a combination of macroscopic and microscopic observations and the speed at which they grow.

tests, are also available for diagnosing certain types of
mycoses.

Mycoses are most effectively treated with antifungal
agents like nystatin, amphotericin B, or 5-fluorocytosine
(discussed in Chapter 9). Because these chemotherapeutic agents may be toxic to humans, they are prescribed
with due consideration and caution.

Dimorphic Fungi. A few
fungi, including some human
pathogens, can live either as
yeasts or as moulds, depending
on growth conditions. This
phenomenon is called *dimorphism*, and the organisms are
referred to as *dimorphic fungi* (Fig. 5-13). When grown in
vitro at body temperature (37°C), dimorphic fungi exist
as unicellular yeasts and produce yeast colonies. Within
the human body (in vivo), dimorphic fungi exist as yeasts.
However, when grown in vitro at room temperature
(25°C), dimorphic fungi exist as moulds, producing
mould colonies (mycelia). Dimorphic fungi that cause
human diseases include *Histoplasma capsulatum* (which
causes histoplasmosis), *Sporothrix schenckii* (which causes
sporotrichosis), *Coccidioides immitis* (which causes coccidioidomycosis), and *Blastomyces dermatitidis* (which causes
blastomycosis).

> Dimorphic fungi can live either as yeasts or as moulds, depending on growth conditions.

FIGURE 5-13. Dimorphism. Photomicrographs illustrating the dimorphic fungus, *H. capsulatum*, being grown at 25°C (left photo) and at 37°C (right photo). (From Schaeter M, et al., eds. Mechanisms of Microbial Disease, 3rd ed. Philadelphia: Lippincott Williams & Wilkins, 1999.)

LICHENS

Nearly everyone has seen lichens, usually while hiking in the woods. They appear as colored, often circular patches on tree trunks and rocks. A **lichen** is actually a combination of two organisms—an alga (or a cyanobacterium) and a fungus—living together in such a close relationship that they appear to be one organism. Close relationships of this type are referred to as symbiotic relationships and the partners in the relationship are referred to as symbionts. A lichen represents a particular type of symbiotic relationship known as mutualism—a relationship in which

> A lichen is a combination of two organisms: an alga (or a cyanobacterium) and a fungus.

both parties benefit (discussed further in Chapter 10). The alga or cyanobacterium in a lichen is sometimes referred to as the photobiont (the photosynthetic partner in the relationship), and the fungus is referred to as the mycobiont. There are about 20,000 different species of lichens. Lichens may be gray, brown, black, orange, various shades of green, and other colors, depending on the specific combination of alga and fungus. Foliose lichens are leaflike, whereas crustose lichens appear as a crust on the rock or tree trunk surface (Fig. 5-14). Other lichens may be shrubby (fruticose lichens) or gelatinous. Lichens are classified as protists. They are not associated with human disease, but some substances produced by lichens have been shown to have antibacterial properties.

SLIME MOULDS

Slime moulds, which are found in soil and on rotting logs, have both fungal and protozoal characteristics and very interesting life cycles. Some slime moulds (known as cellular slime moulds) start out in life as independent amebae, ingesting bacteria and fungi by phagocytosis. When they run out of food, they fuse together to form a motile, multicellular form known as a slug, which is only about 0.5 mm long. The slug then becomes a fruiting body, consisting of a stalk and a spore cap. Spores produced within the spore cap become disseminated, and from each spore emerges an ameba. Cellular slime moulds represent cell differentiation at the lowest level, and scientists are studying them in an attempt to determine how some of the cells in the slug know that they are to become part of the stalk, how others know that they are to become part of the spore cap, and still others know that they are to differentiate into spores within the spore cap. Other slime moulds, known as plasmodial (or acellular) slime moulds, also produce stalks and spores, but their life cycles differ somewhat from those of cellular slime moulds. In the life cycle of a plasmodial slime mould, haploid cells fuse to become diploid cells, which

FIGURE 5-14. Lichens. ([A] Courtesy of http://www. en.wikipedia.org; [B] Photograph by PG Engelkirk.)

FIGURE 5-15. Slime mould growing on the forest floor. (Photograph by PG Engelkirk.)

develop into very large masses of motile, multinucleated protoplasm, each such mass being known as a plasmodium (Fig. 5-15). Some taxonomists classify slime moulds as fungi, whereas others classify them as protists. They are not known to cause human disease.

> ## ON THE CD-ROM
> - Terms Introduced in This Chapter
> - Review of Key Points
> - Insight: Microbes in the News: "Sick Building Syndrome" (Black Mould in Buildings)
> - Increase Your Knowledge
> - Critical Thinking
> - Additional Self-Assessment Exercises

SELF-ASSESSMENT EXERCISES

After studying this chapter, answer the following multiple-choice questions.

1. Which of the following statements about algae and fungi is (are) true?
   a. Algae are photosynthetic, whereas fungi are not.
   b. Algal cell walls contain cellulose, whereas fungal cell walls do not.
   c. Fungal cell walls contain chitin, whereas algal cell walls do not.
   d. all of the above

2. All of the following are algae except:
   a. desmids.
   b. diatoms.
   c. dinoflagellates.
   d. sporozoa.

3. All of the following are fungi except:
   a. moulds.
   b. *Paramecium*.
   c. *Penicillium*.
   d. yeasts.

4. A protozoan may possess any of the following except:
   a. cilia.
   b. flagella.
   c. hyphae.
   d. pseudopodia.

5. Which one of the following terms is not associated with fungi?
   a. conidia
   b. hyphae
   c. mycelium
   d. pellicle

6. All of the following terms can be used to describe hyphae except:
   a. aerial and reproductive.
   b. septate and aseptate.
   c. sexual and asexual.
   d. vegetative.

7. A lichen usually represents a symbiotic relationship between which of the following pairs?
   a. a fungus and an ameba
   b. a yeast and an ameba
   c. an alga and a cyanobacterium
   d. an alga and a fungus

8. A stigma is a:
   a. light-sensing organelle.
   b. primitive mouth.
   c. thickened membrane.
   d. type of plastid.

9. If a dimorphic fungus is causing a respiratory infection, which of the following might be seen in a sputum specimen from that patient?
   a. amebae
   b. conidia
   c. hyphae
   d. yeasts

10. Which one of the following is not a fungus?
    a. *Aspergillus*
    b. *Candida*
    c. *Penicillium*
    d. *Prototheca*

6

BIOCHEMISTRY: THE CHEMISTRY OF LIFE

LEARNING OBJECTIVES

AFTER STUDYING THIS CHAPTER, YOU SHOULD BE ABLE TO:

- Name the four main categories of biochemical molecules discussed in this chapter
- State the major differences among trioses, tetroses, pentoses, hexoses, and heptoses
- Describe each of the following: monosaccharides, disaccharides, and polysaccharides, and cite two examples of each
- Compare and contrast a dehydration synthesis reaction and a hydrolysis reaction, and cite an example of each
- Differentiate among covalent, glycosidic, and peptide bonds
- Discuss the roles of enzymes in metabolism
- Define the following terms: apoenzyme, cofactor, coenzyme, holoenzyme, substrate
- Cite three important differences between the structures of DNA and RNA
- State the major differences between DNA nucleotides and RNA nucleotides
- Define what is meant by "the Central Dogma"
- Describe the processes of DNA replication, transcription, and translation

INTRODUCTION

Some students are surprised to learn that they must study chemistry as part of a microbiology course. The reason why chemistry is an important component of a microbiology course is the answer to the question, "What exactly is a microorganism?" A microbe can be thought of as a "bag" of chemicals that interact with each other in various ways. Even the bag itself is composed of chemicals. Everything a microorganism is and does relates to chemistry. The various ways microorganisms function and survive in their environment depend on their chemical makeup. The same things are true about the cells that make up any living organisms—including human beings; these cells, too, can be thought of as bags of chemicals.

> Cells can be thought of as "bags" of chemicals. Even the bags themselves are composed of chemicals.

To understand microbial cells and how they function, one must have a basic knowledge of the chemistry of atoms, molecules, and compounds. CD-ROM Appendix 3: "Basic Chemistry Concepts" contains such information. Students having little or no background in chemistry should study the material in CD-ROM Appendix 3 before attempting to learn the material in this chapter. CD-ROM Appendix 3 can serve as a review for students who have already studied basic chemistry, either in a biology course or in an introductory chemistry course. Your instructor will inform you as to whether the material in CD-ROM Appendix 3 is "testable."

Even the most simple procaryotic cells consist of very large molecules (*macromolecules*), such as deoxyribonucleic acid (DNA), ribonucleic acid (RNA), proteins, lipids, and polysaccharides, as well as many combinations of these macromolecules that combine to

> Cells contain many large biological molecules, known as macromolecules. Macromolecules include DNA, RNA, proteins, lipids, and polysaccharides.

make up structures like capsules, cell walls, cell membranes, and flagella. These macromolecules can be broken down into smaller units or "building blocks," such as monosaccharides (simple sugars), fatty acids, amino acids, and nucleotides. The macromolecules and building blocks found in cells are collectively referred to as *biological molecules*. The building blocks can be broken down into even smaller molecules such as water, carbon dioxide, ammonia, sulfides, and phosphates, which in turn can be broken down into atoms of carbon (C), hydrogen (H), oxygen (O), nitrogen (N), sulfur (S), phosphorus (P), etc.

Organic chemistry is the study of compounds that contain carbon; **inorganic chemistry** involves all other chemical reactions; **biochemistry** is the chemistry of living cells. Basic inorganic chemistry is introduced in CD-ROM Appendix 3: "Basic Chemistry Concepts"; organic chemistry and biochemistry are discussed in this chapter.

Only when all these molecules and compounds are in place and working together properly can the cell function like a well-managed factory. As in industry, a cell must have the appropriate machinery, regulatory molecules (enzymes) to control its activities, fuel (nutrients or light) to provide energy, and raw materials (nutrients) for manufacturing essential end products.

Everything that a microorganism is and does involves biochemistry. Biochemicals make up the structure of a microorganism, and a multitude of biochemical reactions take

> Everything that a cell is and does involves biochemistry.

place within the microorganism. What is true for microbes is also true for every other living organism. The characteristics that distinguish living organisms from inanimate objects—(a) their complex and highly organized structure; (b) their ability to extract, transform, and use energy from their environment; and (c) their capacity for precise self-replication and self-assembly—all result from the nature, function, and interaction of biomolecules. Because biochemistry is a branch of organic chemistry, a brief introduction to organic chemistry will be presented first.

ORGANIC CHEMISTRY

Organic compounds are compounds that contain carbon, and organic chemistry is that branch of the science of chemistry that specializes in the study of organic compounds. The term *organic* is somewhat misleading, as it implies that all these compounds are produced by or are in some way related to living organisms. This is not true.

> Organic compounds are compounds that contain carbon. Although many organic compounds are produced by or related to living organisms, some are not.

Although some organic compounds are associated with living organisms, many are not. A typical *Escherichia coli* cell contains more than 6,000 different kinds of organic compounds, including about 3,000 different proteins and approximately the same number of different molecules of nucleic acid. Proteins make up about 15% of the total weight of an *E. coli* cell, whereas nucleic acids, polysaccharides, and lipids make up about 7%, 3%, and 2%, respectively.

Organic chemistry is a broad and important branch of chemistry, involving the chemistry of fossil fuels (petroleum and coal), dyes, drugs, paper, ink, paints, plastics, gasoline, rubber tires, food, and clothing. The number of compounds that contain carbon far exceeds the number of compounds that do not contain carbon. Some carbon-containing compounds are very large and complex, some containing thousands of atoms.

Carbon Bonds

In our current understanding of life, carbon is the primary requisite for all living systems. The element carbon exists in three forms or allotropes: amorphous carbon, graphite, and diamond.

1. **Amorphous carbon** is also known as lampblack, gas black, channel black, and carbon black. It is the black soot that forms when a material containing carbon is burned with insufficient oxygen for it to burn completely. It is used to make inks, paints, rubber products, and the cores of dry cell batteries.
2. **Graphite** is one of the softest materials known. It is primarily used as a lubricant, although in a form called coke, is used in the production of steel. The black material in "lead" pencils is actually graphite.
3. **Diamond** is one of the hardest substances known. Naturally occurring diamonds are used for jewelry, whereas artificially produced diamonds are used to make diamond-tipped saw blades.

These three forms of carbon have dramatically different physical properties, making it difficult to believe that they are truly the same element. Carbon atoms have a valence of four, meaning that a carbon atom can bond to four other atoms. For convenience, the carbon atom is illustrated in this text with the symbol C and four bonds.

$$-\overset{|}{\underset{|}{C}}-$$

The uniqueness of carbon lies in the ability of its atoms to bond to each other to form a multitude of compounds. The variety of carbon compounds increases still more when atoms of other elements also attach in different ways to the carbon atom.

There are three ways in which carbon atoms can bond to each other: **single bond**, **double bond**, and **triple bond**. In the following illustrations, each line between the carbon atoms represents a pair of shared electrons (known as a *covalent bond*). In a carbon–carbon single bond, the two carbon atoms share one pair of electrons; in a carbon–carbon double bond, two pairs of electrons; and in a carbon–carbon triple bond, three pairs of electrons. Covalent bonds are typical of the compounds of carbon and are the bonds of primary importance in organic chemistry. Organic chemistry is sometimes defined as the chemistry of carbon and its covalent bonds.

> Organic chemistry is sometimes defined as the chemistry of carbon and its covalent bonds.

| Single bond | Double bond | Triple bond |

When atoms of other elements attach to available bonds of carbon atoms, compounds are formed. For example, if only hydrogen atoms are bonded to the available bonds, compounds called hydrocarbons are formed. In other words, a **hydrocarbon** is an organic molecule that contains only carbon and hydrogen atoms. Just a few of the many hydrocarbon compounds are shown in Figure 6-1.

> Hydrocarbons are organic compounds that contain only carbon and hydrogen.

When more than two carbons are linked together, longer molecules are formed. A series of many carbon atoms bonded together is referred to as a *chain*. Long-chain carbon compounds are usually liquids or solids, whereas short-chain carbon compounds, such as the hydrocarbons shown in Figure 6-1, are gases.

Cyclic Compounds

Carbon atoms may link to carbon atoms to close the chain, forming *rings* or *cyclic compounds*. An example is

FIGURE 6-1. Simple hydrocarbons.

FIGURE 6-2. The benzene ring.

benzene, which has six carbons and six hydrogens, as shown in Figure 6-2. Although benzene contains six carbon atoms, other ring structures contain fewer or more carbon atoms, and some compounds contain fused rings (e.g., double- or triple-ringed compounds).

BIOCHEMISTRY

Biochemistry is the study of biology at the molecular level and can, thus, be thought of as the chemistry of life or the chemistry of living organisms. Not only is biochemistry a branch of biology, but it is also a branch of organic chemistry. Biochemistry involves the study of the biomolecules that are present within living organisms. These biomolecules are usually large molecules (called *macromolecules*) and include carbohydrates, lipids, proteins, and nucleic acids. Other examples of biomolecules are vitamins, enzymes, hormones, and energy-carrying molecules, such as adenosine triphosphate (ATP).

> Biochemistry involves the study of biomolecules, and can be thought of as both a branch of chemistry and a branch of biology.

Humans obtain their nutrients from the foods they eat. The carbohydrates, fats, nucleic acids, and proteins contained in these foods are digested, and their components are absorbed into the blood and carried to every cell in the body. Within cells, these components are then broken down and rearranged. In this way, the compounds necessary for cell structure and function are synthesized. Microorganisms also absorb their essential nutrients into the cell by various means, to be described in Chapter 7. These nutrients are then used in metabolic reactions as sources of energy and as building blocks for enzymes, structural macromolecules, and genetic materials.

Carbohydrates

Carbohydrates are biomolecules composed of carbon, hydrogen, and oxygen, in the ratio of 1:2:1, or simply CH_2O. Glucose, fructose, sucrose, lactose, maltose, starch, cellulose, and glycogen are all examples of carbohydrates.

> Carbohydrates are biomolecules that are composed of carbon, hydrogen, and oxygen in the ratio of 1:2:1.

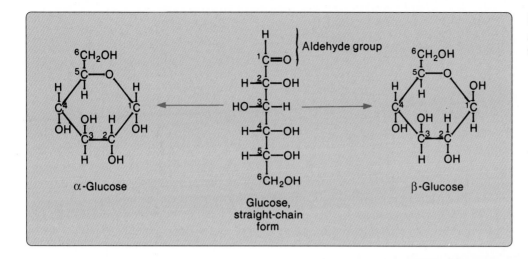

FIGURE 6-3. Glucose.
All three forms may exist in equilibrium in solution.

Monosaccharides

The simplest carbohydrates are sugars, and the smallest sugars (or simple sugars) are called **monosaccharides** (Greek *mono* meaning "one"; *sakcharon* meaning "sugar"). The "one" refers to the number of rings; in other words, monosaccharides are sugars composed of only one ring. The most important monosaccharide in nature is **glucose** ($C_6H_{12}O_6$), which may occur as a chain or in alpha or beta ring configurations, as shown in Figure 6-3. Monosaccharides may contain from three to nine carbon atoms (Table 6-1), although most of them contain five or six. A three-carbon monosaccharide is called a **triose**; one containing

> The simplest carbohydrates are simple sugars or monosaccharides. Trioses, pentoses, and hexoses are examples of monosaccharides.

four carbons is called a **tetrose**; five, a **pentose**; six, a **hexose**; seven, a **heptose**; eight, an **octose**; and nine, a **nonose**. Ribose and deoxyribose are pentoses that are found in RNA and DNA, respectively. Glucose (also called *dextrose*) is a hexose. Octoses and nonoses are quite rare.

Glucose, the main source of energy for body cells, is found in most sweet fruits and in blood. The glucose carried in the blood to the cells is oxidized to produce the energy-carrying molecule ATP, with its high-energy phosphate bonds. ATP molecules are the main source of the energy that is used to drive most metabolic reactions. Galactose and fructose are other examples of hexoses. Fructose (Fig. 6-4), the sweetest of the monosaccharides, is found in fruits and honey.

Disaccharides

Disaccharides (*di* meaning "two") are double-ringed sugars that result from the combination of two monosaccharides. The synthesis of a disaccharide from two monosaccharides by removal of a water molecule is called a **dehydration**

> Sucrose, lactose, and maltose are examples of disaccharides.

TABLE 6-1		Monosaccharides
NUMBER OF CARBON ATOMS	**GENERAL NAME**	**EXAMPLES**
3	Triose	Glyceraldehyde (glycerose), dihydroxyacetone
4	Tetrose	Erythrose
5	Pentose	Ribose, deoxyribose, arabinose, xylose, ribulose
6	Hexose	Glucose, fructose, galactose, mannose
7	Heptose	Sedoheptulose, mannoheptulose
8	Octose	Octoses have been synthetically prepared; they do not occur in nature
9	Nonose	Neuraminic acid

FIGURE 6-4. Fructose in straight-chain form. Fructose may also exist in the ring form shown in Figure 6-5.

FIGURE 6-5. The dehydration synthesis and hydrolysis of sucrose.

Glucose   Fructose   Sucrose   Water

synthesis reaction (Fig. 6-5). The bond holding the two monosaccharides together is called a **glycosidic bond**; it is a type of covalent bond. Glucose is the major constituent of disaccharides. Sucrose (table sugar) is a sweet disaccharide made by joining together a glucose molecule and a fructose molecule. Sucrose comes from sugar cane, sugar beets, and maple sugar. Lactose (milk sugar) and maltose (malt sugar) are also disaccharides. Lactose is made by joining together a molecule of glucose and a molecule of galactose. People who lack the digestive enzyme lactase, needed to split lactose into its monosaccharide components, are said to be lactose intolerant. Maltose is made by combining two molecules of glucose.

Disaccharides react with water in a process called a **hydrolysis reaction**, which causes them to break down into two monosaccharides:

$$\text{disaccharide} + H_2O \rightarrow \text{two monosaccharides}$$
$$\text{sucrose} + H_2O \rightarrow \text{glucose} + \text{fructose}$$
$$\text{lactose} + H_2O \rightarrow \text{glucose} + \text{galactose}$$
$$\text{maltose} + H_2O \rightarrow \text{glucose} + \text{glucose}$$

Peptidoglycan (mentioned in Chapter 3) is a complex macromolecular network found in the cell walls of all members of the domain *Bacteria*. Peptidoglycan consists of a repeating disaccharide, attached by polypeptides (proteins) to form a lattice that surrounds and protects the entire bacterial cell. Several antibiotics (including penicillin) prevent the final cross-linking of the rows of disaccharides, thus weakening the cell wall and leading to lysis (bursting) of the bacterial cell. Although most members of the domain *Archaea* have cell walls, their cell walls do not contain peptidoglycan.

Carbohydrates composed of three monosaccharides are called **trisaccharides**; those composed of four are called **tetrasaccharides**; those composed of five are called **pentasaccharides**; and so on, until one comes to polysaccharides.

Polysaccharides

The definition of a **polysaccharide** varies from one reference book to another, with some stating that a polysaccharide consists of more than six monosaccharides, others stating more than eight, and others stating more than ten. Poly means "many," and in reality, most polysaccharides contain many monosaccharides—up to hundreds or even thousands of monosaccharides. Thus, in this book, polysaccharides are defined as carbohydrate polymers containing many monosaccharides.

Examples include starch and glycogen, which are composed of hundreds of repetitive glucose units held together by different types of covalent bonds, known as glycosidic bonds (or glycosidic linkages). Glucose is the major constituent of polysaccharides. Polysaccharides are examples of **polymers**—molecules consisting of many similar subunits. Some of these molecules are so large that they are insoluble in water. In the presence of the proper enzymes or acids, polysaccharides may be hydrolyzed or broken down into disaccharides, and then finally into monosaccharides (Fig. 6-6).

Polysaccharides serve two main functions. One is to store energy that can be used when the external food supply is low. The common storage molecule in animals is **glycogen**, which is found in the liver and in muscles. In plants, glucose is stored as **starch** and is found in potatoes and other vegetables and seeds. Some algae store starch, whereas bacteria contain glycogen granules as a reserve nutrient supply. The other function of polysaccharides is to provide a "tough" molecule for structural support and protection. Many bacteria produce polysaccharide capsules, which protect the bacteria from being phagocytized (eaten) by white blood cells.

Cellulose is another example of a polysaccharide. Plant and algal cells have cellulose cell walls to provide support and shape as well as protection against the environment. Cellulose is insoluble in water and indigestible for humans and most animals. Some protozoa, fungi, and bacteria have enzymes that will break the β-glycosidic bonds linking the glucose units in cellulose. Some of these microorganisms (saprophytes) are able to disintegrate dead plants in the soil, and others (parasites) live in the digestive organs of herbivores (plant eaters). Protozoa in the gut of termites digest the cellulose in the wood that

Polysaccharides can be defined as carbohydrates that contain many monosaccharides.

Polysaccharides, such as glycogen, starch, and cellulose, are examples of polymers—molecules consisting of many similar subunits. In the case of polysaccharides, the repeating subunits are monosaccharides.

Bacterial cell walls contain peptidoglycan, a complex macromolecule consisting of a repeating disaccharide, attached by proteins.

FIGURE 6-6. The hydrolysis of starch.

the termites eat. Fibers of cellulose extracted from certain plants are used to make paper, cotton, linen, and rope. These fibers are relatively rigid, strong, and insoluble because they consist of 100 to 200 parallel strands of cellulose. Starch and glycogen are easily digested by animals because they possess the digestive enzyme that hydrolyzes the α-glycosidic bonds that link the glucose units into long, helical, or branched polymers (Fig. 6-7).

When polysaccharides combine with other chemical groups (amines, lipids, and amino acids), extremely complex macromolecules are formed that serve specific purposes. Glucosamine and galactosamine (amine derivatives of glucose and galactose, respectively) are important constituents of the supporting polysaccharides in connective tissue fibers, cartilage, and chitin. Chitin is the main component of the hard outer covering of insects, spiders, and crabs, and is also found in the cell walls of fungi. The main portion of the rigid cell wall of bacteria consists of amino sugars and short polypeptide chains that combine to form the peptidoglycan layer.

> Bacterial cell walls contain peptidoglycan, algal cell walls contain cellulose, and fungal cell walls contain chitin. Peptidoglycan, cellulose, and chitin are examples of polysaccharides.

Lipids

Lipids constitute an important class of biomolecules. Most lipids are insoluble in water but soluble in fat solvents, such as ether, chloroform, and benzene. Lipids are essential constituents of almost all living cells.

Fatty Acids

Fatty acids can be thought of as the building blocks of lipids. Fatty acids are long-chain carboxylic acids that are insoluble in water. **Saturated fatty acids** contain only single bonds between the carbon atoms. Fats containing saturated fatty acids are usually solids at room temperature. **Monounsaturated fatty acids** (such as those found in butter, olives, and peanuts) have one double bond in the carbon chain. **Polyunsaturated fatty acids** (such as those found in soybeans, safflowers, sunflowers, and corn) contain two or more double bonds. Most fats containing unsaturated fatty acids are liquids at room temperature. The terms saturated, monounsaturated, and polyunsaturated fatty acids are often heard in discussions about human diet. Certain fatty acids, called **essential fatty acids**, cannot be synthesized in the human body and, thus, must be provided in the diet.

> Whereas monosaccharides are the building blocks of carbohydrates, fatty acids are the building blocks of lipids.

For purposes of discussion, lipids can be classified into the following categories (Fig. 6-8):

- Waxes
- Fats and oils
- Phospholipids
- Glycolipids
- Steroids
- Prostaglandins and leukotrienes

> Waxes, fats, oils, phospholipids, glycolipids, steroids, prostaglandins, and leukotrienes are all examples of lipids.

FIGURE 6-7. The difference between cellulose and starch.

β (beta) linkage (alternating "up and down") in cellulose

α (alpha) linkage (no alternation) in starch

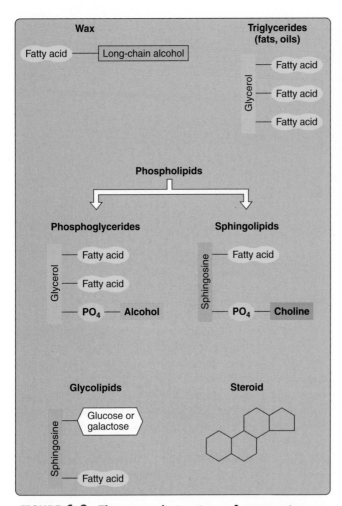

FIGURE 6-8. The general structure of some categories of lipids.

feathers of animals and birds provide a waterproof coating. Lanolin, a mixture of waxes obtained from wool, is used in hand and body lotions to aid in retention of water, thus softening the skin. The waxes that are present in the cell walls of *Mycobacterium tuberculosis* (the causative agent of tuberculosis) are responsible for several interesting characteristics of this bacterium. For example, should an *M. tuberculosis* cell be phagocytized by a phagocytic white blood cell (a phagocyte), the waxes protect the cell from being digested. This enables the bacterial cell to survive and multiply within the phagocyte. Also, the waxes in the cell walls of *M. tuberculosis* make the organism difficult to stain, and, once stained, the waxes make it difficult to remove the stain from the cell. In the acid-fast staining procedure, for example, it is necessary to heat the carbolfuchsin dye to drive it into the cell; once the cell has been stained, the waxes prevent decolorization of the cell when a mixture of acid and alcohol is applied. Because the cell does not decolorize in the presence of acid, the organism is described as being acid-fast.

Fats and Oils

Fats and **oils** are the most common types of lipids. Fats and oils are also known as **triglycerides**, because they are composed of glycerol (a three-carbon alcohol) and three fatty acids (Fig. 6-9). Fats are triglycerides that are solid at room temperature. Most fats come from animal sources; examples include the fats found in meat, whole milk, butter, and cheese. Most oils are triglycerides that are liquid at room temperature. The most commonly used oils come from plant sources. Olive oil and peanut oil are monounsaturated oils, whereas oils from corn, cottonseed, safflower, and sunflower are polyunsaturated.

Phospholipids

Phospholipids contain glycerol, fatty acids, a phosphate group, and an alcohol. There are two types: *glycerophospholipids* (also called *phosphoglycerides*) and *sphingolipids*.

Cell membranes consist of a lipid bilayer, composed of two rows of phospholipids, arranged tail-to-tail.

Glycerophospholipids are the most abundant lipids in cell membranes. The basic structure of a cell membrane

Waxes

A **wax** consists of a saturated fatty acid and a long-chain alcohol. Wax coatings on the fruits, leaves, and stems of plants help to prevent loss of water and damage from pests. Waxes on the skin, fur, and

Waxes in the cell walls of *M. tuberculosis* (the causative agent of tuberculosis) protect phagocytized *M. tuberculosis* cells from being digested.

FIGURE 6-9. The synthesis of a fat.

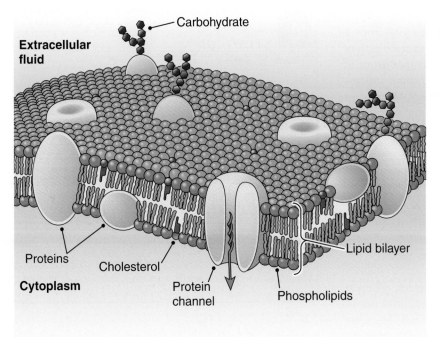

FIGURE 6-10. The lipid bilayer structure of cell membranes, showing the hydrophilic heads and hydrophobic tails of phospholipid molecules (blue). Cell membranes also contain protein molecules (pink), which have been described as resembling icebergs floating in a sea of lipids. (From Cohen BJ. *Memmler's The Human Body in Health and Disease.* 11th Ed. Philadelphia: Lippincott Williams & Wilkins, 2009.)

is a lipid bilayer, consisting of two rows of phospholipids, arranged tail-to-tail (Fig. 6-10). The hydrophobic tails, lacking an affinity for water molecules, point toward each other, enabling them to get as far away from water as possible. The hydrophilic heads, being able to associate with water molecules, project to the inner and outer surfaces of the membrane. Two other types of lipids are also found in eucaryotic cell membranes: steroids (primarily cholesterol, in animal cells) and glycolipids. The cell membrane also contains proteins, which have been described as "icebergs floating in a sea of lipids."

In addition to phospholipids, the outer membrane of Gram-negative bacterial cell walls contains lipoproteins and lipopolysaccharide (LPS). As the name implies, LPS consists of a lipid portion and a polysaccharide portion. The lipid portion is called lipid-A or endotoxin. When endotoxin is present in the human bloodstream, it can cause very serious physiologic conditions (e.g., fever and septic shock). The cell walls of Gram-positive bacteria do not contain LPS.

> When present in the human bloodstream, lipids found in the cell walls of Gram-negative bacteria can cause serious physiologic conditions in humans, such as fever and shock.

Lecithins and cephalins are glycerophospholipids that are found in brain and nerve tissues as well as in egg yolks, wheat germ, and yeast.

Sphingolipids are phospholipids that contain an 18-carbon alcohol called sphingosine rather than glycerol. Sphingolipids are found in brain and nerve tissues. One of the most abundant sphingolipids is sphingomyelin, which makes up the white matter of the myelin sheath that coats nerve cells.

Glycolipids

Glycolipids are abundant in the brain and in the myelin sheaths of nerves. Some glycolipids contain glycerol plus two fatty acids and a monosaccharide. Cerebrosides and gangliosides are examples of glycolipids; both are found in the human nervous system. A person's blood group (A, B, AB, or O) is determined by the particular glycolipids that are present on the surface of that person's red blood cells.

Steroids

Steroids are rather complex, four-ringed structures. Steroids include cholesterol, bile salts, fat-soluble vitamins, and steroid hormones. Cholesterol is a component of cell membranes, myelin sheath, and brain and nerve tissue. Bile salts are synthesized in the liver from cholesterol and stored in the gallbladder. The fat-soluble vitamins are vitamins A, D, E, and K.[a] Steroid hormones include male sex hormones (testosterone and androsterone) and female sex hormones (estrogens such as estradiol and progesterone). The adrenal corticosteroids (aldosterone and cortisone) are steroid hormones produced by the adrenal glands, one of which is located at the top of each kidney.

---

[a] Water-soluble vitamins (the eight B vitamins and vitamin C) dissolve easily in water, and are readily excreted from the body. Fat-soluble vitamins are absorbed through the intestinal tract with the help of lipids, and are more likely to accumulate in the body than are water-soluble vitamins.

Prostaglandins and Leukotrienes

Prostaglandins and **leukotrienes** are derived from a fatty acid called *arachidonic acid*. Both have a wide variety of effects on body chemistry. They act as mediators of hormones, lower or raise blood pressure, cause inflammation, and induce fever. Leukotrienes are produced in leukocytes (for which they are named), but also occur in other tissues. Leukotrienes can produce long-lasting muscle contractions, especially in the lungs, where they cause asthma-like attacks.

Proteins

Proteins are among the most essential chemicals in all living cells, referred to by some scientists as "the substance of life." Some proteins are the structural | Proteins contain carbon, hydrogen, oxygen, nitrogen, and sometimes sulfur.

components of membranes, cells, and tissues, whereas others are enzymes and hormones that chemically control the metabolic balance within both the cell and the entire organism. All proteins are polymers of amino acids; however, they vary widely in the number of amino acids present and in the sequence of amino acids as well as their size, configuration, and functions. Proteins contain carbon, hydrogen, oxygen, nitrogen, and sometimes sulfur.

Amino Acid Structure

A total of 23 different **amino acids** have been found in proteins, 20 primary or naturally occurring amino acids plus 3 secondary amino acids (derived from primary amino acids). | Proteins are polymers that are composed of amino acids (i.e., amino acids are the building blocks of proteins).

Each amino acid is composed of carbon, hydrogen, oxygen, and nitrogen; 3 of the amino acids also have sulfur atoms in the molecule. Humans can synthesize certain amino acids, but not others. Those that cannot be synthesized (called **essential amino acids**) must be ingested as part of our diets. The term *essential amino acids* is somewhat misleading, however, in view of the fact that *all* of the amino acids are necessary for protein synthesis. Because we cannot manufacture the essential amino acids, it is *essential* that they be included in our diets.

The general formula for amino acids is shown in Figure 6-11. In this figure, the "R" group represents any

STUDY AID

Proteins

Proteins can be thought of as "strings of beads." The beads are amino acids. Proteins may contain as few as two amino acids to as many as 5,000 or more. The sequence of amino acids is referred to as the primary structure of a protein.

STUDY AID
Names of Amino Acids

Alanine (1°)	Glutamic acid (1°)	Isoleucine (1°, E)	Serine (1°)
Arginine (1°, E*)	Glutamine (1°)	Leucine (1°, E)	Threonine (1°, E)
Asparagine (1°)	Glycine (1°)	Lysine (1°, E)	Tryptophan (1°, E)
Aspartic (1°)	Histidine (1°, E*)	Methionine (1°, E)	Tyrosine acid (1°)
Cysteine (1°)	Hydroxylysine (2°)	Phenylalanine (1°, E)	Valine (1°, E)
Cystine (2°)	Hydroxyproline (2°)	Proline (1°)	

Key: *1°*, a primary amino acid; *2°*, a secondary amino acid; *E*, an essential amino acid; *E**, additional essential amino acid in infants

of the 23 groups that may be substituted into that position to build the various amino acids. For instance, "H" in place of the "R" represents the amino acid glycine, and "CH₃" in that position results in the structural formula for the amino acid alanine.

The thousands of different proteins in the human body are composed of a great variety of amino acids in various quantities and arrangements. The number of proteins that can be synthesized is virtually unlimited. Proteins are not limited by the number of different amino acids, just as the number of words in a written language is not limited by the number of letters in the alphabet. The actual number of proteins produced by an organism and the amino acid sequence of those proteins are determined by the particular genes present on the organism's chromosome(s).

Protein Structure

When water is removed, by dehydration synthesis, amino acids become linked together by a covalent bond, referred to as a **peptide bond** (as shown in Fig. 6-12). A **dipeptide** is formed by bonding two amino acids, whereas the bonding of three amino acids forms a **tripeptide**. A chain

FIGURE 6-11. The basic structure of an amino acid.

FIGURE 6-12. The formation of a dipeptide. R indicates any amino acid side chain.

(polymer) consisting of more than three amino acids is referred to as a **polypeptide**. Polypeptides are said to have *primary protein structure*—a linear sequence of amino acids in a chain (Fig. 6-13).

Most polypeptide chains naturally twist into helices or sheets as a result of the charged side chains protruding from the carbon–nitrogen backbone of the molecule. This helical or sheetlike configuration is referred to as *secondary protein structure* and is found in fibrous proteins. Fibrous proteins are long, threadlike molecules that are insoluble in water. They make up keratin (found in hair, nails, wool, horns,

> The monosaccharides in carbohydrates are joined together by glycosidic bonds. The amino acids in proteins are joined together by peptide bonds. Glycosidic bonds and peptide bonds are examples of covalent bonds.

feathers), collagen (in tendons), myosin (in muscles), and the microtubules and microfilaments of cells.

Because a long coil can become entwined by folding back on itself, a polypeptide helix may become globular (Fig. 6-13). In some areas the helix is retained, but other areas curve randomly. This globular, *tertiary protein structure* is stabilized not only by hydrogen bonding but also by disulfide bond cross-links between two sulfur groups (S–S). This three-dimensional configuration is characteristic of enzymes, which work by fitting on and into specific molecules (see the next section). Other examples of globular proteins include many hormones (e.g., insulin), albumin in eggs, and hemoglobin and fibrinogen in blood. Globular proteins are soluble in water.

When two or more polypeptide chains are bonded together by hydrogen and disulfide bonds, the resulting

FIGURE 6-13. Protein structure. (A) Primary structure (the sequence of amino acids). **(B)** Secondary structure (a helix). **(C)** Tertiary structure (globular). **(D)** Quaternary structure (four polypeptide chains).

structure is referred to as *quaternary protein structure* (Fig. 6-13). For instance, hemoglobin consists of four globular myoglobins. The size, shape, and configuration of a protein are specific for the function it must perform. If the amino acid sequence and, thus, the configuration of hemoglobin in red blood cells is not perfect, the red blood cells may become distorted and assume a sickle shape (as in sickle cell anemia). In this state, they are unable to carry the oxygen that is necessary for cellular metabolism. Myoglobin, the oxygen-binding protein found in skeletal muscles, was the first protein to have its primary, secondary, and tertiary structure defined by scientists.

Enzymes

Enzymes are protein molecules[b] produced by living cells as "instructed" by genes on the chromosomes. Enzymes are referred to as **biological catalysts**—biologic molecules that **catalyze** metabolic reactions. A

> Enzymes are proteins that function as biological catalysts, meaning that they catalyze (speed up) metabolic reactions.

catalyst is defined as an agent that speeds up a chemical reaction without being consumed in the process. In some cases, a particular metabolic reaction will not occur at all in the absence of an enzyme catalyst. Almost every reaction in the cell requires the presence of a specific enzyme. Although enzymes influence the direction of the reaction and increase its rate of reaction, they do not provide the energy needed to activate the reaction.

Some protein molecules function as enzymes all by themselves. Other proteins (called **apoenzymes**) can only function as enzymes (i.e., can only catalyze a chemical reaction) after they link up with a nonprotein **cofactor**. Some apoenzymes require metal ions (e.g., Ca^{2+}, Fe^{2+}, Mg^{2+}, Cu^{2+}) as cofactors, whereas others require vitamin-type compounds (called **coenzymes**), such as vitamin C, flavin-adenine dinucleotide (FAD), and nicotinamide-adenine dinucleotide (NAD). The combination of the apoenzyme plus the cofactor is called a **holoenzyme** (a "whole" enzyme); the holoenzyme can function as an enzyme.

$$apoenzyme + cofactor = holoenzyme$$
$$(a\ functional\ enzyme)$$

Enzymes are usually named by adding the ending "-ase" to the word, indicating the compound or types of compounds on which an enzyme acts or exerts its effect. For example, proteases, carbohydrases, and lipases are families of enzymes that exert their effects on proteins, carbohydrates, and lipids, respectively. The specific molecule on which an enzyme acts is referred to as that enzyme's **substrate**. Each enzyme has a particular substrate on which it exerts its effect; thus, enzymes are said to be very specific. Although most enzymes end in "-ase," some do not; lysozyme and hemolysins are examples.

> **STUDY AID**
> *Examples of Enzymes*
>
> | | |
> |---|---|
> | Catalase | Lysozyme |
> | Coagulase | Oxidase |
> | DNA polymerase | Peptidases |
> | DNAse | Proteases |
> | Hemolysin | RNA polymerase |
> | Lipases | RNAse |

Some toxins and other poisonous substances cause damage to the human body by interfering with the action of certain necessary enzymes. For example, cyanide poison binds to the iron and copper ions in the cytochrome systems of the mitochondria of eucaryotic cells. As a result, the cells cannot use oxygen to synthesize ATP, which is essential for energy production, and they soon die.

Proteins, including enzymes, may be denatured (structurally altered) by heat or certain chemicals. In a denatured protein, the bonds that hold the molecule in a tertiary structure are broken. With these bonds broken, the protein is no longer functional. Enzymes are discussed further in Chapter 7.

Nucleic Acids

Function

Nucleic acids—DNA and RNA—comprise the fourth major group of biomolecules in living cells. In addition to the elements C, H, O, and N, DNA and RNA also contain P (phosphorus).

> Nucleic acids contain C, H, O, N, and P.

Nucleic acids play extremely important roles in a cell; they are critical to the proper functioning of a cell. DNA is the "hereditary molecule"—the molecule that contains the genes and genetic code. DNA makes up the major portion of chromosomes. The information in DNA must flow to the rest of the cell for the cell to function properly; this flow of information is accomplished by RNA molecules. RNA molecules participate in the conversion of the genetic code into proteins and other gene products.

Structure

The building blocks of nucleic acid polymers are called **nucleotides**. These are more complex monomers (single molecular units that can be repeated to form a polymer) than amino acids, which are the building blocks of proteins.

> The building blocks of nucleic acids are called nucleotides, each of which contains three components: a nitrogenous base, a pentose, and a phosphate group.

---

[b] Certain RNA molecules, called ribozymes, have been shown to have enzymatic activity. However, because most enzymes are proteins, enzymes are discussed in this book as if all of them were proteins.

HISTORICAL NOTE

The Discovery of the Hereditary Molecule

In 1944, Oswald T. Avery and his colleagues at the Rockefeller Institute wrote one of the most important papers ever published in biology. In that paper, they announced their discovery that DNA, not proteins as had earlier been suspected, is the molecule that contains genetic information (i.e., that DNA is the hereditary molecule). They made this discovery while repeating Frederick Griffith's 1928 transformation experiments (see Chapter 7). Whereas Griffith's experiments involved mice, Avery's group conducted in vitro experiments. The importance of this discovery was not fully appreciated at the time, and Avery and his colleagues did not receive a Nobel Prize. Additional evidence that DNA is the molecule that contains genetic information was provided by Alfred Hershey and Martha Chase in 1952. Their work involved a bacteriophage that infects *E. coli*. In 1969, Hershey shared a Nobel Prize with Max Delbrück and Salvador Luria for their discoveries involving the genetic structure and replication of bacteriophages.

STUDY AID

Nucleotides

Three Parts to Every Nucleotide	Four DNA Nucleotides (Deoxyribonucleotides)	Four RNA Nucleotides (Ribonucleotides)
1. Nitrogenous base	Adenine (a purine)	Adenine (a purine)
	Guanine (a purine)	Guanine (a purine)
	Cytosine (a pyrimidine)	Cytosine (a pyrimidine)
	Thymine (a pyrimidine)	Uracil (a pyrimidine)
2. Pentose	Deoxyribose	Ribose
3. Phosphate group	Phosphate group	Phosphate group

Nucleotides consist of three subunits: a nitrogen-containing (nitrogenous) base, a five-carbon sugar (pentose), and a phosphate group, joined together, as shown in Figure 6-14.

The building blocks of DNA are called **DNA nucleotides**; they contain a nitrogenous base, deoxyribose, and a phosphate group. The building blocks of RNA are called **RNA nucleotides**; they contain a nitrogenous base, ribose, and a phosphate group.

> The building blocks of DNA are called DNA nucleotides, whereas the building blocks of RNA are called RNA nucleotides.

As previously stated, there are two kinds of nucleic acids in cells: DNA and RNA. DNA contains deoxyribose as its pentose, whereas RNA contains ribose as its pentose. There are

> The three types of RNA in a cell are messenger RNA (mRNA), ribosomal RNA (rRNA), and transfer RNA (tRNA).

three types of RNA, which are named for the function they serve: *messenger RNA* (mRNA), *ribosomal RNA* (rRNA), and *transfer RNA* (tRNA).

The five nitrogenous bases in nucleic acids are adenine (A), guanine (G), thymine (T), cytosine (C), and uracil (U). Thymine is found in DNA, but not in RNA. Uracil is found in RNA, but not in DNA. The other three bases (A, G, C) are present in both DNA and RNA. Both A and G are **purines** (double-ring structures), whereas T, C, and U are pyrimidines (single-ring structures; Fig. 6-15).

> The nitrogenous bases adenine, guanine, and cytosine are found in both DNA and RNA. However, thymine is found only in DNA and uracil is found only in RNA.

The nucleotides join together (via covalent bonds) between their sugar and phosphate groups to form very long polymers—100,000 or more monomers long—as shown in Figure 6-16.

DNA Structure

For a double-stranded DNA molecule to form, the nitrogenous bases on the two separate strands must bond

FIGURE 6-14. Two nucleotides, each consisting of a nitrogenous base (A or T), a five-carbon sugar (S), and a phosphate group (P).

STUDY AID

Purines and Pyrimidines

Here is one way to remember the difference between purines and pyrimidines. Think of the double-ring structure of a purine (adenine or guanine) as being "pure and un-CUT." The single-ring pyrimidines can be thought of as being "CUT," where the "C" stands for cytosine, the "U" stands for uracil, and the "T" stands for thymine.

FIGURE 6-15. The pyrimidines and purines found in DNA and RNA. Note that pyrimidines are single-ring structures, whereas purines are double-ring structures.

FIGURE 6-17. Base pairs that occur in double-stranded DNA molecules. Note that A and T are connected by two hydrogen bonds, whereas G and C are connected by three hydrogen bonds. The arrows represent the points at which the bases are bonded to deoxyribose molecules.

together. Because of the size and bonding attraction between the two strands, A (a purine) always bonds with T (a pyrimidine) via two hydrogen bonds, and G (a purine) always bonds with C (a pyrimidine) via three hydrogen bonds (Fig. 6-17). (A–T and G–C are known as "base pairs.") The bonding forces of the double-stranded polymer cause it to assume the shape of a double α-helix, which is similar to a right-handed spiral staircase (Fig. 6-18).

> Within a double-stranded DNA molecule, A in one strand always bonds with T in the complimentary strand, and G in one strand always bonds with C in the complimentary strand. A–T and G–C are known as base pairs.

DNA Replication

When a cell is preparing to divide, all the DNA molecules in the chromosomes of that cell must duplicate, thereby ensuring that the same genetic information is passed on to both daughter cells. This process is called

 HISTORICAL NOTE

The Discovery of the Structure of DNA

In the early 1950s, an American named James Watson and an Englishman named Francis Crick published two extremely important papers. The first (published in 1953) proposed a double-stranded, helical structure for DNA (a "double helix"), and the second (published in 1954) proposed a method by which a DNA molecule could copy (replicate) itself exactly, so that identical genetic information could be passed on to each daughter cell. The idea for the double-helical structure was based on an x-ray diffraction photograph of crystallized DNA that Watson had seen in the London laboratory of Maurice Wilkins. The now famous photograph had been produced by Rosalind Franklin, an x-ray crystallographer who worked in Wilkins's lab. Watson, Crick, and Wilkins received a Nobel Prize in Chemistry in 1962 for their contributions to our understanding of DNA. Franklin did not share the prize because she had died before 1962; the Nobel Prize is not awarded posthumously.

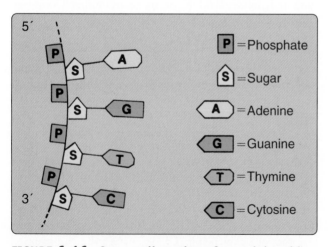

FIGURE 6-16. One small section of a nucleic acid polymer.

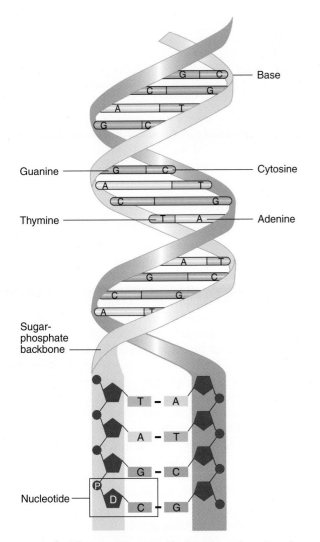

FIGURE 6-18. Double-stranded DNA molecule, also referred to as a double helix.

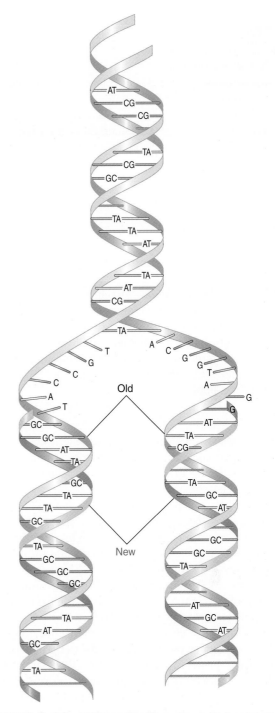

FIGURE 6-19. DNA replication. See text for details.

DNA replication. It occurs by separation of the DNA strands and the building of complementary strands by the addition of the correct DNA nucleotides, as indicated in Figure 6-19. The point on the mole- | The most important enzyme taking part in DNA replication is DNA polymerase (DNA-dependent DNA polymerase).

cule where DNA replication starts is called the *replication fork.* The most important enzyme required for DNA replication is **DNA polymerase** (also known as DNA-dependent DNA polymerase). Other enzymes are also required, including DNA helicase and DNA topoisomerase (which initiate the separation of the two strands of the DNA molecule), primase (which synthesizes a short RNA primer), and DNA ligase (which connects fragments of newly synthesized DNA).

STUDY AID

Major Differences Between DNA and RNA
DNA is double-stranded, whereas RNA is single-stranded.
DNA contains deoxyribose, whereas RNA contains ribose.
DNA contains thymine, whereas RNA contains uracil.

The duplicated DNA of the chromosomes can then be separated during cell division, so that each daughter cell contains the same number of chromosomes, the same genes, and the same amount of DNA as in the parent cell (except during meiosis, the reduction division by which ova and sperm cells are produced in eucaryotes). There are subtle differences between DNA replication in procaryotes and eucaryotes; these differences are beyond the scope of this book.

Gene Expression

As you learned in Chapter 3, a gene is a particular segment of a DNA molecule or chromosome. A gene contains the instructions (the "recipe" or "blueprint") that will enable a cell to make what is known as a *gene product* (in some cases, more than one gene product). The **genetic code** contains four "letters" (the letters that stand for the four nitrogenous bases found in DNA): "A" for adenine, "G" for guanine, "C" for cytosine, and "T" for thymine. It is the sequence of these four bases that spell out the instructions for a particular gene product.

> The genetic code consists of four letters: A, T, G, and C.

Although most genes code for proteins (meaning that each gene contains the instructions for the production of a particular protein), some code for rRNA and tRNA molecules. However, because the vast majority of gene products are proteins, gene products are discussed in this chapter as if all of them are proteins.

The Central Dogma. It was Francis Crick who, in 1957, proposed what is referred to as the **Central Dogma** to explain the flow of genetic information within a cell:

$$DNA \rightarrow mRNA \rightarrow protein$$

The Central Dogma (also known as the "one gene–one protein hypothesis") states that:

1. The genetic information contained in one gene of a DNA molecule is used to make one molecule of mRNA by a process known as transcription.

2. The genetic information in that mRNA molecule is then used to make one protein by a process known as translation.[c]

When the information in a gene has been used by the cell to make a gene product, the gene that codes for that particular gene product is said to have been *expressed*. All the genes on the chromosome are not being expressed at any given time. That would be a terrible waste of energy! For example, it would not be logical for a cell to produce a particular enzyme if that enzyme was not actually needed. Genes that are expressed at all times are called **constitutive genes**. Those that are expressed only when the gene products are needed are called **inducible genes**.

> Genes that are expressed at all times are called constitutive genes, whereas those that are expressed only when the gene products are needed are called inducible genes.

Transcription. When a cell is stimulated (by need) to produce a particular protein, the DNA of the appropriate gene is activated to unwind temporarily from its helical configuration. This unwinding exposes the bases, which then attract the bases of free RNA nucleotides, and an mRNA molecule begins to be assembled alongside one of the strands of the unwound DNA. Thus, one of the DNA strands has served as a template, or pattern (referred to as the *DNA template*), and has coded for a complementary mirror image of its structure in the mRNA molecule. On the growing mRNA molecule, an A will be introduced opposite a T on the DNA molecule, a G opposite a C, a C opposite a G, and a U opposite an A (see the Study Aid on page 99). Remember that there is no T in

> The process by which the information in a single gene is use to make an mRNA molecule is known as transcription.

---

[c] At the time the Central Dogma was proposed, it was thought that a particular gene codes for only one protein. It is now known that a gene can code for more than one protein, depending on several factors (including the manner in which the gene is transcribed and whether or not the final gene product is cut into several proteins).

RNA molecules. This process is called **transcription** because the genetic code from the DNA molecule is transcribed to produce an mRNA molecule. After the mRNA has been synthesized over the length of the gene, it is released from the DNA strand to carry the message to the cytoplasm and direct the synthesis of a particular protein.

The primary enzyme involved in transcription is called **RNA polymerase** (also known as DNA-dependent RNA polymerase). Located along the DNA template are various nucleotide sequences known as "traffic signals" that let the RNA polymerase know where to start and stop the transcription process (i.e., the traffic signals are the starting and stopping points for each gene). Each mRNA molecule contains the same genetic information that was contained in the gene on the DNA template. Note, however, that the genetic code in the mRNA molecule is made up of RNA nucleotides, whereas the genetic code in the DNA template is made up of DNA nucleotides. The information in the mRNA molecule will then be used to synthesize one or more proteins.

In eucaryotes, transcription occurs within the nucleus. The newly formed mRNA molecules then travel through the pores of the nuclear membrane, out into the cytoplasm, where they take up positions on the protein "assembly line." Ribosomes, which are composed of proteins and rRNA, attract the mRNA molecules. In eucaryotic cells, ribosomes are usually attached to endoplasmic reticulum membranes.

In procaryotes, transcription occurs in the cytoplasm. Ribosomes attach to the mRNA molecules as they are being transcribed at the DNA; thus, transcription and translation (protein synthesis) may occur simultaneously.

Translation (Protein Synthesis). The base sequence of the mRNA molecule is read or interpreted in groups of three bases, called *codons*. The sequence of a codon's three bases is the code that determines which amino acid is inserted in that position in the protein being synthesized. Also located on the mRNA molecule are various codons that act as start and stop signals.

Before they can be used to build a protein molecule, amino acids must first be "activated." Each amino acid is activated by attaching to an appropriate tRNA molecule, which then carries (transfers) the amino acid from the cytoplasmic matrix to the site of protein assembly. The enzyme responsible for attaching amino acids to their corresponding tRNA molecules is amino acyl-tRNA synthetase.

The three-base sequence of the codon determines which tRNA brings its specific amino acid to the ribosome, because the tRNA molecule contains an **anticodon**: a three-base sequence that is complementary to, or attracted to, the codon of the mRNA. For example, the tRNA with the anticodon base sequence UUU carries the amino acid lysine to the mRNA codon AAA. Similarly, the mRNA codon CCG codes for the tRNA anticodon GGC, which carries the amino acid proline. The following chart illustrates the sequence of three bases (GGC) in the DNA template that codes for a particular codon (CCG) in mRNA, which, in turn, attracts a particular anticodon (GGC) on the tRNA carrying a specific amino acid (proline).

DNA Template	mRNA (Codon)	tRNA (Anticodon)	Amino Acid
G	C	G	
G	C	G	Proline
C	G	C	

The process of translating the message carried by the mRNA, whereby particular tRNAs bring amino acids to be bound together in the proper sequence to make a specific protein, is called **translation** (summarized in Fig. 6-20). In

FIGURE 6-20. Translation (protein synthesis). See text for details.

this context, translation and protein synthesis are synonyms. It should be noted that a eucaryotic cell is constantly producing mRNAs in its nucleus, which direct the synthesis of all the proteins, including metabolic enzymes necessary for the normal functions of that specific type of cell. Also, mRNA and tRNA are short-lived nucleic acids that may be reused many times and then destroyed and resynthesized. The rRNA molecules are made in the dense portion of the nucleus called the nucleolus. Ribosomes last longer in the cell than do mRNA molecules.

As tRNA molecules attach to mRNA while it is sliding over the ribosome, they bring the correct activated amino acids into contact with each other so that peptide bonds are formed and a polypeptide is synthesized. Recent evidence suggests a role for rRNA (a structural component of the ribosome) in the formation of the peptide bonds. As the polypeptide grows and becomes a protein, it folds into the unique shape determined by the amino acid sequence. This characteristic shape allows the protein to perform its specific function. If one of the bases of a DNA gene is incorrect or out of sequence (known as a *mutation*), the amino acid sequence of the gene product will be incorrect and the altered protein configuration may not allow the protein to function properly. For example, some diabetics may not produce a functional insulin molecule because a mutation in one of their chromosomes caused a rearrangement of the bases in the gene that codes for insulin. Such errors are the basis for most genetic and inherited diseases, such as phenylketonuria (PKU), sickle cell anemia, cerebral palsy, cystic fibrosis, cleft lip, clubfoot, extra fingers, albinism, and many other birth defects. Likewise, nonpathogenic microbes may mutate to become pathogens, and pathogens may lose the ability to cause disease by mutation. Mutations are discussed further in Chapter 7.

The relatively new sciences of genetic engineering and gene therapy attempt to repair the genetic damage in some diseases. As yet, the morality of manipulation of human genes has not been resolved by society. However, many genetically engineered microbes are able to pro-duce substances, such as human insulin, interferon, growth hormones, new pharmaceutical agents, and vaccines, that will have a substantial effect on the medical treatment of humans (see Chapter 7).

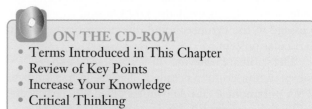

ON THE CD-ROM
• Terms Introduced in This Chapter
• Review of Key Points
• Increase Your Knowledge
• Critical Thinking
• Additional Self-Assessment Exercises

SELF-ASSESSMENT EXERCISES

After studying this chapter, answer the following multiple-choice questions.

1. Which of the following are the building blocks of proteins?
   a. amino acids
   b. monosaccharides
   c. nucleotides
   d. peptides
2. Glucose, sucrose, and cellulose are examples of:
   a. carbohydrates.
   b. disaccharides.
   c. monosaccharides.
   d. polysaccharides.
3. Which of the following nitrogenous bases is *not* found in an RNA molecule?
   a. adenine
   b. guanine
   c. thymine
   d. uracil
4. Which of the following are purines?
   a. adenine and guanine
   b. adenine and thymine
   c. guanine and uracil
   d. guanine and cytosine

5. Which one of the following is *not* found at the site of protein synthesis?
   a. DNA
   b. mRNA
   c. rRNA
   d. tRNA
6. Which of the following statements about DNA is (are) true?
   a. DNA contains thymine but not uracil.
   b. DNA molecules contain deoxyribose.
   c. In a double-stranded DNA molecule, adenine on one strand will be connected to thymine on the complementary strand by two hydrogen bonds.
   d. All of the above statements are true.
7. The amino acids in a polypeptide chain are connected by:
   a. covalent bonds.
   b. glycosidic bonds.
   c. peptide bonds.
   d. both a and c.

8. Which of the following statements about nucleotides is (are) true?
   a. A nucleotide contains a nitrogenous base.
   b. A nucleotide contains a pentose.
   c. A nucleotide contains a phosphate group.
   d. All of the above statements are true.
9. A heptose contains how many carbon atoms?
   a. 4
   b. 5
   c. 6
   d. 7
10. Virtually all enzymes are:
    a. carbohydrates.
    b. nucleic acids.
    c. proteins.
    d. substrates.

7 MICROBIAL PHYSIOLOGY AND GENETICS

CHAPTER OUTLINE

LEARNING OBJECTIVES

AFTER STUDYING THIS CHAPTER, YOU SHOULD BE ABLE TO:

- Define phototroph, chemotroph, autotroph, heterotroph, photoautotroph, chemoheterotroph, endoenzyme, exoenzyme, plasmid, R-factor, "superbug," mutation, mutant, and mutagen
- Discuss the relationships among apoenzymes, coenzymes, and holoenzymes
- Differentiate between catabolism and anabolism
- Explain the role of adenosine triphosphate (ATP) molecules in metabolism
- Briefly describe each of the following: biochemical pathway, aerobic respiration, glycolysis, the Krebs cycle, the electron transport chain, oxidation–reduction reactions, photosynthesis
- Explain the differences among beneficial, harmful, and silent mutations
- Briefly describe each of the following ways in which bacteria acquire genetic information: lysogenic conversion, transduction, transformation, conjugation

MICROBIAL PHYSIOLOGY

Introduction

Physiology is the study of the vital life processes of organisms, especially how these processes normally function in living organisms. *Microbial physiology* concerns the vital life processes of microorganisms. Microorganisms, especially bacteria, are ideally suited for use in studies of the basic metabolic reactions that occur within cells. Bacteria are inexpensive to maintain in the laboratory, take up little space, and reproduce quickly. Their morphology, nutritional needs, and metabolic reactions are easily observable. Of special importance is the fact that species of bacteria can be found that represent each of the nutritional types of organisms on Earth. Scientists can learn a great deal about cells—including human cells—by studying the nutritional needs of bacteria, their metabolic pathways, and why they live, grow, multiply, or die under certain conditions.

> Microbial physiology is the study of the life processes of microorganisms.

Each tiny single-celled bacterium strives to produce more cells like itself, and, as long as water and an adequate nutrient supply are available, it often does so at an alarming rate. Under favorable conditions, in 24 hours, the offspring (progeny) of a single *Escherichia coli* cell would outnumber the entire human population on the Earth! Because some bacteria, fungi, and viruses produce generation after generation so rapidly, they have been used extensively in genetic studies. In fact, most of today's genetic knowledge was and still is being obtained by studying these microorganisms.

Microbial Nutritional Requirements

Studies of bacterial nutrition and other aspects of microbial physiology enable scientists to understand the vital chemical processes that occur within every living cell, including those of the human body. All living protoplasm contains six major chemical elements: carbon, hydrogen, oxygen, nitrogen, phosphorus, and sulfur. Other elements, usually required in lesser amounts, include sodium, potassium, chlorine, magnesium, calcium, iron, iodine, and some trace elements. Combinations of all these elements make up the vital macromolecules of life, including carbohydrates, lipids, proteins, and nucleic acids.

To build necessary cellular materials, every organism requires a source (or sources) of energy, a source (or sources) of carbon, and additional nutrients. Those materials that organisms are unable to synthesize, but are required for the building of macromolecules and sustaining life, are termed *essential nutrients*. Essential nutrients (e.g., essential amino acids and essential fatty acids) must be continually supplied to an organism for it to survive. Essential nutrients vary from species to species.

> **STUDY AID**
>
> **Nutrients**
> The term *nutrients* refers to the various chemical compounds that organisms—including microorganisms—use to sustain life. Many nutrients are energy sources; organisms will obtain energy from these chemicals by breaking chemical bonds. Whenever a chemical bond is broken, energy is released. As nutrients are broken down by enzymatic action, smaller molecules are produced, which are then used by cells as building blocks. Nutrients also serve as sources of carbon, nitrogen, and other elements.

Categorizing Microorganisms According to Their Energy and Carbon Sources

Since the beginning of life on Earth, microorganisms have been evolving, some in different directions than others. Today, there are microbes representing each of the four major nutritional categories (photoautotrophs, photoheterotrophs, chemoautotrophs, chemoheterotrophs; terms defined later in this chapter). Various terms are used to indicate an organism's energy source and carbon source. As you will see, these terms can be used in combination (Table 7-1).

Terms Relating to an Organism's Energy Source

The terms phototroph and chemotroph pertain to what an organism uses as an energy source. **Phototrophs** use light as an energy source. The

TABLE 7-1   Terms Relating to Energy and Carbon Sources

TERMS RELATING TO ENERGY SOURCE	TERMS RELATING TO CARBON SOURCE	
	Autotrophs (organisms that use CO_2 as a carbon source)	Heterotrophs (organisms that use organic compounds other than CO_2 as a carbon source)
Phototrophs (organisms that use light as an energy source)	**Photoautotrophs** (e.g., algae, plants, some photosynthetic, bacteria including cyanobacteria)	**Photoheterotrophs** (e.g., some photosynthetic bacteria)
Chemotrophs[a] (organisms that use chemicals as an energy source)	**Chemoautotrophs** (e.g., some bacteria)	**Chemoheterotrophs** (e.g., protozoa, fungi, animals, most bacteria)

[a]Chemotrophs can be divided into two categories: (1) chemolithotrophs (or simply lithotrophs) are organisms that use inorganic chemicals as an energy source, and (2) chemoorganotrophs (or simply organotrophs) are organisms that use organic chemicals as an energy source.

process by which organisms convert light energy into chemical energy is called *photosynthesis*. **Chemotrophs** use either inorganic or organic chemicals as an energy source. Chemotrophs can be subdivided into two categories: chemolithotrophs and chemoorganotrophs. **Chemolithotrophs** (or simply lithotrophs) are organisms that use inorganic chemicals as an energy source. **Chemoorganotrophs** (or simply organotrophs) are organisms that use organic chemicals as an energy source.

Terms Relating to an Organism's Carbon Source

The terms autotroph and heterotroph pertain to what an organism uses as a carbon source. **Autotrophs** use carbon dioxide (CO_2) as their sole source of carbon. Photosynthetic organisms such as plants, algae, and cyanobacteria are examples of autotrophs. **Heterotrophs** are organisms that use organic compounds other than CO_2 as their carbon source. (Recall that all organic compounds contain carbon.) Humans, animals, fungi, and protozoa are examples of heterotrophs. Both saprophytic fungi, which live on dead and decaying organic matter, and parasitic fungi are heterotrophs. Most bacteria are also heterotrophs.

> Autotrophs use carbon dioxide as their sole source of carbon, whereas heterotrophs use other carbon-containing compounds as their carbon source.

The terms relating to energy source can be combined with the terms relating to carbon source, yielding terms that indicate both an organism's energy source and carbon source. For example, **photoautotrophs** are organisms (such as plants, algae, cyanobacteria, purple and green sulfur bacteria) that use light as an energy source and CO_2 as a carbon source. **Photoheterotrophs**, like purple nonsulfur and green nonsulfur bacteria, use light as an energy source and organic compounds other than CO_2 as a carbon source. **Chemoautotrophs** (such as nitrifying, hydrogen, iron, and sulfur bacteria) use chemicals as an energy source and CO_2 as a carbon source. **Chemoheterotrophs** use chemicals as an energy source and organic compounds other than CO_2 as a carbon source. All animals, all protozoa, all fungi, and most bacteria are chemoheterotrophs. All medically important bacteria are chemoheterotrophs.

Ecology is the study of the interactions between organisms and the world around them. The term *ecosystem* refers to the interactions between living organisms and their nonliving environment. Interrelationships among the different nutritional types are of prime importance in the functioning of the ecosystem. Phototrophs (like algae and plants) are the producers of food and oxygen for chemoheterotrophs (such as animals). Dead plants and animals would clutter the Earth if chemoheterotrophic, saprophytic decomposers (certain fungi and bacteria) did not break down the dead organic matter into small inorganic and organic compounds (carbon dioxide, nitrates, phosphates) in soil, water, and air—compounds that are then used and recycled by chemotrophs. Photoautotrophs contribute energy to the ecosystem by trapping energy from the sun and using it to build organic compounds (carbohydrates, lipids, proteins, and nucleic acids) from inorganic materials in the soil, water, and air. In oxygenic photosynthesis (described later), oxygen is released for use by aerobic organisms, such as animals and humans.

METABOLIC ENZYMES

The term *metabolism* refers to all the chemical reactions that occur within any cell. These chemical reactions are referred to as *metabolic reactions*. The metabolic processes that occur in microbes are similar to those that occur in cells of the human body. Metabolic reactions are enhanced and regulated by enzymes, known as *metabolic enzymes*. A cell can only perform a certain metabolic reaction if it possesses the appropriate metabolic enzyme, and it can only possess that enzyme if the genome of the cell contains the gene that codes for production of that enzyme.

> Metabolism refers to all of the chemical reactions (metabolic reactions) that occur within a living cell.

Biologic Catalysts

As you learned in Chapter 6, enzymes are known as *biologic catalysts*. Enzymes are proteins that catalyze (speed up or accelerate) the rate of biochemical reactions. In some cases, the reaction will not occur at all in the absence of the enzyme. Thus, a complete definition of a biologic catalyst would be a protein that either causes a particular chemical reaction to occur or accelerates it.

> Enzymes are proteins that catalyze (accelerate) biochemical reactions.

Recall that enzymes are very specific. A particular enzyme can only catalyze one particular chemical reaction. In most cases, a particular enzyme can only exert its effect or act on one particular substance—known as the *substrate* for that enzyme. The unique three-dimensional shape of the enzyme enables it to fit the combining site of the substrate, much like a key fits into a lock (Fig. 7-1).

> The substance upon which an enzyme acts is known as that enzyme's substrate.

An enzyme does not become altered during the chemical reaction that it catalyzes. At the conclusion of the reaction, the enzyme is unchanged and is available to drive that reaction over and over. The enzyme moves from substrate molecule to substrate molecule at a rate of several hundred each second, producing a supply of the end product for as long as this particular end product is needed by the cell. However, enzymes do not last indefinitely; they finally degenerate and lose their activity. Therefore, the cell must synthesize and replace these important proteins. Because there are thousands of metabolic reactions continually occurring in the cell, there are thousands of enzymes available to control and direct the

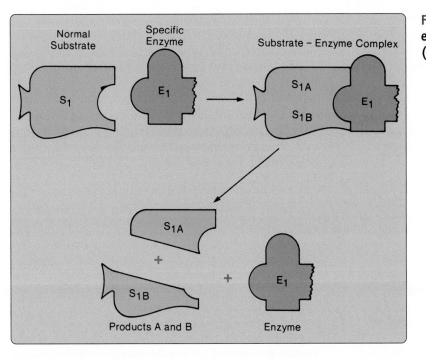

FIGURE 7-1. Action of a specific enzyme (E) breaking down a substrate (S) molecule.

essential metabolic pathways. At any particular time, all the required enzymes need not be present; this situation is controlled by genes on the chromosomes and the needs of the cell, which are determined by the internal and external environments. For example, if no lactose is present in the organism's external environment, the organism does not need the enzyme required to break down lactose.

Enzymes produced within a cell that remain within the cell—to catalyze reactions within the cell—are called *endoenzymes*. The digestive enzymes within phagocytes are good examples of endoenzymes; they are used to digest materials that the phagocytes have ingested. Enzymes produced within a cell that are then released from the cell—to catalyze extracellular reactions—are called *exoenzymes*. Examples of exoenzymes are cellulase and pectinase, which are secreted by saprophytic fungi to digest cellulose and pectin in the external environment (e.g., in rotting leaves on the forest floor). Cellulose and pectin molecules are too large to be absorbed into fungal cells. The exoenzymes cellulase and pectinase break down these large molecules into smaller molecules, which can then be absorbed into the cells.

Hydrolases and polymerases are additional examples of metabolic enzymes. Hydrolases break down macromolecules by the addition of water, in a process called *hydrolysis* or a *hydrolysis reaction*. These hydrolytic processes enable saprophytes to break apart such complex materials as leather, wax, cork, wood, rubber, hair, and some plastics. Some of the enzymes involved in the formation of large polymers like DNA and RNA are called *polymerases*. As was discussed in Chapter 6, DNA polymerase

> Endoenzymes remain within the cell that produced them, whereas exoenzymes leave the cell to catalyze reactions outside of the cell.

is active each time the DNA of a cell is replicated, and RNA polymerase is required for the synthesis of messenger RNA (mRNA) molecules.

As was discussed in Chapter 6, some proteins (called *apoenzymes*) cannot, on their own, catalyze a chemical reaction. An apoenzyme must link up with a cofactor to catalyze a chemical reaction. Cofactors are either mineral ions (e.g., magnesium, calcium, or iron cations) or coenzymes. Coenzymes are small organic, vitamin-type molecules such as flavin-adenine dinucleotide (FAD) and nicotinamide-adenine dinucleotide (NAD). These particular coenzymes participate in the Krebs cycle, which is discussed later in this chapter. Like enzymes, coenzymes do not have to be present in large amounts because they are not altered during the chemical reaction that they catalyze; thus, they are available for use over and over. However, a lack of certain vitamins from which the coenzymes are synthesized will halt all reactions involving that particular coenzyme.

> To catalyze a reaction, an apoenzyme must first link up with a cofactor (either a mineral ion or a coenzyme).

Factors That Affect the Efficiency of Enzymes

Many factors affect the efficiency or effectiveness of enzymes. Certain physical or chemical changes can diminish or completely stop enzyme activity, because enzymes function properly only under optimum conditions. Optimum conditions for enzyme activity include a relatively limited range of pH and temperature as well as the appropriate concentration of enzyme and substrate. Extremes in heat and acidity can denature (or alter) enzymes by breaking the bonds responsible for their three-dimensional shape, resulting in the loss of enzymatic activity.

An enzyme will function at peak efficiency over a particular pH range. If the pH is too high or too low, the enzyme will not function at peak efficiency, and the reaction that the enzyme catalyzes will not proceed at its maximum rate. Likewise, an enzyme will function at peak efficiency over a particular temperature range. If the temperature is too high or too low, the enzyme will not function at peak efficiency, and the reaction that the enzyme catalyzes will not proceed at its maximum rate.

This explains why a particular bacterium grows best at a certain temperature and pH; these are the optimal conditions for the enzymes possessed by that bacterium. The optimal pH and temperature for growth vary from one species to another.

Substrate concentration is another factor that influences the efficiency of an enzyme. If the substrate concentration is too high or too low, the enzyme will not function at peak efficiency, and the reaction that the enzyme catalyzes will not proceed at its maximum rate.

> Enzyme efficiency is influenced by various factors, including pH, temperature, and the concentration of the substrate.

Although certain mineral ions (e.g., calcium, magnesium, and iron) enhance the activity of enzymes by serving as cofactors, other heavy metal ions (e.g., lead, zinc, mercury, and arsenic) usually act as poisons to the cell. These toxic ions inhibit enzyme activity by replacing the cofactors at the combining site of the enzyme, thus inhibiting normal metabolic processes. Some disinfectants containing mineral ions are effective in inhibiting the growth of bacteria in this manner.

Sometimes, a molecule that is similar in structure to the substrate can be used as an inhibitor to deliberately interfere with a particular metabolic pathway. The enzyme binds to the molecule having a similar structure to the substrate, thus, tying the enzyme up, so that it cannot attach to the substrate and cannot catalyze the chemical reaction. If that reaction is essential for the life of the cell, the cell will stop growing and may die. For example, a chemotherapeutic agent, such as a sulfonamide drug, can bind to certain bacterial enzymes, blocking attachment of the enzymes to their substrates and preventing essential metabolites from being formed. This could lead to the death of the bacteria.

METABOLISM

As previously mentioned, the term metabolism refers to all the chemical reactions occurring within a cell. The reactions are referred to as metabolic reactions. A *metabolite* is any molecule that is a nutrient, an intermediary product, or an end product in a metabolic reaction. Within a cell, many metabolic reactions proceed simultaneously, breaking down some compounds and synthesizing (building) others. Most metabolic reactions fall into two categories: catabolism and anabolism.

The term *catabolism* refers to all the catabolic reactions that are occurring in a cell. *Catabolic reactions*, which are described in greater detail in a subsequent section, involve the breaking down of larger molecules into smaller molecules, requiring the breaking of bonds. **Any time that chemical bonds are broken, energy is released. Catabolic reactions are a cell's major source of energy**. Catabolic reactions in bacteria are quite diverse, because energy sources range from inorganic compounds (e.g., sulfide, ferrous ion, hydrogen) to organic compounds (e.g., carbohydrates, lipids, amino acids).

> Catabolic reactions involve the breaking of chemical bonds and the release of energy.

Anabolism refers to all the anabolic reactions that are occurring in a cell. *Anabolic reactions*, which are described in greater detail in a subsequent section, involve the assembly of smaller molecules into larger molecules, requiring the formation of bonds. **Energy is required for bond formation. Once formed, the bonds represent stored energy.** Anabolic reactions tend to be quite similar for all types of cells; the pathways for the biosynthesis of macromolecules do not differ much among organisms. Table 7-2 illustrates the key differences between catabolism and anabolism.

> Anabolic reactions involve the formation of bonds, which requires energy.

The energy that is released during catabolic reactions is used to drive anabolic reactions. A kind of energy balancing act occurs within a cell, with some metabolic reactions releasing energy and other metabolic reactions requiring energy. The energy

> ATP molecules are the major energy-storing or energy-carrying molecules within a cell.

TABLE 7-2	Differences between Catabolism and Anabolism
CATABOLISM	**ANABOLISM**
All the catabolic reactions in a cell	All the anabolic reactions in a cell
Catabolic reactions release energy	Anabolic reactions require energy
Catabolic reactions involve the breaking of bonds; whenever chemical bonds are broken, energy is released	Anabolic reactions involve the creation of bonds; it takes energy to create chemical bonds
Larger molecules are broken down into smaller molecules (sometimes referred to as degradative reactions)	Smaller molecules are bonded together to create larger molecules (sometimes referred to as biosynthetic reactions)

FIGURE 7-2. Adenosine triphosphate (ATP) molecule. As the name implies, ATP molecules contain 3 phosphate groups.

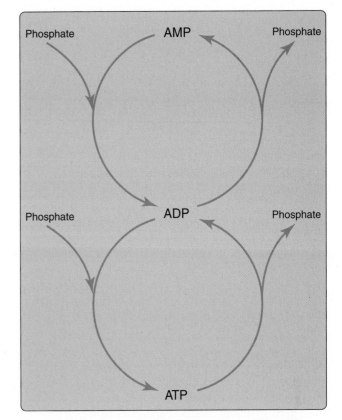

FIGURE 7-3. Interrelationships among ATP, ADP, and AMP molecules.

required by a cell may be trapped from the rays of the sun (as in photosynthesis), or it may be produced by certain catabolic reactions. Then the energy can be temporarily stored within high-energy bonds in special molecules, usually ATP molecules (Fig. 7-2). Although ATP molecules are not the only high-energy compounds found within a cell, they are the most important ones. ATP molecules are the major energy-storing or energy-carrying molecules within a cell.

ATP molecules are found in all cells because they are used to transfer energy from energy-yielding molecules, like glucose, to an energy-requiring reaction. Thus, ATP is a temporary, intermediate molecule. If ATP is not used shortly after it is formed, it is soon hydrolyzed to adenosine diphosphate (ADP), a more stable molecule; the hydrolysis of ATP is an example of a catabolic reaction. If a cell runs out of ATP molecules, ADP molecules can be used as an emergency energy source by the removal of another phosphate group to produce adenosine monophosphate (AMP); the hydrolysis of ADP is also a catabolic reaction. Figure 7-3 illustrates the interrelationships between ATP, ADP, and AMP molecules.

In addition to the energy required for metabolic pathways, energy is also required by the organism for growth, reproduction, sporulation, movement, and the active transport of substances across membranes. Some organisms (e.g., certain planktonic dinoflagellates) even use energy for bioluminescence. They cause a glowing that can sometimes be seen at the surface of an ocean, in a ship's wake, or as waves break on a beach. The value of bioluminescence to these organisms is unclear.

Chemical reactions are essentially energy transformation processes during which the energy that is stored in chemical bonds is transferred to produce new chemical bonds. The cellular mechanisms that release small amounts of energy as the cell needs it usually involve a sequence of catabolic and anabolic reactions.

Catabolism

As previously stated, the term catabolism refers to all the catabolic reactions that occur within a cell. **The key thing about catabolic reactions is that they release energy.** Catabolic reactions are a cell's major source of energy. Catabolic reactions involve the breaking of chemical bonds. Any time chemical bonds are broken, energy is released. The energy produced by catabolic reactions can be used to wiggle flagella and actively transport substances through membranes, but most of the energy produced by catabolic reactions is used to drive anabolic reactions. Unfortunately, some of the energy is lost as heat. Catabolic reactions are often referred to as *degradative reactions*; they degrade larger molecules down into smaller molecules. For example, breaking a disaccharide down into its two original monosaccharides—a hydrolysis reaction—is an example of a catabolic reaction.

> Catabolic reactions release energy because chemical bonds are broken.

Biochemical Pathways

A biochemical pathway is a series of linked biochemical reactions that occur in a stepwise manner, leading from a starting material to an end product (Fig. 7-4).

Glucose is the favorite "food" or nutrient of cells, including microorganisms. **Nutrients should be thought**

FIGURE 7-4. A biochemical pathway. There are four steps in this hypothetical biochemical pathway, in which compound A is ultimately converted to compound E. Compound A is first converted to compound B, which in turn is converted to compound C, which in turn is converted to compound D, which in turn is converted to compound E. Compound A is referred to as the starting material; compounds B, C, and D are referred to as intermediate (or intermediary) products; and compound E is referred to as the end product. A total of four enzymes are required in this pathway. The substrate for enzyme 1 is compound A; the substrate for enzyme 2 is compound B, and so on.

of as energy sources, and chemical bonds should be thought of as stored energy. Whenever the chemical bonds within the nutrients are broken, energy is released.

There are many chemical processes by which glucose is catabolized within cells. Two common processes are the biochemical pathways known as aerobic respiration and fermentation reactions, which will be discussed in this chapter. Additional pathways for catabolizing glucose, such as the Entner-Doudoroff pathway, the pentose phosphate pathway, and anaerobic respiration, will not be described because they are beyond the scope of this book.

Aerobic Respiration of Glucose

The complete catabolism of glucose by the process known as aerobic respiration (or cellular respiration) occurs in three phases, each of which is a biochemical pathway: (a) glycolysis, (b) the Krebs cycle, and (c) the electron-transport chain. Although the first phase—glycolysis—is an anaerobic process, the other two phases require aerobic conditions; hence the name, *aerobic* respiration.

> Aerobic respiration involves (a) glycolysis, (b) the Kreb's cycle, and (c) the electron transport chain.

STUDY AID
A Biochemical Pathway
Think of a biochemical pathway as a journey by car. To drive from city A to city E, you must pass through cities B, C, and D. City A is the starting point. City E is the destination or end point. Cities B, C, and D are intermediate points along the journey.

Glycolysis. Glycolysis, also known as the *glycolytic pathway*, the Embden-Meyerhof pathway, and the Embden-Meyerhof-Parnas pathway, is a nine-step biochemical pathway, involving nine separate biochemical reactions, each of which requires a specific enzyme (Fig. 7-5).

In glycolysis, a six-carbon molecule of glucose is ultimately broken down into two three-carbon molecules of pyruvic acid (also called *pyruvate*). Glycolysis can take place in either the presence or absence of oxygen; oxygen does not participate in this phase of aerobic respiration. Glycolysis produces very little energy—a net yield of only two molecules of ATP. Glycolysis takes place in the cytoplasm of both procaryotic and eucaryotic cells.

Krebs Cycle. The pyruvic acid molecules produced during glycolysis are converted into acetyl-coenzyme A (acetyl-CoA) molecules, which then enter the Krebs cycle (Fig. 7-6).

The Krebs cycle is a biochemical pathway consisting of eight separate reactions, each of which is controlled by a different enzyme. In the first step of the Krebs cycle, acetyl-CoA combines with oxaloacetate to produce citric acid (a tricarboxylic acid); hence, the other names for the Krebs cycle—the citric acid cycle, the tricarboxylic acid cycle, and the TCA cycle. It is referred to as a cycle because at the end of the eight reactions, the biochemical pathway ends up back at its starting point—oxaloacetate. Only two ATP molecules are produced during the Krebs cycle, but several products (e.g., NADH, FADH$_2$, and hydrogen ions) that are formed during the Krebs cycle enter the electron transport chain. (NADH is the reduced form of NAD, and FADH$_2$ is the reduced form of FAD.) In eucaryotic cells, the Krebs cycle and the electron transport chain are located within mitochondria. (Recall from Chapter 3 that mitochondria are referred to as "energy factories" or "power houses.") In procaryotic cells, both the Krebs cycle and the electron transport chain occur at the inner surface of the cell membrane.

Electron Transport Chain. As previously mentioned, certain of the products produced during the Krebs cycle enter the *electron transport chain* (also called the electron transport system or respiratory chain). The electron transport chain consists of a series of oxidation–reduction reactions (described in a subsequent section), whereby energy released as electrons is transferred from one compound to another. These compounds include flavoproteins, quinones, nonheme iron proteins, and cytochromes. Oxygen is at the end of the chain; it is referred to as the final or terminal electron acceptor.

Many different enzymes are involved in the electron transport chain, including cytochrome oxidase (also called cytochrome *c*, or merely oxidase), the enzyme responsible for transferring electrons to oxygen, the final electron acceptor. In the clinical microbiology laboratory, the oxidase test is useful in the identification (speciation) of a Gram-negative bacillus that has been isolated from a

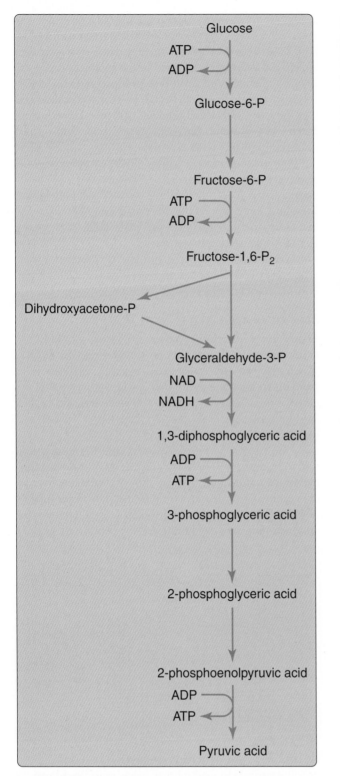

FIGURE 7-5. Glycolysis. Each of the compounds from glucose to fructose-1,6-P_2 contains six-carbon atoms. Fructose-1,6-P_2 is broken into two three-carbon compounds: dihydroxyacetone-P and glyceraldehyde-3-P, each of which is ultimately transformed into a molecule of pyruvic acid. Thus, in glycolysis, one six-carbon molecule of glucose is converted to two three-carbon molecules of pyruvic acid. (See text for additional details.) (From Volk WA, et al. Essentials of Medical Microbiology, 5th ed. Philadelphia: Lippincott-Raven, 1996.)

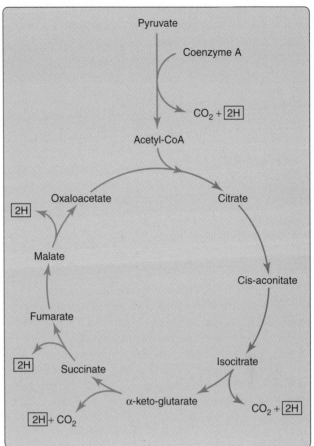

FIGURE 7-6. The Krebs cycle. See text for details.

clinical specimen. Whether or not the organism possesses oxidase is an important clue to the organism's identity.

During the electron transport chain, a large number of ATP molecules (32 in procaryotic cells and 34 in eucaryotic cells) are produced by a process known as oxidative phosphorylation; oxidation referring to a loss of electrons and phosphorylation referring to the conversion of ADP molecules to ATP molecules. The net yield of ATP molecules from the catabolism of one glucose molecule by aerobic respiration is 36 (in procaryotic cells) or 38 (in eucaryotic cells; Table 7-3). That is a great deal of energy from one molecule of glucose. Aerobic respiration is a very efficient system. Aerobic respiration of glucose produces 18 times (procaryotic cells) or 19 times (eucaryotic cells) as much energy than does fermentation of glucose (discussed in a subsequent section).

The breakdown of glucose by aerobic respiration produces 36 ATP molecules in procaryotic cells and 38 ATP molecules in eucaryotic cells.

The chemical equation representing aerobic respiration is:

$$C_6H_{12}O_6 + 6\ O_2 + 38\ ADP + 38\ \textcircled{P} \rightarrow$$
$$6\ H_2O + 6\ CO_2 + 38\ ATP$$

where $\textcircled{P}$ indicates an activated phosphate group.

TABLE 7-3	Recap of the Number of ATP Molecules Produced From One Molecule of Glucose by Aerobic Respiration	
	PROCARYOTIC CELLS	EUCARYOTIC CELLS
Glycolysis	2	2
Krebs cycle	2	2
Electron transport chain	32	34
Total ATP molecules	36	38

The catabolism of glucose by aerobic respiration is just one of many ways in which cells can catabolize glucose molecules. How glucose is utilized by a cell depends on the individual organism, its available nutrient and energy resources, and the enzymes it is able to produce. Some bacteria degrade glucose to pyruvic acid by other metabolic pathways. Also, glycerol, fatty acids from lipids, and amino acids from protein digestion may enter the Krebs cycle to produce energy for the cell when necessary (i.e., when there are insufficient carbohydrates available).

Fermentation of Glucose

The first thing to note about *fermentation* reactions is that they do not involve oxygen; therefore, fermentations usu-

Oxygen does not participate in fermentation reactions.

ally take place in anaerobic environments. The first step in the fermentation of glucose is glycolysis, which occurs exactly as previously described. Remember that glycolysis does not involve oxygen, and very little energy (two ATP molecules) is produced by glycolysis.

The next step in fermentation reactions is the conversion of pyruvic acid into an end product. The particular end product that is produced depends on the specific organism involved. The various end products of fermentation have many industrial applications. For example, certain yeasts (*Saccharomyces* spp.) and bacteria (*Zymomonas* spp.) convert pyruvic acid into ethyl alcohol (ethanol) and CO_2. Such yeasts are used to make wine, beer, other alcoholic beverages, and bread.

A group of Gram-positive bacteria, called *lactic acid bacteria*, convert pyruvic acid to lactic acid. These bacteria are used to make various food products, including cheeses, yogurt, pickles, and cured sausages. In human muscle cells, the lack of oxygen during extreme exertion results in pyruvic acid being converted to lactic acid. The presence of lactic acid in muscle tissue is the cause of soreness that develops in exhausted muscles. Some oral bacteria (e.g., various *Streptococcus* spp.) convert glucose into lactic acid, which then eats away the enamel on our teeth,

leading to tooth decay. The presence of lactic acid bacteria in milk causes the souring of milk into curd and whey.

Some bacteria convert pyruvic acid into propionic acid. *Propionibacterium* spp. are used in the production of Swiss cheese. The propionic acid they produce gives the cheese its characteristic flavor, and the CO_2 that is produced creates the holes. Other end products of fermentation include acetic acid, acetone, butanol, butyric acid, isopropanol, and succinic acid.

Fermentation reactions produce very little energy (approximately two ATP molecules); therefore, they are very inefficient ways to catabolize glucose. Aerobes and facultative anaer-

The breakdown of glucose by fermentation produces only two ATP molecules.

obes are much more efficient in energy production than obligate anaerobes because they are able to catabolize glucose via aerobic respiration.

Oxidation–Reduction (Redox) Reactions

Oxidation–reduction reactions are paired reactions in which electrons are transferred from one compound to another (Fig. 7-7). Whenever an atom, ion, or molecule loses one or

Oxidation reactions involve the loss of an electron, whereas reduction reactions involve the gain of an electron.

more electrons (e^-) in a reaction, the process is called *oxidation*, and the molecule is said to be *oxidized*. The electrons that are lost do not float about at random but, because they are very reactive, attach immediately to another molecule. The resulting gain of one or more electrons by a molecule is called *reduction*, and the molecule is said to be *reduced*. Within the cell, an oxidation reaction is always paired (or coupled) with a

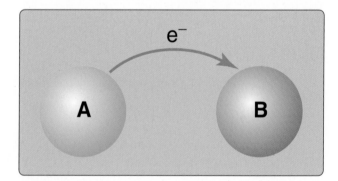

FIGURE 7-7. An oxidation–reduction reaction. In this illustration, an electron has been transferred from compound A to compound B. Two reactions have occurred simultaneously. Compound A has lost an electron (an oxidation reaction), and compound B has gained an electron (a reduction reaction). Oxidation is the loss of an electron. Reduction is the gain of an electron. Compound A has been oxidized, and compound B has been reduced. The term *reduction* relates to the fact that an electron has a negative charge. When compound B receives an electron, its electrical charge is reduced.

reduction reaction, thus the term oxidation–reduction or "redox" reactions. In a redox reaction, the electron donor is referred to as the reducing agent and the electron acceptor is referred to as the oxidizing agent. Thus, in Figure 7-7, compound A is the reducing agent and compound B is the oxidizing agent.

As stated earlier, the electron transport chain consists of a series of oxidation–reduction reactions, whereby energy released as electrons is transferred from one compound to another. Many biologic oxidations are referred to as *dehydrogenation reactions* because hydrogen ions (H^+) as well as electrons are removed. Concurrently, those hydrogen ions must be picked up in a reduction reaction. Many good illustrations are found in the aerobic respiration of glucose, in which the hydrogen ions released during the Krebs cycle enter the electron transport chain. (See "Insight: Why Anaerobes Die in the Presence of Oxygen" on the CD-ROM).

Anabolism

As previously stated, anabolism refers to all the *anabolic reactions* that are occurring in a cell. **Anabolic reactions require energy because chemical bonds are being formed.** It takes energy to create a chemical bond. **Most of the energy required for anabolic reactions is provided by the catabolic reactions that are occurring simultaneously in the cell.** Anabolic reactions are often referred to as biosynthetic reactions. Examples of anabolic reactions include creating a disaccharide from two monosaccharides by dehydration synthesis, the biosynthesis of polypeptides by linking amino acids molecules together, and the biosynthesis of nucleic acid molecules by linking nucleotides together.

Anabolic reactions require energy because chemical bonds are being formed.

Biosynthesis of Organic Compounds

The biosynthesis of organic compounds requires energy and may occur either through photosynthesis (biosynthesis using light energy) or **chemosynthesis** (biosynthesis using chemical energy).

Photosynthesis. In photosynthesis, light energy is converted to chemical energy in the form of chemical bonds. Phototrophs that use CO_2 as their carbon source are called photoautotrophs; examples are algae, plants, cyanobacteria, and certain other photosynthetic bacteria. Phototrophs that use small organic molecules, such as acids and alcohols, to build organic molecules are called photoheterotrophs; some types of bacteria are photoheterotrophs.

The goal of photosynthetic processes is to trap the radiant energy of light and convert it into chemical bond energy in ATP molecules and carbohydrates, particularly glucose, which can then be converted into more ATP molecules at a later time through aerobic respiration. Bacteria that produce oxygen by photosynthesis are called *oxygenic photosynthetic bacteria*, and the process is known as *oxygenic photosynthesis*. The oxygenic photosynthesis reaction is

$$6\,CO_2 + 12\,H_2O \xrightarrow[ATP]{light} C_6H_{12}O_6 + 6\,O_2 + 6\,H_2O + ADP + \textcircled{P}$$

Note that this reaction is almost the reverse of the aerobic respiration reaction; it is nature's way of balancing substrates in the environment. In aerobic respiration, glucose and oxygen are ultimately converted into water and carbon dioxide. In oxygenic photosynthesis, water and carbon dioxide are converted into glucose and oxygen.

Photosynthetic reactions do not always produce oxygen. Purple sulfur bacteria and green sulfur bacteria (which are obligately anaerobic photoautotrophs) are referred to as *anoxygenic photosynthetic bacteria* because their photosynthetic processes do not produce oxygen (*anoxygenic photosynthesis*). These bacteria use sulfur, sulfur compounds (e.g., H_2S gas), or hydrogen gas to reduce CO_2, rather than H_2O.

Bacterial photosynthetic pigments use shorter wavelengths of light, which penetrate deep within a body of water or into mud where it appears to be dark. In the absence of light, some phototrophic organisms may survive anaerobically by the fermentation process alone. Other phototrophic bacteria also have a limited ability to use simple organic molecules in photosynthetic reactions; thus, they become photoheterotrophic organisms under certain conditions.

Chemosynthesis. The chemosynthetic process involves a chemical source of energy and raw materials for synthesis of the metabolites and macromolecules required for growth and function of the organisms. Chemotrophs that use CO_2 as their carbon source are called chemoautotrophs. Examples of chemoautotrophs are a few primitive types of bacteria. You will recall that some archaea are methanogens; they are chemoautotrophs also. Methanogens produce methane in the following manner:

$$4\,H_2 + CO_2 \rightarrow CH_4 + 2\,H_2O$$

Chemotrophs that use organic molecules other than CO_2 as their carbon source are called chemoheterotrophs. Most bacteria, as well as all protozoa, fungi, animals, and humans, are chemoheterotrophs.

BACTERIAL GENETICS

It would be impossible to discuss the genetics of all types of microorganisms in a book of this size. (Recall that some microbes are procaryotic and others are eucaryotic.) Therefore, the following discussion of bacterial genetics will serve as an introduction to the subject of microbial genetics.

Genetics—the study of heredity—involves many topics, some of which (e.g., DNA, genes, the genetic code, chromosomes, DNA replication, transcription, translation) have already been addressed in this book. The topics thus far discussed all relate to molecular genetics—genetics at the molecular level.

An organism's *genotype* (or genome) is its complete collection of genes, whereas an organism's *phenotype* is all the organism's physical traits, attributes, or characteristics. Phenotypic characteristics of humans include hair, eye, and skin color. Phenotypic characteristics of bacteria include the presence or absence of certain enzymes and such structures as capsules, flagella, and pili. An organism's phenotype is dictated by that organism's genotype. **Phenotype is the manifestation of genotype.** For example, an organism cannot produce a particular enzyme unless it possesses the gene that codes for that enzyme. It cannot produce flagella unless it possesses the genes necessary for flagella production.

> An organism's genotype (or genome) is its complete collection of genes, whereas an organism's phenotype is all the physical traits, attributes, or characteristics of an organism.

Most bacteria possess one chromosome, which usually consists of a long, continuous (circular), double-stranded DNA molecule, with no protein on the outside (as is found in eucaryotic chromosomes). A particular segment of the chromosome constitutes a gene. The chromosome can be thought of as a circular strand of genes, all linked together—somewhat like a string of beads. Genes are the fundamental units of heredity that carry the information needed for the special characteristics of each different species of bacteria. **Genes direct all functions of the cell, providing it with its own particular traits and individuality.**

As you learned in Chapter 6, the information in a gene is used by the cell to make an mRNA molecule (via the process known as transcription). Then, the information in the mRNA molecule is used to make a *gene product* (via the process known as translation). Most gene products are proteins, but ribosomal RNA (rRNA) and transfer RNA (tRNA) molecules are also coded for by genes and, therefore, represent other types of gene products. When the information in a gene has been used by the cell to make a gene product, the gene coding for that particular gene product is said to have been *expressed*. All the genes on the chromosome are not being expressed at any given time. That would be a terrible waste of energy! For example, it would be pointless for a cell to produce a particular enzyme if that enzyme was not needed. Genes that are expressed at all times are called *constitutive genes*. Those that are expressed only when the gene products are needed are called *inducible genes*.

> Constitutive genes are expressed at all times, whereas inducible genes are expressed only when needed.

Because there is only one chromosome that replicates just before cell division, identical traits of a species are passed from the parent bacterium to the daughter cells after binary fission has occurred. DNA replication must precede binary fission to ensure that each daughter cell has exactly the same genetic composition as the parent cell.

Mutations

The DNA of any gene on the chromosome is subject to accidental alteration (e.g., the deletion of a base pair), which alters the gene product and perhaps also alters the trait that is controlled by that gene. If the change in the gene alters or eliminates a trait in such a way that the cell does not die or become incapable of division, the altered trait is transmitted to the daughter cells of each succeeding generation. A change in the characteristics of a cell caused by a change in the DNA molecule (genetic alteration) that is transmissible to the offspring is called a *mutation*. There are three categories of mutations: beneficial mutations, harmful (and sometimes lethal) mutations, and silent mutations.

Beneficial mutations, as the name implies, are of benefit to the organism. An example would be a mutation that enables the organism to survive in an environment where organisms without that mutation would die. Perhaps the mutation enables the organism to be resistant to a particular antibiotic.

An example of a *harmful mutation* would be a mutation that leads to the production of a nonfunctional enzyme. A nonfunctional enzyme is unable to catalyze the chemical reaction that it would normally catalyze if it were functional. If it happens to be an enzyme that catalyzes a metabolic reaction essential to the life of the cell, the cell will die. Thus, this is an example of a *lethal mutation*. Not all harmful mutations are lethal.

> Beneficial mutations are of benefit to an organism, whereas harmful mutations result in the production of nonfunctional enzymes. Some harmful mutations are lethal to the organism.

In all likelihood, most mutations are *silent mutations* (or neutral mutations), meaning that they have no effect on the cell. For example, if the mutation causes an incorrect amino acid to be placed near the center of a large, highly convoluted enzyme, composed of hundreds of amino acids, it is doubtful that the mutation would cause any change in the structure or function of that enzyme. If the mutation causes no change in function, it is considered silent.

Most likely, spontaneous mutations (random mutations that occur naturally) occur more or less constantly throughout a bacterial genome. However, some genes are more prone to spontaneous mutations than others. The rate at which spontaneous mutations occur is usually expressed in terms of the frequency at which a mutation will occur in a particular gene. This rate varies from one mutation every 10^4 (10,000) rounds of DNA replication to one mutation every 10^{12} (1 trillion) rounds of DNA replication. The average spontaneous mutation rate is about one mutation every 10^6 (1 million) rounds of DNA replication. In other words, the odds that a spontaneous mutation will occur in a particular gene are about 1 mutation per million cell divisions.

The mutation rate can be increased by exposing cells to physical or chemical agents that affect the chromosome. Such agents are called *mutagens*. In research laboratories, x-rays, ultraviolet light, and radioactive substances, as well as certain chemical agents, are used to increase the mutation rate of bacteria, thus causing more mutations to occur. The organism containing the mutation is called a *mutant*. Bacterial mutants are used in genetic and medical research and in the development of vaccines. The types of mutagenic changes frequently observed in bacteria involve cell shape, biochemical activities, nutritional needs, antigenic sites, colony characteristics, virulence, and drug resistance. Nonpathogenic "live" virus vaccines, such as the Sabin vaccine for polio, are examples of laboratory-induced mutations of pathogenic microorganisms.

> Physical or chemical agents that cause an increased mutation rate are called mutagens.

In a test procedure called the *Ames test* (developed by Bruce Ames in the 1960s), a mutant strain of *Salmonella* is used to learn whether a particular chemical (e.g., a food additive or a chemical used in some type of cosmetic product) is a mutagen. If exposure to the chemical causes a reversal of the organism's mutation (known as a back mutation), then the chemical has been shown to be mutagenic. If the chemical is mutagenic, then it might also be carcinogenic (cancer-causing) and should be tested using laboratory animals or cell cultures. Many substances found to be mutagenic by the Ames test have been shown to be carcinogenic in laboratory animals. Substances that are carcinogenic in laboratory animals might also be carcinogenic in humans.

Ways in Which Bacteria Acquire New Genetic Information

There are at least four additional ways that the genetic composition of bacteria can be changed: lysogenic conversion, transduction, transformation, and conjugation. These are ways in which bacteria acquire new genetic information (i.e., acquire new genes). If the new genes remain in the cytoplasm of the cell, the DNA molecule on which they are located is called a *plasmid* (Fig. 7-8). Because they are not part of the chromosome, plasmids are referred to as extrachromosomal DNA. Many different types of plasmids have been discovered, and information about them all would fill many books. Some plasmids contain many genes, others only a few, but, in all cases, the cell is changed by the acquisition of these genes. Some plasmids replicate simultaneously with chromosomal DNA replication; others replicate independently at various other times. A plasmid that can exist either autonomously (by itself) or can integrate into the chromosome is referred to as an *episome*. Some plasmid genes can be expressed as extrachromosomal genes, but others must integrate into the chromosome before the genes become functional.

Lysogenic Conversion

As mentioned in Chapter 4, there are two categories of bacteriophages (phages): virulent phages and temperate phages. Virulent phages (which were described in Chapter 4) always cause the lytic cycle to occur, ending with the destruction (lysis) of the bacterial cell.

After *temperate phages* (also known as lysogenic phages) inject their DNA into the bacterial cell, the phage DNA integrates into (becomes part of) the bacterial chromosome but does not cause the lytic cycle to occur. This situation—in which the phage genome is present in the cell but is not causing the lytic cycle to occur—is known as *lysogeny*. During lysogeny, all that

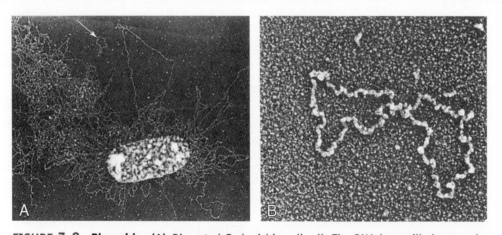

FIGURE 7-8. Plasmids. (A) Disrupted *Escherichia coli* cell. The DNA has spilled out and a plasmid can be seen slightly to the left of top center (arrow). **(B)** Enlargement of a plasmid, which is about 1 μm from side to side. (From Volk WA, et al. Essentials of Medical Microbiology, 4th ed. Philadelphia: JB Lippincott, 1991.)

remains of the phage is its DNA; in this form, the phage is referred to as a *prophage*. The bacterial cell containing the prophage is referred to as a *lysogenic cell* or *lysogenic bacterium*. Each time a lysogenic cell undergoes binary fission, the phage DNA is replicated along with the bacterial DNA and is passed on to each of the daughter cells. Thus, the daughter cells are also lysogenic cells.

Although the prophage does not usually cause the lytic cycle to occur, certain events (e.g., exposure of the bacterial cell to ultraviolet light or certain chemicals) can trigger it to do so. While the prophage is integrated into the bacterial chromosome, the bacterial cell can produce gene products that are coded for by the prophage genes. The bacterial cell

> A lysogenic bacterium is capable of producing one or more new gene products as a result of infection by a temperate bacteriophage.

will exhibit new properties—a phenomenon known as *lysogenic conversion* (or *phage conversion*). In other words, the bacterial cell has been converted as a result of lysogeny and is now able to produce one or more gene products that it previously was unable to produce.

A medically related example of lysogenic conversion involves the disease diphtheria. Diphtheria is caused by a toxin—called diphtheria toxin—that is produced by a Gram-positive bacillus named *Corynebacterium diphtheriae*. Interestingly, the *C. diphtheriae* genome does not normally contain the gene that codes for diphtheria toxin. Only cells of *C. diphtheriae* that contain a prophage can produce diphtheria toxin, because it is actually a phage gene (called the *tox* gene) that codes for the toxin. Strains of *C. diphtheriae* capable of producing diphtheria toxin are called *toxigenic strains*, and those unable to produce the toxin are called *nontoxigenic strains*. A nontoxigenic *C. diphtheriae* cell can be converted to a toxigenic cell as a result of lysogeny. As previously mentioned, conversion as a result of lysogeny is referred to as lysogenic conversion. The phage that infects *C. diphtheriae*—the phage having the *tox* gene in its genome—is called a corynebacteriophage.

Other medically related examples of lysogenic conversion involve *Streptococcus pyogenes*, *Clostridium botulinum*, and *Vibrio cholerae*. Only strains of *S. pyogenes* that carry a prophage are capable of producing erythrogenic toxin—the toxin that causes scarlet fever. Only strains of *C. botulinum* that carry a prophage can produce botulinal toxin, and only strains of *V. cholerae* that carry a prophage can produce cholera toxin. Thus, without being infected by bacteriophages, these bacteria could not cause scarlet fever, botulism, and cholera, respectively. A recap of bacteriophage terminology can be found in Table 7-4.

TABLE 7-4	Recap of Bacteriophage Terminology
TERM	**MEANING**
Bacteriophage (or phage)	A virus that infects bacteria
Lysogenic cell (or lysogenic bacterium)	A bacterial cell with bacteriophage DNA integrated into its chromosome
Lysogenic conversion	When a bacterial cell has acquired new phenotypic characteristics as a result of lysogeny
Lysogeny	When the bacteriophage DNA is integrated into the bacterial chromosome; the bacteriophage DNA replicates along with the chromosome
Lytic cycle	The sequence of events in the multiplication of a virulent bacteriophage; ends with lysis of the bacterial cell
Prophage	The name given to the bacteriophage when all that remains of it is its DNA, integrated into the bacterial chromosome
Temperate bacteriophage (or lysogenic bacteriophage)	A bacteriophage whose DNA integrates into the bacterial chromosome but does not cause the lytic cycle to occur
Virulent bacteriophage	A bacteriophage that always causes the lytic cycle to occur

Transduction

Transduction also involves bacteriophages. Transduction means "to carry across." Some bacterial genetic material may be carried across from one bacterial cell to another by a bacterial virus. This phenomenon may occur after infection of a bacterial cell by a temperate bacteriophage. The viral DNA combines with the bacterial chromosome, becoming a prophage. If a stimulating chemical, heat, or ultraviolet light activates the prophage, it begins to produce new viruses via the production of phage DNA and proteins. As the chromosome disintegrates, small pieces of bacterial DNA may remain attached to the maturing phage DNA. During the assembly of the virus particles, one or more bacterial genes may be incorporated into some of the mature bacteriophages. When all the phages are released by cell lysis, they proceed to infect other cells, some injecting bacterial genes as well as viral genes. Thus, bacterial genes that are attached to the phage DNA are carried to new cells by the virus. As explained on this book's CD-ROM (see "A Closer Look at Transduction"), there are two types of transduction: generalized transduction and specialized transduction. Generalized transduction is illustrated in Figure 7-9.

> Only small segments of DNA are transferred from cell to cell by transduction compared with the amount that can be transferred by transformation and conjugation.

Transformation

In *transformation*, a bacterial cell becomes genetically transformed after the uptake of DNA fragments ("naked DNA") from the environment (Fig. 7-10). Transformation experiments, performed by Oswald Avery and his colleagues, proved that DNA is indeed the genetic material (see Historical Note on page 116). In those experiments, a DNA extract from encapsulated, pathogenic *Streptococcus pneumoniae* (referred to as *S. pneumoniae* type 1) was added to a broth culture of nonencapsulated, nonpathogenic *S. pneumoniae* (referred to as *S. pneumoniae* type 2). Thus, at the beginning of the experiment, there were no live encapsulated bacteria in the culture. After incubation, however, live type 1 (encapsulated) bacteria were recovered from the culture. How was that possible? The only possible explanation was that some of the live type 2 bacteria must have taken up (absorbed) some of the type 1 DNA from the broth. Type 2 bacteria that absorbed pieces of type 1 DNA containing the gene(s) for capsule production were now able to produce capsules. In other words, type 2 (nonencapsulated) bacteria were converted to type 1 (encapsulated) bacteria as a result of the uptake of the genes that code for capsule production.

> In transformation, a bacterial cell becomes genetically transformed following uptake of DNA fragments ("naked DNA") from the environment.

Transformation is probably not widespread in nature. In the laboratory, it has been demonstrated to occur in

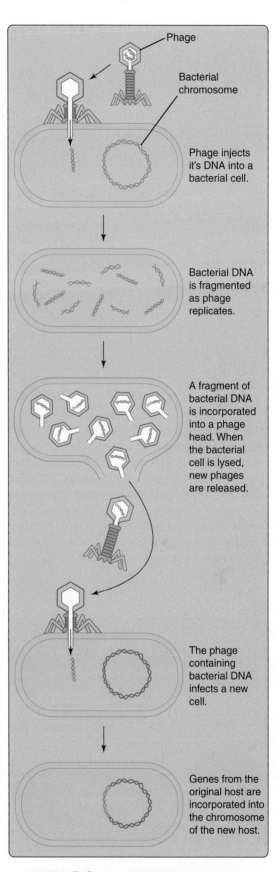

Phage

Bacterial chromosome

Phage injects it's DNA into a bacterial cell.

Bacterial DNA is fragmented as phage replicates.

A fragment of bacterial DNA is incorporated into a phage head. When the bacterial cell is lysed, new phages are released.

The phage containing bacterial DNA infects a new cell.

Genes from the original host are incorporated into the chromosome of the new host.

FIGURE 7-9. Generalized transduction.

1. Naked DNA fragments from disintegrated cells in the area of a competent recipient cell.

2. Entry of naked DNA into competent cell

3. Recombination

One or more DNA fragments integrate into the host cell chromosome. The resultant recombinant cell is said to have been genetically transformed. It can now express the foreign genes it has received and pass them on to its progeny.

DNA that has not recombined is broken down by enzymes.

FIGURE 7-10. Transformation.

several genera including *Bacillus*, *Escherichia*, *Haemophilus*, *Pseudomonas*, and *Neisseria*. Transformations have even been shown to occur between two different species (e.g., between *Staphylococcus* and *Streptococcus*). Extracellular pieces of DNA molecules can only penetrate the cell wall and cell membrane of certain bacteria. The ability to absorb naked DNA into the cell is referred to as *competence*, and bacteria capable of taking up naked DNA molecules are said to be *competent bacteria*.

HISTORICAL NOTE
Transformation and the Discovery of the "Hereditary Molecule"
Transformation was first demonstrated in 1928 by the British physician Frederick Griffith and his colleagues, performing experiments with *S. pneumoniae* and mice. Although the experiments demonstrated that bacteria could take up genetic material from the external environment and, thus, be transformed, it was not known at that time what molecule actually contained the genetic information. It was not until 1944 that Oswald Avery, Colin MacLeod, and Maclyn McCarthy, who also experimented with *S. pneumoniae*, first demonstrated that DNA was the molecule that contained genetic information. Whereas Griffith's experiments were conducted in vivo, Avery's experiments were conducted in vitro. Experiments conducted in 1952 by Alfred Hershey and Martha Chase, using *E. coli* and bacteriophages, confirmed that DNA carried the genetic code.

Some competent bacterial cells have incorporated DNA fragments from certain animal viruses (e.g., cowpox), retaining the latent virus genes for long periods. This knowledge may have some importance in the study of viruses that remain latent in humans for many years before they finally cause disease, as may be the case in Parkinson disease. These human virus genes may hide in the bacteria of the indigenous microflora until they are released to cause disease.

Conjugation
The transfer of genetic material by the process known as conjugation was discovered by Joshua Lederberg and Edward Tatum in 1946, while experimenting with *E. coli*. Conjugation involves a specialized type of

On conjugation, genetic material, usually in the form of a plasmid, is transferred through a hollow sex pilus from a donor cell to a recipient cell.

STUDY AID
Beware of Similar Sounding Terms
The terms **transcription, translation, transduction, and transformation** all sound similar, but each refers to a different phenomenon. **Transcription** and **translation** (both of which were discussed in Chapter 6) relate to the Central Dogma—the flow of genetic information within a cell. **Transduction** and **transformation** are ways in which bacteria acquire new genetic information (i.e., ways in which bacteria acquire new genes).

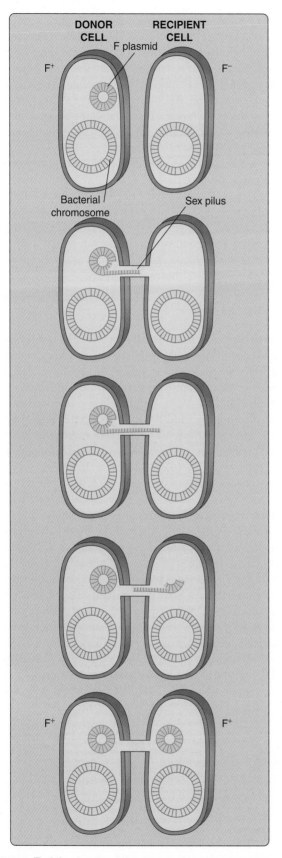

DONOR CELL   **RECIPIENT CELL**

F plasmid

F^+ F^-

Bacterial chromosome   Sex pilus

F^+ F^+

FIGURE 7-11. Conjugation. Note that the donor cell does not lose its plasmid in the process.

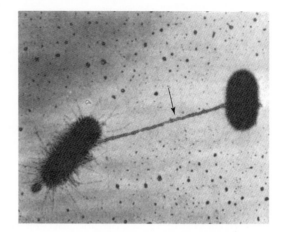

FIGURE 7-12. Conjugation in *Escherichia coli*. The donor cell (the cell on the left, possessing numerous short pili) is connected to the recipient cell by a sex pilus (arrow). (From Volk WA, et al. Essentials of Medical Microbiology, 5th ed. Philadelphia: Lippincott-Raven, 1996.)

pilus called a sex pilus (sometimes referred to as an F pilus or a conjugation bridge). A bacterial cell (called the donor cell or F^+ cell) possessing a sex pilus attaches by means of the sex pilus to another bacterial cell (called the recipient cell or F^- cell). Some genetic material (usually in the form of a plasmid) is then transferred through the hollow sex pilus from the donor cell to the recipient cell (Figures 7-11 and 7-12). Although conjugation has nothing to do with reproduction, the process is sometimes referred to as "bacterial mating," and the terms "male" and "female" cells are sometimes used in reference to the donor and recipient cells, respectively. This type of genetic recombination occurs mostly among species of enteric, Gram-negative bacilli, but has been reported within species of *Pseudomonas* and *Streptococcus* as well. In electron micrographs, microbiologists have observed that sex pili are thicker and longer than other pili.

Although many different genes may be transferred by conjugation, the ones most frequently noted include those coding for antibiotic resistance, colicin (a protein produced by *E. coli* that kills certain other bacteria), and fertility factors (F^+ and Hfr^+), where F stands for fertility and Hfr stands for high frequency of recombination. Check this book's CD-ROM for "A Closer Look at Fertility Factors."

If a plasmid contains multiple genes for antibiotic resistance, the plasmid is referred to as a resistance factor or *R-factor*. A recipient cell that receives an R-factor becomes a multiply drug-resistant organism (referred to by the press as a "superbug"). Superbugs are discussed in detail in Chapter 9.

> A plasmid that contains multiple genes for antibiotic resistance is called a resistance factor or R-factor.

Transduction, transformation, and conjugation are excellent tools for mapping bacterial chromosomes and for studying bacterial and viral genetics. Although all these methods are frequently used in the laboratory, it is believed that they also occur in natural environments under certain circumstances.

GENETIC ENGINEERING

An array of techniques has been developed to transfer eucaryotic genes, particularly human genes, into other easily cultured cells to facilitate the large-scale production of important gene products (proteins, in most cases). This process is known as *genetic engineering* or recombinant DNA technology (see Study Aid). Plasmids are frequently used as vectors or vehicles for inserting genes into cells. Bacteria, yeasts, human leukocytes, macrophages, and fibroblasts have been used as genetically engineered "manufacturing plants" for proteins such as human growth hormone (somatotropin), somatostatin (which inhibits the release of somatotropin), plasminogen-activating factor, insulin, and interferon. For example, the human gene that codes for insulin was inserted into *E. coli* cells, so that those cells and all of their progeny were able to produce human insulin, Somatostatin and insulin were first produced by recombinant DNA technology in 1978.

Many industrial and medical benefits may be derived from genetic engineering research. In agriculture, there is a potential for incorporating nitrogen-fixing capabilities into additional soil microorganisms; to make plants that are resistant to insects, as well as to bacterial and fungal diseases; and to increase the size and nutritional value of foods.

Genetically engineered microorganisms can also be used to clean up the environment (e.g., to get rid of toxic wastes). Consider this hypothetical example. A soil bacterium contains a gene that enables the organism to break oil down into harmless byproducts, but, because the organism cannot survive in salt water, it cannot be used to clean up oil spills at sea. Remove the gene from the soil bacterium, and, using a plasmid vector, insert it into a marine bacterium. Now the marine bacterium has the ability to break down oil and, in large numbers, can be used to clean up oil spills at sea.

In medicine, there is potential for making engineered antibodies, antibiotics, and drugs; for synthesizing important enzymes and hormones for treatment of inherited diseases; and for making vaccines. Such vaccines would contain only part of the pathogen (e.g., the capsid proteins of a virus) to which the person would form protective antibodies (see "Insight: Genetically Engineered Bacteria and Yeasts" on the CD-ROM).

GENE THERAPY

Gene therapy of human diseases involves the insertion of a normal gene into cells to correct a specific genetic or acquired disorder that is being caused by a defective gene. The first gene therapy trials were conducted in the United States in 1990. Viral delivery is currently the most common method for inserting genes into cells, in which specific viruses are selected to target the DNA of specific cells. For example, a virus capable of infecting liver cells would be used to insert a therapeutic gene or genes into the DNA of liver cells. Viruses currently being used or considered for use as vectors include adenoviruses, retroviruses, adeno-associated virus, and herpesviruses. Since 1990, there have been hundreds of human gene therapy trials for many diseases. Nearly all have failed because of the difficulties of inserting a working gene into cells without causing harmful side effects. Nevertheless, scientists remain hopeful that genes will someday be regularly prescribed as "drugs" in the treatment of certain diseases (e.g., autoimmune diseases, sickle cell anemia, cancer, certain liver and lung diseases, cystic fibrosis, heart disease, hemoglobin defects, hemophilia, muscular dystrophy, and various immune deficiencies). In the future, synthetic vectors, rather than viruses, may be used to insert genes into cells.

STUDY AID

Recombinant DNA Technology vs.
Genetic Engineering

Although these terms are frequently used interchangeably, there is a difference between them. **Recombinant DNA (rDNA) technology** can be thought of as the process by which rDNA is produced. This involves inserting a molecule or portion of a molecule of DNA into a different molecule or portion of a different molecule of DNA. The two molecules combine to form a single molecule, and the product is referred to as rDNA. **Genetic engineering** can be thought of as the process by which rDNA is used to modify an organism's genome—often to enable that organism to produce a particular gene product that it previously was unable to produce or to accomplish a task that it previously was unable to accomplish. Both processes—production of rDNA and genetic engineering—are illustrated in Figure 7-13.

ON THE CD-ROM
- Terms Introduced in This Chapter
- Review of Key Points
- Insight
  - Why Anaerobes Die in the Presence of Oxygen
  - Genetically Engineered Bacteria and Yeasts
- Increase Your Knowledge
- Critical Thinking
- Additional Self-Assessment Exercises

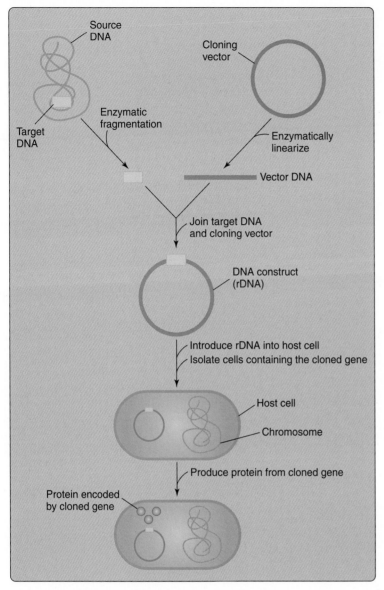

FIGURE 7-13. Recombinant DNA technology and genetic engineering. Plasmids are the most widely used vectors, but bacteriophages, artificial bacterial and yeast chromosomes, and disabled retroviruses have also been used.

SELF-ASSESSMENT EXERCISES

After studying this chapter, answer the following multiple-choice questions.

1. Which of the following characteristics do animals, fungi, and protozoa have in common?
   a. They obtain their carbon from carbon dioxide.
   b. They obtain their carbon from inorganic compounds.
   c. They obtain their energy and carbon atoms from chemicals.
   d. They obtain their energy from light.

2. Most ATP molecules are produced during which phase of aerobic respiration?
   a. electron transport chain
   b. fermentation
   c. glycolysis
   d. Krebs cycle

3. Which of the following processes does not involve bacteriophages?
   a. lysogenic conversion
   b. lytic cycle
   c. transduction
   d. transformation

4. In transduction, bacteria acquire new genetic information in the form of:
   a. bacterial genes.
   b. naked DNA.
   c. R-factors.
   d. viral genes.

5. The process whereby naked DNA is absorbed into a bacterial cell is known as:
   a. transcription.
   b. transduction.
   c. transformation.
   d. translation.

6. In lysogenic conversion, bacteria acquire new genetic information in the form of:
   a. bacterial genes.
   b. naked DNA.
   c. R-factors.
   d. viral genes.
7. Saprophytic fungi are able to digest organic molecules outside of the organism by means of:
   a. apoenzymes.
   b. coenzymes.
   c. endoenzymes.
   d. exoenzymes.
8. The process by which a nontoxigenic *Corynebacterium diphtheriae* cell is changed into a toxigenic cell is called:
   a. conjugation.
   b. lysogenic conversion.
   c. transduction.
   d. transformation.

9. Which of the following does (do) not occur in anaerobes?
   a. anabolic reactions
   b. catabolic reactions
   c. electron transport chain
   d. fermentation reactions
10. Proteins that must link up with a cofactor to function as an enzyme are called:
   a. apoenzymes.
   b. coenzymes.
   c. endoenzymes.
   d. holoenzymes.

CONTROLLING MICROBIAL GROWTH IN VITRO

8

LEARNING OBJECTIVES

AFTER STUDYING THIS CHAPTER, YOU SHOULD BE ABLE TO:

- List several factors that affect the growth of microorganisms
- Describe the following types of microorganisms: psychrophilic, mesophilic, thermophilic, halophilic, haloduric, alkaliphilic, acidophilic, and piezophilic
- List three in vitro sites where microbial growth is encouraged
- Differentiate among enriched, selective, and differential media and cite two examples of each
- Explain the importance of using "aseptic technique" in the microbiology laboratory
- Describe the three types of incubators that are used in the microbiology laboratory
- Draw a bacterial growth curve and label its four phases

- Cite two reasons why bacteria die during the death phase
- Name three ways in which obligate intracellular pathogens can be cultured in the laboratory
- List three in vitro sites where microbial growth must be inhibited
- Differentiate among sterilization, disinfection, and sanitization
- Differentiate between bactericidal and bacteriostatic agents
- Explain the processes of pasteurization and lyophilization
- List several physical methods used to inhibit the growth of microorganisms
- Cite three ways in which disinfectants kill microorganisms
- Identify several factors that can influence the effectiveness of disinfectants
- Explain briefly why the use of antibiotics in animal feed and household products is controversial

INTRODUCTION

In certain locations, such as within microbiology laboratories, the growth[a] of microbes is encouraged; in other words, scientists *want* them to grow. In other locations—such as on hospital wards, in intensive care units, in operating rooms, in kitchens, bathrooms, and restaurants—it is necessary or desirable to *inhibit* the growth of microbes. Both concepts, encouraging and inhibiting the in vitro growth of microbes, are discussed in this chapter. (Recall from Chapter 1 that, as used in this book, *in vitro* refers to events that occur outside the body, whereas *in vivo* refers to events that occur inside the body.) Before discussing these concepts, however, various factors that affect the growth of microbes are examined.

FACTORS THAT AFFECT MICROBIAL GROWTH

Microbial growth is affected by many different environmental factors, including the availability of nutrients and moisture, temperature, pH, osmotic pressure, barometric pressure, and composition of the atmosphere. These environmental factors affect microorganisms in our daily lives and play important roles in the control of microorganisms in laboratory, industrial, and hospital settings. Whether scientists wish to encourage or inhibit the growth of microorganisms, they must first understand the fundamental needs of microbes.

Availability of Nutrients

As discussed in Chapter 7, all living organisms require nutrients—the various chemical compounds that organisms use to sustain life. Therefore, to survive in a particular environment, appropriate nutrients must be available. Many nutrients are energy sources; organisms will obtain energy from these chemicals by breaking chemical bonds. Nutrients also serve as sources of carbon, oxygen, hydrogen, nitrogen, phosphorus, and sulfur as well as other elements (e.g., sodium, potassium, chlorine, magnesium, calcium, trace elements such as iron, iodine, zinc) that are usually required in lesser amounts. About two dozen of the approximately 92 naturally occurring elements are essential to life.[b]

Moisture

On Earth, water is essential for life as we know it. Cells consist of anywhere between 70% and 95% water. All living organisms require water to carry out their normal metabolic processes,

> Water is essential for life, as we know it. Cells are composed of between 70% and 95% water.

and most will die in environments containing too little moisture. There are certain microbial stages (e.g., bacterial endospores, protozoan cysts), however, that can survive the complete drying process (**desiccation**). The organisms contained within the spores and cysts are in a dormant or resting state; if they are placed in a moist, nutrient-rich environment, they will grow and reproduce normally.

Temperature

Every microorganism has an optimum growth temperature—the temperature at which the organism grows best. Every microorganism also has a minimum growth temperature,

> Every microorganism has an optimal, a minimum, and a maximum growth temperature.

below which it ceases to grow, and a maximum growth temperature, above which it dies. The temperature range (i.e., the range of temperatures from the minimum growth temperature to the maximum growth temperature) at which an organism grows can differ greatly from one microbe to another. To a large extent, the temperature and pH ranges over which an organism grows best are determined by the enzymes present within the organism. As discussed in Chapter 7, enzymes have optimum temperature and pH ranges at which they operate at peak efficiency. If an organism's enzymes are operating at peak efficiency, the organism will be metabolizing and growing at its maximum rate.

Microorganisms that grow best at high temperatures are called **thermophiles** (meaning organisms that love heat).

> Thermophiles are organisms that "love" high temperatures.

Thermophiles can be found in hot springs, compost pits, and silage as well as in and near hydrothermal vents at the bottom of the ocean (check this book's CD-ROM for "A Closer Look at Hydrothermal Vents"). Thermophilic cyanobacteria, certain other types of bacteria, and algae cause many of the colors observed in the near-boiling hot springs found in Yellowstone National Park. Organisms that favor temperatures above 100°C are referred to as hyperthermophiles (or extreme thermophiles). The highest temperature at which a bacterium has been found living is around 113°C; it was an archaeon named *Pyrolobus fumarii*.

Microbes that grow best at moderate temperatures are called **mesophiles**. This group includes most of the species that grow on plants and animals and in warm soil and water. Most pathogens and members of the indigenous microflora are mesophilic, because they grow best at normal body temperature (37°C).

Psychrophiles prefer cold temperatures. They thrive in cold ocean water. At high altitudes, algae (often pink) can be seen living on snow. Ironically, the optimum growth temperature of one group of psychrophiles (called **psychrotrophs**) is refrigerator temperature (4°C); perhaps you encountered some of these microbes

> Psychrophiles are organisms that "love" cold temperatures.

---

[a] The word "growth" is used in this chapter to mean proliferation or multiplication.

[b] Scientists continue to debate the actual number of naturally occurring elements, but most would agree that the number lies between 88 and 94.

TABLE 8-1	Categories of Bacteria on the Basis of Growth Temperature		
CATEGORY	MINIMUM GROWTH TEMPERATURE	OPTIMUM GROWTH TEMPERATURE	MAXIMUM GROWTH TEMPERATURE
Thermophiles	25°C	50°–60°C	113°C
Mesophiles	10°C	20°–40°C	45°C
Psychrophiles	−5°C	10°–20°C	30°C

(bread molds, for example) the last time you cleaned out your refrigerator. Microorganisms that prefer warmer temperatures, but can tolerate or endure very cold temperatures and can be preserved in the frozen state, are known as **psychroduric organisms**. Fecal material left by early Arctic explorers contained psychroduric *Escherichia coli* that survived the Arctic temperatures. Refer to Table 8-1 for the temperature ranges of psychrophilic, mesophilic, and thermophilic bacteria.

pH

The term "pH" refers to the hydrogen ion concentration of a solution and, thus, the acidity or alkalinity of the solution (see CD-ROM Appendix 3: "Basic Chemistry Concepts"). Most microorganisms prefer a neutral or slightly alkaline growth medium (pH 7.0–7.4), but *acidophilic* microbes (**acidophiles**), such as those that can live in the stomach and in pickled foods, prefer a pH of 2 to 5. Fungi prefer acidic environments. Acidophiles thrive in highly acidic environments, such as those created by the production of sulfurous gases in hydrothermal vents and hot springs as well as in the debris produced from coal mining. **Alkaliphiles** prefer an alkaline environment (pH >8.5), such as is found inside the intestine (pH ~9), in soils laden with carbonate, and in so-called soda lakes. *Vibrio cholerae*—the bacterium that causes cholera—is the only human pathogen that grows well above pH 8.

> Acidophiles prefer acidic environments, whereas alkaliphiles prefer environments that are alkaline.

Osmotic Pressure and Salinity

Osmotic pressure is the pressure that is exerted on a cell membrane by solutions both inside and outside the cell. When cells are suspended in a solution, the ideal situation is that the pressure inside the cell is equal to the pressure of the solution outside the cell. Substances dissolved in liquids are referred to as solutes. When the concentration of solutes in the environment outside of a cell is greater than the concentration of solutes inside the cell, the solution in which the cell is suspended is said to be **hypertonic**. In such a situation, whenever possible, water leaves the cell by osmosis

> Cells lose water and shrink when placed into a hypertonic solution.

in an attempt to equalize the two concentrations. **Osmosis** is defined as the movement of a solvent (e.g., water), through a permeable membrane, from a solution having a lower concentration of solute to a solution having a higher concentration of solute. If the cell is a human cell, such as a red blood cell (erythrocyte), the loss of water causes the cell to shrink; this shrinkage is called **crenation** and the cell is said to be **crenated**. If the cell is a bacterial cell, having a rigid cell wall, the cell does not shrink. Instead, the cell membrane and cytoplasm shrink away from the cell wall. This condition, known as **plasmolysis**, inhibits bacterial cell growth and multiplication. Salts and sugars are added to certain foods as a way of preserving them. Bacteria that enter such hypertonic environments will die as a result of desiccation.

When the concentration of solutes outside a cell is less than the concentration of solutes inside the cell, the solution in which the cell is suspended is said to be **hypotonic**. In such a situation, whenever possible, water enters the cell in an attempt to equalize the two concentrations. If the cell is a human cell, such as an erythrocyte, the increased water within the cell causes the cell to swell. If sufficient water enters, the cell will burst (lyse). In the case of erythrocytes, this bursting is called **hemolysis**. If a bacterial cell is placed in a hypotonic solution (such as distilled water), the cell may not burst (because of the rigid cell wall), but the fluid pressure within the cell increases greatly. This increased pressure occurs in cells having rigid cell walls such as plant cells and bacteria. If the pressure becomes so great that the cell ruptures, the escape of cytoplasm from the cell is referred to as **plasmoptysis**.

> Cells swell up, and sometimes burst, when placed into a hypotonic solution.

When the concentration of solutes outside a cell equals the concentration of solutes inside the cell, the solution is said to be **isotonic**. In an isotonic environment, excess water neither leaves nor enters the cell and, thus, no plasmolysis or plasmoptysis occurs; the cell has normal turgor (fullness). Refer to Figure 8-1 for a comparison of the effects of various solution concentrations on bacteria and red blood cells.

Sugar solutions for jellies and pickling brines (salt solutions) for meats preserve these foods by inhibiting the growth of most microorganisms. However, some types of

Isotonic solution   **Hypotonic solution**   **Hypertonic solution**

Plasmoptysis / Hemolysis
of bacteria / (red blood cell)

Plasmolysis / Crenation of
of bacteria / red blood cel

FIGURE 8-1. Changes in osmotic pressure. No change in pressure occurs within the cell in an isotonic solution. Internal pressure is increased in a hypotonic solution, resulting in swelling of the cell. Internal pressure is decreased in a hypertonic solution, resulting in shrinking of the cell. (*Arrows* indicate the direction of water flow. The larger the arrow, the greater the amount of water flowing in that direction.)

molds and bacteria can survive and even grow in a salty environment.

Those microbes that actually prefer salty environments (such as the concentrated salt water found in the Great Salt Lake and solar salt evaporation ponds) are called **halophilic**, *halo* referring to "salt" and *philic* meaning "to love." Microbes that live in the ocean, such as *V. cholerae* (mentioned earlier) and other *Vibrio* species, are halophilic. Organisms that do not prefer to live in salty environments but are capable of surviving there (such as *Staphylococcus aureus*) are referred to as **haloduric organisms**.

Barometric Pressure

Most bacteria are not affected by minor changes in barometric pressure. Some thrive at normal atmospheric pressure (about 14.7 pounds per square inch [psi]). Others, known as **piezophiles**, thrive deep in the ocean and in oil wells, where the atmospheric pressure is very high. Some archaea, for example, are piezophiles, capable of living in the deepest parts of the ocean. Check this book's CD-ROM for "A Closer Look at Barometric Pressure."

> Microorganisms that prefer salty environments are called halophiles.

Gaseous Atmosphere

As discussed in Chapter 4, microorganisms vary with respect to the type of gaseous atmosphere that they require. For example, some microbes (obligate aerobes) prefer the same atmosphere that humans do (i.e., about 20%–21% oxygen and 78%–79% nitrogen, with all other atmospheric gases combined representing less than 1%). Although microaerophiles also require oxygen, they require reduced concentrations of oxygen (around 5% oxygen). Obligate anaerobes are killed by the presence of oxygen. Thus, in nature, the types and concentrations of gases present in a particular environment determine which species of microbes are able to live there. To grow a particular microorganism in the laboratory, it is necessary to provide the atmosphere that it requires. For example, to obtain maximum growth in the laboratory, capnophiles require increased concentrations of carbon dioxide (usually from 5%–10% carbon dioxide).

ENCOURAGING THE GROWTH OF MICROBES IN VITRO

There are many reasons why the growth of microbes is encouraged in microbiology laboratories. For example, technologists and technicians who work in clinical microbiology laboratories must be able to isolate microorganisms from clinical specimens and grow them on culture

STUDY AID

-Phile

The suffix *-phile* means to love something. For example, acidophiles are organisms that love acidic conditions; therefore, they live in acidic environments. Alkaliphiles live in alkaline environments. Halophiles live in salty environments. Piezophiles (formerly called barophiles) live in environments where there is high barometric pressure, such as at the bottom of the ocean. Thermophiles prefer hot temperatures. Mesophiles prefer moderate temperatures. Psychrophiles prefer cold temperatures. Microaerophiles live in environments containing reduced concentrations of oxygen (around 5% oxygen). Capnophiles grow best in environments rich in carbon dioxide.

media so they can then gather information that will enable identification of any pathogens that are present. In microbiology research laboratories, scientists must culture microbes so that they can learn more about them, harvest antibiotics and other microbial products, test new antimicrobial agents, and produce vaccines. Microbes must also be cultured in genetic engineering laboratories and in the laboratories of certain food and beverage companies, as well as other industries.

Many different types of microbes can be cultured (grown) in vitro, including viruses, bacteria, fungi, and protozoa. In this chapter, emphasis is placed on culturing bacteria. Culturing other types of microbes will be mentioned only briefly.

Culturing Bacteria in the Laboratory

In many ways, modern microbiology laboratories resemble those of 50, 100, or even 150 years ago. Today's laboratories still use many of the same basic tools that were used in the past. For example, microbiologists still use compound light microscopes, Petri dishes containing solid culture media, tubes containing liquid culture media, Bunsen burners, wire inoculating loops, bottles of staining reagents, and incubators. However, a closer inspection will reveal many modern, commercially available products and instruments that would have been inconceivable in the days of Louis Pasteur and Robert Koch.

HISTORICAL NOTE
Culturing Bacteria in the Laboratory
The earliest successful attempts to culture microorganisms in a laboratory setting were made by Ferdinand Cohn (1872), Joseph Schroeter (1875), and Oscar Brefeld (1875). Robert Koch described his culture techniques in 1881. Initially, Koch used slices of boiled potatoes on which to culture bacteria, but he later developed both liquid and solid forms of artificial media. Gelatin was initially used as a solidifying agent in Koch's culture media, but in 1882, Fanny Hesse, the wife of Dr. Walther Hesse—one of Koch's assistants—suggested the use of agar. Frau Hesse (as she is most commonly called) had been using agar in her kitchen for many years as a solidifying agent in fruit and vegetable jellies. Another of Koch's assistants, Richard Julius Petri, invented glass Petri dishes in 1887 for use as containers for solid culture media and bacterial cultures. The Petri dishes in use today are virtually unchanged from the original design, except that most of today's laboratories use plastic, presterilized, disposable Petri dishes. In 1878, Joseph Lister became the first person to obtain a pure culture of a bacterium (*Streptococcus lactis*) in a liquid medium. As a result of their ability to obtain pure cultures of bacteria in their laboratories, Louis Pasteur and Robert Koch made significant contributions to the germ theory of disease.

Bacterial Growth

With respect to humans, the term *growth* refers to an increase in size; for example, going from a tiny newborn baby to a large adult. Although bacteria do increase in size before cell division, *bacterial growth* refers to an increase in the *number* of organisms rather than an increase in their size. Thus, with respect to bacteria, *growth* refers to their proliferation or multiplication. When each bacterial cell reaches its optimum size, it divides by binary fission (bi meaning "two") into two daughter cells (i.e., each bacterium simply splits in half to become two identical cells). (Recall from Chapter 3 that DNA replication must occur before binary fission occurs, so that each daughter cell has exactly the same genetic makeup as the parent cell.) On solid medium, binary fission continues through many generations until a colony is produced. A bacterial colony is a mound or pile of bacteria containing millions of cells. Binary fission continues for as long as the nutrient supply, water, and space allow and ends when the nutrients are depleted or the concentration of cellular waste products reaches a toxic level. The division of staphylococci by binary fission is shown in Figure 8-2.

The time it takes for one cell to become two cells by binary fission is called the **generation time**. The generation time varies from one bacterial species to another. In the laboratory, under ideal growth conditions, *E. coli*, *V. cholerae*,

> Throughout this book, the term *bacterial growth* refers to the proliferation or multiplication of bacteria.

> Bacteria multiply by binary fission. The time it takes a particular bacterial species to undergo binary fission is called that organism's generation time.

FIGURE 8-2. Binary fission of staphylococci. (Courtesy of Ray Rupel.)

Staphylococcus spp., and *Streptococcus* spp. all have a generation time of about 20 minutes, whereas some *Pseudomonas* and *Clostridium* spp. may divide every 10 minutes, and *Mycobacterium tuberculosis* may divide only every 18 to 24 hours. Bacteria with short generation times are referred to as rapid growers, whereas those with long generation times are referred to as slow growers.

The growth of microorganisms in the body, in nature, or in the laboratory is greatly influenced by temperature, pH, moisture content, available nutrients, and the characteristics of other organisms present. Therefore, the number of bacteria in nature fluctuates unpredictably because these factors vary with the seasons, rainfall, temperature, and time of day.

In the laboratory, however, a pure culture of a single species of bacteria can usually be maintained if the appropriate growth medium and environmental conditions are provided. The temperature, pH, and proper atmosphere are quite easily controlled to provide optimum conditions for growth. Appropriate nutrients must be provided in the growth medium, including an appropriate energy and carbon source. Some bacteria, described as being *fastidious*, have complex nutritional requirements. Often, special mixtures of vitamins and amino acids must be added to the medium to culture these fastidious organisms. Some organisms will not grow at all on artificial culture; these include obligate intracellular pathogens, such as viruses, rickettsias, and chlamydias. To propagate obligate intracellular pathogens in the laboratory, they must be inoculated into live animals, embryonated chicken eggs, or cell cultures. Other microorganisms that will not grow on artificial media include *Treponema pallidum* (the causative agent of syphilis) and *Mycobacterium leprae* (the causative agent of leprosy).

> Microorganisms that are difficult to grow in the laboratory are said to be fastidious.

Culture Media

The media (sing., medium) that are used in microbiology laboratories to culture bacteria are referred to as **artificial media** or **synthetic media**, because they do not occur naturally; rather, they are prepared in the laboratory. There are a number of ways of categorizing the media that are used to culture bacteria.

One way to classify culture media is based on whether the exact contents of the media are known. A **chemically defined medium** is one in which all the ingredients are known; this is because the medium was prepared in the laboratory by adding a certain number of grams of each of the components (e.g., carbohydrates, amino acids, salts). A **complex medium** is one in which the exact contents are not known. Complex media contain ground up or digested extracts from animal organs (e.g., hearts, livers, brains), fish, yeasts, and plants, which provide necessary nutrients, vitamins, and minerals.

Culture media can also be categorized as liquid or solid. Liquid media (also known as broths) are contained in tubes and are thus often referred to as tubed media. Solid media are prepared by adding agar to liquid media and then pouring the media into tubes or Petri dishes, where the media solidifies. Bacteria are then grown on the surface of the agar-containing solid media. Agar is a complex polysaccharide that is obtained from a red marine alga; it is used as a solidifying agent, much like gelatin is used as a solidifying agent in the kitchen.

An **enriched medium** is a broth or solid medium containing a rich supply of special nutrients that promotes the growth of fastidious organisms. It is usually prepared by adding extra nutrients to a medium called nutrient agar. Blood agar (nutrient agar plus 5% sheep red blood cells) and chocolate agar (nutrient agar plus powdered hemoglobin) are examples of solid enriched media that are used routinely in the clinical bacteriology laboratory. Blood agar is bright red, whereas chocolate agar is brown (the color of chocolate). Although both of these media contain hemoglobin, chocolate agar is considered to be more enriched than blood agar because the hemoglobin is more readily accessible in chocolate agar. Chocolate agar is used to culture important, fastidious, bacterial pathogens, like *Neisseria gonorrhoeae* and *Haemophilus influenzae*, which will not grow on blood agar.

> Blood agar and chocolate agar are examples of enriched media.

A **selective medium** has added inhibitors that discourage the growth of certain organisms without inhibiting growth of the organism being sought. For example, MacConkey agar inhibits growth of Gram-positive bacteria and thus is selective for Gram-negative bacteria. Phenylethyl alcohol (PEA) agar and colistin–nalidixic acid (CNA) agar inhibit growth of Gram-negative bacteria and thus are selective for Gram-positive bacteria. Thayer-Martin agar and Martin-Lewis agar (chocolate agars containing extra nutrients plus several antimicrobial agents) are selective for *N. gonorrhoeae*. Only salt-tolerant (haloduric) bacteria can grow on mannitol salt agar (MSA).

> A selective medium is used to discourage the growth of certain organisms without inhibiting growth of the organism being sought.

A **differential medium** permits the differentiation of organisms that grow on the medium. For example, Mac-Conkey agar is frequently used to differentiate among various Gram-negative bacilli that are isolated from fecal specimens. Gram-negative bacteria capable of fermenting lactose (an ingredient of MacConkey agar) produce pink colonies, whereas those that are unable to ferment lactose produce colorless colonies (Fig. 8-3). Thus, MacConkey agar differ-

> A differential medium allows one to readily differentiate among the various types of organisms that are growing on the medium.

FIGURE 8-3. Bacterial colonies on MacConkey agar, which is a selective and differential medium.
It is selective for Gram-negative bacteria, meaning that only Gram-negative bacteria will grow on this medium. Colonies of lactose-fermenters (pink colonies) and nonlactose-fermenters (clear colonies) can be seen. (From Winn WC Jr, et al. Koneman's Color Atlas and Textbook of Diagnostic Microbiology, 6th ed. Philadelphia: Lippincott Williams & Wilkins, 2006.)

FIGURE 8-5. Colonies of beta-hemolytic *Streptococcus pyogenes* on a blood agar plate. The clear zones (β-hemolysis) surrounding the colonies are caused by enzymes (hemolysins) that lyse the red blood cells in the agar. (Note: Information about the Greek alphabet can be found in Appendix D.) (From Winn WC Jr, et al. Koneman's Color Atlas and Textbook of Diagnostic Microbiology, 6th ed. Philadelphia: Lippincott Williams & Wilkins, 2006.)

entiates between lactose-fermenting (LF) and nonlactose-fermenting (NLF) Gram-negative bacteria. Mannitol salt agar is used to screen for *S. aureus*; not only will *S. aureus* grow on MSA, but it turns the originally pink medium to yellow because of its ability to ferment mannitol (Fig. 8-4). In a sense, blood agar is also a differential medium because it is used to determine the type of hemolysis (alteration or destruction of red blood cells) that the bacterial isolate produces (Fig. 8-5).

FIGURE 8-4. Mannitol salt agar, a selective and differential medium, is used to screen for *Staphylococcus aureus*. Any bacteria capable of growing in a 7.5% sodium chloride concentration will grow on this medium, but *S. aureus* will turn the medium yellow because of its ability to ferment the mannitol in the medium. The organism growing on the upper section of the plate is unable to ferment mannitol, but the organism growing on the lower section is a mannitol fermenter. (From Koneman E, et al. Color Atlas and Textbook of Diagnostic Microbiology, 5th ed. Philadelphia: Lippincott Williams & Wilkins, 1997.)

The various categories of media (enriched, selective, differential) are not mutually exclusive. For example, as just seen, blood agar is enriched and differential. MacConkey agar and MSA are selective and differential. PEA and CNA are enriched and selective: they are blood agars to which selective inhibitory substances have been added. Thayer-Martin and Martin-Lewis agars are highly enriched and highly selective.

Thioglycollate broth (THIO) is a very popular liquid medium for use in the bacteriology laboratory. THIO supports the growth of all categories of bacteria from obligate aerobes to obligate anaerobes. How is this possible? Within the tube of THIO there is a concentration gradient of dissolved oxygen. The concentration of oxygen decreases with depth. The concentration of oxygen in the broth at the top of the tube is about 20% to 21%. At the bottom of the tube, there is no oxygen in the broth. Organisms will grow only in that part of the broth where the oxygen concentration meets their needs (Fig. 8-6). For example, microaerophiles will grow where there is around 5% oxygen, and obligate anaerobes will only grow at the very bottom of the tube where there is no oxygen. Facultative anaerobes can grow anywhere in the tube. (Recall that facultative anaerobes can live in the presence or absence of oxygen.)

Inoculation of Culture Media

In clinical microbiology laboratories, culture media are routinely inoculated with clinical specimens (i.e., specimens that have been collected from patients suspected of having infectious diseases). **Inoculation** of a liquid medium involves adding a portion of the specimen to the medium. Inoculation of a solid or plated medium involves the use of a sterile inoculating loop

FIGURE 8-6. Thioglycollate broth contains a concentration gradient of dissolved oxygen, ranging from 20% to 21% O₂ at the top of the tube to 0% O₂ at the bottom of the tube. A particular bacterium will grow only in that part of the broth containing the concentration of oxygen that it requires.

to apply a portion of the specimen to the surface of the medium; a process commonly referred to as *streaking* (Fig. 8-7). The proper method of inoculating plated media to obtain well-isolated colonies is described in CD-ROM Appendix 5: "Clinical Microbiology Laboratory Procedures."

FIGURE 8-7. The proper method of inoculating the surface of an agar plate. The plate is held in the palm of one hand. The other hand is used to lightly drag the inoculating loop over the surface of the solid culture medium. The inoculating loop is held in much the same manner as a small camel-hair paint brush is held by an artist when applying paint to the surface of a canvas.

Importance of Using "Aseptic Technique"

Individuals working in a microbiology laboratory must practice what is known as **aseptic technique** and must understand its importance. Aseptic technique is practiced to prevent (a) microbiology professionals from becoming infected, (b) contamination of their work environment, and (c) contamination of clinical specimens, cultures, and subcultures. For example, when inoculating plated media, it is important to keep the Petri dish lid in place at all times, except for the few seconds that it takes to inoculate the specimen to the surface of the culture medium. Every additional second that the lid is off provides an opportunity for airborne organisms (e.g., bacterial and fungal spores) to land on the surface of the medium, where they will then grow. Such unwanted organisms are referred to as **contaminants**, and the plate is said to be *contaminated*. Of equal importance is to maintain the sterility of the media before inoculation and to avoid touching the agar surface with fingertips or other nonsterile objects. Inoculating media within a biologic safety cabinet (BSC) minimizes the possibility of contamination and protects the laboratory worker from becoming infected with the organism(s) that he or she is working with. BSCs are further discussed in CD-ROM Appendix 4: "Responsibilities of the Clinical Microbiology Laboratory."

> Aseptic technique is practiced in the microbiology laboratory to prevent infection of individuals and contamination of the work environment, clinical specimens, and cultures.

Incubation

After media are inoculated, they must be incubated (i.e., they must be placed into a chamber [called an *incubator*] that contains the appropriate atmosphere and moisture level and is set to maintain the appropriate temperature). This is called **incubation**. To culture most human pathogens, the incubator is set at 35°C to 37°C. Three types of incubators are used in a clinical microbiology laboratory:

> The three types of incubators used in the microbiology laboratory are CO₂ incubators, non-CO₂ incubators, and anaerobic incubators.

1. A CO_2 (carbon dioxide) incubator is an incubator to which a cylinder of CO_2 is attached. CO_2 is periodically introduced into the incubator to maintain a CO_2 concentration of about 5% to 10%. Such an incubator is used to isolate capnophiles (organisms that grow best in atmospheres containing increased CO_2). It is important to keep in mind that a CO_2 incubator contains oxygen (about 15%–20%) in addition to CO_2. Thus, a CO_2 incubator is *not* an anaerobic incubator.
2. A non-CO_2 incubator is an incubator containing room air; thus, it contains about 20% to 21% oxygen.
3. An anaerobic incubator is an incubator containing an atmosphere devoid of oxygen.

Once a particular species of bacteria has been isolated from a clinical specimen, it can be separated from any other organisms that were present in the specimen and can be grown as a pure culture. The term *pure culture* refers to the fact that there is only one bacterial species present. The changes in a bacterial population over an extended period follow a definite predictable pattern that can be shown by plotting the population growth curve on a graph (discussed later in this chapter).

> A pure culture is a culture that contains only one species of organism.

Bacterial Population Counts

Microbiologists sometimes need to know how many bacteria are present in a particular liquid at any given time (e.g., to determine the degree of bacterial contamination in drinking water, milk, and other foods). The microbiologist may (a) determine the total number of bacterial cells in the liquid (the total number would include both viable and dead cells) or (b) determine the number of viable (living) cells.

Various types of instruments are available to determine the total number of cells (e.g., a spectrophotometer could be used). In a spectrophotometer, a beam of light is passed through the liquid. When no bacteria are present in the liquid, the liquid is clear, and a large amount of light passes through. As bacteria increase in number, the liquid becomes turbid (cloudy), and less light passes through. Turbidity increases (i.e., the solution becomes more cloudy) as the number of organisms increases; therefore, the amount of transmitted light decreases as the bacteria increase in number. Formulas are available to equate the amount of transmitted light to the concentration of organisms in the liquid, which is usually expressed as the number of organisms per milliliter (mL) of suspension.

The **viable plate count** is used to determine the number of viable bacteria in a liquid sample, such as milk, water, ground food diluted in water, or a broth culture. In this procedure, serial dilutions of the sample are prepared, and then 0.1-mL or 1-mL aliquots (portions) are inoculated onto plates of nutrient agar. After overnight incubation, the number of colonies are counted. (Usually, a plate containing 30–300 colonies is used.) To determine the concentration of bacteria in the original sample, the number of colonies must be multiplied by the dilution factor(s). For example, if 220 colonies were counted on an agar plate that had been inoculated with a 1.0-mL sample of a 1:10,000 dilution, there were $220 \times 10,000 = 2,200,000$ bacteria/mL of the original material at the time the dilutions were made and cultured. If, however, 220 colonies were counted on an agar plate that had been inoculated with a 0.1-mL sample of a 1:10,000 dilution, there were $220 \times 10 \times 10,000 = 22,000,000$ bacteria/mL of the original material at the time the dilutions were made and cultured.

In the clinical microbiology laboratory, a viable cell count is an important part of a urine culture. (The technique is described in Chapter 13.) The number of viable bacteria per milliliter of a urine specimen is used as an indicator of a urinary tract infection (UTI). As explained in Chapter 13, high colony counts may also be caused by contamination of the urine specimen with indigenous microflora during specimen collection or failure to refrigerate the specimen between collection and transport to the laboratory.

Bacterial Population Growth Curve

A **population growth curve** for any particular species of bacterium may be determined by growing a pure culture of the organism in a liquid medium at a constant temperature. Samples of the culture are collected at fixed intervals (e.g., every 30 minutes), and the number of viable organisms in each sample is determined. The data are then plotted on logarithmic graph paper. The graph in Figure 8-8 was obtained by plotting the logarithm ($\log_{10}$) of the number of viable bacteria (on the vertical or *y*-axis) against the incubation time (on the horizontal or *x*-axis). (If you are not familiar with logarithms, refer to a math book.)

> A bacterial population growth curve consists of four phases: a lag phase, a log phase, a stationary phase, and a death phase.

The growth curve consists of the following four phases:

1. The first phase of the growth curve is the **lag phase** (**A** in Fig. 8-8), during which the bacteria absorb nutrients, synthesize enzymes, and prepare for cell division. The bacteria do not increase in number during the lag phase.
2. The second phase of the growth curve is the **logarithmic growth phase** (also known as the **log phase** or exponential growth phase; **B** in Fig. 8-8). In the log phase, the bacteria multiply so rapidly that the number of organisms doubles with each generation time

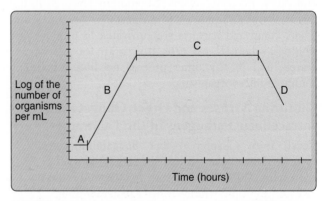

FIGURE 8-8. A population growth curve of living organisms. The logarithm of the number of bacteria per milliliter of medium is plotted against time. **(A)** Lag phase. **(B)** Logarithmic growth phase. **(C)** Stationary phase. **(D)** Death phase. See text for details.

(i.e., the number of bacteria increases exponentially). Growth rate is the greatest during the log phase. The log phase is always brief, unless the rapidly dividing culture is maintained by constant addition of nutrients and frequent removal of waste products. When plotted on logarithmic graph paper, the log phase appears as a steeply sloped straight line.

3. As the nutrients in the liquid medium are used up and the concentration of toxic waste products from the metabolizing bacteria build up, the rate of division slows, such that the number of bacteria that are dividing equals the number that are dying. The result is the **stationary phase** (**C** in Fig. 8-8). It is during this phase that the culture is at its greatest population density.

4. As overcrowding occurs, the concentration of toxic waste products continues to increase and the nutrient supply decreases. The microorganisms then die at a rapid rate; this is the **death phase** or **decline phase** (**D** in Fig. 8-8). The culture may die completely, or a few microorganisms may continue to survive for months. If the bacterial species is a sporeformer, it will produce spores to survive beyond this phase. When cells are observed in old cultures of bacteria in the death phase, some of them look different from healthy organisms seen in the log phase. As a result of unfavorable conditions, morphologic changes in the cells may appear. Some cells undergo involution and assume various shapes, becoming long, filamentous rods or branching or globular forms that are difficult to identify. Some develop without a cell wall and are referred to as protoplasts, spheroplasts, or L-phase variants (L-forms). When these involuted forms are inoculated into a fresh nutrient medium, they usually revert to the original shape of the healthy bacteria.

Many industrial and research procedures depend on the maintenance of an essential species of microorganism. These are continuously cultured in a controlled environment called a *chemostat* (Fig. 8-9), which regulates the supply of nutrients and the removal of waste products and excess microorganisms. Chemostats are used in industries where yeast is grown to produce beer and wine, where fungi and bacteria are cultivated to produce antibiotics, where *E. coli* cells are grown for genetic research, and in any other process needing a constant source of microorganisms.

Culturing Viruses and Other Obligate Intracellular Pathogens in the Laboratory

Recall from Chapter 4 that obligate intracellular pathogens are microbes that can only survive and multiply within living cells (called host cells). Obligate intracellular pathogens include viruses and two groups of Gram-negative bacteria—rickettsias and chlamydias. Because

Obligate intracellular pathogens can be propagated in the laboratory using embryonated chicken eggs, laboratory animals, or cell cultures.

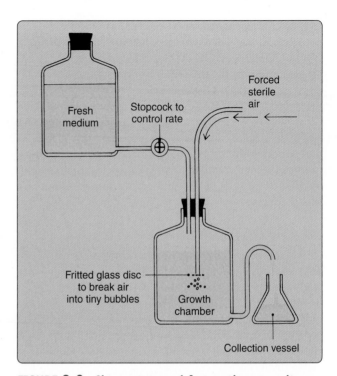

FIGURE 8-9. Chemostat used for continuous cultures. Rates of growth can be controlled either by controlling the rate at which new medium enters the growth chamber or by limiting a required growth factor in the medium.

obligate intracellular pathogens will not grow on artificial (synthetic) media, they present a challenge to laboratorians when large numbers of the organisms are required for diagnostic or research purposes (e.g., development of vaccines and new drugs). To grow such organisms in the laboratory, they must be inoculated into embryonated chicken eggs, laboratory animals, or cell cultures.

In the virology laboratory, cell cultures are primarily used for the propagation of viruses. Because a given virus can only attach to and infect cells that bear appropriate cell receptors, it is necessary to maintain several different types of cell lines in the virology laboratory. Examples of cell lines are kidney cells from monkeys, rabbits, or humans, human and mink lung cells, and various cancer cell lines. After appropriate cells are inoculated with a clinical specimen suspected of containing a specific type of virus, the cells are incubated for several days, and then examined microscopically. If present, a given virus will cause specific morphologic alterations to the cells. These changes are called cytopathic effect (CPE). Examples of CPE include rounding, swelling, and shrinking or cells, or cells may become granular, glassy, vacuolated, or fused (illustrated in Fig. 13-17 in Chapter 13). Viruses can then be identified, based upon the particular type of CPE that they cause in a specific cell line.

Culturing Fungi in the Laboratory

Fungi (including yeasts, molds, and dimorphic fungi) will grow on and in various solid and liquid culture media. There is no one medium that is best for all medically important fungi. Examples of solid culture media used to grow fungi include brain–heart infusion (BHI) agar, BHI agar with blood, and Sabouraud dextrose agar (SDA). Antibacterial agents are often added to the media to suppress the growth of bacteria. The low pH of SDA (pH 5.6) inhibits the growth of most bacteria; thus, SDA is selective for fungi. Laboratory personnel must exercise caution when culturing fungi, because the spores of certain fungi are highly infectious. Because of the potential danger, a Class II biologic safety cabinet must be used.

Culturing Protozoa in the Laboratory

Most clinical microbiology laboratories do not culture protozoa, but techniques are available for culturing protozoa in reference and research laboratories. Examples of protozoa that can be cultured in vitro are amebae (e.g., *Acanthamoeba* spp., *Balamuthia* spp., *Entamoeba histolytica*, *Naegleria fowleri*), *Giardia lamblia*, *Leishmania* spp., *Toxoplasma gondii*, *Trichomonas vaginalis*, and *Trypanosoma cruzi*. Of these protozoa, it is of greatest importance to culture *Acanthamoeba*, *Balamuthia*, and *N. fowleri* in a clinical microbiology laboratory. These amebae can cause serious (often fatal) infections of the central nervous system—infections that are difficult to diagnose by other methods. Parasitic protozoa are further discussed in Chapter 21.

INHIBITING THE GROWTH OF MICROBES IN VITRO

In certain environments, it is necessary or desirable to inhibit the growth of microbes. In hospitals, nursing homes, and other healthcare institutions, for example, it is necessary to inhibit the growth of pathogens so that they will not infect patients, staff members, or visitors. Other environments in which it is necessary or desirable to inhibit microbial growth include food and beverage processing plants, restaurants, kitchens, and bathrooms.

Definition of Terms

Before discussing the various methods used to destroy or inhibit the growth of microbes, a number of terms should be understood as they apply to microbiology.

Sterilization

Sterilization involves the destruction or elimination of *all* microbes, including cells, spores, and viruses. When something is *sterile*, it is devoid of microbial life. In healthcare facilities, sterilization of objects can be accomplished by physical or chemical methods. Dry heat, autoclaving (steam under pressure), ethylene oxide gas, and various liquid chemicals (such as formaldehyde) are the principal sterilizing agents in healthcare facilities. In some situations, certain types of radiation (e.g., ultraviolet light and gamma rays) are also used. These techniques are discussed later in this chapter.

> Sterilization involves the destruction or elimination of *all* microbes.

Disinfection, Pasteurization, Disinfectants, Antiseptics, and Sanitization

Disinfection describes the elimination of most or all pathogens (except bacterial spores) from nonliving objects. In healthcare settings, objects usually are disinfected by liquid chemicals or wet pasteurization. The heating process developed by Pasteur to kill microbes in wine—*pasteurization*—is a method of disinfecting liquids. Pasteurization is used today to eliminate pathogens from milk and most other beverages. It should be remembered that pasteurization is not a sterilization procedure, because not all microbes are destroyed.

> Disinfection involves the elimination of most or all pathogens (except bacterial spores) from nonliving objects.

Chemicals used to disinfect inanimate objects, such as bedside equipment and operating rooms, are called **disinfectants**. Disinfectants do not kill spores (i.e., they are not sporicidal). Because they are strong chemical substances, disinfectants cannot be used on living tissue. **Antiseptics** are solutions used to disinfect skin and other living tissues. **Sanitization** is the reduction of microbial populations to levels considered safe by public health standards, such as those applied to restaurants.

Microbicidal Agents

The suffix *-cide* or *-cidal* refers to "killing," as in the words homicide, suicide, and genocide. General terms like **germicidal agents** (*germicides*), **biocidal agents** (*biocides*), and **microbicidal agents** (*microbicides*) are disinfectants or antiseptics that kill microbes. **Bactericidal agents** (*bactericides*) specifically kill bacteria, but not necessarily bacterial endospores. Because spore coats are thick and resistant to the effects of many disinfectants, **sporicidal agents** are required to kill bacterial endospores. **Fungicidal agents** (*fungicides*) kill fungi, including fungal spores. **Algicidal agents** (*algicides*) are used to kill algae in swimming pools and hot tubs. **Viricidal agents** (or *virucidal agents*) destroy viruses. **Pseudomonicidal agents** kill *Pseudomonas* species, and **tuberculocidal agents** kill *M. tuberculosis*.

> Agents having the suffix "-cidal" kill organisms, whereas agents having the suffix "-static" merely inhibit their growth and reproduction.

Microbistatic Agents

A **microbistatic agent** is a drug or chemical that inhibits reproduction of microorganisms, but does not necessarily kill them. A **bacteriostatic agent** is one that specifically inhibits the metabolism and reproduction of bacteria. Some of the drugs used to treat bacterial diseases are bacteriostatic, whereas others are bactericidal. Freeze-drying (lyophilization) and rapid freezing (using liquid nitrogen) are microbistatic techniques that are used to preserve microbes for future use or study.

Lyophilization is a process that combines dehydration (drying) and freezing. Lyophilized materials are frozen in a vacuum; the container is then sealed to maintain the inactive state. This freeze-drying method is widely used in industry to preserve foods, antibiotics, antisera, microorganisms, and other biologic materials. It should be remembered that lyophilization cannot be used to kill microorganisms, but, rather, is used to prevent them from reproducing and to store them for future use.

> Lyophilization is a good method of preserving microorganisms for future use.

Sepsis, Asepsis, Aseptic Technique, Antisepsis, and Antiseptic Technique

Sepsis refers to the presence of pathogens in blood or tissues, whereas **asepsis** means the absence of pathogens. The two general categories of aseptic technique—medical and surgical asepsis—are described in detail in Chapter 12. Various techniques, collectively referred to as **aseptic techniques**, are used to eliminate and exclude pathogens. Earlier in this chapter, you learned of the importance of using aseptic technique in the microbiology laboratory when inoculating culture media. In other areas of the hospital, aseptic techniques include hand hygiene[c]; the use of sterile gloves, masks, and gowns; sterilization of surgical instruments and other equipment; and the use of disinfectants and antiseptics. **Antisepsis** is the prevention of infection. **Antiseptic technique**, developed by Joseph Lister in 1867, refers to the use of antiseptics. Antiseptic technique is a type of aseptic technique. Lister used dilute carbolic acid (phenol) to cleanse surgical wounds and equipment and a carbolic acid aerosol to prevent harmful microorganisms from entering the surgical field or contaminating the patient.

Sterile Technique

Sterile technique is practiced when it is necessary to exclude *all* microorganisms from a particular area, so that the area will be sterile. In Chapter 12, you will learn how sterile technique is used in areas of the hospital such as the operating room.

Using Physical Methods to Inhibit Microbial Growth

The methods used to destroy or inhibit microbial life are either physical or chemical, and sometimes both types are used. Physical methods commonly used in hospitals, clinics, and laboratories to destroy or control pathogens include heat, the combination of heat and pressure, desiccation, radiation, sonic disruption, and filtration. Each of these methods will now be briefly discussed.

Heat

Heat is the most practical, efficient, and inexpensive method of sterilization of those inanimate objects and materials that can withstand high temperatures. Because of these advantages, it is the means most frequently used.

> Heat is the most common type of sterilization for inanimate objects able to withstand high temperatures.

Two factors—*temperature* and *time*—determine the effectiveness of heat for sterilization. There is considerable variation from organism to organism in their susceptibility to heat; pathogens usually are more susceptible than nonpathogens. Also, the higher the temperature, the shorter the time required to kill the organisms. The **thermal death point (TDP)** of any particular species of microorganism is the lowest temperature that will kill all the organisms in a standardized pure culture within a specified period. The **thermal death time (TDT)** is the length of time necessary to sterilize a pure culture at a specified temperature.

In practical applications of heat for sterilization, one must consider the material in which a mixture of microorganisms and their spores may be found. Pus, feces, vomitus, mucus, and blood contain proteins that serve as a protective coating to insulate the pathogens; when these substances are present on bedding, bandages, surgical instruments, and syringes, very high temperatures are required to destroy vegetative (growing) microorganisms and spores. In practice, the most effective procedure is to wash away the protein debris with strong soap, hot water, and a disinfectant, and then sterilize the equipment or materials with heat.

Dry Heat. Dry-heat baking in a thermostatically controlled oven provides effective sterilization of metals, glassware, some powders, oils, and waxes. These items must be baked at 160°C to 165°C for 2 hours or at 170°C to 180°C for 1 hour. An ordinary oven of the type found in most homes may be used if the temperature remains constant. The effectiveness of dry-heat sterilization depends on how deeply the heat penetrates throughout the material, and the items to be baked must be positioned so that the hot air circulates freely among them.

Incineration (burning) is an effective means of destroying contaminated disposable materials. An incinerator must never be overloaded with moist or protein-laden materials, such as feces, vomitus, or pus, because the contaminating microorganisms within these moist substances may not be destroyed if the heat does not readily penetrate and burn them. Flaming the surface of metal forceps and wire bacteriologic loops is an effective way to kill microorganisms and, for many years, was a common laboratory procedure. Flaming is accomplished by briefly holding the end of the loop or forceps in the inner, hottest portion of a gas flame (Fig. 8-10). Open flames are dangerous, however, and, for this reason, are

---

[c] The term "hand hygiene" refers to handwashing; the use of alcohol-based gels, rinses, and foams; keeping fingernails clean and short; and not wearing artificial fingernails or rings.

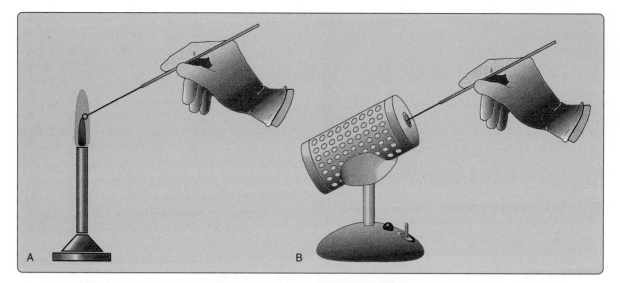

FIGURE 8-10. Dry-heat sterilization. (A) Flaming a wire inoculating loop in a Bunsen burner flame. **(B)** Sterilizing a wire inoculating loop using an electrical heating device.

rarely used in modern microbiology laboratories, in which sterile, disposable, plastic inoculating loops are primarily used. Today, whenever wire inoculating loops are used, heat sterilization is usually accomplished using electrical heating devices (Fig. 8-10).

Moist Heat. Heat applied in the presence of moisture, as in boiling or steaming, is faster and more effective than dry heat, and can be accomplished at a lower temperature; thus, it is less destructive to many materials that otherwise would be damaged at higher temperatures. Moist heat causes proteins to coagulate (as occurs when eggs are hard boiled). Because cellular enzymes are proteins, they are inactivated by moist heat, leading to cell death.

The vegetative forms of most pathogens are quite easily destroyed by boiling for 30 minutes. Thus, clean articles made of metal and glass, such as syringes, needles, and simple instruments, may be disinfected by boiling for 30 minutes. Because the temperature at which water boils is lower at higher altitudes, water should always be boiled for longer times at high altitudes. Boiling is not always effective, however, because heat-resistant bacterial endospores, mycobacteria, and viruses may be present. The endospores of the bacteria that cause anthrax, tetanus, gas gangrene, and botulism, as well as hepatitis viruses, are especially heat resistant and often survive boiling. Also, because thermophiles thrive at high temperatures, boiling is not an effective means of killing them.

An **autoclave** is like a large metal pressure cooker that uses steam under pressure to completely destroy all microbial life (Fig. 8-11). The increased pressure raises the temperature above the temperature of boiling water (i.e., >100°C), and forces the steam into the materials being sterilized.

Autoclaves should be set to run 20 minutes at a pressure of 15 psi and a temperature of 121.5°C.

Autoclaving at a pressure of 15 psi, at a temperature of 121.5°C, for 20 minutes, kills vegetative microorganisms, bacterial endospores, and viruses, as long as they are not protected by pus, feces, vomitus, blood, or other proteinaceous substances. Some types of equipment and certain materials, such as rubber, which may be damaged by high temperatures, can be autoclaved at lower temperatures for longer periods. The timing must be carefully determined based on the contents and compactness of the load. All articles must be properly packaged and arranged within the autoclave to allow steam to penetrate each package completely. Cans should remain open, bottles covered loosely with foil or cotton, and instruments wrapped in cloth. Sealed containers should not be autoclaved. Pressure-sensitive autoclave tape

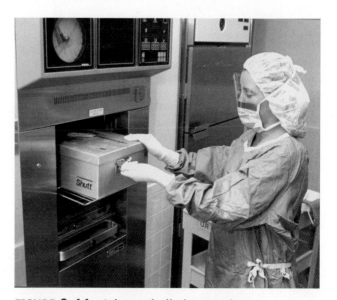

FIGURE 8-11. A large, built-in autoclave. (Courtesy of Scott & White Hospital, Temple, TX.)

FIGURE 8-12. Pressure-sensitive autoclave tape showing dark stripes after sterilization.
(From Volk WA, et al. Essentials of Medical Microbiology, 4th ed. Philadelphia: JB Lippincott, 1991.)

(Fig. 8-12) and commercially available strips or solutions containing bacterial spores (Fig. 8-13) can be used as quality-control measures to ensure that autoclaves are functioning properly. After autoclaving, the spores are tested to see whether they were killed.

FIGURE 8-13. Biological indicator used to monitor the effectiveness of steam sterilization. Sealed ampules containing bacterial spores suspended in a growth medium are placed in the load to be sterilized. Following sterilization, the ampules are incubated at 35°C. If the spores were killed, there will be no change in the color of the medium; it will remain purple. If the spores were not killed, acid production by the organisms will cause the medium to change from purple to yellow. (Courtesy of Fisher Scientific.)

Home canning conducted without the use of a pressure cooker does not destroy the endospores of bacteria—notably the anaerobe, *Clostridium botulinum*. Occasionally, local newspapers report cases of food poisoning resulting from the ingestion of *C. botulinum* toxins in improperly canned fruits, vegetables, and meats. Botulism food poisoning is preventable by properly washing and pressure cooking (autoclaving) food.

An effective way to disinfect clothing, bedding, and dishes is to use hot water (>60°C) with detergent or soap and to agitate the solution around the items. This combination of heat, mechanical action, and chemical inhibition is deadly to most pathogens.

Cold

Most microorganisms are not killed by cold temperatures and freezing, but their metabolic activities are slowed, greatly inhibiting their growth. Refrigeration merely slows the growth of most microorganisms; it does not completely inhibit growth. Slow freezing causes ice crystals to form within cells and may rupture the cell membranes and cell walls of some bacteria; hence, slow freezing should not be used as a way to preserve or store bacteria. Rapid freezing, using liquid nitrogen, is a good way to preserve foods, biologic specimens, and bacterial cultures. It places bacteria into a state of suspended animation. Then, when the temperature is raised above the freezing point, the organisms' metabolic reactions speed up and the organisms begin to reproduce again.

Persons who are involved in the preparation and preservation of foods must be aware that thawing foods allows bacterial spores in the foods to germinate and microorganisms to resume growth. Consequently, refreezing of thawed foods is an unsafe practice, because it preserves the millions of microbes that might be present, leading to rapid deterioration of the food when it is rethawed. Also, if the endospores of *C. botulinum* or *C. perfringens* were present, the viable bacteria would begin to produce the toxins that cause food poisoning.

Desiccation

For many centuries, foods have been preserved by drying. However, even when moisture and nutrients are lacking, many dried microorganisms remain viable, although they cannot reproduce. Foods, antisera, toxins, antitoxins, antibiotics, and pure cultures of microorganisms are often preserved by lyophilization—the combined use of freezing and drying (discussed previously).

In the hospital or clinical environment, healthcare professionals should keep in mind that dried viable pathogens may be present in dried matter, including blood, pus, fecal material, and dust that are found on floors, in bedding, on clothing, and in wound dressings. Should these dried materials be disturbed, such as by dry dusting, the microbes would be easily transmitted through the air or by contact. They would then grow rapidly if they settled in a suitable moist, warm nutrient environment such as a wound or a burn. Therefore, important precautions that must be observed include wet mopping of floors, damp dusting of furniture, rolling bed linens and towels carefully, and proper disposal of wound dressings.

Radiation

The sun is not a particularly reliable disinfecting agent because it kills only those microorganisms that are exposed to direct sunlight. The rays of the sun include the long infrared (heat) rays, the visible light rays, and the shorter ultraviolet (UV) rays. The UV rays, which do not penetrate glass and building materials, are effective only in the air and on surfaces. They do, however, penetrate cells and, thus, can cause damage to DNA. When this occurs, genes may be so severely damaged that the cell dies (especially unicellular microorganisms) or is drastically changed.

In practice, a UV lamp (often called a germicidal lamp) is useful for reducing the number of microorganisms in the air. Its main component is a low-pressure mercury vapor tube. Such lamps are found in newborn nurseries, operating rooms, elevators, entryways, cafeterias, and classrooms, where they are incorporated into louvered ceiling fixtures designed to radiate UV light across the top of the room without striking people in the room. Sterility may also be maintained by having a UV lamp placed in a hood or cabinet containing instruments, paper and cloth equipment, liquid, and other inanimate articles. Many biologic materials, such as sera, antisera, toxins, and vaccines, are sterilized with UV rays.

Those whose work involves the use of UV lamps must be particularly careful not to expose their eyes or skin to the rays, because they can cause serious burns and cellular damage. Because UV rays do not penetrate cloth, metals, and glass, these materials may be used to protect persons working in a UV environment. It has been shown that skin cancer can be caused by excessive exposure to the UV rays of the sun; thus, extensive suntanning is harmful.

X-rays and gamma and beta rays of certain wavelengths from radioactive materials may be lethal or cause mutations in microorganisms and tissue cells because they damage DNA and proteins within those cells. Studies performed in radiation research laboratories have demonstrated that these radiations can be used for the prevention of food spoilage, sterilization of heat-sensitive surgical equipment, preparation of vaccines, and treatment of some chronic diseases such as cancer, all of which are very practical applications for laboratory research. The U.S. Food and Drug Administration approved the use of gamma rays (from cobalt-60) to process chickens and red meat in 1992 and 1997, respectively. Since then, gamma rays have been used by some food

FIGURE 8-14. International symbol for irradiated food. (Courtesy of the United States Department of Agriculture.)

processing plants to kill pathogens (like *Salmonella* and *Campylobacter* spp.) in chickens; the chickens are labeled "irradiated" and marked with the green international symbol for irradiation (Fig. 8-14).

Ultrasonic Waves

In hospitals, medical clinics, and dental clinics, ultrasonic waves are a frequently used means of cleaning delicate equipment. Ultrasonic cleaners consist of tanks filled with liquid solvent (usually water); the short sound waves are then passed through the liquid. The sound waves mechanically dislodge organic debris on instruments and glassware. Glassware and other articles that have been cleansed in ultrasonic equipment must be washed to remove the dislodged particles and solvent and are then sterilized by another method before they are used. Following cleaning of their instruments, most dental professionals sterilize them using steam under pressure (autoclave), chemical (formaldehyde) vapor, or dry heat (e.g., 160°C for 2 hours).

Filtration

Filters of various pore sizes are used to filter or separate cells, larger viruses, bacteria, and certain other microorganisms from the liquids or gases in which they are suspended. Filters with tiny pore sizes (called micropore filters) are used in laboratories to filter bacteria and viruses out of liquids. The variety of filters is large and includes sintered glass (in which uniform particles of glass are fused), plastic films, unglazed porcelain, asbestos, diatomaceous earth, and cellulose membrane filters. Small quantities of liquid can be filtered through a filter-containing syringe, but large quantities require larger apparatuses.

> Microbes, even those as small as viruses, can be removed from liquids using filters having appropriate pore sizes.

A cotton plug in a test tube, flask, or pipette is a good filter for preventing the entry of microorganisms. Dry gauze and paper masks prevent the outward passage of microbes from the mouth and nose, at the same time protecting the wearer from inhaling airborne pathogens and foreign particles that could damage the lungs. Biologic safety cabinets contain high-efficiency particulate air (HEPA) filters to protect workers from contamination. HEPA filters are also located in operating rooms and patient rooms to filter the air that enters or exits the room.

Gaseous Atmosphere

In limited situations, it is possible to inhibit growth of microorganisms by altering the atmosphere in which they are located. Because aerobes and microaerophiles require oxygen, they can be killed by placing them into an atmosphere devoid of oxygen or by removing oxygen from the environment in which they are living. Conversely, obligate anaerobes can be killed by placing them into an atmosphere containing oxygen or by adding oxygen to the environment in which they are living. For instance, wounds likely to contain anaerobes are lanced (opened) to expose them to oxygen. Another example is gas gangrene, a deep wound infection that causes rapid destruction of tissues. Gas gangrene is caused by various anaerobes in the genus *Clostridium*. In addition to debridement of the wound (removal of necrotic tissue) and the use of antibiotics, gas gangrene can be treated by placing the patient in a hyperbaric (increased pressure) oxygen chamber or in a room with high oxygen pressure. As a result of the pressure, oxygen is forced into the wound, providing oxygen to the oxygen-starved tissue and killing the clostridia.

Using Chemical Agents to Inhibit Microbial Growth

Disinfectants

Chemical disinfection refers to the use of chemical agents to inhibit the growth of pathogens, either temporarily or permanently. The mechanism by which various disinfectants kill cells varies from one type of disinfectant to another. Various factors affect the efficiency or effectiveness of a disinfectant (Fig. 8-15), and these factors must be taken into consideration whenever a disinfectant is used. These factors include the following:

- Prior cleaning of the object or surface to be disinfected
- The organic load that is present, meaning the presence of organic matter (e.g., feces, blood, vomitus, pus) on the materials being treated
- The bioburden, meaning the type and level of microbial contamination
- The concentration of the disinfectant
- The contact time, meaning the amount of time that the disinfectant must remain in contact with the organisms in order to kill them (see this book's CD-ROM for "A Closer Look at Contact Time")
- The physical nature of the object being disinfected (e.g., smooth or rough surface, crevices, hinges)
- Temperature and pH

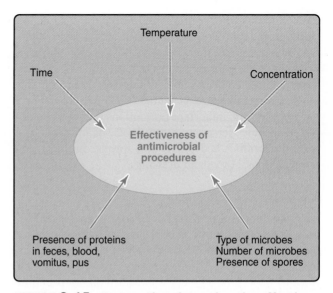

FIGURE 8-15. Factors that determine the effectiveness of any antimicrobial procedure.

Directions for preparing the proper dilution of a disinfectant must be followed carefully, because too weak or too strong a concentration is usually less effective than the proper concentration. (Information about preparing dilutions can be found on this book's CD-ROM.) The items to be disinfected must first be washed to remove any proteinaceous material in which pathogens may be hidden. Although the washed article may then be clean, it is not safe to use until it has been properly disinfected. Healthcare personnel need to understand an important limitation of chemical disinfection—that many disinfectants that are effective against pathogens in the controlled conditions of the laboratory may be ineffective in the actual hospital or clinical environment. Furthermore, the stronger and more effective antimicrobial chemical agents are of limited usefulness because of their destructiveness to human tissues and certain other substances.

Almost all bacteria in the vegetative state, as well as fungi, protozoa, and most viruses, are susceptible to many disinfectants, although the mycobacteria that cause tuberculosis and leprosy, bacterial endospores, pseudomonads (*Pseudomonas* spp.), fungal spores, and hepatitis viruses are notably resistant (see Table 8-2). Therefore, chemical disinfection should never be attempted when it is possible to use proper physical sterilization techniques.

The disinfectant most effective for each situation must be chosen carefully. Chemical agents used to disinfect respiratory therapy equipment and thermometers must destroy all pathogenic bacteria, fungi, and viruses that may be found in sputum and saliva. One must be particularly aware of the oral and respiratory pathogens, including *M. tuberculosis*; species of *Pseudomonas*, *Staphylococcus*, and *Streptococcus*; the various fungi that cause candidiasis, blastomycosis, coccidioidomycosis, and histoplasmosis; and all respiratory viruses.

TABLE 8-2	Degree of Resistance of Microbes to Disinfection and Sterilization
LEVEL OF RESISTANCE	**MICROBES**
High	Prions, bacterial spores, coccidia, mycobacteria
Intermediate	Nonlipid or extremely small viruses, fungi
Low	Vegetative bacteria, lipid, or medium-sized viruses

Note: Coccidia is a category of protozoan parasites. Vegetative bacteria are bacteria that are actively metabolizing and multiplying (as opposed to spores, which are dormant and possess a thick spore coat).

Because most disinfection methods do not destroy all bacterial endospores that are present, any instrument or dressing used in the treatment of an infected wound or a disease caused by sporeformers must be autoclaved or incinerated. Gas gangrene, tetanus, and anthrax are examples of diseases caused by sporeformers that require the healthcare worker to take such precautions. Formaldehyde and ethylene oxide, when properly used, are highly destructive to spores, mycobacteria, and viruses. Certain articles are heat sensitive and cannot be autoclaved or safely washed before disinfection; such articles are soaked for 24 hours in a strong detergent and disinfectant solution, washed, and then sterilized in an ethylene oxide autoclave. The use of disposable equipment whenever possible in these situations helps to protect patients and healthcare personnel.

The effectiveness of a chemical agent depends to some extent on the physical characteristics of the article on which it is used. A smooth, hard surface is readily disinfected, whereas a rough, porous, or grooved surface is not. Thought must be given to selection of the most suitable germicide for cleaning patient rooms and all other areas where patients are treated.

The most effective antiseptic or disinfectant should be chosen for the specific purpose, environment, and pathogen or pathogens likely to be present. The characteristics of an ideal chemical antimicrobial agent include the following:

- It should have a wide or broad antimicrobial spectrum, meaning that it should kill a wide variety of microorganisms.
- It should be fast-acting, meaning that the contact time should be short.
- It should not be affected by the presence of organic matter (e.g., feces, blood, vomitus, pus).
- It must be nontoxic to human tissues and noncorrosive and nondestructive to materials on which it is used (for instance, if a tincture [e.g., alcohol–water solution] is being used, evaporation of the alcohol solvent can cause a 1% solution to increase to a 10% solution, and at this concentration, it may cause tissue damage).

- It should leave a residual antimicrobial film on the treated surface.
- It must be soluble in water and easy to apply.
- It should be inexpensive and easy to prepare, with simple, specific directions.
- It must be stable both as a concentrate and as a working dilution, so that it can be shipped and stored for reasonable periods.
- It should be odorless.

How do disinfectants kill microorganisms? Some disinfectants (e.g., surface-active soaps and detergents, alcohols, phenolic compounds) target and destroy cell membranes. Others (e.g., halogens, hydrogen peroxide, salts of heavy metals, formaldehyde, ethylene oxide) destroy enzymes and structural proteins. Others attack cell walls or nucleic acids. Some of the disinfectants that are commonly used in hospitals are discussed in Chapter 12.

The effectiveness of phenol as a disinfectant was demonstrated by Joseph Lister in 1867, when it was used to reduce the incidence of infections after surgical procedures. The effectiveness of other disinfectants is compared with that of phenol using the *phenol coefficient test*. To perform this test, a series of dilutions of phenol and the experimental disinfectant are inoculated with the test bacteria, *Salmonella typhi* and *S. aureus*, at 37°C. The highest dilutions (lowest concentrations) that kill the bacteria after 10 minutes are used to calculate the phenol coefficient.

Antiseptics

Most antimicrobial chemical agents are too irritating and destructive to be applied to mucous membranes and skin. Those that may be used safely on human tissues are called antiseptics. An antiseptic merely reduces the number of organisms on a surface; it does not penetrate pores and hair follicles to destroy microorganisms residing there. To remove organisms lodged in pores and folds of the skin, healthcare personnel use an antiseptic soap and scrub with a brush. To prevent resident indigenous microflora from contaminating the surgical field, surgeons wear sterile gloves on freshly scrubbed hands, and masks and hoods to cover their face and hair. Also, an antiseptic is applied at the site of the surgical incision to destroy local microorganisms.

Controversies Relating to the Use of Antimicrobial Agents in Animal Feed and Household Products

It has been estimated that approximately 40% of the antibiotics manufactured in the United States are used in animal feed. The reason is obvious: to prevent infectious diseases in farm animals—infections that could lead to huge economic loses for farmers and ranchers. The problem is that when antibiotics are fed to an animal, the antibiotics kill any indigenous microflora organisms that are susceptible to the antibiotics. But what survives? Any organisms that are resistant to the antibiotics. Having less competition now for space and nutrients, these drug-resistant organisms multiply and become the predominant organisms of the animal's indigenous microflora. These drug-resistant organisms are then transmitted in the animal's feces or food products (e.g., eggs, milk, meat) obtained from the animal. Many multidrug-resistant *Salmonella* strains—strains that cause disease in animals and humans—developed in this manner. The use of antibiotic-containing animal feed is quite controversial. Microbiologists concerned about ever-increasing numbers of drug-resistant bacteria are currently attempting to eliminate or drastically reduce the practice of adding antibiotics to animal feed.

Another controversy concerns the antimicrobial agents that are being added to toys, cutting boards, hand soaps, antibacterial kitchen sprays, and many other household products. The antimicrobial agents in these products kill any organisms that are susceptible to these drugs, but what survives? Any organisms that are resistant to these agents. These drug-resistant organisms then multiply and become the predominant organisms in the home. Should a member of the household become infected with these drug-resistant and multidrug-resistant organisms, the infection will be more difficult to treat. Concerned microbiologists are currently attempting to eliminate or drastically reduce the practice of adding antimicrobial agents to household products.

Another argument against the use of antimicrobial agents in the home concerns proper development of the immune system. Many scientists believe that children must be exposed to all sorts of microorganisms during their growth and development so that their immune systems will develop correctly and be capable of properly responding to pathogens in later years. The use of household products containing antimicrobial agents might be eliminating the very organisms that are essential for proper maturation of the immune system.

ON THE CD-ROM
- Terms Introduced in This Chapter
- Review of Key Points
- Insight: Microbes in Our Food
- Insight: Inhibiting the Growth of Pathogens in Our Kitchens
- Increase Your Knowledge
- Critical Thinking
- Additional Self-Assessment Exercises

SELF-ASSESSMENT EXERCISES

After studying this chapter, answer the following multiple-choice questions.

1. It would be necessary to use a tuberculocidal agent to kill a particular species of:
   a. *Clostridium*.
   b. *Mycobacterium*.
   c. *Staphylococcus*.
   d. *Streptococcus*.
2. Pasteurization is an example of what kind of technique?
   a. antiseptic
   b. disinfection
   c. sterilization
   d. surgical aseptic
3. The combination of freezing and drying is known as:
   a. desiccation.
   b. lyophilization.
   c. pasteurization.
   d. tyndallization.
4. Organisms that live in and around hydrothermal vents at the bottom of the ocean are:
   a. acidophilic, psychrophilic, and halophilic.
   b. halophilic, alkaliphilic, and psychrophilic.
   c. halophilic, psychrophilic, and piezophilic.
   d. halophilic, thermophilic, and piezophilic.
5. When placed into a hypertonic solution, a bacterial cell will:
   a. take in more water than it releases.
   b. lyse.
   c. shrink.
   d. swell.
6. To prevent *Clostridium* infections in a hospital setting, what kind of disinfectant should be used?
   a. fungicidal
   b. pseudomonicidal
   c. sporicidal
   d. tuberculocidal
7. Sterilization can be accomplished by use of:
   a. an autoclave.
   b. antiseptics.
   c. medical aseptic techniques.
   d. pasteurization.

8. The goal of medical asepsis is to kill _____, whereas the goal of surgical asepsis is to kill _____.
   a. all microorganisms . . . . . pathogens
   b. bacteria . . . . . bacteria and viruses
   c. nonpathogens . . . . . pathogens
   d. pathogens . . . . . all microorganisms

9. Which of the following types of culture media is selective *and* differential?
   a. blood agar
   b. MacConkey agar
   c. phenylethyl alcohol agar
   d. Thayer-Martin agar

10. All the following types of culture media are enriched and selective except:
    a. blood agar.
    b. colistin–nalidixic acid agar.
    c. phenylethyl alcohol agar.
    d. Thayer-Martin agar.

9

CONTROLLING MICROBIAL GROWTH IN VIVO USING ANTIMICROBIAL AGENTS

LEARNING OBJECTIVES

AFTER STUDYING THIS CHAPTER, YOU SHOULD BE ABLE TO:

- Identify the characteristics of an ideal antimicrobial agent
- Compare and contrast chemotherapeutic agents, antimicrobial agents, and antibiotics as to their intended purpose
- State the five most common mechanisms of action of antimicrobial agents
- Differentiate between bactericidal and bacteriostatic agents
- State the difference between narrow-spectrum and broad-spectrum antimicrobial agents
- Identify the four most common mechanisms by which bacteria become resistant to antimicrobial agents
- State what the initials "MRSA" and "MRSE" stand for
- Define the following terms: β-lactam ring, β-lactam antibiotics, β-lactamase
- Name two major groups of bacterial enzymes that destroy the β-lactam ring
- State six actions that clinicians or patients can take to help in the war against drug resistance
- Explain what is meant by empiric therapy
- List six factors that a clinician would take into consideration before prescribing an antimicrobial agent for a particular patient
- State three undesirable effects of antimicrobial agents

- Explain what is meant by a "superinfection" and cite three diseases that can result from superinfections
- Explain the difference between synergism and antagonism with regard to antimicrobial agents

INTRODUCTION

Chapter 8 contained information regarding the control of microbial growth in vitro. Another aspect of controlling the growth of microorganisms involves the use of drugs to treat (and, hopefully, to cure) infectious diseases; in other words, using drugs to control the growth of microbes in vivo.

Although we most often hear the term *chemotherapy* used in conjunction with cancer (i.e., cancer chemotherapy), *chemotherapy* actually refers to the use of any chemical (drug) to treat any disease or condition. The chemicals (drugs) used to treat diseases are referred to as chemotherapeutic agents. By definition, a *chemotherapeutic agent* is *any* drug used to treat *any* condition or disease.

> A chemotherapeutic agent is *any* drug used to treat *any* condition or disease.

For thousands of years, people have been discovering and using herbs and chemicals to cure infectious diseases. Native witch doctors in Central and South America long ago discovered that the herb, ipecac, aided in the treatment of dysentery, and that a quinine

HISTORICAL NOTE
The Father of Chemotherapy

The true beginning of modern chemotherapy came in the late 1800s when Paul Ehrlich, a German chemist, began his search for chemicals (referred to as "magic bullets") that would destroy bacteria, yet would not damage normal body cells. By 1909, he had tested more than 600 chemicals, without success. Finally, in that year, he discovered an arsenic compound that proved effective in treating syphilis. Because this was the 606th compound Ehrlich had tried, he called it "Compound 606." The technical name for Compound 606 is arsphenamine and the trade name was Salvarsan. Until the availability of penicillin in the early 1940s, Salvarsan and a related compound—Neosalvarsan—were used to treat syphilis. Ehrlich also found that rosaniline was useful for treating African trypanosomiasis.

STUDY AID
Clarifying Drug Terminology

Imagine that all *chemotherapeutic agents* are contained within one very large wooden box. Within that large box are many smaller boxes. Each of the smaller boxes contains drugs to treat one particular category of diseases. For example, one of the smaller boxes contains drugs to treat cancer; these are called cancer chemotherapeutic agents. Another of the smaller boxes contains drugs to treat hypertension (high blood pressure). Another of the smaller boxes contains drugs to treat infectious diseases; these are called *antimicrobial agents*. Now imagine that the box containing antimicrobial agents contains even smaller boxes. One of these very small boxes contains drugs to treat bacterial diseases; these are called *antibacterial agents*. Another of these very small boxes contains drugs to treat fungal diseases; these are called *antifungal agents*. Other very small boxes contain drugs to treat protozoal diseases (*antiprotozoal agents*) and drugs to treat viral infections (*antiviral agents*). To appropriately treat a particular disease, a clinician[b] must select a drug from the appropriate box. To treat a fungal infection, for example, the clinician must select a drug from the box containing antifungal agents.

extract of cinchona bark was effective in treating malaria. During the 16th and 17th centuries, the alchemists of Europe searched for ways to cure smallpox, syphilis, and many other diseases that were rampant during that period of history. Many of the mercury and arsenic chemicals that were used frequently caused more damage to the patient than to the pathogen.

The chemotherapeutic agents used to treat infectious diseases are collectively referred to as antimicrobial agents.[a] Thus, an *antimicrobial agent* is any chemical (drug) used to treat an infectious disease, either by inhibiting or killing pathogens in vivo. Drugs used to treat bacterial diseases are called *antibacterial agents*, whereas those used to treat fungal diseases are called *antifungal agents*. Drugs used to treat protozoal diseases are called *antiprotozoal agents*, and those used to treat viral diseases are called *antiviral agents*.

> The chemotherapeutic agents used to treat infectious diseases are collectively referred to as antimicrobial agents.

Some antimicrobial agents are antibiotics. By definition, an *antibiotic* is a substance produced by a microorganism that is effective in killing or inhibiting the growth of other microorganisms. Although all antibiotics are antimicrobial agents, not all antimicrobial agents are antibiotics; therefore, the terms

> An antibiotic is a substance produced by a microorganism that is effective in killing or inhibiting the growth of other microorganisms.

are not synonyms and care should be taken to use the terms correctly.

Antibiotics are produced by certain moulds and bacteria, usually those that live in soil. The antibiotics produced by soil organisms give them a selective advantage in the struggle for the available nutrients in the soil. Penicillin and cephalosporins are examples of antibiotics produced by moulds; bacitracin, erythromycin, and chloramphenicol are examples of antibiotics produced by bacteria. Although originally produced by microorganisms, many antibiotics are now synthesized or manufactured in pharmaceutical laboratories. Also, many antibiotics have been chemically modified to kill a wider variety of pathogens or reduce side effects; these modified antibiotics are called *semisynthetic antibiotics*. Semisynthetic antibiotics include semisynthetic penicillins, such as ampicillin and carbenicillin. Antibiotics are primarily antibacterial agents and are thus used to treat bacterial diseases.

> Antibiotics are primarily antibacterial agents and are thus used to treat bacterial diseases.

---

[a] Technically, an antumicrobial agent is *any* chemical agent that kills or inhibits the growth of microbes. However, throughout this book, the term is used in reference to drugs that are used to treat infectious diseases.

[b] The term *clinician* is used throughout this book to refer to a physician or other healthcare professional who is authorized to make diagnoses and prescribe medications.

HISTORICAL NOTE

The First Antibiotics

In 1928, **Alexander Fleming**, a Scottish bacteriologist, accidentally discovered the first antibiotic when he noticed that growth of contaminant *Penicillium notatum* mould colonies on his culture plates was inhibiting the growth of *Staphylococcus* bacteria (Fig. 9-1). Fleming gave the name "penicillin" to the inhibitory substance being produced by the mould. He found that broth cultures of the mould were not toxic to laboratory animals and that they destroyed staphylococci and other bacteria. He speculated that penicillin might be useful in treating infectious diseases caused by these organisms. As was stated by Kenneth B. Raper in 1978, "Contamination of his *Staphylococcus* plate by a mould was an accident; but Fleming's recognition of a potentially important phenomenon was no accident, for Pasteur's observation that 'chance favors the prepared mind' was never more apt than with Fleming and penicillin."

During World War II, two biochemists, **Sir Howard Walter Florey** and **Ernst Boris Chain**, purified penicillin and demonstrated its effectiveness in the treatment of various bacterial infections. By 1942, the U.S. drug industry was able to produce sufficient penicillin for human use, and the search for other antibiotics began. (Earlier—in 1935—a chemist named **Gerhard Domagk** discovered that the red dye, Prontosil, was effective against streptococcal infections in mice. Further research demonstrated that Prontosil was degraded or broken down in the body into sulfanilamide, and that sulfanilamide [a sulfa drug] was the effective agent. Although sulfanilamide is an antimicrobial agent, it is not an antibiotic because it is not produced by a microorganism.) In 1944, **Selman Waksman** and his colleagues isolated streptomycin (the first antituberculosis drug) and subsequently discovered antibiotics such as chloramphenicol, tetracycline, and erythromycin in soil samples. It was Waksman who first used the term "antibiotic." For their outstanding contributions to medicine, these investigators—Ehrlich, Fleming, Florey, Chain, Waksman, and Domagk—were all Nobel Prize recipients at various times.

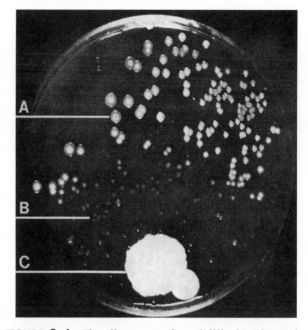

FIGURE 9-1. The discovery of penicillin by Alexander Fleming. (A) Colonies of *Staphylococcus aureus* (a bacterium) are growing well in this area of the plate. **(B)** Colonies are poorly developed in this area of the plate because of an antibiotic (penicillin) being produced by the colony of *P. notatum* (a mould) shown at **C**. (This photograph originally appeared in the *British Journal of Experimental Pathology* in 1929.) (From Winn WC Jr., et al. Koneman's Color Atlas and Textbook of Diagnostic Microbiology, 6th ed. Philadelphia: JB Lippincott, 2006.)

Unfortunately, most antimicrobial agents have some side effects, produce allergic reactions, or permit development of resistant mutant pathogens.

HOW ANTIMICROBIAL AGENTS WORK

To be acceptable, an antimicrobial agent must inhibit or destroy the pathogen without damaging the host. To accomplish this, the agent must target a metabolic process or structure possessed by the pathogen but not possessed by the host (i.e., the infected person).

The five most common mechanisms of action of antimicrobial agents are as follows:

- Inhibition of cell wall synthesis
- Damage to cell membranes
- Inhibition of nucleic acid synthesis (either DNA or RNA synthesis)
- Inhibition of protein synthesis
- Inhibition of enzyme activity

ANTIBACTERIAL AGENTS

Sulfonamide drugs inhibit production of folic acid (a vitamin) in those bacteria that require *p*-aminobenzoic acid

CHARACTERISTICS OF AN IDEAL ANTIMICROBIAL AGENT

The ideal antimicrobial agent should:

- Kill or inhibit the growth of pathogens
- Cause no damage to the host
- Cause no allergic reaction in the host
- Be stable when stored in solid or liquid form
- Remain in specific tissues in the body long enough to be effective
- Kill the pathogens before they mutate and become resistant to it

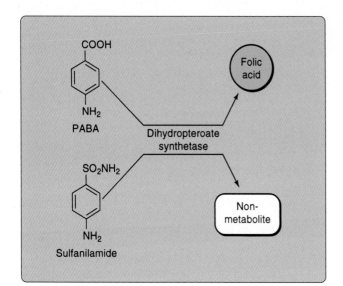

FIGURE 9-2. The effect of sulfonamide drugs. See text for details.

(PABA) to synthesize folic acid. Because the sulfonamide molecule is similar in shape to the PABA molecule, bacteria attempt to metabolize sulfonamide to produce folic acid (Fig.

> Bacteriostatic drugs inhibit growth of bacteria, whereas bactericidal agents kill bacteria.

9-2). However, the enzymes that convert PABA to folic acid cannot produce folic acid from the sulfonamide molecule. Without folic acid, bacteria cannot produce certain essential proteins and finally die. Sulfa drugs, therefore, are called competitive inhibitors; that is, they inhibit growth of microorganisms by competing with an enzyme required to produce an essential metabolite. Sulfa drugs are *bacteriostatic*, meaning that they inhibit growth of bacteria (as opposed to a *bactericidal agent*, which kills bacteria). Cells of humans and animals do not synthesize folic acid from PABA; they get folic acid from the food they eat. Consequently, they are unaffected by sulfa drugs.

In most Gram-positive bacteria, including streptococci and staphylococci, penicillin interferes with the synthesis and cross-linking of peptidoglycan, a component of bacterial cell walls. Thus, by inhibiting cell wall synthesis, penicillin destroys the bacteria. Why doesn't penicillin also destroy human cells? Because human cells do not have cell walls.

There are other antimicrobial agents that have a similar action; they inhibit a specific step that is essential to the microorganism's metabolism and, thereby, cause its destruction. Antibiotics like vancomycin, which de-

stroys only Gram-positive bacteria, and colistin and nalidixic acid, which destroy only Gram-negative bacteria, are referred to as *narrow-spectrum antibiotics*. Those that are destructive to both Gram-positive and Gram-negative bacteria are called *broad-spectrum antibiotics*. Examples of broad-spectrum antibiotics are ampicillin, chloramphenicol, and tetracycline. Tables 9-1 and 9-2 contain information about some of the antimicrobial drugs most frequently used to treat bacterial infections.

> Narrow spectrum antibiotics kill *either* Gram-positive or Gram-negative bacteria, whereas broad spectrum antibiotics kill *both* Gram-positives and Gram-negatives.

Antimicrobial agents work well against bacterial pathogens because the bacteria (being procaryotic) have different cellular structures and metabolic pathways that can be disrupted or destroyed by drugs that do not damage the eucaryotic host's cells. As mentioned earlier, bactericidal agents kill bacteria, whereas bacteriostatic agents stop them from growing and dividing. Bacteriostatic agents should only be used in patients whose host defense mechanisms (Chapters 15 and 16) are functioning properly (i.e., only in patients whose bodies are capable of killing the pathogen once its multiplication is stopped). Bacteriostatic agents should not be used in immunosuppressed or leukopenic patients (patients having an abnormally low number of white blood cells). Some of the mechanisms by which antibacterial agents kill or inhibit bacteria are shown in Table 9-2.

Virtually all of the antibacterial agents currently available either kill bacteria or inhibit their growth. Researchers are attempting to develop antibacterial agents that target bacterial virulence factors, rather than targeting the pathogens themselves. Bacterial virulence factors include various harmful substances, like toxins and enzymes, produced by bacteria. Virulence factors are discussed in detail in Chapter 14.

Some Major Categories of Antibacterial Agents

Penicillins. Penicillins are referred to as β-lactam drugs because their molecular structure includes a four-sided ring structure known as a β-lactam ring (shown in Figure 9-3).[c] Penicillins interfere with the synthesis of bacterial cell walls and have maximum effect on bacteria that are actively dividing. They are bactericidal drugs. Except for drug-resistant strains, penicillin G is effective against Gram-positive cocci (e.g., *Staphylococcus aureus*, *Streptococcus pneumoniae*, *Streptococcus pyogenes*), Gram-positive bacilli (e.g., *Bacillus anthracis*, *Corynebacterium diphtheriae*), Gram-negative cocci (e.g., *Neisseria gonorrhoeae*, *Neisseria meningitidis*), some anaerobic bacteria (e.g., *Clostridium perfringens*), and some spirochetes (e.g., *Treponema*

STUDY AID
Spelling Tip
Note that the word bacteriostatic contains an "o," whereas the word bactericidal does not.

---

[c] The symbol "β" is the Greek letter "beta." The complete Greek alphabet can be found in Appendix D.

TABLE 9-1	Antibacterial Agents Listed by Class or Category	
CLASS/CATEGORY	DESCRIPTION/SOURCE	EXAMPLES OF ANTIBACTERIAL AGENTS WITHIN THE CLASS OR CATEGORY
Penicillins[a]	Naturally occurring penicillins; produced by moulds in the genus *Penicillium*	Benzylpenicillin (penicillin G), phenoxymethyl penicillin (penicillin V)
	Semisynthetic penicillins: broad-spectrum aminopenicillins	Amoxicillin, ampicillin
	Semisynthetic penicillins: broad-spectrum carboxypenicillins	Carbenicillin, ticarcillin
	Semisynthetic penicillins: broad-spectrum ureidopenicillins	Azlocillin, mezlocillin, piperacillin
	Semisynthetic penicillins: penicillinase-resistant penicillins	Cloxacillin, dicloxacillin, methicillin, nafcillin
	Penicillin + β-lactamase inhibitor	Amoxicillin-clavulanic acid (Augmentin), ampicillin-sulbactam (Unasyn), piperacillin-tazobactam (Zosyn), ticarcillin-clavulanic acid (Timentin)
Cephalosporins[a]	Derivatives of fermentation products of the mould, *Cephalosporium* (*Acremonium*)	Narrow-spectrum (first-generation) cephalosporins: cefazolin, cephalothin, cephapirin, cephradine; first-generation cephalosporins have good activity against Gram-positive bacteria and relatively modest activity against Gram-negative bacteria
		Expanded-spectrum (second-generation) cephalosporins: cefamandole, cefonicid, cefuroxime; second-generation cephalosporins have increased activity against Gram-negative bacteria
		Cephamycins (second-generation cephalosporins): cefmetazole, cefotetan, cefoxitin
		Broad-spectrum (third-generation) cephalosporins: cefoperazone, cefotaxime, ceftazidime, ceftizoxime, ceftriaxone; third-generation cephalosporins are less active against Gram-positive bacteria than first- and second-generation cephalosporins but are more active against members of the Enterobacteriaceae family and *Pseudomonas aeruginosa*
		Extended-spectrum (fourth-generation) cephalosporin: cefepime; fourth-generation cephalosporins have increased activity against Gram-negative bacteria
Monobactam[a]	Synthetic drug	Aztreonam
Carbapenems[a]	Imipenem is a semisynthetic derivative of thienamycin, produced by *Streptomyces* spp.	Ertapenem, imipenem, meropenem
Aminocyclitol	Produced by *Streptomyces spectabilis*	Spectinomycin, trospectinomycin
Aminoglycosides	Naturally occurring antibiotics or semisynthetic derivatives from *Micromonospora* spp. or *Streptomyces* spp.	Amikacin, gentamicin, kanamycin, netilmicin, streptomycin, tobramycin
Ansamycin	Semisynthetic antibiotic derived from compounds produced by *Streptomyces mediterranei*	Rifampin

TABLE 9-1	Antibacterial Agents Listed by Class or Category (continued)	
CLASS/CATEGORY	**DESCRIPTION/SOURCE**	**EXAMPLES OF ANTIBACTERIAL AGENTS WITHIN THE CLASS OR CATEGORY**
Quinolones	Synthetic drugs	Cinoxacin, garenoxacin, nalidixic acid
Fluoroquinolones	Synthetic drugs	Ciprofloxacin, clinafloxacin, enoxacin, fleroxacin, gatifloxacin, gemifloxacin, grepafloxacin, levofloxacin, lomefloxacin, moxifloxacin, norfloxacin, ofloxacin, sparfloxacin, trovafloxacin
Macrolides	Erythromycin is produced by *Streptomyces erythraeus*; the others are natural analogs of erythromycin or semisynthetic antibiotics	Azithromycin, clarithromycin, dirithromycin, erythromycin
Ketolides	Semisynthetic derivative of erythromycin	Telithromycin
Tetracyclines	Tetracycline is produced by *Streptomyces rimosus*; the others are semisynthetic antibiotics	Doxycycline, minocycline, tetracycline
Lincosamide	Clindamycin is a semisynthetic antibiotic	Clindamycin
Glycopeptide	Produced by *Streptomyces orientales*	Vancomycin
Lipopeptide	Semisynthetic antibiotic	Teicoplanin
Streptogramins	Produced by *Streptomyces* spp.	Quinupristin-dalfopristin
Oxazolidinone	Synthetic drug	Linezolid
Sulfonamides	Synthetic drugs derived from sulfanilamide	Sulfacetamide, sulfadiazine, sulfadoxine, sulfamethizole, sulfamethoxazole (SMX), sulfisoxazole, trisulfapyrimidine (triple sulfa)
Trimethroprim	Synthetic drug	Used alone or in combination with SMX (the combination is also called co-trimoxazole)
Polypeptides	Originally produced by *Bacillus polymyxa* Originally produced by *Bacillus licheniformis* (formerly named *Bacillus subtilis*)	Polymyxins: polymyxin B, polymixin E (colistin) Bacitracin
Phenicol	Originally produced by *Streptomyces venezuelae*	Chloramphenicol
Nitroimidazole	Synthetic drug	Metronidazole
Nitrofuran	Synthetic drug	Nitrofurantoin
Fosfomycin	Originally produced by *Streptomyces* spp.	

Sources: Winn WC Jr, et al. Koneman's Color Atlas and Textbook of Diagnostic Microbiology. 6th ed. Philadelphia: Lippincott Williams & Wilkins, 2006. Yao JDC, Moellering RC Jr. Antibacterial Agents. In: Murray PR, Baron EJ, Jorgensen JH, et al., eds. Manual of Clinical Microbiology. 8th ed. Washington, DC: ASM Press, 2003.

[a]β-lactam antibiotics (i.e., antibiotics that contain a β-lactam ring).

TABLE 9-2   Antibacterial Agents Listed by Mechanism of Action

MODE OF ACTION	AGENT	SPECTRUM OF ACTIVITY	BACTERICIDAL OR BACTERIOSTATIC
Inhibition of cell wall synthesis	Aztreonam	Gram-negative bacteria	Bactericidal
	Bacitracin (also disrupts cell membranes)	Broad spectrum[a]	Bactericidal
	Carbapenem	Broad spectrum	Bactericidal
	Cephalosporins	Broad spectrum	Bactericidal
	Daptomycin	Broad spectrum	Bactericidal
	Fosfomycin	Broad spectrum	Bactericidal
	Penicillins and semisynthetic penicillins	Broad spectrum	Bactericidal
	Vancomycin	Gram-positive bacteria	Bactericidal
Inhibition of protein synthesis	Aminoglycosides	Primarily Gram-negative bacteria and *Staphylococcus aureus*; not effective against anaerobes	Bactericidal
	Chloramphenicol	Broad spectrum	Bacteriostatic
	Clindamycin	Most Gram-positive bacteria and some Gram-negative bacteria; highly active against anaerobes	Bacteriostatic or bactericidal, depending upon drug concentration and bacterial species
	Erythromycin and other macrolides	Most Gram-positive bacteria and some Gram-negative bacteria	Bacteriostatic (usually); bactericidal at higher concentrations
	Ketolides	Broad spectrum	Bacteriostatic
	Linezolid	Gram-positive bacteria	Bacteriostatic
	Mupirocin	Broad spectrum	Bacteriostatic
	Streptogramins	Primarily Gram-positive bacteria	Bactericidal
	Tetracyclines	Broad-spectrum and some intracellular bacterial pathogens	Bacteriostatic
Inhibition of nucleic acid synthesis	Rifampin	Gram-positive and some Gram-negative bacteria (e.g., *Neisseria meningitidis*)	Bactericidal
	Quinolones and fluoroquinolones (e.g., ciprofloxacin, levofloxacin, moxifloxacin)	Broad spectrum	Bactericidal
Destruction of DNA	Metronidazole	Effective against anaerobes	Bactericidal
Disruption of cell membranes	Polymyxin B and polymyxin E (colistin)	Gram-negative bacteria	Bactericidal
Inhibition of enzyme activity	Sulfonamides	Primarily Gram-positive bacteria and some Gram-negative bacteria	Bacteriostatic
	Trimethoprim	Gram-positive and many Gram-negative bacteria	Bacteriostatic

[a]Effective against both Gram-positive and Gram-negative bacteria, but spectrum may vary with the individual antimicrobial agent.

FIGURE 9-3. Sites of β-lactamase attack on penicillin and cephalosporin molecules. See p. 153 for details.

pallidum). Some extended-spectrum penicillins are used to treat infections caused by Gram-negative bacilli.

Cephalosporins. The cephalosporins are also β-lactam antibiotics and, like penicillin, are produced by moulds. Also like penicillins, cephalosporins interfere with cell wall synthesis and are bactericidal. The cephalosporins are classified as first-, second-, third-, and fourth-generation cephalosporins (Table 9-3). The first-generation agents are active primarily against Gram-positive bacteria. Second-generation cephalosporins have increased activity against Gram-negative bacteria, and third-generation cephalosporins have even greater activity against Gram-negatives (including *Pseudomonas aeruginosa*). Cefepime is a fourth-generation cephalosporin with activity against both Gram-positives and Gram-negatives, including *P. aeruginosa*).

Tetracyclines. Tetracyclines are broad-spectrum drugs that exert their effect by targeting bacterial ribosomes. They are bacteriostatic. Tetracyclines are effective against a wide variety of bacteria, including chlamydias, mycoplasmas, rickettsias, *Vibrio cholerae*, and spirochetes like *Borrelia* spp. and *T. pallidum*.

Aminoglycosides. Aminoglcosides are bactericidal broad-spectrum drugs that inhibit bacterial protein synthesis. Aminoglycosides are effective against a wide variety of aerobic Gram-negative bacteria, but are ineffective against anaerobes. They are used to treat infections with members of the family Enterobacteriaceae (e.g., *Escherichia coli* and *Enterobacter, Klebsiella, Proteus, Serratia,* and *Yersinia* spp.), as well as *P. aeruginosa* and *V. cholerae*.

Macrolides. Macrolides inhibit protein synthesis. They are considered bacteriostatic at lower doses and bactericidal at higher doses. The macrolides include erythromycin, clarithromycin, and azithromycin. They are effective against chlamydias, mycoplasmas, *T. pallidum*, and *Legionella* spp.

Fluoroquinolones. Fluoroquinolones are bactericidal drugs that inhibit DNA synthesis. The most commonly used fluoroquinolone, ciprofloxacin, is effective against members of the family Enterobacteriaceae and *P. aeruginosa*.

Multidrug Therapy

In some cases, a single antimicrobial agent is not sufficient to destroy all the pathogens that develop during the course of a disease; thus, two or more drugs may be used simultaneously to kill all the pathogens and to prevent resistant mutant pathogens from emerging. In tuberculosis, for example, in which multidrug-resistant strains of *Mycobacterium tuberculosis* are frequently encountered, four drugs (isoniazid, rifampin, pyrazinamide, and ethambutol) are routinely prescribed, and as many as 12 drugs may be required for especially resistant strains.

Synergism versus Antagonism

The use of two antimicrobial agents to treat an infectious disease sometimes produces a degree of pathogen killing that is far greater than that achieved by either drug alone. This is known as *synergism*. Synergism is a good thing! Many urinary, respiratory, and gastrointestinal infections respond particularly well to a combination of trimethoprim and sulfamethoxazole, a combination referred to as co-trimoxazole; brand names include Bactrim and Septra.

When the use of two antimicrobial agents to treat an infectious disease produces a degree of pathogen killing that is far greater than that achieved by either drug alone, the phenomenon is known as synergism.

There are situations, however, when two drugs are prescribed (perhaps by two different clinicians who are treating the patient's infection) that actually work against each other. This is known as *antagonism*. The extent of pathogen killing is less than that achieved by either drug alone. Antagonism is a bad thing!

When the use of two drugs produces an extent of pathogen killing that is less than that achieved by either drug alone, the phenomenon is known as antagonism.

TABLE 9-3	Cephalosporin Antibiotics	

The more useful drugs are shown in **bold print.**
Gram-positive bacteria are in blue print.
Gram-negative bacteria are in red print.

GENERATION	NAME OF DRUG	THERAPEUTIC APPLICATIONS
First	*Cefazolin*	*Staphylococcus aureus* *
	Cefadroxil	*Staphylococcus epidermidis*
	Cephalexin	*Streptococcus pneumoniae*
	Cephalothin	*Streptococcus pyogenes*
	Cephapirin	Anaerobic Gram-positive cocci
	Cephadine	*Escherichia coli*
		Klebsiella pneumoniae
		Proteus mirabilis
Second	*Cefacior*	*S. pneumoniae*
	Cefamandole	*S. pyogenes*
	Cefonicid	Anaerobic Gram-positive cocci
	Cefmetazole	*Neisseria gonorrhoeae*
	Cefotetan	*Enterobacter aerogenes*
	Cefoxitin	*E. coli*
	Cefuroxime	*K. pneumoniae*
	Cefuroxime axetil	*P. mirabilis*
		Haemophilus influenzae
Third	Cefdinir	*N. gonorrhoeae*
	Cefixime	*E. aerogenes*
	Cefoperazone	*E. coli*
	Cefotaxime	*K. pneumoniae*
	Ceftazidime	*P. mirabilis*
	Cefibuten	*H. influenzae*
	Ceftizoxime	*Pseudomonas aeruginosa*
	Ceftriaxone	

*Except for methicillin-resistant *S. aureus* (MRSA) strains. (Modified from Harvey RA, et al. Lippincott's Illustrated Reviews: Microbiology, 2nd ed. Philadelphia: Lipincott Williams & Wilkins, 2007.)

ANTIFUNGAL AGENTS

It is much more difficult to use antimicrobial drugs against fungal and protozoal pathogens, because they are eucaryotic cells; thus, the drugs tend to be more toxic to the patient. Most antifungal agents work in one of three ways:

Antifungal and antiprotozoal drugs tend to be more toxic to the patient because, like the infected human, they are eucaryotic organisms.

- By binding with cell membrane sterols (e.g., nystatin and amphotericin B)
- By interfering with sterol synthesis (e.g., clotrimazole and miconazole)
- By blocking mitosis or nucleic acid synthesis (e.g., griseofulvin and 5-flucytosine)

Examples of antifungal agents are shown in Table 9-4.

ANTIPROTOZOAL AGENTS

Antiprotozoal drugs are usually quite toxic to the host and work by (a) interfering with DNA and RNA synthesis (e.g., chloroquine, pentamidine, and quinacrine), or (b) interfering with protozoal metabolism (e.g., metronidazole; brand name Flagyl). Table 9-5 lists several antiprotozoal drugs and the protozoal diseases they are used to treat.

ANTIVIRAL AGENTS

Antiviral agents are the newest weapons in antimicrobial methodology. Until recent years, there were no drugs for the treatment of viral diseases. Antiviral agents are particularly difficult to develop and use because viruses are produced within host cells. A few drugs have been found to be effective in certain viral infections; these work by

TABLE 9-4	Antifungal Agents
DRUG[a]	FUNGAL DISEASE(S) THAT THE DRUG IS USED TO TREAT
Amphotericin B	Aspergillosis, blastomycosis, invasive candidiasis, coccidioidomycosis, cryptococcosis, fusariosis, histoplasmosis, mucormycosis, paracoccidioidomycosis, penicilliosis, systemic sporotrichosis
Atovaquone	*Pneumocystis* pneumonia
Echinocandins	Aspergillosis, candidiasis
Fluconazole	Blastomycosis; oropharyngeal, esophageal, and invasive candidiasis; coccidioidomycosis, cryptococcosis, fusariosis, histoplasmosis, sporotrichosis
Flucytosine	Candidiasis, chromoblastomycosis, cryptococcosis
Griseofulvin	Dermatomycosis (less toxic drugs are available, however)
Itraconazole	Aspergillosis, blastomycosis, invasive candidiasis, coccidioidomycosis, cryptococcosis, histoplasmosis, paracoccidioidomycosis, penicilliosis, pseudallescheriasis, scedosporiosis, cutaneous or systemic sporotrichosis
Ketoconazole	Blastomycosis, coccidioidomycosis, histoplasmosis, paracoccidioidomycosis
Terbinafine	Dermatomycosis
Trimethoprim-sulfamethoxazole	*Pneumocystis* pneumonia
Voriconazole	Aspergillosis, invasive candidiasis, scedosporiasis

[a]Note: This information is provided solely to acquaint readers of this book with the names of some antifungal agents and should not be construed as advice regarding recommended therapy.

inhibiting viral replication within cells. Some antiviral agents are listed in Table 9-6.

The first antiviral agent effective against human immunodeficiency virus (HIV) (the causative agent of acquired immune deficiency syndrome or acquired immunodeficiency syndrome [AIDS])—zidovudine (also known as azidothymidine [AZT])—was introduced in 1987. A variety of additional drugs for the treatment of HIV infection were introduced subsequently. Certain of these antiviral agents are administered simultaneously, in combinations referred to as "cocktails." Unfortunately, such cocktails are quite expensive and some strains of HIV have become resistant to some of the drugs.

DRUG RESISTANCE

"Superbugs"

These days, it is quite common to hear about drug-resistant bacteria, or "superbugs," as they have been labeled by the press. Although "superbug" can refer to an organism that is resistant to only one antimicrobial agent, the term usually refers to multiply drug-resistant organisms (i.e., organisms that are resistant to more than one antimicrobial agent). Infections caused by superbugs

are much more difficult to treat. Especially troublesome superbugs include:

- Methicillin-resistant *S. aureus* (MRSA) and methicillin-resistant *Staphylococcus epidermidis* (MRSE). These strains are resistant to all antistaphylococcal drugs except vancomycin and one or two more recently developed drugs (e.g., Synercid and Zyvox). Some strains of *S. aureus*, called vancomycin-intermediate *S. aureus* (VISA), have developed resistance to the usual dosages of vancomycin, necessitating the use of higher doses to treat infections caused by these organisms. Recently, strains of *S. aureus* (called vancomycin-resistant *S. aureus* or VRSA strains) have been isolated that are resistant to even the highest practical doses of vancomycin. *S. aureus* is a very common cause of healthcare-associated infections[d] (Figure 9-4).
- Vancomycin-resistant *Enterococcus* spp. (VRE). These strains are resistant to most antienterococcal drugs, including vancomycin. *Enterococcus* spp. are common causes of healthcare-associated infections, especially urinary tract infections.

[d] The term *healthcare-associated infections* refers to infections acquired by individuals while they are hospitalized or within other types of healthcare facilities. Healthcare-associated infections are discussed in detail in Chapter 12.

TABLE 9-5   Antiprotozoal Agents

DRUG[a]	PROTOZOAL DISEASE(S) THAT THE DRUG IS USED TO TREAT
Amphotericin B	Primary amebic meningoencephalitis, mucocutaneous leishmaniasis
Artemisinin derivatives	Multidrug-resistant *Plasmodium falciparum* malaria
Benznidazole	American trypanosomiasis (Chagas' disease)
Chloroquine phosphate or quinidine gluconate or quinine dihydrochloride	Malaria (except for chloroquine-resistant *P. falciparum* malaria and chloroquine-resistant *Plasmodium vivax* malaria)
Clindamycin plus quinine	Babesiosis
Diloxanide furoate	Amebiasis
Eflornithine	African trypanosomiasis (with or without CNS involvement)
Furazolidone	Giardiasis
Halofantrine	Chloroquine-resistant *P. falciparum* malaria
Iodoquinol	Amebiasis, balantidiasis, *Dientamoeba fragilis* infection
Mefloquine	Chloroquine-resistant *P. falciparum* and *P. vivax* malaria
Melarsoprol	African trypanosomiasis (with CNS involvement)
Metronidazole	Amebiasis, giardiasis, trichomoniasis
Nifurtimox	American trypanosomiasis (Chagas' disease)
Nitazoxanide	Giardiasis in children and cryptosporidiosis
Paromomycin	Amebiasis, cryptosporidiosis, *D. fragilis* infection, cutaneous leishmaniasis
Pentamidine Isethionate	African sleeping sickness (without CNS involvement), leishmaniasis
Primaquine phosphate	Malaria
Proguanil hydrochloride	Malaria
Pyrimethamine plus sulfadiazine	*P. falciparum* malaria, toxoplasmosis
Quinacrine hydrochloride	Giardiasis
Quinidine gluconate	*P. falciparum* malaria
Quinine	Malaria
Spiramycin	Toxoplasmosis
Stibogluconate sodium	Visceral, cutaneous, and mucocutaneous leishmaniasis
Suramin	African trypanosomiasis (with no CNS involvement)
Tetracycline hydrochloride	Balantidiasis, *Dientamoeba fragilis* infection; can be used with quinine or quinidine for *P. falciparum* malaria
Tinidazole	Amebiasis, giardiasis, trichomoniasis
Trimethoprim-sulfamethoxazole	Cyclosporiasis, isosporiasis

[a]This information is provided solely to acquaint the reader with the names of some antiprotozoal agents and should not be construed as advice regarding recommended therapy.
CNS, central nervous system.

TABLE 9-6	Antiviral Agents
VIRUS/VIRAL INFECTION(S)	**ANTIVIRAL AGENTS**[a]
Herpes simplex infections	Acyclovir, cidofovir, famciclovir, fomivirsen, foscarnet, ganciclovir, penciclovir, valacyclovir, valganciclovir, vidarabine
Respiratory viruses	Amantadine (influenza A virus), oseltamivir (influenza A and B viruses), ribavirin (respiratory syncytial virus, influenza A and B viruses, parainfluenza virus), rimantadine (influenza A virus), zanamivir (influenza A and B viruses)
HIV: nucleoside reverse transcriptase inhibitors	Abacavir, didanosine, lamivudine, stavudine, tenofovir, zalcitabine, zidovudine (AZT, ZDV)
HIV: nonnucleoside reverse transcriptase inhibitors	Delavirdine, efavirenz, nevirapine
HIV: protease inhibitors	Amprenavir, indinavir, lopinavir, nelfinavir, ritonavir, saquinavir

[a]This information is provided solely to acquaint the reader with the names of some antiviral agents and should not be construed as advice regarding recommended therapy.

- Multidrug-resistant *M. tuberculosis* (MDR-TB). These strains are resistant to the two most effective first-line therapeutic drugs—isoniazid and rifampin. Extensively drug-resistant strains, called XDR-TB are also resistant to the most effective second-line therapeutic drugs—fluoroquinolones and at least one of the following: amikacin, kanamycin, capreomycin. Some drug-resistant strains of *M. tuberculosis* are resistant to *all* antitubercular drugs and combinations of these drugs. Patients infected with these strains may have a lung or section of lung removed—just as in the pre-antibiotic days—and many will die. Tuberculosis remains one of the major killers worldwide.
- Multidrug-resistant strains of *Acinetobacter baumannii*, *Burkholderia cepacia*, *E. coli*, *Klebsiella pneumoniae*, *N. gonorrhoeae*, *Pseudomonas* spp., *Ralstonia pickettii*, *Salmonella* spp., *Shigella* spp., and *Stenotrophomonas maltophilia*.
- β-Lactamase–producing strains of *S. pneumoniae* and *Haemophilus influenzae* (β-lactamases are discussed later in the chapter). Some strains of these pathogens have become multiply resistant.
- Carbapenemase-producing *K. pneumoniae*. These strains produce a β-lactamase that destroys penicillins, cephalosporins, aztreonam, carbapenemes, and other antibiotics.

It is important to note that bacteria are not the only microorganisms that have developed resistance to drugs. Certain viruses (including HIV, herpes simplex viruses, and influenza viruses), fungi (both yeasts and moulds), parasitic protozoa, and helminths have also become drug-resistant. Parasitic protozoa that have become drug-resistant include strains of *Plasmodium falciparum*, *Trichomonas vaginalis*, *Leishmania* spp., and *Giardia lamblia*.

> Although the term *superbug* most often refers to multiply resistant bacteria, other types of microbes (e.g., viruses, fungi, protozoa) have also become multiply drug resistant.

How Bacteria Become Resistant to Drugs

How do bacteria become resistant to antimicrobial agents? Some bacteria are naturally resistant to a particular antimicrobial agent because they lack the specific target site for that drug (e.g., mycoplasmas have no cell walls and are, therefore, resistant to any drugs that interfere with cell wall synthesis). Other bacteria are naturally resistant because the drug is unable to cross the organism's cell wall or cell membrane and, thus, cannot reach its site of action (e.g., ribosomes). Such resistance is known as *intrinsic resistance*.

It is also possible for bacteria that were once susceptible to a particular drug to become resistant to it; this is called *acquired resistance*. Bacteria usually acquire resistance to antibiotics and other antimicrobial agents by one of four mechanisms, each of which is shown in Table 9-7 and briefly described in this list:

- Before a drug can enter a bacterial cell, molecules of the drug must first bind (attach) to proteins on the surface of the cell; these protein molecules are called *drug-binding sites*. A chromosomal mutation can result in an alteration in the structure of the drug-binding site, so that the drug is no longer able to bind to the cell. If the drug cannot bind to the cell, it cannot enter the cell, and the organism is, therefore, resistant to the drug.
- To enter a bacterial cell, a drug must be able to pass through the cell wall and cell membrane. A chromosomal mutation can result in an alteration in the structure of the cell membrane, which in turn can change the permeability of the membrane. If the drug is no longer

MRSA FACT SHEET

What is MRSA?

MRSA is methicillin-resistant *Staphylococcus aureus*, a potentially dangerous type of staph bacteria that is resistant to certain antibiotics and may cause skin and other infections. As with all regular staph infections, recognizing the signs and receiving treatment for MRSA skin infections in the early stages reduces the chances of the infection becoming severe. MRSA is spread by:

> Having direct contact with another person's infection
> Sharing personal items, such as towels or razors, that have touched infected skin
> Touching surfaces or items, such as used bandages, contaminated with MRSA

What are the signs and symptoms?

Most staph skin infections, including MRSA, appear as a bump or infected area on the skin that may be:

> Red
> Swollen
> Painful
> Warm to the touch
> Full of pus or other drainage
> Accompanied by a fever

What if I suspect an MRSA skin infection?

Cover the area with a bandage and contact your healthcare professional. It is especially important to contact your healthcare professional if signs and symptoms of an MRSA skin infection are accompanied by a fever.

How are MRSA skin infections treated?

Treatment for MRSA skin infections may include having a healthcare professional drain the infection and, in some cases, prescribe an antibiotic. Do not attempt to drain the infection yourself – doing so could worsen or spread it to others. If you are given an antibiotic, be sure to take all of the doses (even if the infection is getting better), unless your healthcare professional tells you to stop taking it.

How can I protect my family from MRSA skin infections?

> Know the signs of MRSA skin infections and get treated early
> Keep cuts and scrapes clean and covered
> Encourage good hygiene such as cleaning hands regularly
> Discourage sharing of personal items such as towels and razors

© Bernard Cohen, MD, Dermatlas; www.dermatlas.org   http://phil.cdc.gov

For more information, please call 1-800-CDC-INFO or visit www.cdc.gov/MRSA.

Developed with support from the CDC Foundation through an educational grant from Pfizer Inc.

FIGURE 9-4. MRSA fact sheet. (From the Centers for Disease Control and Prevention, http://www.cdc.gov/mrsa)

able to pass through the cell membrane, it cannot reach its target (e.g., a ribosome or the DNA of the cell), and the organism is now resistant to the drug.

• Another way in which bacteria become resistant to a certain drug is by developing the ability to produce an enzyme that destroys or inactivates the drug. Because enzymes are coded for by genes, a bacterial cell would have to acquire a new gene for the cell to be able to produce an enzyme that it never before produced. The primary way in which bacteria acquire new genes is by

TABLE 9-7	Mechanisms by which Bacteria Become Resistant to Antimicrobial Agents
MECHANISM	**EFFECT**
A chromosomal mutation that causes a change in the structure of a drug binding site	The drug cannot bind to the bacterial cell
A chromosomal mutation that causes a change in cell membrane permeability	The drug cannot pass through the cell membrane and thus cannot enter the cell
Acquisition (by conjugation, transduction or transformation) of a gene that enables the bacterium to produce an enzyme that destroys or inactivates the drug	The drug is destroyed or inactivated by the enzyme
Acquisition (by conjugation, transduction, or transformation) of a gene that enables the bacterium to produce a multidrug-resistance (MDR) pump	The drug is pumped out of the cell before it can damage or kill the cell

conjugation (Chapter 7). Often, a plasmid containing such a gene is transferred from one bacterial cell (the donor cell) to another bacterial cell (the recipient cell) during conjugation. For example, many bacteria have become resistant to penicillin because they have acquired the gene for penicillinase production during conjugation. (Penicillinase is described in the following section.) A plasmid containing multiple genes for drug resistance is called a *resistance factor* (R-factor). A recipient cell that receives an R-factor becomes multidrug-resistant (i.e., it becomes a superbug). Bacteria can also acquire new genes by transduction (whereby bacteriophages carry bacterial DNA from one bacterial cell to another) and transformation (the uptake of naked DNA from the environment). (Transduction and transformation were discussed in Chapter 7.)

- A fourth way in which bacteria become resistant to drugs is by developing the ability to produce multidrug-resistance (MDR) pumps (also known as MDR transporters or efflux pumps). An MDR pump enables the cell to pump drugs out of the cell before the drugs can damage or kill the cell. The genes encoding these pumps are often located on plasmids that bacteria receive during conjugation. Bacteria receiving such plasmids become multidrug-resistant (i.e., they become resistant to several drugs).

Thus, bacteria can acquire resistance to antimicrobial agents as a result of chromosomal mutation or the acquisition of new genes by transduction, transformation, and, most commonly, by conjugation.

β-Lactamases

At the heart of every penicillin and cephalosporin molecule is a double-ringed structure, which in penicillins resembles a "house and garage" (see Fig. 9-3).

The "garage" is called the β-lactam ring. Some bacteria produce enzymes that destroy the β-lactam ring; these enzymes are known as β-lactamases. When the β-lactam ring is destroyed, the antibiotic no longer works. Thus, an organism that produces a β-lactamase is resistant to antibiotics containing the β-lactam ring (collectively referred to as β-lactam antibiotics or β-lactams).

There are two types of β-lactamases: penicillinases and cephalosporinases. *Penicillinases* destroy the β-lactam ring in penicillins; thus, an organism that produces penicillinase is resistant to penicillins. *Cephalosporinases* destroy the β-lactam ring in cephalosporins; thus, an organism that produces cephalosporinase is resistant to cephalosporins. Some bacteria produce both types of β-lactamases.

To combat the effect of β-lactamases, drug companies have developed special drugs that combine a β-lactam antibiotic with a β-lactamase inhibitor (e.g., clavulanic acid, sulbactam, or tazobactam). The β-lactam inhibitor irreversibly binds to and inactivates the β-lactamase, thus enabling the companion drug to enter the bacterial cell and disrupt cell wall synthesis. Some of these special combination drugs are:

- Clavulanic acid (clavulanate) combined with amoxicillin (brand name, Augmentin)
- Clavulanic acid (clavulanate) combined with ticarcillin (Timentin)
- Sulbactam combined with ampicillin (Unasyn)
- Tazobactam combined with piperacillin (Zosyn)

A β-lactam antibiotic is an antibiotic that contains a β-lactam ring in its molecular structure.

Penicillinases and cephalosporinases are examples of β-lactamases; they destroy the β-lactam ring in penicillins and cephalosporins, respectively.

Bacteria can acquire resistance to antimicrobial agents as a result of chromosomal mutation or the acquisition of new genes by transduction, transformation, and, most commonly, by conjugation.

SOME STRATEGIES IN THE WAR AGAINST DRUG RESISTANCE

- Education is crucial—education of healthcare professionals and, in turn, education of patients.
- Patients should never pressure clinicians to prescribe antimicrobial agents. Parents must stop demanding antibiotics every time they have a sick child. The majority of sore throats and many respiratory infections are caused by viruses, and viruses are unaffected by antibiotics. Because viruses are not killed by antibiotics, patients and parents should not expect antibiotics when they or their children have viral infections. Instead of demanding antibiotics from clinicians, they should be asking *why* one is being prescribed.
- It is important that clinicians not allow themselves to be pressured by patients. They should prescribe antibiotics only when warranted (i.e., only when there is a demonstrated need for them). Whenever possible, clinicians should collect a specimen for culture and have the Clinical Microbiology Laboratory perform susceptibility testing (Chapter 13) to determine which antimicrobial agents are likely to be effective.
- Clinicians should prescribe an inexpensive, narrow-spectrum drug whenever the laboratory results demonstrate that such a drug effectively kills the pathogen. According to Dr. Stuart B. Levy,[e] by some estimates, at least half of current antibiotic use in the United States is inappropriate—antibiotics are either not indicated at all or they are incorrectly prescribed as the wrong drug, the wrong dosage, or the wrong duration. Another study[f] demonstrated that colds, other upper respiratory infections, and bronchitis accounted for 21% of all antibiotic prescriptions in 1992, although these conditions typically do not benefit from antibiotics.
- Patients must take their antibiotics in the exact manner in which they are prescribed. Healthcare professionals should emphasize this to patients and do a better job explaining exactly how medications should be taken.
- It is critical that clinicians prescribe the appropriate amount of antibiotic necessary to cure the infection. Then, unless instructed otherwise, patients must take *all* their pills—even after they are feeling better. Again, this must be explained and emphasized. If treatments are cut short, there is selective killing of only the most susceptible members of a bacterial population. The more resistant variants are left behind to multiply and cause a new infection.
- Patients should always destroy any excess medications and should never keep antibiotics in their medicine cabinet. Antimicrobial agents, including antibiotics, should be taken only when prescribed and only under a clinician's supervision.
- Unless prescribed by a clinician, antibiotics should never be used in a prophylactic manner—such as to avoid "traveler's diarrhea" when traveling to a foreign country. Taking antibiotics in that manner actually *increases* the chances of developing traveler's diarrhea. The antibiotics kill some of the beneficial indigenous intestinal flora, eliminating the competition for food and space, making it easier for pathogens to gain a foothold.
- Healthcare professionals must practice good infection prevention and control procedures (Chapter 12). Frequent and proper handwashing is essential to prevent the transmission of pathogens from one patient to another. Healthcare professionals should monitor for important pathogens (such as MRSA) within healthcare settings and always isolate patients infected with multidrug-resistant pathogens.

EMPIRIC THERAPY

In some cases, a clinician must initiate therapy before laboratory results are available. This is referred to as *empiric therapy*. In an effort to save the life of a patient, it is sometimes necessary for the clinician to "guess" the most likely pathogen and the drug most likely to be effective. It will be an "educated guess," based on the clinician's prior experiences with the particular type of infectious disease that the patient has. Before writing a prescription for a certain antimicrobial agent, several factors must be taken into consideration by the clinician; some of these are in the following list:

- If the laboratory has reported the identity of the pathogen, the clinician can refer to a "pocket chart" that is available in most hospitals. This pocket chart, published by the Clinical Microbiology Laboratory, contains antimicrobial susceptibility test data that have been accumulated during the past year. The pocket chart provides important information regarding drugs to which various bacterial pathogens were susceptible and resistant (Fig. 9-5).
- Is the patient allergic to any antimicrobial agents? Obviously, it would be unwise to prescribe a drug to which the patient is allergic.
- What is the age of the patient? Certain drugs are contraindicated in very young or very old patients.
- Is the patient pregnant? Certain drugs are known to be or suspected to be teratogenic (i.e., they cause birth defects).
- Is the patient an inpatient or outpatient? Certain drugs can only be administered intravenously and, therefore, cannot be prescribed for outpatients.
- If the patient is an inpatient, the clinician must prescribe a drug that is available in the hospital pharmacy (i.e., a drug that is listed in the hospital formulary).
- What is the site of the patient's infection? If the patient has cystitis (urinary bladder infection), the clinician

[e] Levy SB. The Antibiotic Paradox: How the Misuse of Antibiotics Destroys Their Curative Powers, 2nd ed. Cambridge, MA: Perseus Publishing, 2002.

[f] Gonzales R, et al. Antibiotic prescribing for adults with colds, upper respiratory tract infections, and bronchitis by ambulatory care patients. JAMA 1997;278:901–904.

	E. coli	P. aeruginosa	Klebsiella	Proteus mirabilis	Enterobacter	Proteus sp.	Serratia	Citrobacter
Total isolates	615	371	253	193	107	33	40	56
Percent Sensitive								
Ampicillin	55	1	3	58	3	15	22	7
Carbenicillin	59	88	2	59	74	91	93	24
Timentin	87	81	88	99	82	97	98	93
Piperacillin	65	91	84	68	89	94	100	96
Cefazolin	95	1	83	97	11	18	0	76
Cefotetan	100	1	100	100	77	100	100	97
Ceftriaxone	100	80	100	100	90	100	100	98
Ceftazidime	100	98	95	100	86	97	100	98
Amikacin	100	100	100	100	100	100	100	100
Gentamicin	100	88	89	93	100	92	100	97
Tobramycin	100	89	94	92	100	94	100	100
Tetracycline	84	3	78	4	97	41	41	93
Trimeth-Sulfa	84	2	75	83	96	88	100	90
Nitrofurantoin	100	1	89	21	95	92	0	100
Ciprofloxacin	100	74	80	85	100	97	100	100

FIGURE 9-5. Pocket chart for aerobic Gram-negative bacteria. Illustrated here is the type of chart that clinicians carry in their pockets for use as a quick reference whenever empiric therapy is necessary. The pocket chart, which is prepared by the medical facility's Clinical Microbiology Laboratory, shows the percentage of particular organisms that were susceptible to the various drugs that were tested. The following is an example of how the pocket chart is used. A clinician is informed that *Pseudomonas aeruginosa* has been isolated from his or her patient's blood culture, but the antimicrobial susceptibility testing results on that isolate will not be available until the following day. Because therapy must be initiated immediately, the clinician refers to the pocket chart and sees that amikacin is the most appropriate drug to use (of the 371 strains of *P. aeruginosa* tested, 100% were susceptible to amikacin). (As mentioned in the text, other factors would be taken into consideration by the clinician *before* prescribing amikacin for this patient.) According to the pocket chart, which drug would be the second choice, if amikacin is not available in the hospital pharmacy? Answer: ceftazidime (98%). (Note: This chart is included for educational purposes only. It should not actually be used in a clinical setting.)

might prescribe a drug that concentrates in the urine. Such a drug is rapidly removed from the blood by the kidneys, and high concentrations of the drug are achieved in the urinary bladder. To treat a brain abscess, the clinician would select a drug capable of crossing the blood-brain barrier.

- What other medications is the patient taking or receiving? Some antimicrobial agents will cross-react with certain other drugs, leading to a drug interaction that could be harmful to the patient.
- What other medical problems does the patient have? Certain antimicrobial agents are known to have toxic side effects (e.g., nephrotoxicity, hepatotoxicity, ototoxicity).

For example, a clinician would not prescribe a nephrotoxic drug to a patient who has prior kidney damage.

- Is the patient leukopenic or immunocompromised? If so, it would be necessary to use a bactericidal agent to treat the patient's bacterial infection, rather than a bacteriostatic agent. Recall that bacteriostatic agents should only be used in patients whose host defense mechanisms are functioning properly (i.e., only in patients whose bodies are capable of killing the pathogen once its multiplication is stopped). A leukopenic patient has too few white blood cells to kill the pathogen, and the immune system of an immunocompromised patient would be unable to kill the pathogen.

- The cost of the various drugs is also a major consideration. Whenever possible, clinicians should prescribe less costly, narrow-spectrum drugs, rather than expensive, broad-spectrum drugs.

Although the patient's weight will influence the dosage of a particular drug, it is usually not taken into consideration when deciding which drug to prescribe.

UNDESIRABLE EFFECTS OF ANTIMICROBIAL AGENTS

Listed below are some of the many reasons why antimicrobial agents should not be used indiscriminately.

- Whenever an antimicrobial agent is administered to a patient, organisms within that patient that are susceptible to the agent will die, but resistant ones will survive. This is referred to as selecting for resistant organisms (Fig. 9-6). The resistant organisms then multiply, become dominant, and can be transmitted to other people. To prevent the overgrowth of resistant organisms, sometimes several drugs, each with a different mode of action, are administered simultaneously.
- The patient may become allergic to the agent. For example, penicillin G in low doses often sensitizes those who are prone to allergies; when these persons receive a second dose of penicillin at some later date, they may have a severe reaction known as anaphylactic shock, or they may break out in hives.
- Many antimicrobial agents are toxic to humans, and some are so toxic that they are administered only for serious diseases for which no other agents are available. One such drug is chloramphenicol, which, if given in high doses for a long period, may cause a very severe type of anemia called aplastic anemia. Another is streptomycin, which can damage the auditory nerve and cause deafness. Other drugs are hepatotoxic or nephrotoxic, causing liver or kidney damage, respectively.
- With prolonged use, broad-spectrum antibiotics may destroy the normal flora of the mouth, intestine, or vagina. The person no longer has the protection of the indigenous microflora and thus becomes much more susceptible to infections caused by opportunists or secondary invaders.

Prolonged antibiotic use can lead to population explosions of microorganisms that are resistant to the antibiotic(s) being used. Such overgrowths are known as "superinfections."

The resultant overgrowth by such organisms is referred to as a *superinfection*. A superinfection can be thought of as a "population explosion" of organisms that are usually present only in small numbers. For example, the prolonged use of oral antibiotics can result in a superinfection of *Clostridium difficile* in the colon, which can lead to such diseases as antibiotic-associated diarrhea (AAD) and pseudomembranous colitis (PMC). Yeast vaginitis often follows antibacterial therapy because many bacteria of the vaginal flora were destroyed, leading to a superinfection of the indigenous yeast, *Candida albicans*.

FIGURE 9-6. Selecting for drug-resistant organisms. (A) Indigenous microflora of a patient before initiation of antibiotic therapy. Most members of the population are susceptible (indicated by S) to the antibiotic to be administered; very few are resistant (indicated by R). (B) After antibiotic therapy has been initiated, the susceptible organisms are dead; only a few resistant organisms remain. (C) As a result of decreased competition for nutrients and space, the resistant organisms multiply and become the predominant organisms in the patient's indigenous microflora. (The same type of selection process occurs when farm animals are fed antibiotic-containing feed and when antimicrobial-containing products [e.g., toys, cutting boards] are used in our homes. Both of these topics were discussed in Chapter 8.)

CONCLUDING REMARKS

In recent years, microorganisms have developed resistance at such a rapid pace that many people, including many scientists, are beginning to fear that science is losing the war against pathogens. Some strains of pathogens have arisen that are resistant to all known drugs; examples include certain strains of *M. tuberculosis* (the bacterium that causes tuberculosis), *Plasmodium* spp. (the protozoa that cause malaria), and *S. aureus* (the bacterium that causes many different types of infections, including pneumonia and postsurgical wound infections). To win the war against drug resistance, more prudent use of currently available drugs, the discovery of new drugs, and the development of new vaccines will all be necessary. Unfortunately, as someone once said, "When science builds a better mousetrap, nature builds a better mouse." To learn more about antibiotic resistance, the book by Dr. Stuart Levy (previously cited) is highly recommended.

Fortunately, antimicrobial agents are not the only in vivo weapons against pathogens. Operating within our bodies are various systems that function to kill pathogens and protect us from infectious diseases. These systems, collectively referred to as host defense systems, are discussed in Chapters 15 and 16.

 SOMETHING TO THINK ABOUT

The following quotation is from a book published in 2000, but the words are as true today as when they were written. "The promise of antibiotics seems to be fading. We are faced today with a rising tide of antibiotic-resistant microbes that cause serious disease. In some rare cases, the microbes are untouchable by modern medicine, resistant to every single antibiotic in our armamentarium. Patients infected with these resistant microbes are dying, much as people did before Fleming brought us his historic discovery. Some fear we may be returning to an era that we thought was past—an era without the benefit of modern antibiotics."

(From Needham C, et al. Intimate Strangers: Unseen Life on Earth. Washington, DC: ASM Press, 2000.)

ON THE CD-ROM
- Terms Introduced in This Chapter
- Review of Key Points
- Increase Your Knowledge
- Critical Thinking
- Additional Self-Assessment Exercises

SELF-ASSESSMENT EXERCISES

After studying this chapter, answer the following multiple-choice questions.

1. Which of the following is *least* likely to be taken into consideration when deciding which antibiotic to prescribe for a patient?
   a. patient's age
   b. patient's underlying medical conditions
   c. patient's weight
   d. other medications that the patient is taking

2. Which of the following is *least* likely to lead to drug resistance in bacteria?
   a. a chromosomal mutation that alters cell membrane permeability
   b. a chromosomal mutation that alters the shape of a particular drug-binding site
   c. receiving a gene that codes for an enzyme that destroys a particular antibiotic
   d. receiving a gene that codes for the production of a capsule

3. Which of the following is *not* a common mechanism by which antimicrobial agents kill or inhibit the growth of bacteria?
   a. damage to cell membranes
   b. destruction of capsules
   c. inhibition of cell wall synthesis
   d. inhibition of protein synthesis

4. Multidrug therapy is always used when a patient is diagnosed as having:
   a. an infection caused by MRSA.
   b. diphtheria.
   c. strep throat.
   d. tuberculosis.

5. Which of the following terms or names has *nothing* to do with the use of two drugs simultaneously?
   a. antagonism
   b. Salvarsan
   c. Septra
   d. synergism

6. Which of the following is *not* a common mechanism by which antifungal agents work?
   a. by binding with cell membrane sterols
   b. by blocking nucleic acid synthesis
   c. by dissolving hyphae
   d. by interfering with sterol synthesis

7. Which of the following scientists discovered penicillin?
   a. Alexander Fleming
   b. Paul Ehrlich
   c. Selman Waksman
   d. Sir Howard Walter Florey

8. Which of the following scientists is considered to be the "Father of Chemotherapy?"
   a. Alexander Fleming
   b. Paul Ehrlich
   c. Selman Waksman
   d. Sir Howard Walter Florey

9. All the following antimicrobial agents work by inhibiting cell wall synthesis except:
   a. cephalosporins.
   b. chloramphenicol.
   c. penicillin.
   d. vancomycin.

10. All the following antimicrobial agents work by inhibiting protein synthesis except:
   a. chloramphenicol.
   b. erythromycin.
   c. imipenem.
   d. tetracycline.

Environmental and Applied Microbiology

10 MICROBIAL ECOLOGY AND MICROBIAL BIOTECHNOLOGY

CHAPTER OUTLINE

LEARNING OBJECTIVES

AFTER STUDYING THIS CHAPTER, YOU SHOULD BE ABLE TO:

- Define ecology, human ecology, and microbial ecology
- List three categories of symbiotic relationships
- Differentiate between mutualism and commensalism and give an example of each
- Cite an example of a parasitic relationship
- Discuss the beneficial and harmful roles of the indigenous microflora of the human body
- Describe biofilms and their impact on human health
- Outline the nitrogen cycle; include the meanings of the terms nitrogen-fixation, nitrification, denitrification, and ammonification in the description
- Name 10 foods that require microbial activity for their production
- Define biotechnology and cite four examples of how microbes are used in industry
- Define bioremediation and cite an example

INTRODUCTION

The science of *ecology* is the systematic study of the interrelationships that exist between organisms and their environment. If you were to take a course in human ecology, you would study the interrelationships between humans and the world around them—the nonliving world as well as the living world. *Microbial ecology* is the study of the numerous interrelationships between microorganisms and the world around them; how microbes interact with other microbes, how microbes interact with organisms other than microbes, and how microbes interact with the nonliving world around them. Interactions between microorganisms and animals, plants, other microbes, soil, and our atmosphere have far-reaching effects on our lives. We are all aware of the diseases caused by pathogens (Chapters 17 through 21), but this is only one example of the many ways that microbes interact with humans. Most relationships between humans and microbes are beneficial rather than harmful. Although the "bad guys" get most of the attention in the news media, our microbial allies far outnumber our microbial enemies.

Microorganisms interact with humans in many ways and at many levels. The most intimate association that we have with microorganisms is their presence both on and within our bodies. Additionally, microbes play important roles in agriculture, various industries, disposal

> Microbial ecology is the study of the numerous interrelationships between microorganisms and the world around them.

of industrial and toxic wastes, sewage treatment, and water purification. Microbes are essential in the fields of biotechnology, bioremediation, genetic engineering, and gene therapy (genetic engineering and gene therapy were discussed in Chapter 7).

SYMBIOTIC RELATIONSHIPS INVOLVING MICROORGANISMS

Symbiosis

Symbiosis, or a *symbiotic relationship*, is defined as the living together or close association of two dissimilar organisms (usually two different species). The organisms that live together in such a relationship are referred to as *symbionts*. Some symbiotic relationships (called mutualistic relationships) are beneficial to *both* symbionts, others (commensalistic relationships) are beneficial to only one symbiont, and others (parasitic relationships) are harmful to one symbiont. Many microorganisms participate in symbiotic relationships. Various symbiotic relationships involving microbes are discussed in subsequent sections; some are illustrated in Figure 10-1.

> Symbiosis is defined as the living together or close association of two dissimilar organisms (usually two different species).

Neutralism

The term *neutralism* is used to describe a symbiotic relationship in which neither symbiont is affected by the relationship. In other words, neutralism reflects a situation in which different microorganisms occupy the same ecologic niche, but have absolutely no effect on each other.

Commensalism

A symbiotic relationship that is beneficial to one symbiont and of no consequence (i.e., is neither beneficial nor harmful) to the other is called *commensalism*. Many of the organisms in the indigenous microflora of humans are considered to be commensals. The relationship is of obvious benefit to the microorganisms (they are provided nutrients and "housing"), but the microorganisms have no effect on the host. A *host* is defined as a living organism that harbors another living organism. One example of a commensal, illustrated in Figure 10-1, is the tiny mite called *Demodex*, which lives within hair follicles and sebaceous glands, especially those of the eyelashes and eyebrows.

> Commensalism is a symbiotic relationship that is beneficial to one symbiont and of no consequence (i.e., is neither beneficial nor harmful) to the other.

Mutualism

Mutualism is a symbiotic relationship that is beneficial to both symbionts (i.e., the relationship is mutually beneficial). Humans have a mutualistic relationship with many of the microorganisms of their indigenous microflora. An example is the intestinal bacterium *Escherichia coli*, which obtains nutrients from food materials ingested by the host and produces vitamins (such as vitamin K) that are used by the host. Vitamin K is a blood-clotting factor that is essential to humans. Also, some members of our indigenous microflora prevent colonization by pathogens and overgrowth by opportunistic pathogens (discussed further in a following section entitled "Microbial Antagonism").

> Mutualism is a symbiotic relationship that is beneficial to both symbionts (i.e., the relationship is mutually beneficial).

As another example of a mutualistic relationship, consider the protozoa that live in the intestine of termites. Termites eat wood, but they cannot digest wood. Fortunately for them, the protozoa that live in their intes-

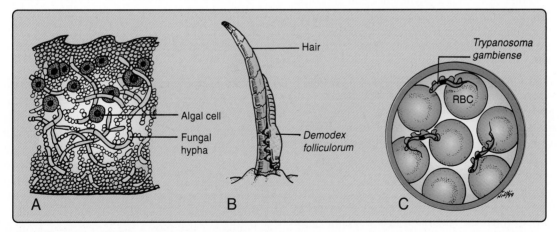

FIGURE 10-1. Various symbiotic relationships. (A) A lichen is an example of a mutualistic relationship (i.e., a relationship that is beneficial to both symbionts). **(B)** The tiny *Demodex* mites that live in human hair follicles are examples of commensals. **(C)** The flagellated protozoan that causes African sleeping sickness is a parasite (*RBC*, red blood cell).

tinal tract break down the large molecules in wood into smaller molecules which can be absorbed and used as nutrients by the termites. In turn, the termite provides food and a warm, moist place for the protozoa to live. Without these protozoa, the termites would die of starvation.

The lichens that you see as colored patches on rocks and tree trunks are further examples of mutualism. As discussed in Chapter 5, a lichen is composed of an alga (or a cyanobacterium) and a fungus, living so closely together that they appear to be one organism. The fungus uses some of the energy that the alga produces by photosynthesis (recall that fungi are not photosynthetic), and the chitin in the fungal cell walls protects the alga from desiccation. Thus, both symbionts benefit from the relationship.

Parasitism

Parasitism is a symbiotic relationship that is beneficial to one symbiont (the parasite) and detrimental to the other symbiont (the host). Being detrimental to the host does not necessarily mean that the parasite causes disease. In some cases, a host can harbor a parasite, without the parasite causing harm to the host. "Smart'" parasites do not cause disease, but rather take only the nutrients they need to exist. The especially "dumb" parasites kill their hosts; then they must either find a new host or die. Nonetheless, certain parasites always cause disease, and some cause the death of the host. For example, the protozoan illustrated

> Parasitism is a symbiotic relationship that is beneficial to one symbiont (the parasite) and detrimental to the other symbiont (the host).

in Figure 10-1—*Trypanosoma gambiense*—is the parasite that causes African sleeping sickness, a human disease that often causes death of the host. Parasites are discussed further in Chapter 21.

A change in conditions can cause one type of symbiotic relationship to shift to another type. For example, conditions can cause a mutualistic or commensalistic relationship between humans and their indigenous microflora to shift to a parasitic, disease-causing (pathogenic) relationship. Recall that many of the microbes of our indigenous microflora are opportunistic pathogens (opportunists), awaiting the opportunity to cause disease. Conditions that may enable an opportunist to cause disease include burns, lacerations, surgical procedures, or diseases that debilitate (weaken) the host or interfere with host defense mechanisms. Immunosuppressed individuals are especially susceptible to opportunistic pathogens. Opportunists can also cause disease in otherwise healthy persons if they gain access to the blood, urinary bladder, lungs, or other organs and tissues of those individuals.

INDIGENOUS MICROFLORA OF HUMANS

A person's *indigenous microflora* or *indigenous microbiota* (sometimes referred to as "normal flora") includes all of the microbes (bacteria, fungi, protozoa, and viruses) that reside on and within that person (Fig. 10-2). It has been estimated that our bodies are composed of about 10 trillion cells (including nerve cells, muscle cells, and epithelial cells), and that we have about 10 times that many microbes that live on and within our bodies (10 × 10 trillion = 100 trillion). It has also been estimated that our indigenous microflora is composed of between 500 and 1,000 different species!

> A person's indigenous microflora or indigenous microbiota (sometimes referred to as "normal flora") includes all of the microbes (bacteria, fungi, protozoa, and viruses) that reside on and within that person.

SOMETHING TO THINK ABOUT

"I would like to point out that we depend on more than the activity of some 30,000 genes encoded in the human genome. Our existence is critically dependent on the presence of upwards of 1000 bacterial species (the exact number is unknown because many are uncultivable) living in and on us; the oral cavity and gastrointestinal tracts contain particularly rich and active populations. Thus, if truth be known, human life depends on an additional 2 to 4 million genes, mostly uncharacterized. Until the synergistic activities between humans (and other animals) with their obligatory commensals has been elucidated, an understanding of human biology will remain incomplete." (Julian Davies, Science Magazine, 2001;291:2316.)

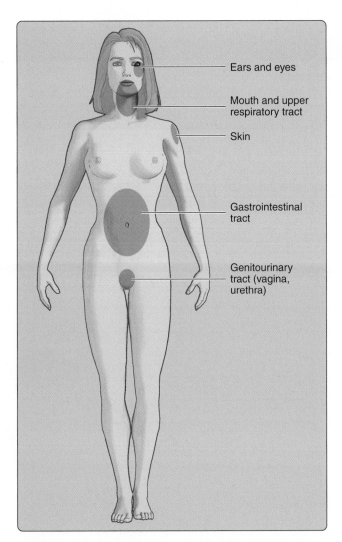

FIGURE 10-2. Areas of the body where most of the indigenous microflora reside: skin, mouth, ears, eyes, upper respiratory tract, gastrointestinal tract, and genitourinary tract.

A fetus has no indigenous microflora. During and after delivery, a newborn is exposed to many microorganisms from its mother, food, air, and virtually everything that touches the infant. Both harmless and helpful microbes take up residence on the baby's skin, at all body openings, and on mucous membranes that line the digestive tract (mouth to anus) and the genitourinary tract. These moist, warm environments provide excellent conditions for growth. Conditions for proper growth (moisture, pH, temperature, nutrients) vary throughout the body; thus, the types of resident flora differ from one anatomic site to another. Blood, lymph, spinal fluid, and most internal tissues and organs are normally free of microorganisms (i.e., they are sterile). Table 10-1 lists microorganisms frequently found on and within the human body.

In addition to the resident microflora, transient microflora take up temporary residence on and within humans. The body is constantly exposed to microorganisms from the external environment; these transient microbes frequently are attracted to moist, warm body areas. These microbes are only temporary for many reasons: they may be washed from external areas by bathing; they may not be able to compete with the resident microflora; they may fail to survive in the acidic or alkaline environment of the site; they may be killed by substances produced by resident microflora; or they may be flushed away by bodily excretions or secretions (such as urine, feces, tears, and perspiration). Many microbes are unable to colonize (inhabit) the human body because they do not find the body to be a suitable host.

Destruction of the resident microflora disturbs the delicate balance established between the host and its microorganisms. For example, prolonged therapy with certain antibiotics often destroys many of the intestinal microflora. Diarrhea is usually the result of such an imbalance, which in turn leaves the body more susceptible to secondary invaders. When the number of usual resident microbes is greatly reduced, opportunistic invaders can more easily establish themselves within those areas. One important opportunist usually found in small numbers near body openings is the yeast, *Candida albicans*, which, in the absence of sufficient numbers of other resident microflora, may grow unchecked in the mouth, vagina, or lower intestine, causing the disease *candidiasis* (also known as moniliasis). Such an overgrowth or population explosion of an organism that is usually present in low numbers is referred to as a *superinfection*.

Microflora of the Skin

The resident microflora of the skin consists primarily of bacteria and fungi—as many as 300 different species, depending on the anatomical location. The number of different types of microbes varies greatly from body part to body part and from person to person. Although the skin is constantly exposed to air, many of the bacteria that live on the skin are anaerobes; in fact, anaerobes actually outnumber aerobes. Anaerobes live in the deeper layers of skin, hair follicles, and sweat and sebaceous glands. The most common bacteria on the skin are species of *Staphylococcus* (especially *S. epidermidis* and other coagulase-negative staphylococci[a]), *Corynebacterium*, and *Propionibacterium*. The number and variety of microorganisms present on the skin depends on many factors, such as the:

> The most common bacteria on the skin are *Staphylococcus*, *Corynebacterium*, and *Propionibacterium* spp.

- Anatomical location
- Amount of moisture present
- pH

---

[a] Coagulase is an enzyme that causes clot formation. In the clinical microbiology laboratory, the coagulase test is used to differentiate *Staphylococcus aureus* (which produces coagulase and is referred to as being coagulase-positive) from other species of *Staphylococcus* (which do not produce coagulase and are referred to as being coagulase-negative).

TABLE 10-1	Anatomic Locations of Bacteria and Yeasts Found as Indigenous Microflora of Humans					
	SKIN	MOUTH	NOSE AND NASOPHARYNX	OROPHARYNX	GI TRACT	GU TRACT
Anaerobic Gram-negative cocci	−	+	−	−	−	−
Anaerobic Gram-positive cocci	−	+	−	+	+	+
Bacteroides spp.	±	+	−	+	+	+
Candida spp.	+	±	−	−	−	+
Clostridium spp.	+	−	−	−	+	+
Diphtheroids	+	−	+	+	−	+
Enterobacteriaceae[a]	−	−	−	−	+	±
Enterococcus spp.	−	±	±	−	+	+
Fusobacterium spp.	−	±	±	+	+	−
Haemophilus spp.	−	−	+	+	−	−
Lactobacillus spp.	+	+	−	−	−	+
Micrococcus spp.	+	−	−	−	−	−
Neisseria meningitidis	−	−	±	±	−	−
Prevotella/Porphyromonas spp.	−	+	−	+	−	−
Staphylococcus spp.	+	+	+	+	+	+
Streptococcus spp.	±	+	+	+	−	−

+, commonly present; ±, less commonly present; −, absent

[a]Sometimes referred to as enteric bacilli (includes *Escherichia, Klebsiella, Proteus* spp.)

- Temperature
- Salinity
- Presence of chemical wastes such as urea and fatty acids
- Presence of other microbes, which may be producing toxic substances

Moist, warm conditions in hairy areas of the body where there are many sweat and oil glands, such as under the arms and in the groin area, stimulate the growth of many different microorganisms. Dry, calloused areas of skin have few bacteria, whereas moist folds between the toes and fingers support many bacteria and fungi. The surface of the skin near mucosal openings of the body (the mouth, eyes, nose, anus, and genitalia) is inhabited by bacteria present in various excretions and secretions.

Frequent washing with soap and water removes most of the potentially harmful transient microorganisms harbored in sweat, oil, and other secretions from moist body parts, as well as the dead epithelial cells on which they feed. Proper hygiene also serves to remove odorous organic materials present in perspiration, sebum (sebaceous gland secretions), and microbial metabolic byproducts. Healthcare professionals must be particularly careful to keep their skin and clothing as free of transient microbes as possible to help prevent personal infections and to avoid transferring pathogens to patients. These individuals should always keep in mind that most infections after burns, wounds, and surgery result from the growth of resident or transient skin microflora in these susceptible areas.

Microflora of the Ears and Eyes

The middle ear and inner ear are usually sterile, whereas the outer ear and the auditory canal contain the same types of microorganisms as are found on the skin. When a person coughs, sneezes, or blows his or her nose, these microbes may be carried along the eustachian tube and into the middle ear where they can cause infection. Infection can also develop in the middle ear when the eustachian tube does not open and close properly to maintain correct air pressure within the ear.

The external surface of the eye is lubricated, cleansed, and protected by tears, mucus, and sebum. Thus, continual production of tears and the presence of the enzyme lysozyme and other antimicrobial substances found in tears greatly reduce the numbers of indigenous microflora organisms found on the eye surfaces.

Microflora of the Respiratory Tract

The respiratory tract can be divided into the upper respiratory tract and the lower respiratory tract. The upper respiratory tract consists of the nasal passages and the throat (pharynx). The lower respiratory tract consists of the larynx (voice box), trachea, bronchi, bronchioles, and lungs.

The nasal passages and throat have an abundant and varied population of microorganisms, because these areas provide moist, warm mucous membranes that furnish excellent conditions for microbial growth. Many microorganisms found in the healthy nose and throat are harmless. Others are opportunistic pathogens, which have the potential to cause disease under certain circumstances. Some people—known as healthy *carriers*—harbor virulent (disease-causing) pathogens in their nasal passages or throats, but do not have the diseases associated with them, such as diphtheria, meningitis, pneumonia, and whooping cough. Although these carriers are unaffected by these pathogens, carriers can transmit them to susceptible persons.

The lower respiratory tract is usually free of microbes because the mucous membranes and lungs have defense mechanisms (described in Chapter 15) that efficiently remove invaders.

Microflora of the Oral Cavity (Mouth)

The anatomy of the oral cavity (mouth) affords shelter for numerous anaerobic and aerobic bacteria. Anaerobic microorganisms flourish in gum margins, crevices between the teeth, and deep folds (crypts) on the surface of the tonsils. Bacteria thrive especially well in particles of food and in the debris of dead epithelial cells around the teeth. Food remaining on and between teeth provides a rich nutrient medium for growth of the many oral bacteria. Carelessness in dental hygiene allows growth of these bacteria, with development of dental caries (tooth decay), gingivitis (gum disease), and more severe periodontal diseases.

The list of microbes that have been isolated from healthy human mouths reads like a manual of the major groups of microbes. It includes Gram-positive and Gram-negative bacteria (both cocci and bacilli), spirochetes, and sometimes yeasts, mouldlike organisms, protozoa, and viruses. The bacteria include species of *Actinomyces, Bacteroides, Borrelia, Corynebacterium, Fusobacterium, Haemophilus, Lactobacillus, Neisseria, Porphyromonas, Prevotella, Propionibacterium, Staphylococcus, Streptococcus, Treponema,* and *Veillonella.* The most common organisms in the indigenous microflora of the mouth are various species of α-hemolytic streptococci. The bacterium most often implicated in the formation of plaque is *Streptococcus mutans.*

> The most common organisms in the indigenous microflora of the mouth are various species of α-hemolytic streptococci.

Microflora of the Gastrointestinal Tract

The gastrointestinal (GI) tract (or digestive tract) consists of a long tube with many expanded areas designed for digestion of food, absorption of nutrients, and elimination of undigested materials. Excluding the oral cavity and pharynx, which have already been discussed, the GI tract includes the esophagus, stomach, small intestine, large intestine (colon), and anus. Accessory glands and organs of the GI system include the salivary glands, pancreas, liver, and gallbladder.

Gastric enzymes and the extremely acidic pH (approximately pH 1.5) of the stomach usually prevent growth of indigenous microflora, and most transient microbes (i.e., microbes consumed in foods and beverages) are killed as they pass through the stomach. There is one bacterium—a Gram-negative bacillus named *Helicobacter pylori*—that lives in some people's stomachs and is a common cause of ulcers. A few microbes, enveloped by food particles, manage to pass through the stomach during periods of low acid concentration. Also, when the amount of acid is reduced in the course of diseases such as stomach cancer, certain bacteria may be found in the stomach.

Few microflora usually exist in the upper portion of the small intestine (the duodenum) because bile inhibits their growth, but many are found in the lower parts of the small intestine (the jejunum and ileum).

The colon contains the largest number and variety of microorganisms of any colonized area of the body. It has been estimated that as many as 500 to 600 different species—primarily bacteria—live there. Because the colon is anaerobic, the bacteria living there are obligate, aerotolerant, and facultative anaerobes. Bacteria found in the gastrointestinal tract include species of *Actinomyces, Bacteroides, Clostridium, Enterobacter, Enterococcus, Escherichia, Klebsiella, Lactobacillus, Proteus, Pseudomonas, Staphylococcus,* and *Streptococcus.*

> The colon contains as many as 500 to 600 different species—primarily bacteria.

Also, many fungi, protozoa, and viruses can live in the colon. Many of the microflora of the colon are opportunists, causing disease only when they gain access to other areas of the body (e.g., urinary bladder, bloodstream, or lesion of some type), or when the usual balance among the microorganisms is upset. *E. coli* is a good example. All humans have *E. coli* bacteria in their colon. They are opportunists, usually causing us no problems at all, but they can cause urinary tract infections (UTIs) when they gain access to the urinary bladder. In fact, *E. coli* is the most common cause of UTIs.

Many microbes are removed from the GI tract as a result of defecation. It has been estimated that about 50% of the fecal mass consists of bacteria.

Microflora of the Genitourinary Tract

The genitourinary (GU) tract (or urogenital tract) consists of the urinary tract (kidneys, ureters, urinary bladder, and urethra) and the various parts of the male and female reproductive systems.

The healthy kidney, ureters, and urinary bladder are sterile. However, the distal urethra (that part of the urethra farthest from the urinary bladder) and the external opening of the urethra harbor many microbes, including bacteria, yeasts, and viruses. As a rule, these organisms do not invade the bladder because the urethra is periodically flushed by acidic urine. Frequent urination helps to prevent UTIs. However, persistent, recurring UTIs often develop when there is an obstruction or narrowing of the urethra, which allows the invasive organisms to multiply. The most frequent causes of urethral infection (urethritis)—*Chlamydia trachomatis*, *Neisseria gonorrhoeae*, and mycoplasmas—are easily introduced into the urethra by sexual intercourse.

The reproductive systems of both men and women are usually sterile, with the exception of the vagina; here, the microflora varies with the stage of sexual development. During puberty and after menopause, vaginal secretions are alkaline, supporting the growth of various diphtheroids, streptococci, staphylococci, and coliforms (*E. coli* and closely related enteric Gram-negative bacilli). Through the childbearing years, vaginal secretions are acidic (pH 4.0–5.0), encouraging the growth mainly of lactobacilli, along with a few α-hemolytic streptococci, staphylococci, diphtheroids, and yeasts. Bacteria found in the vagina include species of *Actinomyces*, *Bacteroides*, *Corynebacterium*, *Klebsiella*, *Lactobacillus*, *Mycoplasma*, *Proteus*, *Pseudomonas*, *Staphylococcus*, and *Streptococcus*.

The metabolic byproducts of lactobacilli, especially lactic acid, inhibit growth of the bacteria associated with bacterial vaginosis (BV). Factors that lead to a decrease in the number of lactobacilli in the vaginal microflora can lead to an overgrowth of other bacteria (e.g., *Bacteroides* spp., *Mobiluncus* spp., *Gardnerella vaginalis*, and anaerobic cocci), which in turn can lead to BV. Likewise, a decrease in the number of lactobacilli can lead to an overgrowth of yeasts, which in turn can lead to yeast vaginitis.

STUDY AID
"Vaginitis" versus "Vaginosis"

The similarly sounding terms *vaginitis* and *vaginosis* both refer to vaginal infections. The suffix "-itis" refers to inflammation, and inflammation usually involves the influx of white blood cells known as polymorphonuclear cells (PMNs). Thus, a vaginal infection involving inflammation and the influx of PMNs is referred to as vaginitis. In bacterial vaginosis (BV), there is a watery, noninflammatory discharge, lacking white blood cells (WBCs). Thus, the difference between vaginitis and vaginosis boils down to the presence or absence of WBCs. Whereas vaginitis is usually caused by one particular pathogen, BV is a synergistic infection.

BENEFICIAL AND HARMFUL ROLES OF INDIGENOUS MICROFLORA

Humans derive many benefits from their indigenous microflora, some of which have already been mentioned. Some nutrients, particularly vitamins K and B$_{12}$, pantothenic acid, | Certain of our intestinal bacteria are beneficial to us in that they produce useful vitamins and other nutrients.

pyridoxine, and biotin, are obtained from secretions of certain intestinal bacteria. Evidence also indicates that indigenous microbes provide a constant source of irritants and antigens to stimulate the immune system. This causes the immune system to respond more readily by producing antibodies to foreign invaders and substances, which in turn enhances the body's protection against pathogens. The mere presence of large numbers of microorganisms at certain anatomic locations is beneficial, in that they prevent pathogens from colonizing those locations.

Microbial Antagonism

The term *microbial antagonism* means "microbes versus microbes" or "microbes against microbes." Many of the microbes of our indigenous microflora serve a beneficial role by preventing other microbes from becoming established in or colonizing a particular anatomic | Many members of our indigenous microflora serve a beneficial role by preventing other microbes from becoming established in or colonizing a particular anatomic location.

location. For example, the huge numbers of bacteria in our colons accomplish this by occupying space and consuming nutrients. "Newcomers" (including pathogens that we have ingested) cannot gain a foothold because of the intense competition for space and nutrients.

Other examples of microbial antagonism involve the production of antibiotics and bacteriocins. As discussed in Chapter 9, many bacteria and fungi produce antibiotics. Recall that an antibiotic is a substance produced by one microorganism that kills or inhibits the growth of another microorganism. (Actually, the term antibiotic is usually reserved for those substances produced by bacteria and fungi that have been found useful in treating infectious diseases.) Some bacteria produce proteins called bacteriocins which kill other bacteria. An example is colicin, a bacteriocin produced by *E. coli*.

Opportunistic Pathogens

As you know, many members of the indigenous microflora of the human body are opportunistic pathogens (opportunists), which can be thought of as organisms that are hanging around, waiting for the opportunity to cause infections. Take *E. coli* for example. Huge numbers of *E. coli* live in our intestinal tract, | Opportunistic pathogens (opportunists) can be thought of as organisms that are hanging around, awaiting the opportunity to cause infections.

causing us no problems whatsoever on a day-to-day basis. They do possess the potential to be pathogenic, however, and can cause serious infections should they find their way to a site such as the urinary bladder, bloodstream, or wound. Other especially important opportunistic pathogens in the human indigenous microflora include other members of the family *Enterobacteriaceae*, *Staphylococcus aureus*, and *Enterococcus* spp.

Biotherapeutic Agents

When the delicate balance among the various species in the population of indigenous microflora is upset by antibiotics, other types of chemotherapy, or changes in pH, many complications may result. Certain microorganisms may flourish out | Bacteria and yeasts that are ingested to reestablish and stabilize the microbial balance within our bodies are called biotherapeutic agents or probiotics.

of control, such as *C. albicans* in the vagina, leading to yeast vaginitis. Also, diarrhea and pseudomembranous colitis may occur as a result of overgrowth of *Clostridium difficile* in the colon. Cultures of *Lactobacillus* in yogurt or in medications may be prescribed to reestablish and stabilize the microbial balance. Bacteria and yeasts used in this manner are called *biotherapeutic agents* (or probiotics).[b] Other microorganisms that have been used as biotherapeutic agents include *Bifidobacterium* spp., nonpathogenic *Enterococcus* spp., and *Saccharomyces* spp. (yeasts).

MICROBIAL COMMUNITIES (BIOFILMS)

We often read about one particular microbe as being the cause of a certain disease or as playing a specific role in nature. In reality, it is rare to find an ecologic niche in which only one type of microbe is present | In nature, microbes are often organized into complex and persistant communities of assorted organisms called biofilms.

or only one microbe is causing a particular effect. In nature, microbes are often organized into what are known as *biofilms*—complex and persistant communities of assorted microbes. Bacterial biofilms are virtually everywhere; examples include dental plaque, the slippery coating on a rock in a stream, and the slime that accumulates on the inner walls of various types of pipes and tubing. A bacterial biofilm consists of a variety of different species of bacteria plus a gooey extracellular matrix that the bacteria secrete, composed of polysaccharides, proteins, and nucleic acids. The bacteria grow in tiny clusters—called *microcolonies*—that are separated by a network of water channels. The fluid that flows through these channels bathes the microcolonies with dissolved nutrients and carries away waste products.

Biofilms have medical significance. They form on bones, heart valves, tissues, and inanimate objects such as artificial heart valves, catheters, and prosthetic implants. Biofilms have been implicated in diseases such as endocarditis, cystic fibrosis, middle ear infections, | Biofilms have been implicated in diseases such as endocarditis, cystic fibrosis, middle ear infections, kidney stones, periodontal disease, and prostate infections.

kidney stones, periodontal disease, and prostate infections. It has been estimated that perhaps as many as 60% of human infections are due to biofilms. Microbes commonly associated with biofilms on indwelling medical devices include the yeast *C. albicans* and bacteria such as *S. aureus*, coagulase-negative staphylococci, *Enterococcus* spp., *Klebsiella pneumoniae*, and *Pseudomonas aeruginosa*.

Dental plaque consists of a community of microorganisms attached to various proteins and glycoproteins adsorbed onto tooth surfaces. If the plaque is not removed, substances produced by these organisms can penetrate the tooth enamel, leading to cavities, and eventually causing soft tissue disease.

Biofilms are very resistant to antibiotics, disinfectants, and certain types of host defense mechanisms. Antibiotics that, in the laboratory, have been shown to be effective against pure cultures of organisms within biofilms may be ineffective against those same organisms within an actual biofilm. Let's take penicillin as an example. Penicillin is an antibiotic that prevents bacteria from producing cell walls. In the laboratory, penicillin may kill actively growing cells of a particular organism, but it does not kill any cells of that organism within the biofilm that are not growing (i.e., that are not actively building cell walls). Also, any penicillinases (discussed in Chapter 9) being produced by organisms within the biofilm will inactivate the penicillin molecule, and will thus protect other organisms within the biofilm from the effects of penicillin. Therefore, some bacteria that are present within the biofilm protect other species of bacteria within the biofilm. Biofilms are also protected from antimicrobial agents as a result of decreased penetration or diffusion of the agents into the biofilms.

---

[b] Probiotics should not be confused with prebiotics. Whereas probiotics are microorganisms, prebiotics are food ingredients with the capacity to improve health when metabolized by intestinal bacteria.

Another example of how bacteria within a biofilm cooperate with each other involves nutrients. In some biofilms, bacteria of different species cooperate to break down nutrients that any single species cannot break down by itself. In some cases, one species within a biofilm feeds on the metabolic wastes of another.

Biofilms are resistant to certain types of host defense mechanisms. For example, it is difficult for leukocytes to penetrate biofilms, and those that do penetrate seem less efficient | **Bacteria within biofilms are protected from antibiotics and certain types of host defense mechanisms.**

at phagocytizing bacteria within the biofilm. Although the macrophages and leukocytes cannot ingest the bacteria, they do become activated and secrete toxic compounds that cause damage to nearby healthy host tissues. This phenomenon has been referred to as *frustrated phagocytosis*. The biofilms also appear to suppress the ability of phagocytes to kill any biofilm bacteria that they do manage to ingest.

Research has shown that bacteria within biofilms produce many different types of proteins that those same organisms do not produce when they are grown in pure culture. Some of these proteins are involved in the formation of the extracellular matrix and microcolonies. It is thought that bacteria in biofilms can communicate with each other. Experiments with *P. aeruginosa* have demonstrated that when a sufficient number of cells accumulate, the concentration of certain signaling molecules becomes high enough to trigger changes in the activity of dozens of genes. Whereas in the past, scientists studied ways to control individual species of bacteria, they are now concentrating their efforts on ways to attack and control biofilms.

Synergism (Synergistic Infections)

Sometimes, two (or more) microorganisms may "team up" to produce a disease that neither could cause by itself. This is referred to as *synergism* or a *synergistic relationship*. The diseases are referred to as *synergistic infections*, polymicrobial infections, or mixed infections. For example, certain oral bacteria can work together to cause a serious oral disease called acute necrotizing ulcerative gingivitis (ANUG; also known as Vincent | **When two or more microbes "team up" to produce a disease that neither could cause by itself, the phenomenon is referred to as synergism or a synergistic relationship, and the diseases they cause are referred to as synergistic infections, polymicrobial infections, or mixed infections.**

disease and "trench mouth"). Similarly, the disease known as BV is the result of the combined efforts of several different species of bacteria.

AGRICULTURAL MICROBIOLOGY

There are many uses for microorganisms in agriculture. They are used extensively in the field of genetic

engineering to create new or genetically altered plants. Such genetically engineered plants might grow larger, be better tasting, or be more resistant to insects, plant diseases, or extremes in temperature. Some microorganisms are used as pesticides. Many microorganisms are decomposers, which return minerals and other nutrients to soil. In addition, microorganisms play major roles in elemental cycles, such as the carbon, oxygen, nitrogen, phosphorous, and sulfur cycles.

Role of Microbes in Elemental Cycles

Bacteria are exceptionally adaptable and versatile. They are found on the land, in all waters, in every animal and plant, and even inside other microorganisms (in which case they are referred to as *endosymbionts*). Some bacteria and fungi serve a valuable function by recycling back into the soil the nutrients from dead, decaying animals and plants, as was briefly discussed in Chapter 1. Free-living fungi and bacteria that decompose dead organic matter into inorganic materials are called saprophytes. The inorganic nutrients that are returned to the soil are used by chemotrophic bacteria and plants for synthesis of biologic molecules necessary for their growth. The plants are eaten by animals, which eventually die and are recycled again with the aid of saprophytes. The cycling of elements by microorganisms is sometimes referred to as biogeochemical cycling.

Good examples of the cycling of nutrients in nature are the nitrogen, carbon, oxygen, sulfur, and phosphorus cycles, in which microorganisms play very important roles. In the | **The nitrogen cycle involves nitrogen-fixing bacteria, nitrifying bacteria, and denitrifying bacteria.**

nitrogen cycle (Fig. 10-3), free atmospheric nitrogen gas (N_2) is converted by *nitrogen-fixing bacteria* and cyanobacteria into ammonia (NH_3) and the ammonium ion (NH_4^+). Then, chemolithotrophic soil bacteria, called *nitrifying bacteria*, convert ammonium ions into nitrite ions (NO_2^-) and nitrate ions (NO_3^-). Plants then use the nitrates to build plant proteins; these proteins are eaten by animals, which then use them to build animal proteins.

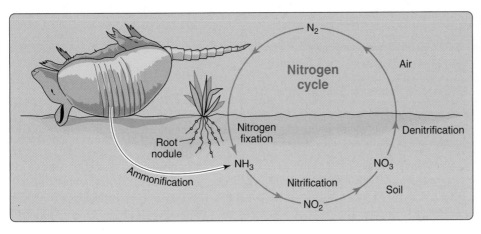

FIGURE 10-3. The nitrogen cycle. See text for details.

Excreted nitrogen-containing animal waste products (such as urea in urine) are converted by certain bacteria to ammonia by a process known as *ammonification*. Also, dead plant and animal nitrogen-containing debris and fecal material are transformed by saprophytic fungi and bacteria into ammonia, which in turn is converted into nitrites and nitrates for recycling by plants. To replenish the free nitrogen in the air, a group of bacteria called *denitrifying bacteria* convert nitrates to atmospheric nitrogen gas (N_2). The cycle goes on and on.

Some nitrogen-fixing bacteria (e.g., *Rhizobium* and *Bradyrhizobium* spp.) live in and near the root nodules of plants called legumes, such as alfalfa, clover, peas, soybeans, and peanuts (Fig. 10-4). These plants are often used in crop-rotation techniques by farmers to return nitrogen compounds to the soil for use as nutrients by cash crops. Nitrifying soil bacteria include *Nitrosomonas*, *Nitrosospira*, *Nitrosococcus*, *Nitrosolobus*, and *Nitrobacter* spp. Denitrifying bacteria include certain species of *Pseudomonas* and *Bacillus*.

Other Soil Microorganisms

In addition to the bacteria that play essential roles in elemental cycles, there are a multitude of other microorganisms in soil—bacteria (including cyanobacteria), fungi (primarily moulds), algae, protozoa, viruses, and viroids. Many of the soil microorganisms are decomposers.

A variety of human pathogens live in soil, including various *Clostridium* spp. (e.g., *Clostridium tetani*, the causative agent of tetanus; *Clostridium botulinum*, the causative agent of botulism; and the various *Clostridium* spp. that cause gas gangrene). The spores of *Bacillus anthracis* (the causative agent of anthrax) may also be present in soil, where they can remain viable for many years. Various yeasts (e.g., *Cryptococcus neoformans*) and fungal spores present in soil may cause human diseases after inhalation of the dust that results from overturning dirt.

> The spores of many human pathogens can be found in soil, including those of *Clostridium* spp., *Bacillus anthracis*, and *Cryptococcus neoformans*.

The types and amounts of microorganisms living in soil depend on many factors, including the amount of decaying organic material, available nutrients, moisture content, amount of oxygen available, pH, temperature, and the presence of waste products of other microbes.

Infectious Diseases of Farm Animals

Farmers, ranchers, and agricultural microbiologists are concerned about the many infectious diseases of farm animals—diseases that may be

> Microbes cause many diseases of farm animals, wild animals, zoo animals, and domestic pets.

FIGURE 10-4. Root nodules of legumes. (A) Soybean root nodules, which contain nitrogen-fixing *Rhizobium* bacteria. **(B)** Nitrogen-fixing bacteria (arrows) can be seen in this cross section of a soybean root nodule. (Courtesy of **[A]** http://en.wikipedia.org and **[B]** http://commons.wikimedia.org.)

TABLE 10-2	Infectious Diseases of Farm Animals
CATEGORY	**DISEASES**
Prion diseases	Bovine spongiform encephalopathy ("mad cow disease"), scrapie
Viral diseases	Blue tongue (sore muzzle), bovine viral diarrhea (BVD), equine encephalomyelitis (sleeping sickness), equine infectious anemia, foot-and-mouth disease, infectious bovine rhinotracheitis, influenza, rabies, swine pox, vesicular stomatitis, warts
Bacterial diseases	Actinomycosis ("lumpy jaw"), anthrax, blackleg, botulism, brucellosis ("Bang's disease), campylobacteriosis, distemper (strangles), erysipelas, foot rot, fowl cholera, leptospirosis, listeriosis, mastitis, pasteurellosis, pneumonia, redwater (bacillary hemoglobinuria), salmonellosis, tetanus ("lock jaw"), tuberculosis, vibriosis
Fungal diseases	Ringworm
Protozoal diseases	Anaplasmosis, bovine trichomoniasis, cattle tick fever (babesiosis), coccidiosis, cryptosporidiosis

caused by a wide variety of pathogens (e.g., viruses, bacteria, protozoa, fungi, and helminths). Not only is there the danger that some of these diseases could be transmitted to humans (discussed in Chapter 11), but these diseases are also of obvious economic concern to farmers and ranchers. Fortunately, vaccines are available to prevent many of these diseases. Although a discussion of these diseases is beyond the scope of this introductory microbiology book, it is important for microbiology students to be aware of their existence. (Likewise, microbiology students should realize that there are many infectious diseases of wild animals, zoo animals, and domestic pets; topics that, because of space limitations, also cannot be addressed in this book.) Table 10-2 lists a few of the many infectious diseases of farm animals and the causative agents of those diseases.

Microbial Diseases of Plants

Microbes cause thousands of different types of plant diseases, often resulting in huge economic losses. Most plant diseases are caused by fungi, viruses, viroids, and bacteria. Not only are living plants attacked and destroyed, but microbes (primarily fungi) also cause the rotting of stored grains and other crops. Plant diseases have interesting names such as blights, cankers, galls, leaf spots, mildews, mosaics, rots, rusts, scabs, smuts, and wilts. Three especially infamous plant diseases are Dutch elm disease (which, since its importation into the United States in 1930, has destroyed about 70% of the elm trees in North America), late blight of potatoes (which resulted in the Great Potato Famine in Ireland, 1845–1849), and wheat rust (which destroys tons of wheat annually). Table 10-3 contains the names of a few of the many plant diseases caused by microorganisms.

> Microbes cause thousands of different types of plant diseases, with names such as blights, cankers, galls, leaf spots, mildews, mosaics, rots, rusts, scabs, smuts, and wilts.

MICROBIAL BIOTECHNOLOGY

The United Nations Convention on Biological Diversity defines biotechnology as "any technological application that uses biological systems, living organisms, or derivatives thereof, to make or modify products or processes for specific use." Although not all areas of biotechnology involve microbes, microbes are used in many aspects of biotechnology. Some examples are listed here:

> Biotechnology is defined as "any technological application that uses biological systems, living organisms, or derivatives thereof, to make or modify products or processes for specific use."

- **Production of therapeutic proteins.** Human genes are introduced (usually by transformation) into bacteria and yeasts. Such genetically engineered microorganisms have been used to produce therapeutic proteins such as human insulin, human growth hormone, human tissue plasminogen activator, interferon, and hepatitis B vaccine.
- **Production of DNA vaccines.** DNA vaccines (also called gene vaccines) are presently only experimental. To prepare a DNA vaccine, a particular pathogen gene (let's use as an example the gene that codes for a specific protein on a pathogen's surface) is inserted into a plasmid (*E. coli* plasmids have been used). Copies of the plasmid are then injected (usually intramuscularly) into a person's tissue. After cells within that tissue internalize the plasmids, the cells produce copies of the gene product (the pathogen's surface protein in this example). The person's immune system then produces antibodies against that gene product, and the antibodies protect the person from infection with that pathogen. The various ways in which antibodies protect us from pathogens are discussed in Chapter 16.

TABLE 10-3	Examples of Plant Diseases Caused by Microorganisms		
DISEASE	**PATHOGEN**	**DISEASE**	**PATHOGEN**
Bean mosaic disease	Virus	Late blight of potatoes	Fungus (a water mold)
Black spot of roses	Fungus	Mushroom root rot	Fungus
Blue mold of tobacco	Fungus (a water mold)	Potato spindle tuber	Viroid
Brown patch of lawns	Fungus	Powdery mildews	Fungi
Chestnut blight	Fungus	Tobacco mosaic disease	Virus
Citrus exocortis	Viroid	Various leaf spots	Bacteria and fungi
Cotton root rot	Fungus	Various rots	Fungi
Crown gall	Bacteria	Various rusts	Fungi
Downy mildew of grapes	Fungus (a water mold)	Various smuts	Fungi
Dutch elm disease	Fungus	Wheat mosaic disease	Virus
Ergot	Fungus	Wheat rust	Fungus

- **Production of vitamins.** Bacteria can be used as sources of vitamins B_2 (riboflavin), B_7 (biotin), B_9 (folic acid), B_{12}, and K_2.
- **Use of microbial metabolites as antimicrobial agents and other types of therapeutic agents.** Penicillins and cephalosporins are examples of antibiotics produced by fungi. Bacitracin, chloramphenicol, erythromycin, polymyxin B, streptomycin, tetracycline, and vancomycin are examples of antibiotics produced by bacteria. Recall that antibiotics were discussed in Chapter 9. Other microbial metabolites have been used as anticancer drugs, immunosuppressants, and herbicides.
- **Agricultural applications.**
  - Certain microbial metabolites have microbicidal, herbicidal, insecticidal, or nematocidal activities. For example, a soil bacterium named *Bacillus subtilis* secretes compounds with antifungal, antibacterial, and insecticidal activities.
  - Bacterial plasmids are used to introduce foreign genes into plants. Plants containing foreign genes are referred to as transgenic plants. Transgenic plants have been produced that are tolerant of or resistant to harsh environments, herbicides, insect pests, and viral, bacterial, fungal, and nematode pathogens. For example, *Bacillus thuringiensis* is a bacterium that produces toxins capable of killing various plant pathogens (e.g., caterpillar larvae). The genes that code for these toxins can be introduced into plants, thus protecting the plants from damage caused by these larvae. Tobacco, cotton, and tomato plants have been protected in this manner.

- **Food technology.**
  - Microorganisms are used in the production of foods such as acidophilus milk, bread, butter, cocoa, coffee, cottage cheese, cultured buttermilk, fish sauces, green olives, kimchi (from cabbage), meat products (e.g., country-cured hams, sausage, salami), olives, pickles, poi (fermented taro root), sauerkraut, sour cream, soy sauce, tofu, various ripened cheeses (e.g., Brie, Camembert, Cheddar, Colby, Edam, Gouda, Gruyere, Limburger, Muenster, Parmesan, Romano, Roquefort, Swiss), vinegar, and yogurt.
  - Yeasts are used in the production of alcoholic beverages, such as ale, beer, bourbon, brandy, cognac, rum, rye whiskey, sake (rice wine), Scotch whiskey, vodka, and wine.
  - Microbes are used in the commercial production of amino acids (e.g., alanine, aspartate, cysteine, glutamate, glycine, histidine, lysine, methionine, phenylalanine, tryptophan) for use in the food industry.
  - Algae and fungi are used as a source of single-cell protein for animal and human consumption.
- **Production of chemicals.** Microbes can be used in the large-scale production of acetic acid, acetone, butanol, citric acid, ethanol, formic acid, glycerol, isopropanol, and lactic acid, as well as biofuels such as hydrogen and methane.
- **Biomining.** Microbes have been used in the mining of arsenic, cadmium, cobalt, copper, nickel, uranium, zinc, and other metals by a process known as leaching or bioleaching.
- **Bioremediation.** The term *bioremediation* refers to the use of microorganisms to clean up various types of wastes, including industrial wastes and other pollutants

(e.g., herbicides and pesticides). Some of the microbes used in this manner have been genetically engineered to digest specific wastes. For example, genetically engineered, petroleum-digesting bacteria were used to clean up the 11 million–gallon oil spill in Prince William Sound, Alaska, in 1989. At a government defense plant in Savannah River, Georgia, scientists have used naturally occurring bacteria known as methanotrophs to remove highly toxic solvents such as trichloroethylene and tetrachloroethylene (collectively referred to as TCEs) from the soil. The methanotrophs, which normally consume methane in the environment, were more or less "tricked" into decomposing the TCEs. In addition, microbes are used extensively in composting, sewage treatment, and water purification (see Chapter 11).

- **Other.**
  - Microbial enzymes used in industry include amylases, cellulase, collagenase, lactase, lipase, pectinase, and proteases.
  - Two amino acids produced by microbes are used in the artificial sweetener called aspartame (NutraSweet).

ON THE CD-ROM
- Terms Introduced in This Chapter
- Review of Key Points
- Insight
  - How Bacteria Communicate with Each Other
- Increase Your Knowledge
- Critical Thinking
- Additional Self-Assessment Exercises

SELF-ASSESSMENT EXERCISES

After studying this chapter, answer the following multiple-choice questions.

1. A symbiont could be a(n):
   a. commensal.
   b. opportunist.
   c. parasite.
   d. all of the above
2. The greatest number and variety of indigenous microflora of the human body live in or on the:
   a. colon.
   b. genitourinary tract.
   c. mouth.
   d. skin.

3. *Escherichia coli* living in the human colon can be considered to be a(n):
   a. endosymbiont.
   b. opportunist.
   c. symbiont in a mutualistic relationship.
   d. all of the above
4. Which of the following sites of the human body does not have indigenous microflora?
   a. bloodstream
   b. colon
   c. distal urethra
   d. vagina
5. Which of the following would be present in highest numbers in the indigenous microflora of the human mouth?
   a. α-hemolytic streptococci
   b. β-hemolytic streptococci
   c. *Candida albicans*
   d. *Staphylococcus aureus*
6. Which of the following would be present in highest numbers in the indigenous microflora of the skin?
   a. *C. albicans*
   b. coagulase-negative staphylococci
   c. *Enterococcus* spp.
   d. *E. coli*
7. The indigenous microflora of the external ear canal is most like the indigenous microflora of the:
   a. colon.
   b. mouth.
   c. skin.
   d. distal urethra.
8. Which of the following are *least* likely to play a role in the nitrogen cycle?
   a. indigenous microflora
   b. nitrifying and denitrifying bacteria
   c. nitrogen-fixing bacteria
   d. bacteria living in the root nodules of legumes
9. Microorganisms are used in which of the following industries?
   a. antibiotic
   b. chemical
   c. food, beer, and wine
   d. all of the above
10. The term that best describes a symbiotic relationship in which two different microorganisms occupy the same ecologic niche, but have absolutely no effect on each other is:
    a. commensalism.
    b. mutualism.
    c. neutralism.
    d. parasitism.

EPIDEMIOLOGY AND PUBLIC HEALTH

11

CHAPTER OUTLINE

LEARNING OBJECTIVES

AFTER STUDYING THIS CHAPTER, YOU SHOULD BE ABLE TO:

- Define epidemiology
- Differentiate among infectious, communicable, and contagious diseases; cite an example of each
- Differentiate between the incidence of a disease and the prevalence of a disease
- Distinguish among sporadic, endemic, nonendemic, epidemic, and pandemic diseases
- Name three diseases that are currently considered to be pandemics
- List, in the proper order, the six components of the chain of infection
- Identify three examples of living reservoirs and three examples of nonliving reservoirs
- List five modes of infectious disease transmission
- List four examples of potential biological warfare (BW) or bioterrorism agents
- Outline the steps involved in water treatment
- Explain what is meant by a coliform count and state its importance

EPIDEMIOLOGY

Introduction

Both **pathology** and **epidemiology** can be loosely defined as the study of disease, but they involve different aspects of disease. Whereas a pathologist studies the structural and functional manifestations of disease and is involved in diagnosing diseases in individuals, an *epidemiologist* studies the factors that determine the frequency, distribution, and determinants of diseases in human populations. With respect to infectious diseases, these factors include the characteristics of various pathogens; susceptibility of different human populations resulting from overcrowding, lack of immunization, nutritional status, inadequate sanitation procedures, and other factors; locations (reservoirs) where pathogens are lurking; and the various ways in which infectious diseases are transmitted. It could be said that epidemiologists are concerned with the who,

> Epidemiology is the study of factors that determine the frequency, distribution, and determinants of diseases in human populations, and ways to prevent, control, or eradicate diseases in populations.

what, where, when, and why of infectious diseases: Who becomes infected? What pathogens are causing the infections? Where do the pathogens come from? When do certain diseases occur? Why do some diseases occur in certain places but not in others? How are pathogens transmitted? Do some diseases occur only at certain times of the year? If so, why? Epidemiologists also develop ways to prevent, control, or eradicate diseases in populations. Epidemiologists are concerned with *all* types of diseases—not just infectious diseases. However, only infectious diseases are discussed in this chapter.

SPOTLIGHTING EPIDEMIOLOGISTS

Epidemiologists are scientists who specialize in the study of disease and injury patterns (incidence and distribution patterns) in populations, and ways to prevent or control diseases and injuries. Epidemiologists study virtually all types of diseases, including heart, hereditary, communicable, and zoonotic diseases and cancer. In some ways, epidemiologists are like disease detectives, gathering and piecing together clues to determine what causes a particular disease, why it occurs only at certain times, and why certain people in a population get the disease while others do not. Quite often, epidemiologists are called on to track down the cause of epidemics and figure out how to stop them. Data collection and statistical analysis of data are among the many duties of epidemiologists.

Epidemiologists have various educational backgrounds. Some are physicians, with specialization in epidemiology or public health. Others have a Doctor of Philosophy degree (PhD or DPhil), a Master of Science or Master of Public Health degree (MS or MPH), or a Bachelor of Science degree (e.g., RN degree) plus specialized training in epidemiology. Many epidemiologists are employed at public health agencies and healthcare institutions. The Centers for Disease Control and Prevention (CDC) employs many epidemiologists, and offers a 2-year, postgraduate course to train health professionals as Epidemic Intelligence Service (EIS) officers. EIS officers, many of whom are employed at state health departments, conduct epidemiologic investigations, research, and public health surveillance. To learn more about the EIS, visit this CDC web site: http://www.cdc.gov/eis.

Epidemiologic Terminology

It sometimes seems like epidemiologists speak a language all their own. They frequently use terms such as communicable, contagious, and zoonotic diseases; the incidence, morbidity rate, prevalence, and mortality rate of a particular disease; and adjectives such as sporadic, endemic,

epidemic, and pandemic to describe the status of a particular infectious disease in a given population. The following sections briefly examine these terms.

Communicable and Contagious Diseases

As previously stated, an infectious disease (infection) is a disease that is caused by a pathogen. If the infectious disease is transmissible from one human to another (i.e., person to person), it is called a **communicable disease**. Although it might seem like splitting hairs, a **contagious disease** is defined as a communicable disease that is *easily transmitted* from one person to another. Example: Assume that you are in the front row of a movie theater. One person seated in the back row has gonorrhea and another has influenza, both of which are communicable diseases. The person with influenza is coughing and sneezing throughout the movie, creating an aerosol of influenza viruses. Thus, even though you are seated far away from the person with influenza, you might very well develop influenza as a result of inhalation of the aerosols produced by that person. Influenza is a contagious disease. On the other hand, you would not contract gonorrhea as a result of your movie-going experience. Gonorrhea is not a contagious disease.

Zoonotic Diseases

Infectious diseases that humans acquire from animal sources are called **zoonotic diseases** or **zoonoses** (sing., zoonosis). These diseases are discussed later in this chapter.

Incidence and Morbidity Rate

The **incidence** of a particular disease is defined as the number of new cases of that disease in a defined population during a specific time period, for example, the number of new cases of hantavirus pulmonary syndrome (HPS) in the United States during 2009. The incidence of a disease is similar to the **morbidity rate** for that disease, which is usually expressed as the number of new cases of a particular disease that occurred during a specified time period per a specifically defined population (usually per 1,000, 10,000, or 100,000 population), for example, the number of new cases of a particular disease in 2009 per 100,000 U.S. population.

STUDY AID
Infectious versus Communicable Diseases
Infectious diseases (infections) are diseases caused by pathogens. **Communicable diseases** are infectious diseases that can be transmitted from one human to another (i.e., person to person). **Contagious diseases** are communicable diseases that are *easily transmitted* from one person to another.

Prevalence

There are two types of **prevalence**: period prevalence and point prevalence. The **period prevalence** of a particular disease is the number of cases of the disease existing in a given population during a specific time period (e.g., the total number of cases of gonorrhea that existed in the U.S. population during 2009). The **point prevalence** of a particular disease is the number of cases of the disease existing in a given population at a particular moment in time (e.g., the number of cases of malaria in the U.S. population at this moment).

Mortality Rate

Mortality refers to death. The **mortality rate** (also known as the *death rate*) is the ratio of the number of people who died of a particular disease during a specified time period per a specified population (usually per 1,000, 10,000, or 100,000 population); for example, the number of people who died of a particular disease in 2009 per 100,000 U.S. population.

Sporadic Diseases

A **sporadic disease** is a disease that occurs only occasionally (sporadically) within the population of a particular geographic area. In the United States, sporadic diseases include botulism, cholera, gas gangrene, plague, tetanus, and typhoid fever. Quite often, certain diseases occur only sporadically because they are kept under control as a result of immunization programs and sanitary conditions. It is possible for outbreaks of these controlled diseases to occur, however, whenever vaccination programs and other public health programs are neglected.

> A sporadic disease is a disease that occurs only occasionally (sporadically) within the population of a particular geographic area, whereas an endemic disease is a disease that is always present within that population.

Endemic Diseases

Endemic diseases are diseases that are always present within the population of a particular geographic area. The number of cases of the disease may fluctuate over time, but the disease never dies out completely. Endemic infectious diseases of the United States include bacterial diseases such as tuberculosis (TB), staphylococcal and streptococcal infections, sexually transmitted diseases (STDs) like gonorrhea and syphilis, and viral diseases such as the common cold, influenza, chickenpox, and mumps. In some parts of the United States, plague (caused by a bacterium called *Yersinia pestis*) is endemic among rats, prairie dogs, and other rodents, but is not endemic among humans. Plague in humans is only occasionally observed in the United States, and is, therefore, a sporadic disease. The actual incidence of an endemic disease at any particular time depends on a balance among several factors, including the environment, genetic susceptibility of the population, behavioral factors, number of people who are immune, virulence of the pathogen, and reservoir or source of infection.

Epidemic Diseases

Endemic diseases may on occasion become **epidemic diseases**. An epidemic (or outbreak) is defined as a greater than usual number of cases of a disease in a particular region, usually occurring within a relatively short period of time. An epidemic does not necessarily involve a large number of people, although it might. If a dozen people develop staphylococcal food poisoning shortly after their return from a church picnic, then that constitutes an epidemic—a small one, to be sure, but an epidemic nonetheless.

> Epidemic diseases are diseases that occur in a greater than usual number of cases in a particular region, and usually occur within a relatively short period of time.

Listed here are a few of the epidemics that have occurred in the United States within the past 35 years:

- **1976.** An epidemic of a respiratory disease (Legionnaires' disease or legionellosis) occurred during an American Legion convention in Philadelphia, Pennsylvania. It resulted in approximately 220 hospitalizations and 34 deaths. The pathogen (a Gram-negative bacillus named *Legionella pneumophila*) was present in the water being circulated through the air-conditioning system of the hotel where the affected Legionnaires were staying. Aerosols of the organism were inhaled by

---

HISTORICAL NOTE

The Broad Street Pump

In the mid-19th century, a British physician by the name of John Snow designed and conducted an epidemiologic investigation of a cholera outbreak in London. He carefully compared households affected by cholera with households that were unaffected, and concluded that the primary difference between them was their source of drinking water. At one point in his investigation, he ordered the removal of the handle of the Broad Street water pump, thus helping to end an epidemic that had killed more than 500 people. People were unable to pump (and, therefore, unable to drink) the contaminated water. Snow published a paper, *On the Communication of Cholera by Impure Thames Water*, in 1884, and a book, *On the Mode of Communication of Cholera*, in 1885. He concluded that cholera was spread via fecally contaminated water. The water at the Broad Street pump was being contaminated with sewage from the adjacent houses (Fig. 11-1). Snow is considered by many to be the "Father of Epidemiology."

FIGURE 11-1. *Thames Water,* **an etching by William Heath, c. 1828.** This etching is a satire on the contamination of the water supply. A London commission reported in 1828 that the Thames River water at Chelsea was "charged with the contents of the great common-sewers, the drainings of the dunghills and laystalls, [and] the refuse of hospitals, slaughterhouses, and manufactures." (Zigrosser C. Medicine and the Artist [Ars Medica]. New York: Dover Publications, Inc., 1970. By permission of the Philadelphia Museum of Art.)

occupants of some of the rooms in the hotel. Subsequent epidemics of legionellosis have occurred in other hotels, hospitals, cruise ships, and supermarkets. The supermarket outbreaks were associated with the misting of vegetables. Virtually all epidemics of legionellosis have involved contaminated water or colonized water pipes and aerosols containing the pathogen.

- **1992–1993.** An epidemic involving *Escherichia coli* O157:H7-contaminated hamburger meat occurred in the Pacific northwest. It resulted in approximately 500 diarrheal cases, 45 cases of kidney failure as a result of hemolytic uremic syndrome (HUS), and the death of several young children. *E. coli* O157:H7 is a particularly virulent serotype of *E. coli*; it is also known as enterohemorrhagic *E. coli*. In this epidemic, the source of the *E. coli* was cattle feces. The ground beef used to make the hamburgers had been contaminated with cattle feces during the slaughtering process. The hamburgers had not been cooked long enough, or at a high enough temperature, to kill the bacteria.
- **1993.** An epidemic of hantavirus pulmonary syndrome (HPS) occurred on Native American reservations in the Four Corners region (where the borders of Colorado, New Mexico, Arizona, and Utah all meet). It resulted in approximately 50 to 60 cases, including

28 deaths. The particular hantavirus strain (now called *Sin Nombre virus*) was present in the urine and feces of deer mice, some of which had gained entrance to the homes of villagers. Aerosols of the virus were produced when residents swept up house dust containing the rodent droppings. The pathogen was then inhaled by individuals in those homes.

- **1993.** An epidemic of cryptosporidiosis (a diarrheal disease) occurred in Milwaukee, Wisconsin. It resulted from drinking water that was contaminated with the oocysts of *Cryptosporidium parvum* (a protozoan parasite). This epidemic is described more fully later in this chapter.
- **2002.** An epidemic of West Nile virus (WNV) infections occurred throughout the United States. More than 4,100 human cases occurred that year, resulting in 284 deaths. In addition, more than 16,000 birds died as a result of WNV infections, and more than 14,500 horses were infected with WNV during 2002. The 2002 WNV epidemic was the largest recognized arboviral meningoencephalitis epidemic in the Western Hemisphere and the largest WNV meningoencephalitis epidemic ever recorded. However, the 2003 WNV epidemic was even worse, with a total of 9,862 cases and 264 deaths. WNV epidemics occur each year in the United States.

- **Waterborne disease outbreaks.** Such outbreaks occur annually in the United States, associated both with drinking water and water that is not intended for drinking. The CDC (described later in the chapter) have presented data associated with 28 waterborne disease outbreaks (WBDOs) that occurred during 2005 and 2006.[a] Of these, 20 were associated with drinking water that caused illness among an estimated 612 persons and four deaths. Etiologic agents were identified in 18 of the 20 outbreaks: 12 were associated with bacteria (135 cases; four deaths), three with viruses (212 cases; no deaths), two with parasites (51 cases; no deaths), and one with a combination of bacteria and viruses (139 cases; no deaths). Ten of the bacterial WBDOs and all four deaths were caused by *Legionella*. *Campylobacter* and/or *E. coli* were involved in the other two bacterial WBDOs. Viral causes included norovirus and hepatitis A virus. Protozoan parasite causes included *Giardia* and *Cryptosporidium*.

- **Foodborne disease outbreaks.** Over 200 known diseases can be transmitted through food, caused by microbes (viruses, bacteria, parasites, prions) or toxins and metals. Investigators at the CDC[b] have estimated that foodborne diseases cause approximately 76 million illnesses, 325,000 hospitalizations, and 5,000 deaths per year in the United States. More than 75% of illnesses caused by identified pathogens are caused by two bacteria (*Salmonella* and *Listeria* spp.) and one parasite (*Toxoplasma*). The bacteria *Campylobacter jejuni* and *E. coli* O157:H7, the protozoan parasite *Cyclospora cayetanensis*, and norwalk virus are other important microbial causes of foodborne illness.

These and other epidemics have been identified through constant surveillance and accumulation of data by the CDC. Epidemics usually follow a specific pattern, in which the number of cases of a disease increases to a maximum and then decreases rapidly, because the number of susceptible and exposed individuals is limited.

Epidemics may occur in communities that have not been previously exposed to a particular pathogen. People from populated areas who travel into isolated communities frequently introduce a new pathogen to susceptible inhabitants of that community, after which the disease spreads rapidly. Over the years, there have been many such examples. The syphilis epidemic in Europe in the early 1500s might have been caused by a highly virulent spirochete carried back from the West Indies by Columbus' men in 1492. Also, measles, smallpox, and TB introduced to Native Americans by early explorers and settlers almost destroyed many tribes.

In communities in which normal sanitation practices are relaxed, allowing fecal contamination of water supplies and food, epidemics of typhoid fever, cholera, giardiasis, and dysentery often occur. Visitors to these communities should be aware that they are especially susceptible to these diseases, because they never developed a natural immunity by being exposed to them during childhood.

Influenza ("flu") epidemics occur in many areas during certain times of the year and involve most of the population because the immunity developed in prior years is usually temporary. Thus, the disease recurs each year among those who are not revaccinated or naturally resistant to the infection. Epidemics of influenza cause approximately 20,000 deaths per year in the United States.

Ebola virus has caused several epidemics of hemorrhagic fever in Africa (Sudan and the Republic of the Congo in 1976; Sudan in 1979; the Republic of the Congo in 1995; Gabon in 1994 and 1996; Uganda in 2000; several outbreaks in Gabon and the Republic of the Congo between 2001 and 2003). The 2000 outbreak in Uganda (425 cases, 224 deaths) was the largest Ebola epidemic ever recorded. Between 25% and 90% of infected patients have died in these epidemics. The source of the virus is not yet known.

In a hospital setting, a relatively small number of infected patients can constitute an epidemic. If a higher than usual number of patients on a particular ward should suddenly become infected by a particular pathogen, this would constitute an epidemic, and the situation must be brought to the attention of the Hospital Infection Control Committee (discussed in Chapter 12).

Pandemic Diseases

A **pandemic disease** is a disease that is occurring in epidemic proportions in many countries simultaneously—sometimes worldwide. The 1918 Spanish flu pandemic was the most devastating pandemic of the 20th century, and is the catastrophe against which all modern pandemics are measured. That pandemic killed more than 20 million people worldwide, including 500,000 in the United States. Almost every nation on Earth was affected. Influenza pandemics are often named for the point of origin or first recognition, such as the Taiwan flu, Hong Kong flu, London flu, Port Chalmers flu, and the Russian flu.

According to the World Health Organization (WHO), infectious diseases are responsible for approximately half the deaths that occur in developing countries; approximately half of those are caused by three infectious diseases—human immunodeficiency virus/acquired immunodeficiency syndrome (HIV/AIDS),

> A pandemic disease is a disease that is occurring in epidemic proportions in many countries simultaneously— sometimes worldwide.

> Collectively, HIV/AIDS, TB, and malaria cause more than 300 million illnesses and more than 5 million deaths per year.

---

[a] *Morbidity and Mortality Weekly Report (MMWR)* 57 (SS09): 39–62, 2008.
[b] *Emerging Infectious Diseases* 5 (No. 5): Sep–Oct, 1999.

FIGURE 11-2. Common modes of HIV transmission.
(From Harvey RA et al. Lippincott's Illustrated Reviews:
Microbiology. 2nd ed. Philadelphia: Lippincott Williams &
Wilkins, 2007.)

tuberculosis, and malaria—each of which is currently occurring in pandemic proportions. Collectively, these
three diseases cause more than 300 million illnesses and
more than 5 million deaths per year.

HIV/AIDS Although the first documented evidence of
HIV infection in humans can be traced to an African
serum sample collected in 1959, it is possible that humans were infected with HIV before that date. The
AIDS epidemic began in the United States around 1979,
but the epidemic was not detected until 1981. It was not
until 1983 that the virus that causes AIDS was discovered. HIV is thought to have been transferred to humans
from other primates (chimpanzees in the case of HIV-1,
and sooty mangabeys [a type of Old World monkey] in
the case of HIV-2). Common modes of HIV transmission are shown in Figure 11-2. Additional information
about AIDS can be found in Chapter 18 . The following
statistics, which should prove sobering to anyone who
thought that AIDS was "on the run," were obtained from
the WHO and CDC web sites (http://www.who.int/en/;
http://www.cdc.gov):

* The total number of people living with HIV, worldwide, in 2007 is estimated to be 33.2 million. Table
  11-1 shows the distribution of HIV-infected individuals in 2007.
* An estimated 2.5 million people worldwide acquired
  HIV infection in 2007. Approximately 68% of these
  cases occurred in sub-Saharan Africa.
* The global AIDS pandemic killed an estimated 2.1
  million people worldwide in 2007 (over 5,700 AIDS
  deaths per day). Approximately 76% of these deaths
  occurred in sub-Saharan Africa.
* As of December 2007, a total of 1,051,875 U.S. cases
  had been reported to the CDC, with 37,503 of those
  cases reported during 2006.
* As of December 2007, the total number of U.S. deaths
  of persons with AIDS was 562,793, with 14,110 of
  those deaths occurring in 2007.
* According to the CDC, an estimated 455,636 persons
  in the United States were living with HIV/AIDS at the
  end of 2007.

TABLE 11-1	Estimated Number of People Living with HIV Infection/AIDS at the End of 2007
GEOGRAPHIC AREA	**ESTIMATED NUMBER**
Sub-Saharan Africa	22.5 million
South and Southeast Asia	4.0 million
Latin America	1.6 million
Eastern Europe and Central Asia	1.6 million
East Asia	800,000
North America	1.3 million
Western and Central Europe	760,000
North Africa and Middle East	380,000
Caribbean	230,000
Oceania	75,000

Source: World Health Organization (WHO), Geneva (http://www.who.int/en/).

Tuberculosis. Another current pandemic is TB. To complicate matters, many strains of *Mycobacterium tuberculosis* (the bacterium that causes TB) have developed resistance to the drugs that are used to treat TB. TB caused by these strains is known as *multidrug-resistant tuberculosis* (MDR-TB), or in some cases, *extensively drug-resistant tuberculosis* (XDR-TB). Some strains of *M. tuberculosis* have developed resistance to every drug and every combination of drugs that has ever been used to treat TB. MDR-TB and XDR-TB are present in virtually all regions of the world, including the United States. According to the WHO, China and the countries of the former Soviet Union have the highest occurrence rates of MDR-TB. Additional information about TB can be found in Chapter 19 . The following statistics were obtained from the WHO and CDC web sites:

- Among infectious diseases, TB remains the second leading killer of adults in the world, with approximately 2 million TB-related deaths each year.
- TB is a worldwide pandemic. The highest rates per capita are in Africa (28% of all TB cases), but half of all new cases are in Asian countries.
- Worldwide, there were an estimated 9.2 million new TB cases in 2006.
- Overall, 2 billion people, equal to one third of the world's population, are currently infected with *M. tuberculosis*. There were an estimated 14.4 million active cases of TB in 2006, including an estimated 0.5 million cases of MDR-TB.
- Someone in the world becomes newly infected with *M. tuberculosis* every second.
- Excluding individuals infected with HIV, 10% of people who are infected with *M. tuberculosis* become sick with active TB at some time during their life. People living with HIV are at a much greater risk.

- Left untreated, each person with active TB can infect on average between 10 and 15 people a year.
- TB is a leading killer among people infected with HIV. Worldwide, about 200,000 people with HIV die from TB every year, most of them in Africa.
- During 2006, TB caused an estimated 1.7 million deaths worldwide, equal to about 4,650 deaths per day. The vast majority of TB deaths are in the developing world, with more than half occurring in Asia.
- In 2007, 13,299 new U.S. cases of TB were reported to the CDC. The CDC reported a total of 644 U.S. TB deaths in 2006.

Malaria. Malaria is the world's most important tropical parasitic disease, killing more people than any other communicable disease, except TB. Additional information about malaria can be found in Chapter 21. The following statistics were obtained from the WHO and CDC web sites:

- About half of the world's population (3.3 billion people) live in malaria-endemic areas and one fifth of the world's population (1.2 billion people) live in areas with a high risk of malaria.
- Africa has the largest number of people living in areas with a high risk of malaria, followed by the Southeast Asia region.
- There were an estimated 247 million malaria cases worldwide in 2006, of which 91% (230 million cases) were caused by *Plasmodium falciparum*.
- An estimated 1 million people die of malaria annually.
- One in five (20%) of all childhood deaths in Africa are caused by malaria. In Africa, malaria causes one child to die every 30 seconds.
- In 2002, malaria was the fourth leading cause of death in children in developing countries (after perinatal conditions, lower respiratory infections, and diarrheal diseases).
- During 2007, 1,408 new U.S. cases of malaria were reported to the CDC. All of these cases were deemed to be imported, meaning that the infection was acquired outside of the United States and its territories.
- Mosquito-borne malaria does occur in the United States. Between 1957 and 2003, 63 such outbreaks have occurred. In virtually all cases, the mosquito vectors became infected by biting persons who had acquired malaria outside the United States.

INTERACTIONS AMONG PATHOGENS, HOSTS, AND ENVIRONMENTS

Whether or not an infectious disease occurs depends on many factors, some of which are listed here:

1. Factors pertaining to the pathogen:
   - The virulence of the pathogen (Virulence will be discussed in Chapter 14 ; for now, think of virulence

as a measure or degree of pathogenicity; some pathogens are more virulent than others.)

- A way for the pathogen to enter the body (i.e., Is there a portal of entry?)
- The number of organisms that enter the body (i.e., Will there be a sufficient number to cause infection?)

Whether or not an infectious disease occurs depends on many factors, including those pertaining to the pathogen, those pertaining to the host, and those pertaining to the environment.

2. Factors pertaining to the host (i.e., the person who may become infected):
   - The person's health status (e.g., Is the person hospitalized? Does he or she have any underlying illnesses? Has the person undergone invasive medical or surgical procedures or catheterization? Does he or she have any prosthetic devices?)
   - The person's nutritional status
   - Other factors pertaining to the susceptibility of the host (e.g., age, lifestyle [behavior], socioeconomic level, occupation, travel, hygiene, substance abuse, immune status [immunizations or previous experience with the pathogen])

3. Factors pertaining to the environment:
   - Physical factors such as geographic location, climate, heat, cold, humidity, and season of the year.
   - Availability of appropriate reservoirs (discussed later in this chapter), intermediate hosts (discussed in Chapter 21), and vectors (discussed later in this chapter)
   - Sanitary and housing conditions; adequate waste disposal; adequate healthcare
   - Availability of potable (drinkable) water

CHAIN OF INFECTION

There are six components in the infectious disease process (also known as the *chain of infection*). They are illustrated in Figure 11-3 and are briefly described here:

The six components in the chain of infection are (a) a pathogen, (b) a reservoir of infection, (c) a portal of exit, (d) a mode of transmission, (e) a portal of entry, and (f) a susceptible host.

1. There must first be a pathogen. As an example, let us assume that the pathogen is a cold virus.
2. There must be a source of the pathogen (i.e., a reservoir). In Figure 11-3, the infected person on the right ("Andy") is the reservoir. Andy has a cold.
3. There must be a portal of exit (i.e., a way for the pathogen to escape from the reservoir). When Andy blows his nose, cold viruses get onto his hands.
4. There must be a mode of transmission (i.e., a way for the pathogen to travel from Andy to another person). In Figure 11-3, the cold virus is being transferred by direct contact between Andy and his friend ("Bob")— by shaking hands.
5. There must be a portal of entry (i.e., a way for the pathogen to gain entry into Bob). When Bob rubs his nose, the cold virus is transferred from his hand to the mucous membranes of his nose.
6. There must be a susceptible host. For example, Bob would not be a susceptible host (and would, therefore, not develop a cold) if he had previously been infected by that particular cold virus and had developed immunity to it.

FIGURE 11-3. The six components in the infectious disease process; also known as the chain of infection.

STRATEGIES FOR BREAKING THE CHAIN OF INFECTION

To prevent infections from occurring, measures must be taken to break the chain of infection at some point (link) in the chain. Strategies for breaking the chain of infection are discussed in detail in Chapter 12. Some of the broad goals are to:

- Eliminate or contain the reservoirs of pathogens or curtail the persistence of a pathogen at the source
- Prevent contact with infectious substances from exit pathways
- Eliminate means of transmission
- Block exposure to entry pathways
- Reduce or eliminate the susceptibility of potential hosts

Some of the specific methods of breaking the chain of infection are:

- Practice effective hand hygiene procedures
- Maintain good nutrition and adequate rest and reduce stress
- Obtain immunizations against common pathogens
- Practice insect and rodent control measures
- Practice proper patient isolation procedures
- Ensure proper decontamination of surfaces and medical instruments
- Dispose of sharps and infectious waste properly
- Use gloves, gowns, masks, respirators, and other personal protective equipment, whenever appropriate to do so
- Use needle safety devices during blood collection

RESERVOIRS OF INFECTION

The sources of microbes that cause infectious diseases are many and varied. They are known as **reservoirs of infection** or simply **reservoirs**. A reservoir is any site where the pathogen can multiply or merely survive until it is transferred to a host. Reservoirs may be living hosts or inanimate objects or materials (Fig. 11-4).

> Reservoirs of infection may be living hosts or inanimate objects or materials.

Living Reservoirs

Living reservoirs include humans, household pets, farm animals, wild animals, certain insects, and certain arachnids (ticks and mites). The human and animal reservoirs may or may not be experiencing illness caused by the pathogens they are harboring.

Human Carriers

The most important reservoirs of human infectious diseases are other humans—people with infectious diseases as well as carriers. A **carrier** is a person who is colonized with a particular pathogen, but the pathogen is not currently causing disease in that person. However, the pathogen can be transmitted from the carrier to others, who may then become ill. There are several types of carriers. **Passive carriers** carry the pathogen without ever having had the disease. An **incubatory carrier** is a person who is capable of transmitting a pathogen during the incubation period of a particular infectious disease. **Convalescent carriers** harbor and can transmit a particular pathogen while recovering from an infectious disease (i.e., during the convalescence period). **Active carriers** have completely recovered from the disease, but continue to harbor the pathogen indefinitely (see the following "Historical Note" for an example). Respiratory secretions or feces are usually the vehicles by which the pathogen is

> A carrier is a person who is colonized with a particular pathogen, but the pathogen is not currently causing disease in that person.

FIGURE 11-4. Reservoirs of infection include soil, dust, contaminated water, contaminated foods, insects, and infected humans, domestic animals, and wild animals. (Reproduced courtesy of Engelkirk PG, et al. Principles and Practice of Clinical Anaerobic Bacteriology. Belmont, CA: Star Publishing Co., 1992.)

HISTORICAL NOTE

"Typhoid Mary": An Infamous Carrier

Mary Mallon was a domestic employee—a cook—who worked in the New York City area in the early 1900s. Mary had recovered from typhoid fever earlier in life. Although no longer ill, she was a carrier. *Salmonella typhi*, the causative agent of typhoid fever, was still living in her gallbladder and passing in her feces. Apparently, Mary's hygienic practices were inadequate, and she would transport the *Salmonella* bacteria via her hands from the restroom to the kitchen, where she then unwittingly introduced them into foods that she prepared. After several typhoid fever outbreaks were traced to her, Mary was offered the choice of having her gallbladder removed surgically or being jailed. She opted for the latter and spent several years in jail. Mary was released from jail after promising never to cook professionally again. However, the lure of the kitchen was too great. She changed her name and resumed her profession in various hotels, restaurants, and hospitals. As in the past, "everywhere that Mary went, typhoid fever was sure to follow." She was again arrested and spent her remaining years quarantined in a New York City hospital. Mary Mallon died in 1938 at the age of 70.

transferred, either directly from the carrier to a susceptible individual or indirectly through food or water. Human carriers are very important in the spread of staphylococcal and streptococcal infections as well as in the spread of hepatitis, diphtheria, dysentery, meningitis, and STDs.

Animals

As previously stated, infectious diseases that humans acquire from animal sources are called zoonotic diseases or zoonoses. Many pets and other animals are important reservoirs of zoonoses. Zoonoses are acquired by direct contact with the animal, by inhalation or ingestion of the pathogen, or by injection of the pathogen by an arthropod vector. Measures for the control of zoonotic diseases include the use of personal protective equipment when handling animals, animal vaccinations, proper use of pesticides, isolation or destruction of infected animals, and proper disposal of animal carcasses and waste products.

> Zoonotic diseases (zoonoses) are infectious diseases that humans acquire from animal sources.

Examples of Zoonoses. Dogs, cats, bats, skunks, and other animals are known reservoirs of rabies. The rabies virus is usually transmitted to a human through the saliva that is injected when one of these rabid animals bites the human. Cat and dog bites often transfer bacteria from the mouths of animals into tissues, where severe infec-

tions may result. Toxoplasmosis, a protozoan disease caused by *Toxoplasma gondii*, can be contracted by ingesting oocysts from cat feces that are present in litter boxes or sand boxes, as well by ingesting cysts that are present in infected raw or undercooked meats. Toxoplasmosis may cause severe brain damage to, or death of, the fetus when contracted by a woman during her first trimester (first 3 months) of pregnancy. The diarrheal disease, salmonellosis, is frequently acquired by ingesting *Salmonella* bacteria from the feces of turtles, other reptiles, and poultry. A variant form of Creutzfeldt-Jakob (CJ) disease in humans, called variant C-J disease, may be acquired by ingestion of prion-infected beef from cows with bovine spongiform encephalopathy (BSE or "mad cow disease"). Persons skinning rabbits can become infected with the bacterium *Francisella tularensis* and develop tularemia. Contact with dead animals or animal hides could result in the inhalation of the spores of *Bacillus anthracis*, leading to inhalation anthrax, or the spores could enter a cut, leading to cutaneous anthrax. Ingestion of the spores could lead to gastrointestinal anthrax. Psittacosis or "parrot fever" is a respiratory infection that may be acquired from infected birds (usually parakeets and parrots).

The most prevalent zoonotic infection in the United States is Lyme disease (discussed under "Arthropods"), one of many arthropod-borne zoonoses. (Arthropod-borne diseases are diseases that are transmitted by arthropods.) Other zoonoses that occur in the United States include anthrax, brucellosis, campylobacteriosis, cryptosporidiosis, echinococcosis, ehrlichiosis, HPS, leptospirosis, pasteurellosis, plague, psittacosis, Q fever, rabies, ringworm, Rocky Mountain spotted fever, salmonellosis, toxoplasmosis, tularemia, and various viral encephalitides (e.g., Western equine encephalitis, Eastern equine encephalitis, St. Louis encephalitis, California encephalitis, WNV encephalitis). Some of the more than 200 known zoonoses are listed in Table 11-2. For a discussion of healthcare-associated zoonoses, see the "Insight" section on this topic under Chapter 12 of this book's CD-ROM.

> There are over 200 known zoonoses—diseases that can be transmitted from animals to humans.

Arthropods

Technically, arthropods are animals, but they are being discussed here separately from other animals because, as a group, they are so commonly associated with human infections. Many different types of arthropods serve as reservoirs of infection, including insects (e.g., mosquitoes, biting flies, lice, fleas), and arachnids (e.g., mites, ticks). When involved in the transmission of infectious diseases, these arthropods are referred to as **vectors**. The arthropod vector may first take a blood meal from an infected person or animal and then transfer the pathogen to a healthy individual. Take Lyme disease, for example, which is the most common arthropod-borne disease in the United States. First, a tick takes a blood

TABLE 11-2	Examples of Zoonotic Diseases			
CATEGORY	**DISEASE**	**PATHOGEN**	**ANIMAL RESERVOIR(S)**	**MODE OF TRANSMISSION**
Viral diseases	Avian influenza ("bird flu")	An influenza virus	Birds	Direct or indirect contact with infected birds
	Equine encephalitis	Various arboviruses	Birds, small mammals	Mosquito bite
	Hantavirus pulmonary syndrome	Hantaviruses	Rodents	Inhalation of contaminated dust or aerosols
	Lassa fever	Lassa virus	Wild rodents	Inhalation of contaminated dust or aerosols
	Marburg disease	Marburg virus	Monkeys	Contact with blood or tissues from infected monkeys
	Rabies	Rabies virus	Rabid dogs, cats, skunks, foxes, wolves, raccoons, coyotes, bats	Animal bite or inhalation
	Yellow fever	Yellow fever virus	Monkeys	*Aedes aegypti* mosquito bite
	West Nile virus encephalitis	West Nile virus	Birds	Mosquito bite
Bacterial diseases	Anthrax	*Bacillus anthracis*	Cattle, sheep, goats	Inhalation, ingestion, entry through cuts, contact with mucous membranes
	Bovine tuberculosis	*Mycobacterium bovis*	Cattle	Ingestion
	Brucellosis	*Brucella* spp.	Cattle, swine, goats	Inhalation, ingestion of contaminated milk, entry through cuts, contact with mucous membranes
	Campylobacter infection	*Campylobacter* spp.	Wild mammals, cattle, sheep, pets	Ingestion of contaminated food and water
	Cat-scratch disease	*Bartonella henselae*	Domestic cats	Cat scratch, bite, or lick
	Ehrlichiosis	*Ehrlichia* spp.	Deer, mice	Tick bite
	Endemic typhus	*Rickettsia typhi*	Rodents	Flea bite
	Leptospirosis	*Leptospira* spp.	Cattle, rodents, dogs	Contact with contaminated animal urine
	Lyme disease	*Borrelia burgdorferi*	Deer, rodents	Tick bite
	Pasteurellosis	*Pasteurella multocida*	Oral cavities of animals	Bites, scratches
	Plague	*Yersinia pestis*	Rodents	Flea bite
	Psittacosis (ornithosis, parrot fever)	*Chlamydophila psittaci*	Parrots, parakeets, other pet birds, pigeons, poultry	Inhalation of contaminated dust and aerosols
	Relapsing fever	*Borrelia* spp.	Rodents	Tick bite
	Rickettsial pox	*Rickettsia akari*	Rodents	Mite bite
	Rocky Mountain spotted fever	*Rickettsia rickettsii*	Rodents, dogs	Tick bite
	Salmonellosis	*Salmonella* spp.	Poultry, livestock, reptiles	Ingestion of contaminated food, handling reptiles
	Scrub typhus	*Orientia tsutsugamushi*	Rodents	Mite bite
	Tularemia	*Francisella tularensis*	Wild mammals	Entry through cuts, inhalation, tick or deer fly bite
	Q fever	*Coxiella burnetii*	Cattle, sheep, goats	Tick bite, air, mild contact with infected animals

(continues)

TABLE 11-2	Examples of Zoonotic Diseases (continued)			
CATEGORY	DISEASE	PATHOGEN	ANIMAL RESERVOIR(S)	MODE OF TRANSMISSION
Fungal diseases	Tinea (ringworm) infections	Various dermatophytes	Various animals including dogs	Contact with infected animals
Protozoal diseases	African trypanosomiasis	Subspecies of *Trypanosoma brucei*	Cattle, wild game animals	Tsetse fly bite
	American trypanosomiasis (Chagas' disease)	*Trypanosoma cruzi*	Numerous wild and, domestic animals including dogs, cats, wild rodents	Trypomastigotes in the feces of reduviid bug are rubbed into bite wound or the eye
	Babesiosis	*Babesia microti*	Deer, mice, voles	Tick bite
	Leishmaniasis	*Leishmania* spp.	Rodents, dogs	Sandfly bite
	Toxoplasmosis	*Toxoplasma gondii*	Cats, pigs, sheep, rarely cattle	Ingestion of oocysts in cat feces or cysts in raw or undercooked meat
Helminth diseases	Echinococcosis (hydatid disease)	*Echinococcus granulosis*	Dogs	Ingestion of eggs
	Dog tapeworm infection	*Dipylidium caninum*	Dogs, cats	Ingestion of flea containing the larval stage
	Rat tapeworm infection	*Hymenolepis diminuta*	Rodents	Ingestion of beetle containing the larval stage

meal from an infected deer or mouse (Fig. 11-5). The tick is now infected with *Borrelia burgdorferi*, the spirochete that causes Lyme disease. Some time later, the tick takes a blood meal from a human and, in the process, injects the bacteria into the human. Ticks are especially notorious vectors. In the United States, there are at least 10 infectious diseases that are transmitted by ticks (see the following "Study Aid"). Other arthropod-borne infectious diseases are shown in Table 11-3. Chapter 21 contains additional information about arthropods.

Nonliving Reservoirs

Nonliving or inanimate reservoirs of infection include air, soil, dust, food, milk, water, and fomites (defined later in the chapter). Air can become contaminated by dust or res-

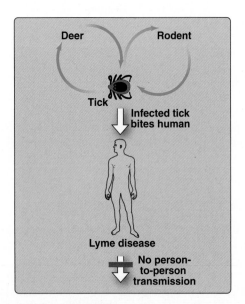

FIGURE 11-5. Transmission of Lyme disease. (From Harvey RA, et al. Lippincott's Illustrated Reviews: Microbiology. 2nd ed. Philadelphia: Lippincott Williams & Wilkins, 2007.)

STUDY AID
Tickborne Diseases of the United States
Viral diseases:
  Colorado tick fever
  Powassan virus encephalitis
Bacterial diseases:
  Human granulocytic ehrlichiosis
  Human monocytic ehrlichiosis
  Lyme disease
  Q fever
  Rocky Mountain spotted fever
  Tickborne relapsing fever
  Tularemia
Protozoal disease:
  Babesiosis
(In addition to serving as vectors in these infectious diseases, ticks can cause tick paralysis.)

TABLE 11-3	Arthropods that Serve as Vectors of Human Infectious Diseases
VECTORS	**DISEASE(S)**
Black flies (*Simulium* spp.)	Onchocerciasis ("river blindness") (H)
Cyclops spp.	Fish tapeworm infection (H), guinea worm infection (H)
Fleas	Dog tapeworm infection (H), endemic typhus (B), murine typhus (B), plague (B)
Lice	Epidemic relapsing fever (B), epidemic typhus (B), trench fever (B)
Mites	Rickettsial pox (B), scrub typhus (B)
Mosquitoes	Dengue fever (V), filariasis ("elephantiasis") (H), malaria (P), viral encephalitis (V), yellow fever (V)
Reduviid bugs	American trypanosomiasis (Chagas' disease) (P)
Sand flies (*Phlebotomus* spp.)	Leishmaniasis (P)
Ticks	Babesiosis (P), Colorado tick fever (V), ehrlichiosis (B), Lyme disease (B), relapsing fever (B), Rocky Mountain spotted fever (B), tularemia (B)
Tsetse flies (*Glossina* spp.)	African trypanosomiasis (P)

B, bacterial disease; *P*, protozoal disease; *H*, helminth disease; *V*, viral disease.

piratory secretions of humans expelled into the air by breathing, talking, sneezing, and coughing. The most highly contagious diseases include colds and influenza, in which the respiratory viruses can be transmitted through the air on droplets of respiratory tract secretions. Air currents and air vents can transport respiratory pathogens throughout healthcare facilities and other buildings. Dust particles can carry spores of certain bacteria and dried bits of human and animal excretions containing pathogens. Bacteria cannot multiply in the air, but can easily be transported by airborne particles to a warm, moist, nutrient-rich site, where they can multiply. Also, some fungal respiratory diseases (e.g., histoplasmosis) are frequently transferred by dust containing yeasts or spores. Soil contains the spores of the *Clostridium* species that cause tetanus, botulism, and gas gangrene. Any of these diseases can follow the introduction of spores into an open wound.

Food and milk may be contaminated by careless handling, which allows pathogens to enter from soil, dust particles, dirty hands, hair, and respiratory secretions. If these pathogens are not destroyed by proper processing and cooking, food poisoning can develop. As stated previously, foodborne diseases cause approximately 76 million illnesses, 325,000 hospitalizations, and 5,000 deaths per year in the United States. Diseases frequently transmitted through foods and water are amebiasis (caused by the ameba, *Entamoeba histolytica*), botulism (caused by the bacterium, *Clostridium botulinum*), cholera (caused by the bacterium, *Vibrio cholerae*), *Clostridium perfringens* food poisoning, infec-

> Air, soil, dust, food, milk, water, and fomites are examples of nonliving or inanimate reservoirs of infection.

tious hepatitis (caused by hepatitis A virus), staphylococcal food poisoning, typhoid fever (caused by the bacterium, *S. typhi*), and trichinosis (a helminth disease, caused by ingesting *Trichinella spiralis* larvae in pork). Other common foodborne and waterborne pathogens are shown in Table 11-4.

Human and animal fecal matter from outhouses, cesspools, and feed lots is often carried into water supplies. Improper disposal of sewage and inadequate treatment of drinking water contribute to the spread of fecal and soil pathogens. **Fomites** are inanimate objects capable of transmitting pathogens. Fomites found within healthcare settings include patients' gowns, bedding, towels, eating and drinking utensils, and hospital equipment, such as bedpans, stethoscopes, latex gloves, electronic thermometers, and electrocardiographic electrodes, which become contaminated by pathogens from the respiratory tract, intestinal tract, or the skin of patients. Even telephones, doorknobs, and computer keyboards can serve as fomites. Great care must be taken by healthcare personnel to prevent transmission of pathogens from living and nonliving reservoirs to hospitalized patients.

MODES OF TRANSMISSION

Healthcare professionals must be thoroughly familiar with the sources (reservoirs) of potential pathogens and pathways for their transfer. A hospital staphylococcal epidemic may begin when aseptic conditions are relaxed and a *Staphylococcus aureus* carrier transmits the pathogen to susceptible patients (e.g., babies, surgical patients, debilitated persons). Such an infection could quickly spread throughout the entire hospital population.

TABLE 11-4	Pathogens Commonly Transmitted via Food and Water[a]	
PATHOGEN	**VEHICLE**	**COMMENTS**
Campylobacter jejuni (bacterium)	Chickens	
Cryptosporidium parvum (protozoan)	Drinking water	Highly resistant to disinfectants used to purify drinking water
Cyclospora cayetanensis (protozoan)	Drinking water, raspberries	
E. coli 0157:H7 (bacterium)	Meats, produce contaminated by manure in growing fields (e.g., sprouts), drinking water	
Giardia lamblia (also called *Giardia intestinalis*) (protozoan)	Drinking water	Moderately resistant to disinfectants used to purify drinking water
Listeria monocytogenes (bacterium)	Soft cheeses and deli meats	
Salmonella enteritidis (bacterium)	Eggs	
Salmonella typhimurium DT-104 (bacterium)	Unpasteurized milk	Resistant to many antibiotics
Shigella spp. (bacteria)	Drinking water	

[a]Additional pathogens transmitted in food and water are mentioned in the text.

The five principal modes by which transmission of pathogens occur are contact (either direct or indirect contact), droplet, airborne, vehicular, and vector transmission (Fig. 11-6 and Table 11-5). Droplet transmission involves the transfer of pathogens via infectious droplets (particles 5 μm in diameter or larger). Droplets may be generated by coughing, sneezing, and even talking. Airborne transmission involves the dispersal of droplet nuclei, which are the residue of evaporated droplets, and are smaller than 5 μm in diameter. Vehicular transmission involves contaminated inanimate objects ("vehicles"), such as food, water, dust, and fomites. Vectors include various types of biting insects and arachnids.

> The five principal modes by which transmission of pathogens occur are contact (either direct or indirect contact), droplet, airborne, vehicular, and vector transmission.

FIGURE 11-6. Modes of disease transmission.

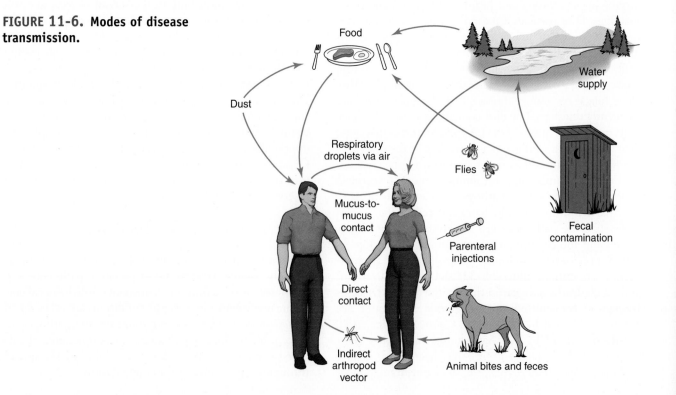

TABLE 11-5	**Common Routes of Transmission of Infectious Diseases**	
ROUTE OF EXIT	**ROUTE OF TRANSMISSION OR ENTRY**	**DISEASES**
Skin	Skin discharge → air → respiratory tract	Chickenpox, colds, influenza, measles, staph and strep infections
	Skin to skin	Impetigo, eczema, boils, warts, syphilis
Respiratory	Aerosol droplet inhalation Nose or mouth → hand or object → nose	Colds, influenza, pneumonia, mumps, measles, chickenpox, tuberculosis
Gastrointestinal	Feces → hand → mouth Stool → soil, food, or water → mouth	Gastroenteritis, hepatitis, salmonellosis, shigellosis, typhoid fever, cholera, giardiasis, amebiasis
Salivary	Direct salivary transfer	Herpes cold sore, infectious mononucleosis, strep throat
Genital secretions	Urethral or cervical secretions Semen	Gonorrhea, herpes, *Chlamydia* infection Cytomegalovirus infection, AIDS, syphilis, warts
Blood	Transfusion or needlestick injury Insect bite	Hepatitis B, cytomegalovirus infection, malaria, AIDS Malaria relapsing fever
Zoonotic	Animal bite Contact with animal carcasses	Rabies Tularemia, anthrax
	Arthropod	Rocky Mountain spotted fever, Lyme disease, typhus, viral encephalitis, yellow fever, malaria, plague

Communicable diseases—infectious diseases that are transmitted from person to person—are most commonly transmitted in the following ways:

- **Direct skin-to-skin contact.** For example, the common cold virus is frequently transmitted from the hand of someone who just blew his or her nose to another person by hand shaking. Within hospitals, this mode of transfer is particularly prevalent, which is why it is so important for healthcare professionals to wash their hands before and after every patient contact. Frequent handwashing will prevent the transfer of pathogens from one patient to another.
- **Direct mucous membrane-to-mucous membrane contact by kissing or sexual intercourse.** Most STDs are transmitted in this manner. STDs include syphilis, gonorrhea, and infections caused by chlamydia, herpes, and HIV. Chlamydial genital infections are especially common in the United States; in fact, they are the most common nationally notifiable infectious diseases in the United States. (Nationally notifiable infectious diseases are discussed later in this chapter.)
- **Indirect contact via airborne droplets of respiratory secretions, usually produced as a result of sneezing or coughing.** Most contagious airborne diseases are caused by respiratory pathogens carried to susceptible people in droplets of respiratory secretions. Some respiratory pathogens may settle on dust particles and be carried long distances through the air and into a building's ventilation or air-conditioning system. Improperly cleaned inhalation therapy equipment can easily transfer these pathogens from one patient to another. Diseases that may be transmitted in this manner include colds, influenza, measles, mumps, chickenpox, smallpox, and pneumonia.
- **Indirect contact via food and water contaminated with fecal material.** Many infectious diseases are transmitted by restaurant food handlers who fail to wash their hands after using the restroom.
- **Indirect contact via arthropod vectors.** Arthropods such as mosquitoes, flies, fleas, lice, ticks, and mites can transfer various pathogens from person to person.
- **Indirect contact via fomites that become contaminated by respiratory secretions, blood, urine, feces, vomitus, or exudates from hospitalized patients.** Fomites such as stethoscopes and latex gloves are sometimes the vehicles by which pathogens are transferred from one patient to another. Examples of fomites are shown in Figure 11-7.
- **Indirect contact via transfusion of contaminated blood or blood products from an ill person or by *parenteral injection* (injection directly into the bloodstream) using nonsterile syringes and needles.** One reason why disposable sterile tubes, syringes, and various other types of single-use hospital equipment have become very popular is that they are effective in preventing bloodborne infections (e.g., hepatitis, syphilis, malaria, AIDS, systemic staphylococcal infections) that result from reuse of equipment. Individuals using illegal intravenous drugs commonly transmit these diseases to each other by sharing needles and syringes, which easily become contaminated with the blood of an infected person.

FIGURE 11-7. Various medical instruments and apparatus that may serve as inanimate vectors of infection (fomites).

Cup

Blood transfusion apparatus

Syringes, needles, and solutions

Surgical equipment

Stethoscope

Eating utensils

Wound dressings

Bedding

PUBLIC HEALTH AGENCIES

Public health agencies at all levels constantly strive to prevent epidemics and to identify and eliminate any that do occur. One way in which healthcare personnel participate in this massive program is by reporting cases of communicable diseases to the proper agencies. They also help by educating the public, explaining how diseases are transmitted, explaining proper sanitation procedures, identifying and attempting to eliminate reservoirs of infection, carrying out measures to isolate diseased persons, participating in immunization programs, and helping to treat sick persons. Through measures such as these, smallpox and poliomyelitis have been totally or nearly eliminated in most parts of the world.

World Health Organization

The WHO, a specialized agency of the United Nations, was founded in 1948. Its missions are to promote technical cooperation for health among nations, carry out programs to control and eradicate diseases, and improve the quality of human life. When an epidemic strikes, such as the 2000 Ebola outbreak in Uganda, teams of epidemiologists are sent to the site to investigate the situation and assist in bringing the outbreak under control. Because of this assistance, many countries have been successful in their fight to control smallpox, diphtheria, malaria, trachoma, and numerous other diseases. At one time, smallpox killed about 40% of those infected and caused scarring and blindness in many others. In 1980, the WHO announced that smallpox had been completely eradicated from the face of the Earth; hence, routine smallpox vaccination is no longer required.[c] More recently, the WHO has been attempting to eradicate polio and dracunculiasis (Guinea worm infection); to eliminate leprosy, neonatal tetanus, and Chagas' disease; and to control onchocerciasis ("river blindness"). WHO's definitions of control, elimination, and eradication of disease are presented in Table 11-6. The WHO is currently attempting to eradicate polio. Thus far, polio has been eradicated from the Western Hemisphere (including the United States). Certification of total eradication requires that no wild poliovirus be found through optimal surveillance for at least 3 years.

Centers for Disease Control and Prevention

In the United States, a federal agency called the U.S. Department of Health and Human Services administers the Public Health Service and CDC, which assist state and local health departments in the application of all aspects of epidemiology. Many microbiologists and epidemiologists work at the CDC headquarters in Atlanta, Georgia. Microbiologists at the CDC are able to work with the most dangerous pathogens known to science because of the elaborate containment facilities that are located there. CDC epidemiologists travel to areas of the United States and elsewhere in the world, wherever and whenever an epidemic is occurring, to investigate and attempt to control the epidemic.

---

[c] Because smallpox virus is a potential bioterrorism agent, public health authorities have authorized the manufacture and stockpiling of smallpox vaccine, to be administered in the event of an emergency.

TABLE 11-6	WHO Definitions of Epidemiologic Terms Relating to Infectious Diseases
TERM	**DEFINITION**
Control of an infectious disease	Ongoing operations or programs aimed at reducing the incidence or prevalence of that disease
Elimination of an infectious disease	The reduction of case transmission to a predetermined very low level (e.g., to a level below one case per million population)
Eradication of an infectious disease	Achieving a status where no further cases of that disease occur anywhere and where continued control measures are unnecessary

When the CDC was first established as the Communicable Disease Center in Atlanta, Georgia, in 1946, its focus was communicable diseases. The two most important infectious diseases in the United States at that time were malaria and typhus. Since then, the CDC's scope has been expanded greatly, and the organization now consists of approximately two dozen offices, centers, and institutes. The CDC's overall mission is "to collaborate to create the expertise, information, and tools that people and communities need to protect their health—through health promotion, prevention of disease, injury and disability, and preparedness for new health threats." (http://www.cdc.gov) One of the CDC centers—the Coordinating Center for Infectious Diseases—coordinates the activities of four National Centers:

• National Center for Immunization and Respiratory Diseases
• National Center for Zoonotic, Vector-Borne, and Enteric Diseases
• National Center for HIV/AIDS, Viral Hepatitis, STD, and TB Prevention
• National Center for Preparedness, Detection, and Control of Infectious Diseases

Certain infectious diseases, referred to as nationally notifiable diseases, must be reported to the CDC by all 50 states.[d] (As of January 2009, there were approximately 64 nationally notifiable diseases; most of them are discussed in Chapters 18 through 21.) Ten of the most common nationally notifiable infectious diseases in the United States are listed in Table 11-7.

The CDC prepares a weekly publication entitled *Morbidity and Mortality Weekly Report* (*MMWR*), which

[d] A notifiable disease is one for which regular, frequent, and timely information regarding individual cases is considered necessary for the prevention and control of the disease. Notifiable disease reporting protects the public's health by ensuring the proper identification and follow-up of cases.

TABLE 11-7	Ten of the Most Common Nationally Notifiable Infectious Diseases in the United States	
RANKING	**DISEASE**	**NUMBER OF U.S. CASES REPORTED (2007)**
1	Genital chlamydial infections	1,108,374
2	Gonorrhea	355,991
3	Salmonellosis	47,995
4	Syphilis (all stages)	40,920
5	Chickenpox	40,146
6	AIDS	37,503
7	Lyme disease	27,444
8	Shigellosis	19,758
9	Giardiasis	19,417
10	Tuberculosis	13,299

Source: Centers for Disease Control (CDC), Atlanta, GA (http://www.cdc.gov).

contains timely information about infectious disease outbreaks in the United States and other parts of the world, as well as cumulative statistics regarding the number of cases of nationally notifiable infectious diseases that have occurred in the United States during the current year. Students of the health sciences are encouraged to read *MMWR*, which is accessible at the CDC web site (http://www.cdc.gov).

Through the efforts of these public health agencies, working with local physicians, nurses, other healthcare professionals, educators, and community leaders, many diseases are no longer endemic in the United States. Some of the diseases that no longer pose a serious threat to U.S. communities include cholera, diphtheria, malaria, polio, smallpox, and typhoid fever.

The prevention and control of epidemics is a never-ending community goal. To be effective, it must include measures to:

- Increase host resistance through the development and administration of vaccines that induce active immunity and maintain it in susceptible persons
- Ensure that persons who have been exposed to a pathogen are protected against the disease (e.g., through injections of gamma globulin or antisera)
- Segregate, isolate, and treat those who have contracted a contagious infection to prevent the spread of pathogens to others
- Identify and control potential reservoirs and vectors of infectious diseases; this control may be accomplished by prohibiting healthy carriers from working in restaurants, hospitals, nursing homes, and other institutions where they may transfer pathogens to susceptible people and by instituting effective sanitation measures to control diseases transmitted through water supplies, sewage, and food (including milk)

BIOTERRORISM AND BIOLOGICAL WARFARE AGENTS

Sad to say, pathogenic microorganisms sometimes wind up in the hands of terrorists and extremists who want to use them to cause harm to others. In times of war, the use of microorganisms in this manner is called **biological warfare** (BW), and the microbes are referred to as **biological warfare agents**. However, the danger does not exist solely during times of war. The possibility that members of terrorist or radical hate groups might use pathogens to create fear, chaos, illness, and death always exists. These people are referred to as biological terrorists or bioterrorists, and the specific pathogens they use are referred to as **bioterrorism agents**.

Four of the pathogens most often discussed as potential BW and bioterrorism agents are *B. anthracis*, *C. botulinum*, smallpox virus (*Variola major*), and *Y. pestis*, the causative

> Four pathogens that are potential BW and bioterrorism agents are *B. anthracis*, *C. botulinum*, *V. major*, and *Y. pestis*.

agents of anthrax, botulism, smallpox, and plague, respectively.

Anthrax

Anthrax is caused by *B. anthracis*, a spore-forming, Gram-positive bacillus. People can develop anthrax in several ways (Fig. 11-8), resulting in three forms of the disease: cutaneous anthrax, inhalation anthrax, and gastrointestinal anthrax. Anthrax infections involve marked hemorrhaging and serous effusions (fluid that has escaped from blood or lymphatic vessels) in various organs and body cavities and are frequently fatal. Of the three forms of anthrax, inhalation anthrax is the most severe, followed by gastrointestinal anthrax and then cutaneous anthrax. Patients with cutaneous anthrax develop lesions (Fig. 11-9). Bioterrorists could disseminate *B. anthracis* spores via aerosols or contamination of food supplies. In the fall of 2001, letters containing *B. anthracis* spores were mailed to several politicians and members of the news media. According to the CDC, a total of 22 cases of anthrax resulted: 11 cases of inhalation anthrax (with five fatalities) and 11 cases of cutaneous anthrax (with no fatalities). Undoubtedly, many additional cases were prevented as a result of prompt prophylactic (preventative) antibiotic therapy.

Botulism

Botulism is a potentially fatal microbial intoxication, caused by botulinal toxin, a neurotoxin produced by *C. botulinum*. *C. botulinum* is a spore-forming anaerobic Gram-positive bacillus. Botulinal toxin may cause nerve damage, visual difficulty, respiratory failure, flaccid paralysis of voluntary muscles, brain damage, coma, and death within a week if untreated. Respiratory failure is the usual cause of death. Bioterrorists could add botulinal toxin to water supplies or food. Botulinal toxin is odorless and tasteless, and only a tiny quantity of the toxin need be ingested to cause a potentially fatal case of botulism. Botulism can also result from entry of *C. botulinum* spores into open wounds.

Smallpox

Smallpox is a serious, contagious, and sometimes fatal viral disease. Patients experience fever, malaise, headache,

FIGURE 11-9. Black anthrax lesion (eschar) on a patient's forearm. The name of the disease comes from the Greek word *anthrax*, which means "coal," in reference to the black skin lesions of anthrax. (Courtesy of James H. Steele and the CDC.)

Although there are no reservoirs for smallpox virus in nature, preserved samples of the virus exist in a few medical research laboratories worldwide. There is always the danger that smallpox virus, or any of the other pathogens mentioned here, could fall into the wrong hands.

Plague

Plague is caused by *Y. pestis*, a Gram-negative coccobacillus. Plague is predominantly a zoonosis and is usually transmitted to humans by flea bite (Fig. 11-11). Plague

FIGURE 11-8. Anthrax transmission. (From Harvey RA, et al. Lippincott's Illustrated Reviews: Microbiology. 2nd ed. Philadelphia: Lippincott Williams & Wilkins, 2007.)

prostration, severe backache, a characteristic skin rash (Fig. 11-10), and occasional abdominal pain and vomiting. Smallpox can become severe, with bleeding into the skin and mucous membranes, followed by death. The last case of smallpox in the United States was in 1949, and the last naturally occurring case in the world was in Somalia in 1977. Since 1980, when the WHO announced that smallpox had been eradicated, most people no longer receive smallpox vaccinations. Thus, throughout the world, huge numbers of people are highly susceptible to the virus.

FIGURE 11-10. Child with smallpox. (Courtesy of Dr. Stan Foster and the CDC.)

can manifest itself in several ways: bubonic plague, septicemic plague, pneumonic plague, and plague meningitis. Bubonic plague is named for the swollen, inflamed, and tender lymph nodes (buboes) that develop. Pneumonic plague, which is highly communicable, involves the lungs. It can result in localized outbreaks or devastating epidemics. Septicemic plague may cause septic shock, meningitis, or death. Patients with plague are depicted in Figure 11-12. Bioterrorists could disseminate *Y. pestis* via aerosols, resulting in numerous severe and potentially fatal pulmonary infections. Pneumonic plague can be transmitted from person to person.

The CDC has classified the etiologic agents of anthrax, botulism, smallpox, and plague as category A bioterrorism agents. Category A agents are those that:

• Pose the greatest possible threat for a bad effect on public health
• May spread across a large area or need public awareness
• Need a great deal of planning to protect the public's health

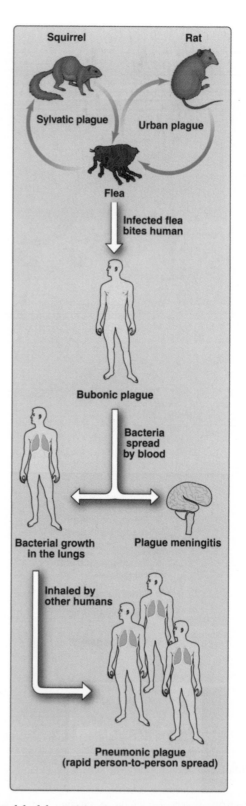

FIGURE 11-11. Epidemiology and pathology of plague. (From Harvey RA, et al. Lippincott's Illustrated Reviews: Microbiology. 2nd ed. Philadelphia: Lippincott Williams & Wilkins, 2007.)

FIGURE 11-12. Gangrenous hand (A) and foot (B) of patients with plague. ([A] Courtesy of Dr. Jack Poland and the CDC. [B] Courtesy of William Archibald and the CDC.)

Other pathogens viewed as potential BW agents are the causative agents of brucellosis, Q fever, tularemia, viral encephalitis, and viral hemorrhagic fevers. Table 11-8 contains a listing of potential bioterrorism agents that, according to the CDC, pose the greatest threats to civilians—pathogens with which public health agencies must be prepared to cope.

To minimize the danger of potentially deadly microorganisms falling into the wrong hands, the U.S. Antiterrorism and Effective Death Penalty Act of 1996

TABLE 11-8	Critical Biological Agent Categories for Public Health Preparedness[a]	
CATEGORY	**BIOLOGICAL AGENT(S)**	**DISEASE**
Category A—Agents having the greatest potential for adverse public health impact; most require broad-based public health preparedness efforts	*Variola major* *Bacillus anthracis* *Yersinia pestis* *Clostridium botulinum* *Francisella tularensis* Filoviruses and arenaviruses (e.g., Ebola virus, Lassa virus)	Smallpox Anthrax Plague Botulism (botulinal toxins) Tularemia Viral hemorrhagic fevers
Category B—Agents having a moderate to high potential for large-scale dissemination or a heightened general public health awareness that could cause mass public fear and civil disruption	*Coxiella burnetii* *Brucella* spp. *Burkholderia mallei* *Burkholderia pseudomallei* Alphaviruses (Venezuela equine, eastern equine, and western equine encephalitis viruses) *Rickettsia prowazekii* Toxins (e.g., ricin [from the castor oil plant], staphylococcal enterotoxin B) *Chlamydophila psittaci* Food safety treats (e.g., *Salmonella* spp., *Escherichia coli* O157:H7) Water safety treats (e.g., *Vibrio cholerae, Cryptosporidium parvum*)	Q fever Brucellosis Glanders Melioidosis Encephalitis Typhus fever Toxic syndromes Psittacosis
Category C—Agents currently not believed to present a high bioterrorism risk to public health, but could emerge as future threats	Emerging threat agents (e.g., Nipah virus, hantavirus)	

[a]From Rotz LD, et al. Public health assessment of potential biological terrorism agents. Emerg Infect Dis 2002;8:225–230 (prepared and published by the National Center for Infectious Diseases, Centers for Disease Control and Prevention, based on unclassified information)

makes the CDC responsible for controlling shipment of select agents—pathogens and toxins—deemed most likely to be used as BW agents. On its web site, the American Society for Microbiology (ASM; http://www.asm.org) offers this definition: "Select agents are microorganisms, biological agents, or biological toxins that have been deemed by the United States Government to be major threats to public safety because they could be used as agents of bioterrorism."

Authorities must constantly be on the alert for possible theft of these pathogens from biological supply houses and legitimate laboratories. In addition, vaccines, antitoxins, and other antidotes must be available wherever the threat of the use of these biological agents is high, as in various potential war zones.

The ASM has recommended that all clinical microbiology laboratories be staffed with persons familiar with the likely agents of bioterrorism and trained to detect, identify, and safely handle these agents. What individuals can do to prepare for bioterrorist attacks is discussed in "Insight: Preparing for a Bioterrorist Attack" on the CD-ROM.

WATER SUPPLIES AND SEWAGE DISPOSAL

Water is the most essential resource necessary for the survival of humanity. The main sources of community water supplies are surface water from rivers, natural lakes, and reservoirs, as well as groundwater from wells. However, two general types of water pollution (i.e., chemical pollution and biological pollution) are present in our society, making it increasingly difficult to provide safe water supplies.

Chemical pollution of water occurs when industrial installations dump waste products into local waters without proper pretreatment, when pesticides are used indiscriminately, and when chemicals are expelled in the air and carried to earth by rain ("acid rain"). The main source of biological pollution is waste products of humans—fecal material and garbage—that swarm with pathogens. The causative agents of cholera, typhoid fever, bacterial and amebic dysentery, giardiasis, cryptosporidiosis, infectious hepatitis, and poliomyelitis can all be spread through contaminated water.

Waterborne epidemics today are the result of failure to make use of available existing knowledge and technology. In those countries that have established safe sanitary procedures for water purification and sewage disposal, outbreaks of typhoid fever, cholera, and dysentery occur only rarely.

In spring 1993, a waterborne epidemic of cryptosporidiosis (a diarrheal disease) affected more than 400,000 people in Milwaukee, Wisconsin. This was the largest waterborne epidemic that has ever occurred in the United States. The oocysts of *C. parvum* (a protozoan parasite) were present in cattle feces, which, when the winter snow melted, were washed off Wisconsin's numerous dairy farms into Lake Michigan. Milwaukee uses the water of Lake Michigan as its drinking water supply. Although the lake water had been treated, the tiny oocysts passed through the filters that were being used at that time. Thus, the *Cryptosporidium* oocysts were present in the city's drinking water, and people became infected when they drank the water. The epidemic caused the death of more than 100 immunosuppressed individuals.

> The largest waterborne epidemic to occur in the United States was an outbreak of cryptosporidiosis in Milwaukee, Wisconsin, in 1993, which affected more than 400,000 people.

Sources of Water Contamination

Rainwater falling over large areas collects in lakes and rivers and, thus, is subject to contamination by soil microbes and raw fecal material. For example, an animal feed lot located near a community water supply source harbors innumerable pathogens, which are washed into lakes and rivers. A city that draws its water from a local river, processes it, and uses it, but then dumps inadequately treated sewage into the river at the other side of town, may be responsible for a serious health problem in another city downstream on the same river. The city downstream must then find some way to rid its water supply of the pathogens. In many communities, untreated raw sewage and industrial wastes are dumped directly into local waters. Also, a storm or a flood may result in contamination of the local drinking water with sewage (Fig. 11-13).

Groundwater from wells also can become contaminated. To prevent such contamination, the well must be dug deep enough to ensure that the surface water is filtered through soil before it reaches the level of the well. Outhouses, septic tanks, and cesspools must be situated in such a way that surface water passing through these areas does not carry fecal microbes directly into the well water. With the growing popularity of trailer homes, a new problem has arisen because of trailer sewage disposal tanks that are located too near a water supply. In some very old cities, where cracked underground water pipes lie alongside leaking sewage pipes, sewage can enter the water pipes, thus contaminating the water just before it enters people's homes.

Water Treatment

Water must be properly treated to make it safe for human consumption. It is interesting to trace the many steps involved in such treatment (Fig. 11-14). The water first is filtered to remove large pieces of debris such as twigs and leaves. Next, the water remains in a holding tank, where additional debris settles to the bottom of the tank; this phase of the process is known as **sedimentation** or **settling**. Alum (aluminum potassium sulfate) is then added to coagulate smaller pieces of debris, which then settle to the bottom; this phase is known as **coagulation** or **flocculation**. The water is then filtered through sand or

FIGURE 11-13. Sources of water contamination.

diatomaceous earth filters to remove the remaining bacteria, protozoan cysts and oocysts, and other small particles. In some water treatment facilities, charcoal filters or membrane filtration systems are also used. Membrane filtration will remove tiny *Giardia lamblia* cysts and *C. parvum* oocysts. Finally, chlorine gas or sodium hypochlorite is added to a final concentration of 0.2 to 1.0 ppm; this kills most remaining bacteria. In some water treatment facilities, ozone (O_3) treatment or ultraviolet (UV) light may be used in place of chlorination.

Small communities in rural areas may be financially unable to construct water treatment plants that incorporate all of these steps. Some may rely on chlorination alone. Unfortunately, the levels of chlorine routinely used for water treatment do not kill some pathogens, such as *Giardia* cysts and *Cryptosporidium* oocysts. Other communities use all the water treatment steps, but fail to use filters having a small enough pore size to trap tiny pathogens such as *Cryptosporidium* oocysts (which are about 4–6 μm in diameter).

In the laboratory, water can be tested for fecal contamination by checking for the presence of coliform bacteria (**coliforms**). Coliforms are *E. coli* and other lactose-fermenting members of the family Enterobacteriaceae,

FIGURE 11-14. Steps in water treatment. (See text for details.)

such as *Enterobacter* and *Klebsiella* spp. These bacteria normally live in the intestinal tracts of animals and humans; thus, their presence in drinking water is an indication that

> Water is considered potable (safe to drink) if it contains 1 coliform or less per 100 mL of water.

the water was fecally contaminated. With respect to the presence of coliforms, water is considered potable (safe to drink) if it contains 1 coliform or less per 100 mL of water.

If one is unsure about the purity of drinking water, boiling it for 20 minutes destroys most pathogens that are present. It can then be cooled and consumed. Boiling will kill *Giardia* cysts and *Cryptosporidium* oocysts, but there are some bacterial spores and viruses that can withstand long periods of boiling. The most common causes of waterborne outbreaks in the United States are *G. lamblia*, *C. parvum*, *E. coli* O157:H7, *Shigella*, and norovirus.

Sewage Treatment

Raw sewage consists mainly of water, fecal material (including intestinal pathogens), and garbage and bacteria from the drains of houses and other buildings. When sewage is adequately treated in a disposal plant, the water it contains can be returned to lakes and rivers to be recycled.

Primary Sewage Treatment

In the sewage disposal plant, large debris is first filtered out (called screening), skimmers remove floating grease and oil, and floating debris is shredded or ground. Then, solid material settles out in a primary sedimentation tank. Flocculating substances can be added to cause other solids to settle out. The material that accumulates at the bottom of the tank is called **primary sludge**.

Secondary Sewage Treatment

The liquid (called primary effluent) then undergoes secondary treatment, which includes aeration or trickling filtration. The purpose of aeration is to encourage the growth of aerobic microbes, which oxidize the dissolved organic matter to CO_2 and H_2O. Trickling filters accomplish the same thing (i.e., conversion of dissolved organic matter to CO_2 and H_2O by microbes), but in a different manner. After either aeration or trickling filtration, the activated sludge is transferred to a settling tank, where any remaining solid material settles out. The remaining liquid (called secondary effluent) is filtered and disinfected (usually by chlorination), so that the effluent water can be returned to rivers or oceans.

Tertiary Sewage Treatment

In some desert cities, where water is in short supply, the effluent water from the sewage disposal plant is further treated (referred to as tertiary sewage treatment), so that it can be returned directly to the drinking water system; this is a very expensive process. Tertiary sewage treatment involves the addition of chemicals, filtration (using fine sand or charcoal), chlorination, and sometimes distillation. In other cities, effluent water is used to irrigate lawns; however, it is expensive to install a separate water system for this purpose. In some communities, the sludge is heated to kill bacteria, then dried and used as fertilizer.

ON THE CD-ROM
- Terms Introduced in This Chapter
- Review of Key Points
- Insight
  - Preparing for a Bioterrorist Attack
- Increase Your Knowledge
- Critical Thinking
- Additional Self-Assessment Exercises

SELF-ASSESSMENT EXERCISES

After studying this chapter, answer the following multiple-choice questions.

1. Which of the following terms best describes chlamydial genital infection in the United States?
   a. arthropod-borne disease
   b. epidemic disease
   c. pandemic disease
   d. sporadic disease
2. Which of the following are considered reservoirs of infection?
   a. carriers
   b. contaminated food and drinking water
   c. rabid animals
   d. all of the above
3. The most common nationally notifiable infectious disease in the United States is:
   a. chlamydial genital infections.
   b. gonorrhea.
   c. the common cold.
   d. TB.
4. Which of the following arthropods is the vector of Lyme disease?
   a. flea
   b. mite
   c. mosquito
   d. tick

5. The most common zoonotic disease in the United States is:
   a. Lyme disease.
   b. plague.
   c. rabies.
   d. Rocky Mountain spotted fever.
6. Which one of the following organisms is *not* one of the four most likely potential BW or bioterrorism agents?
   a. *B. anthracis*
   b. Ebola virus
   c. *V. major*
   d. *Y. pestis*
7. All of the following are major steps in the treatment of a community's drinking water except:
   a. boiling.
   b. filtration.
   c. flocculation.
   d. sedimentation.

8. The largest waterborne epidemic ever to occur in the United States occurred in which of the following cities?
   a. Chicago
   b. Los Angeles
   c. Milwaukee
   d. New York City
9. Typhoid fever is caused by a species of:
   a. *Campylobacter*.
   b. *Escherichia*.
   c. *Salmonella*.
   d. *Shigella*.
10. Which of the following associations is incorrect?
   a. ehrlichiosis . . . tick
   b. malaria . . . mosquito
   c. plague . . . flea
   d. Rocky Mountain spotted fever . . . mite

12 HEALTHCARE EPIDEMIOLOGY

LEARNING OBJECTIVES

AFTER STUDYING THIS CHAPTER, YOU SHOULD BE ABLE TO:

- Differentiate among healthcare-associated, community-acquired, and iatrogenic infections
- List the seven pathogens that most commonly cause healthcare-associated infections
- State the four most common types of healthcare-associated infections
- List six types of patients who are especially vulnerable to healthcare-associated infections
- State the three major contributing factors in healthcare-associated infections
- Differentiate between medical and surgical asepsis
- State the most important and effective way to reduce the number of healthcare-associated infections
- Differentiate between Standard Precautions and Transmission-Based Precautions and state the three types of Transmission-Based Precautions

- Describe the types of patients placed in Protective Environments
- Cite three important considerations in the handling of each of the following in healthcare settings: food, eating utensils, fomites, and sharps
- List six responsibilities of an Infection Control Committee
- Explain three ways in which the Clinical Microbiology Laboratory participates in infection control

INTRODUCTION

Healthcare epidemiology can be defined as the study of the occurrence, determinants, and distribution of health and disease within healthcare settings. Health and disease are the result of complex interactions among pathogens, patients, and

Healthcare epidemiology can be defined as the study of the occurrence, determinants, and distribution of health and disease within healthcare settings.

the healthcare environment. Although the primary focus of healthcare epidemiology is on infection control and preventing healthcare-associated infections (HAIs), healthcare epidemiology includes any activities designed to study and improve patient care outcomes. These activities include surveillance measures, risk reduction programs focused on device and procedure management, policy development and implementation, education of healthcare personnel in infection control practices and procedures, cost–benefit assessment of prevention and control programs, and any measures designed to eliminate or contain reservoirs of infection, interrupt the transmission of infection, and protect patients, healthcare workers, and visitors against infection and disease.

The importance of microbiology to those who work in health-related occupations can never be overemphasized. Whether working in a hospital, medical or dental clinic, long-term care facility, rehabilitation center, or hospice, or caring for sick persons in their homes, all healthcare professionals must follow standardized procedures to prevent the spread of infectious diseases. Thoughtless or careless actions when providing patient care can cause serious infections that otherwise could have been prevented.

HEALTHCARE-ASSOCIATED INFECTIONS

Definitions

Infectious diseases (infections) can be divided into two categories depending on where the person became infected: (a) infections that are acquired *within* hospitals or other healthcare facilities (called **healthcare-associated infections** or HAIs)[a] and (b) infections that are acquired *outside* of healthcare facilities (called **community-acquired infections**). A hospitalized patient could have either type of infection. According to the Centers for Disease Control and Prevention (CDC), community-acquired infections are those that are present or incubating at the time of hospital admission. All other infections are considered HAIs, including those that erupt within 14 days of hospital discharge.

> Community-acquired infections are those that are present or incubating at the time of hospital admission. All other infections are considered HAIs, including those that erupt within 14 days of hospital discharge.

The term "healthcare-associated infection" should not be confused with the term "iatrogenic infection" (iatrogenic literally meaning "physician-induced"). An iatrogenic infection is an infection that results from medical or surgical treatment (i.e., an infection that is *caused* by a surgeon, another physician, or some other healthcare worker). Examples of iatrogenic infections are surgical site infections and urinary tract infections (UTIs) that result from urinary catheterization of patients. Iatrogenic infections are a type of HAI, but not all HAIs are iatrogenic infections.

> An iatrogenic infection is an infection that results from medical or surgical treatment—an infection that is *caused* by a surgeon, another physician, or some other healthcare worker.

Frequency of Healthcare-Associated Infections

It is sad to think that a patient who enters a hospital for one problem could develop an infection while in the hospital and perhaps die of that infection. However, this is an all too common occurrence. In 2002, the estimated number of HAIs in U.S. hospitals was approximately 1.7 million (roughly 5% of hospitalized patients).[b] The estimated number of deaths in 2002, associated with HAIs, was 98,987 (approximately 6% of the patients having HAIs). Of these, the greatest number of deaths (35,967) was caused by pneumonia. HAIs cause significant increases in excess hospital stays and costs for additional treatment.

> In the United States, approximately 5% of hospitalized patients develop HAIs.

Pathogens Most Often Involved in Healthcare-Associated Infections

The hospital environment harbors many pathogens and potential pathogens. Some live on and in healthcare professionals, other hospital employees, visitors to the hospital, and patients themselves. Others live in dust or wet or moist areas like sink drains, showerheads, whirlpool baths, mop buckets, flower pots, and even food from the kitchen. To make matters worse, the bacterial pathogens that are present in hospital settings are usually drug-resistant strains and, quite often, are multidrug-resistant.

The following bacteria are the most common causes of HAIs in the United States:

- **Gram-positive cocci:**
  Staphylococcus aureus (including methicillin-resistant strains of *Staphylococcus aureus* [MRSA])
  Coagulase-negative staphylococci
  Enterococcus spp. (including vancomycin-resistant enterococci)

- **Gram-negative bacilli:**
  Escherichia coli
  Pseudomonas aeruginosa
  Enterobacter spp.
  Klebsiella spp.

---

[a] The CDC recommend use of the term "healthcare-associated infections" for infections acquired within any type of healthcare facility. The term replaces the older term "hospital-acquired infections," and its synonym, "nosocomial infections."

[b] Information source: Klevens RM, et al. Estimating Health Care-Associated Infections and Deaths in U.S. Hospitals, 2002. Public Health Reports 122: 160–166, 2007.

Although some of the pathogens that cause HAIs originate in the external environment, many come from the patients themselves—their own indigenous microflora that enter a surgical incision or otherwise gain entrance to areas of the body other than those where they normally reside. Urinary catheters, for example, provide a "superhighway" for indigenous microflora of the distal urethra to gain access to the urinary bladder.

Approximately 70% of HAIs involve drug-resistant bacteria, which are common in hospitals, nursing homes, and other healthcare settings as a result of the many antimicrobial agents in use there. The drugs place selective pressure on the microbes, meaning that only those that are resistant to the drugs will survive. These resistant organisms then multiply and predominate (refer back to Fig. 9-6).

> Approximately 70% of HAIs involve drug-resistant bacteria.

Pseudomonas infections are especially difficult to treat, as are infections caused by multidrug-resistant *Mycobacterium tuberculosis* (MDR-TB), vancomycin-resistant *Enterococcus* spp. (VRE), and MRSA and methicillin-resistant strains of *Staphylococcus epidermidis* (MRSE). Bacteria are not the only pathogens that have become drug resistant, however. Viruses (such as human immunodeficiency virus [HIV]), fungi (such as various *Candida* spp.), and protozoa (such as malarial parasites) have also developed drug resistance.

In 2001, the CDC launched a campaign to prevent antimicrobial resistance in healthcare settings. Table 12-1 contains the 12 steps recommended by the CDC to prevent antimicrobial resistance among hospitalized adults.

Modes of Transmission

The three principle routes by which pathogens involved in HAIs are transmitted are contact, droplet, and airborne.

Contact Transmission

There are two types of contact transmission:

- In direct contact transmission, pathogens are transferred from one infected person to another person without a contaminated intermediate object or person.
- Indirect contact transmission happens when pathogens are transferred via a contaminated intermediate object or person.

Droplet Transmission

In droplet transmission, respiratory droplets carrying pathogens transmit infection when they travel from the respiratory tract of an infectious individual (e.g., by sneezing or coughing) to susceptible mucosal surfaces of a recipient. Droplets traditionally have been defined as being larger than 5 μm in size.

Airborne Transmission

Airborne transmission occurs with dissemination of either airborne droplet nuclei or small particles containing pathogens. Traditionally, airborne droplets are defined as being less than or equal to 5 μm in size.

> The three most common modes of transmission in healthcare settings are contact, droplet, and airborne transmission.

Most Common Types of Healthcare-Associated Infections

According to the CDC,[c] the four most common types of HAIs in U.S. hospitals are:

> The most common type of HAI in the United States is UTI, followed, in order, by surgical site, lower respiratory tract, and bloodstream infections.

1. **UTIs**, which represent about 32% of all HAIs and cause about 13% of the deaths associated with HAIs
2. **Surgical site infections**, which represent about 22% of all HAIs and cause about 8% of the deaths associated with HAIs
3. **Lower respiratory tract infections (primarily pneumonia)**, which represent about 15% of HAIs and cause about 36% of the deaths associated with HAIs
4. **Bloodstream infections (septicemia)**, which represent about 14% of HAIs and cause about 31% of the deaths associated with HAIs

Other common HAIs are the gastrointestinal diseases caused by *Clostridium difficile*, which are referred to as *C. difficile*-associated diseases.

> *C. difficile* is a common cause of healthcare-associated gastrointestinal infections.

C. difficile (often referred to as "C. diff") is an anaerobic, spore-forming, Gram-positive bacillus. It is a common member of the indigenous microflora of the colon, where it exists in relatively small numbers. Although *C. difficile* produces two types of toxins (an enterotoxin and a cytotoxin), the concentrations of these toxins are too low to cause disease when only small numbers of *C. difficile* are present. However, superinfections of *C. difficile* can occur when a patient receives oral antibiotics that kill off susceptible members of the gastrointestinal flora (superinfections are described in Chapter 9). *C. difficile*, which is resistant to many orally administered antibiotics, then increases in number, leading to increased concentrations of the toxins. The enterotoxin causes a disease known as **antibiotic-associated diarrhea** (AAD). The cytotoxin causes a disease known as **pseudomembranous colitis** (PMC), in which sections of the lining of the colon slough off, resulting in bloody stools. Both AAD and PMC are common in hospitalized patients.

---

[c] Much of the information in this chapter is from Siegel JD, et al. 2007 Guidelines for Isolation Precautions: Preventing Transmission of Infectious Agents in Healthcare Settings, 2007, published by the Centers for Disease Control and Prevention.

TABLE 12-1	Twelve Steps to Prevent Antimicrobial Resistance among Hospitalized Adults
Prevent Infection	
Step 1. Vaccinate	Give influenza vaccine and *Streptococcus pneumoniae* vaccine to at-risk patients before discharge. Healthcare workers should receive the influenza vaccine annually.
Step 2. Get the catheters out	Use catheters only when essential. Use the correct catheter. Use proper insertion and catheter-care protocols. Remove catheters when they are no longer essential.
Diagnose and Treat Infection Effectively	
Step 3. Target the pathogen	Culture the patient. Target empiric therapy to likely pathogens and your facility's antibiogram information. Target definitive therapy to known pathogens and antimicrobial susceptibility test results.
Step 4. Access the experts	Consult infectious disease experts for patients with serious infections.
Use Antimicrobials Wisely	
Step 5. Practice antimicrobial control	Engage in local antimicrobial control efforts.
Step 6. Use local data	Know your facility's antibiogram. Know your patient population.
Step 7. Treat infection, not contamination	Use proper antisepsis for blood and other cultures. Culture the blood, not the skin or catheter hub. Use proper methods to obtain and process all cultures.
Step 8. Treat infection, not colonization	Treat pneumonia, not the tracheal aspirate. Treat bacteremia, not the catheter tip or hub. Treat urinary tract infection, not the indwelling catheter.
Step 9. Know when to say "no" to vancomycin	Treat infection, not contaminants or colonization. Fever in a patient with an intravenous catheter is not a routine indication for vancomycin.
Step 10. Stop antimicrobial treatment	When infection is cured. When cultures are negative and infection is unlikely. When infection is not diagnosed.
Prevent Transmission	
Step 11. Isolate the pathogen	Use standard infection control precautions. Contain infectious body fluids. (Follow Airborne, Droplet, and Contact Precautions.) When in doubt, consult infection control experts.
Step 12. Break the chain of contagion	Stay home when you (the healthcare worker) are sick. Keep your hands clean. Set an example.

Source: Centers for Disease Control (CDC), Atlanta, GA (http://www.cdc.gov/drugresistance/healthcare/ha/12steps_HA.htm). This web site also discusses steps to prevent antimicrobial resistance among dialysis patients, surgical patients, hospitalized children, and long-term care patients.

Healthcare-associated zoonoses are a recently recognized problem in hospitals (see "Insight: Healthcare-Associated Zoonoses" on the CD-ROM). Recall that zoonoses are diseases that are transmissible from animals to humans.

Patients Most Likely To Develop Healthcare-Associated Infections

Patients most likely to develop HAIs are immunosuppressed patients—patients whose immune systems have been weakened by age, underlying diseases, or medical or surgical treatments. Contributing factors include an aging population, increasingly aggressive medical and therapeutic interventions, and an increase in the number of implanted prosthetic devices, organ transplantations, xenotransplantations (the transplantation of animal organs or tissues into humans), and vascular and urinary catheterizations. The highest infection rates are in intensive care unit (ICU)

Immunosuppressed patients are especially likely to develop HAIs.

patients. HAI rates are three times higher in adult and pediatric ICUs than elsewhere in the hospital. Listed here are the most vulnerable patients in a hospital setting:

- Elderly patients
- Women in labor and delivery
- Premature infants and newborns
- Surgical and burn patients
- Patients with diabetes or cancer
- Patients with cystic fibrosis
- Patients having an organ transplant
- Patients receiving treatment with steroids, anticancer drugs, antilymphocyte serum, or radiation
- Immunosuppressed patients (i.e., patients whose immune systems are not functioning properly)
- Patients who are paralyzed or are undergoing renal dialysis or urinary catheterization
- Patients with indwelling devices such as endotracheal tubes, central venous and arterial cathers, and synthetic implants

Major Factors Contributing to Healthcare-Associated Infections

The three major factors that combine to cause HAIs (Fig. 12-1) are:

1. An ever-increasing number of drug-resistant pathogens
2. The failure of healthcare personnel to follow infection control guidelines
3. An increased number of immunocompromised patients

> The three major causes of HAIs are drug-resistant bacteria, the failure of healthcare personnel to follow infection control guidelines, and an increased number of immunocompromised patients.

Additional contributing factors are:

- The indiscriminate use of antimicrobial agents, which has resulted in an increase in the number of drug-resistant and multidrug-resistant pathogens
- A false sense of security about antimicrobial agents, leading to a neglect of aseptic techniques and other infection control procedures
- Lengthy, more complicated types of surgery
- Overcrowding of hospitals and other healthcare facilities, as well as shortages of staff
- Increased use of less-highly trained healthcare workers, who are often unaware of infection control procedures
- Increased use of anti-inflammatory and immunosuppressant agents, such as radiation, steroids, anticancer chemotherapy, and antilymphocyte serum
- Overuse and improper use of indwelling medical devices

Medical devices that support or monitor basic body functions contribute greatly to the success of modern medical treatment. However, by bypassing normal defensive barriers, these devices provide microbes access

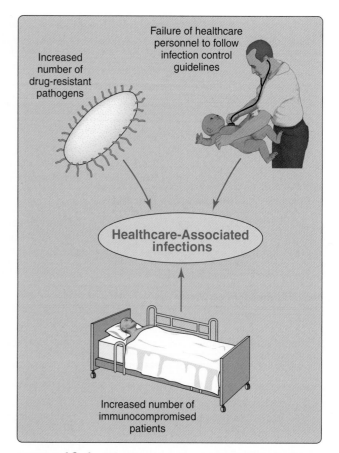

FIGURE 12-1. The three major contributing factors in HAIs.

to normally sterile body fluids and tissues. The risk of bacterial or fungal infection is related to the degree of debilitation of the patient and the design and management of the device. It is advisable to discontinue the use of urinary catheters, vascular catheters, respirators, and hemodialysis on individual patients as soon as medically feasible.

What Can Be Done to Reduce the Number of Healthcare-Associated Infections?

It is critical for all healthcare workers to be aware of the problem of HAIs and to take appropriate measures to minimize the number of such infections that occur within healthcare facilities. The primary way to reduce the number of HAIs is strict compliance with infection control guidelines (these guidelines are described in a subsequent section).

> The primary way to reduce the number of HAIs is strict compliance with infection control guidelines.

Handwashing is the single most important measure to reduce the risks of transmitting pathogens from one patient to another or from one anatomic site to another on the same patient. Handwashing, as it specifically pertains to healthcare personnel, is discussed later in the chapter ("Standard Precautions"). Presented here are common sense, everyday, handwashing guidelines that pertain to everyone:

Wash your hands before you:
- Prepare or eat food
- Treat a cut or wound or tend to someone who is sick
- Insert or remove contact lenses

Wash your hands after you:
- Use the restroom
- Handle uncooked foods, particularly raw meat, poultry, or fish
- Change a diaper
- Cough, sneeze, or blow your nose
- Touch a pet, particularly reptiles and exotic animals
- Handle garbage
- Tend to someone who is sick or injured

Wash your hands in the following manner:
- Use warm or hot running water
- Use soap (preferably an antibacterial soap)
- Wash all surfaces thoroughly, including wrists, palms, back of hands, fingers, and under fingernails (preferably with a nail brush)
- Rub hands together for at least 10 to 15 seconds
- When drying, begin with your forearms and work toward your hands and fingertips, and pat your skin rather than rubbing to avoid chapping and cracking

(These handwashing guidelines were originally published by the Bayer Corporation and the American Society for Microbiology.)

> Handwashing is the single most important measure to reduce the risks of transmitting pathogens from one patient to another or from one anatomic site to another on the same patient.

Other means of reducing the incidence of HAIs include disinfection and sterilization techniques, air filtration, use of ultraviolet lights, isolation of especially infectious patients, and wearing gloves, masks, and gowns whenever appropriate.

INFECTION CONTROL

The term **infection control** pertains to the numerous measures that are taken to prevent infections from occurring in healthcare settings. These pre-

> Infection control measures are designed to break various links in the chain of infection.

ventive measures include actions taken to eliminate or contain reservoirs of infection, interrupt the transmission of pathogens, and protect persons (patients, employees, and visitors) from becoming infected—in short, they are ways to break various links in the chain of infection (refer back to Fig. 11-3).

Ever since the discoveries and observations of Ignaz Semmelweis and Joseph Lister (see the following "Historical Notes") in the 19th century, it has been known that wound contamination is not inevitable and

HISTORICAL NOTE
Contributions of Joseph Lister

Joseph Lister (1827–1912), a British surgeon, made significant contributions in the areas of antisepsis (against infection) and asepsis (without infection). During the 1860s, he instituted the practice of using phenol (carbolic acid) as an antiseptic to reduce microbial contamination of open surgical wounds. Lister routinely applied a dilute phenol solution to all wounds and insisted that anything coming in contact with the wounds (e.g., surgeons' hands, surgical instruments, and wound dressings) be immersed in phenol. In 1870, he instituted the practice of performing surgical procedures within a phenol mist. Although this practice probably killed microbes that were present in the air, it proved unpopular with the surgeons and nurses who inhaled the irritating phenol mist. Later contributions by Lister included such aseptic techniques as steam sterilization of surgical instruments; the use of sterile masks, gloves, and gowns by members of the surgical team; and the use of sterile drapes and gauze sponges in the operating room. Lister's antiseptic and aseptic techniques greatly reduced the incidence of surgical wound infections and surgical mortality. Because phenol is quite caustic and toxic, it was later replaced by other antiseptics.

that pathogens can be prevented from reaching vulnerable areas, a concept referred to as **asepsis**. Asepsis, which literally means *without infection*, in-

> Aseptic techniques are actions taken to prevent infection or break the chain of infection.

cludes any actions (referred to as aseptic techniques) taken to prevent infection or break the chain of infection. Such actions include general cleanliness, frequent and thorough handwashing, isolation of infected patients, disinfection, and sterilization. The techniques used to achieve asepsis depend on the site, circumstances, and environment. There are two main types or categories of asepsis: medical asepsis and surgical asepsis.

Medical Asepsis

Once basic cleanliness is achieved, it is not difficult to maintain asepsis. Medical asepsis, or clean technique, involves procedures and practices that

> Medical asepsis is a clean technique. Its goal is to exclude pathogens.

reduce the number and transmission of pathogens. Medical asepsis includes all the precautionary measures necessary to prevent direct transfer of pathogens from person to person and indirect transfer of pathogens through the air or on instruments, bedding, equipment, and other inanimate objects (fomites). Medical aseptic techniques include frequent and thorough handwashing; personal grooming; wearing of clean masks, gloves, and gowns when appropriate; proper cleaning of supplies and equipment; disinfection; proper disposal of needles, contaminated materials, and infectious waste; and sterilization.

Disinfection

General principles of disinfection were discussed in Chapter 8. Principles of disinfection as they pertain to the healthcare environment are discussed in this section.[d]

Categories of Disinfectants. A few disinfectants will kill bacterial spores with prolonged exposure times (3–12 hours); these are referred to as **chemical sterilants**. Other disinfectants used within healthcare settings are categorized as high-level, intermediate-level, and low-level disinfectants. **High-level disinfectants** kill all microbes (including viruses),[e] except large numbers of bacterial spores. **Intermediate-level disinfectants** might kill mycobacteria, vegetative bacteria, most viruses, and most fungi, but do not necessarily kill bacterial spores. **Low-level disinfectants** kill most vegetative bacteria, some fungi, and some viruses within 10 minutes of exposure. Disinfectants commonly used in healthcare settings are shown in Table 12-2.

Spaulding System for Classification of Instruments and Items for Patient Care. More than 30 years ago, Earle H. Spaulding devised a system of classifying instruments and items for patient care according to the degree of risk for infection that was involved. This system is still used to determine how these items are to be disinfected or sterilized.

- **Critical Items.** Critical items confer a high risk for infection if they are contaminated with *any* microbe. Thus, such objects must be sterile. Critical items include surgical instruments, cardiac and urinary catheters, implants, and ultrasound probes used in sterile body cavities. Items in this category should be purchased as sterile or be sterilized using steam (preferably), ethylene oxide gas, hydrogen peroxide gas plasma, or liquid chemical sterilants.
- **Semicritical Items.** Semicritical items contact mucous membranes or nonintact skin and require high-level disinfection. Semicritical items include respiratory therapy and anesthesia equipment, some endoscopes, laryngoscope blades, esophageal manometry probes, cytoscopes, anorectal manometry catheters, and diaphragm fitting rings. Semicritical items minimally require high-level disinfection using glutaraldehyde, hydrogen peroxide, ortho-phthalaldehyde, or peracetic acid with hydrogen peroxide.

- **Noncritical Items.** Noncritical items are those that come in contact with intact skin, but not mucous membranes. Such items are divided into two subcategories: noncritical patient care items (e.g., bedpans, blood pressure cuffs, crutches, computers) and noncritical environmental surfaces (e.g., bed rails, some food utensils, bedside tables, patient furniture, floors). Low-level disinfectants may be used for noncritical items. Any of the following disinfectants may be used for noncritical items: 70% to 90% ethyl or isopropyl alcohol, sodium hypochlorite (household bleach diluted 1:500), phenolic germicidal detergent solution, iodophor germicidal detergent solution, quaternary ammonium germicidal detergent solution.

Surgical Asepsis

Surgical asepsis, or sterile technique, includes practices used to render and keep objects and areas sterile (i.e., free of microbes). Note the differences between medical and surgical asepsis:

> Surgical asepsis is a sterile technique. Its goal is to exclude all microbes.

- Medical asepsis is a clean technique, whereas surgical asepsis is a sterile technique.
- The goal of medical asepsis is to exclude pathogens, whereas the goal of surgical asepsis is to exclude all microbes.

Surgical aseptic techniques are practiced in operating rooms, in labor and delivery areas, and during invasive procedures. For example, invasive procedures, such as drawing blood, injecting medications, urinary catheter insertion, cardiac catheterization, and lumbar punctures, must be performed using strict surgical aseptic precautions. Other surgical aseptic techniques include surgical scrubbing of hands and fingernails before entering the operating room; wearing sterile masks, gloves, caps, gowns, and shoe covers; using sterile solutions and dressings; using sterile drapes and creating a sterile field; and using heat-sterilized surgical instruments. Methods of sterilization were discussed in Chapter 8.

SPOTLIGHTING PERFUSIONISTS

As stated in the American Medical Association's Health Care Careers Directory, 2008–2009 (available at http://www.ama-assn.org), "Perfusionists are skilled allied health professionals, trained and educated specifically as members of an open-heart, surgical team responsible for the selection, setup, and operation of a mechanical device commonly referred to as the heart-lung machine."

"During open heart surgery, when the patient's heart is immobilized and cannot function in a normal

(continues)

---

[d] Much of the information in this section is from Rutala WA, et al. Guideline for Disinfection and Sterilization in Healthcare Facilities, 2008. Centers for Disease Control and Prevention.

[e] Viruses can be inactivated by some disinfectants, but are not really "killed." Recall that viruses are not actually "alive" to begin with.

fashion while the operation is being performed, the patient's blood is diverted and circulated outside the body through the heart-lung machine and returned again to the patient. In effect, the machine assumes the function of both the heart and lungs."

"The perfusionist is responsible for operating the machine during surgery, monitoring the altered circulatory process closely, taking appropriate corrective action when abnormal situations arise, and keeping both the surgeon and anesthesiologist fully informed."

"In addition to the operation of the heart-lung machine during surgery, perfusionists often function in supportive roles for other medical specialties in operating mechanical devices to assist in the conservation of blood and blood products during surgery, and provide extended, long-term support of patients' circulation outside of the operating room environment."

Information concerning educational requirements and programs, certification, and salary is available at the AMA web site.

Hair at the surgical site must be clipped using an electric shaver and the patient's skin must be thoroughly cleansed and scrubbed with soap and antiseptic. If the surgery is to be extensive, the surrounding area is covered with a sterile plastic film or sterile cloth drapes so that a sterile surgical field is established. The surgeon and all surgical assistants must scrub their hands for 5 to 10 minutes with a disinfectant soap and cover their clothes, mouth, and hair, because these might shed microbes onto the operative site. These coverings include sterile gloves, gowns, caps, masks, and shoe covers (Fig. 12-2). All instruments, sutures, and dressings must be sterile. They are handled only while wearing sterile masks and gloves. As soon as these items become contaminated, they must be thoroughly cleaned and sterilized for reuse or disposed of properly. All needles, syringes, and other sharp items of equipment ("sharps") must be disposed of by placing them into appropriate puncture-proof "sharps containers."

Floors, walls, and all equipment in the operating room must be thoroughly cleaned and disinfected before and after each use. Proper ventilation must be maintained to ensure that fresh, filtered air is circulated throughout the room at all times.

SPOTLIGHTING SURGICAL TECHNOLOGISTS

As stated in the American Medical Association's Health Care Careers Directory, 2008–2009 (available at http://www.ama-assn.org), "Surgical technologists are an integral part of the team of medical practitioners

providing surgical care to patients in a variety of settings." The directory's career description for surgical technologists includes the following duties relating to infection control:

"Surgical technologists . . .

- "Prepare the operating room by selecting and opening sterile supplies. . . . Common duties include operating sterilizers, lights, suction machines, electrosurgical units, and diagnostic equipment."
- "Properly position the patient on the operating table, assist in connecting and applying surgical equipment and/or monitoring devices, and prepare the incision site. [They] have primary responsibility for maintaining the sterile field, being constantly vigilant that almembers of the tram adhere to aseptic technique."
- "Most often function as the sterile member of the surgical team who passes instruments, sutures, and sponges during surgery. After 'scrubbing,' they don sterile gown and gloves and prepare the sterile setup for the appropriate procedure. After other members of the sterile team have scrubbed, they assist them with gowning and gloving and with the application of sterile drapes that isolate the operative site."
- "Anticipate the needs of the surgeons, passing instruments and providing sterile items in an efficient manner."
- "May hold retractors or instruments, sponge or suction the operative site, or cut suture materials as directed by the surgeon. They connect drains and tubing and receive and prepare specimens for subsequent pathologic analysis. They are responsible for preparing and applying sterile dressings following the procedure and may assist in the application of nonsterile dressings, including plaster or synthetic casting materials. After surgery, they prepare the operating room for the next patient."

Information concerning educational requirements and programs, certification, and salary is available at the AMA web site.

Regulations Pertaining to Healthcare Epidemiology and Infection Control

In the United States, there are many different regulations that pertain to healthcare epidemiology and infection control—so many, in fact, that it is not possible to discuss them all in this book this size. One of the most important of these regulations was published in 2001 by the Occupational Safety and Health Administration (OSHA). It is entitled the Bloodborne Pathogen Standard (29 CFR 1910.1030). This standard requires facilities having employees who have occupational exposure to blood or other potentially infectious materials to prepare and update a written plan called the Exposure Control Plan. This plan is designed to eliminate or minimize

TABLE 12-2   Disinfectants Commonly Used in Hospitals

DISINFECTANT	MODE OF ACTION AND SPECTRUM	USES
Alcohols (e.g., 60%–90% solutions of ethyl, isopropyl, and benzyl alcohols)	Cause denaturation of proteins; bactericidal, tuberculocidal, fungicidal, virucidal, but not sporicidal	For disinfection of thermometers, rubber stoppers, external surfaces of stethoscopes, endoscopes, and certain other equipment
Chorine and chlorine compounds (Clorox, Halazone, hypochlorites, Warexin)	Thought to cause inhibition of key enzymatic reactions, protein denaturation, and inactivation of nucleic acids; bactericidal, tuberculocidal, fungicidal, virucidal, sporicidal	For disinfection of countertops, floors, blood spills, needles, syringes; water treatment
Formaldehyde (formalin is 37% formaldehyde by weight)	Alters the structure of proteins and purine bases; bactericidal, tuberculocidal, fungicidal, virucidal, sporicidal	Limited uses because of irritating fumes, pungent odor, and potential carcinogenicity; used for preserving anatomic specimens
Glutaraldehyde	Interferes with DNA, RNA, and protein synthesis; bactericidal, fungicidal, virucidal, sporicidal; relatively slow tuberculocidal activity	For disinfection of medical equipment such as endoscopes, tubing, dialyzers, and anesthesia and respiratory therapy equipment; has a pungent odor and is irritating to eyes, throat, and nose; may cause respiratory irritation, asthma, rhinitis, and contact dermatitis
Hydrogen peroxide	Produces destructive free radicals that attack membrane lipids, DNA, and other essential cell components; bactericidal, tuberculocidal, fungicidal, virucidal, sporicidal	For disinfection of inanimate surfaces; limited clinical use; contact with eyes may cause serious eye damage
Iodine (iodine solutions or tinctures) and iodophors (e.g., povidone-iodine, Wescodyne, Betadine, Isodine, Ioprep, Surgidine)	Thought to disrupt protein and nucleic acid structure and synthesis; bactericidal, tuberculocidal, virucidal; may require prolonged contact times to be fungicidal and sporicidal	Primarily for use as antiseptics; also for disinfection of rubber stoppers, thermometers, endoscopes
Orthophthaldehyde	Mode of action unknown; bactericidal, tuberculocidal, fungicidal, virucidal, sporicidal	Stains skin, clothing, environmental surfaces; limited clinical use
Peracetic acid (peroxyacetic acid)	Thought to disrupt cell wall permeability and alter the structure of proteins; bactericidal, tuberculocidal, fungicidal, virucidal, sporicidal	Used in an automated machine to chemically sterilize immersible medical, surgical, and dental instruments, including endoscopes and arthroscopes; concentrate can cause serious eye and skin damage
Combination of peracetic acid and hydrogen peroxide	Mode of action as described above for hydrogen peroxide and peracetic acid; bactericidal, tuberculocidal, fungicidal, virucidal, but not sporicidal	For disinfection of hemodialyzers
Phenol (carbolic acid) and phenolics (e.g., xylenols, o-phenylphenol, hexylresorcinol, hexachlorophene, cresol, Lysol)	Disrupts cell walls and inactivates essential enzyme systems; bactericidal, tuberculocidal, fungicidal, virucidal, but not sporicidal	For decontamination of the hospital environment, including laboratory surfaces, and for non-critical medical and surgical items; residual disinfectant on porous surfaces may cause tissue irritation
Quaternary ammonium compounds (a variety of organically substituted ammonium compounds, such as dodecyldimethyl ammonium chloride)	Inactivate energy-producing enzymes, denaturation of disruption of cell membranes; bactericidal, fungicidal, and virucidal to lipophilic viruses; generally not tuberculocidal, sporicidal, or virucidal to hydrophilic viruses	For disinfection of noncritical surfaces such as floors, furniture, and walls; should not be used as antiseptics

Additional information about disinfectants can be found in CDC's Guideline for Disinfection and Sterilization in Healthcare Facilities, 2008, available on the CDC web site: http://www.cdc.gov.

FIGURE 12-2.
Healthcare professional donning personal protective equipment (PPE). (A) sterile gown, **(B)** mask, **(C)** gloves. (From McCall RE, Tankersley CM. Phlebotomy Essentials, 4th ed. Philadelphia: Lippincott Williams & Wilkins, 2008.)

employee exposure to pathogens. Other topics addressed in 29 CFR 1910.1030 are:

- Postexposure follow-up
- Recordkeeping for bloodborne pathogens
- Needlestick injuries and other sharps
- Universal precautions
- Latex allergy
- Bloodborne illnesses such as HIV, hepatitis B virus (HBV), and hepatitis C virus (HCV)
- Labelling and signs

(29 CFR 1910.1030 can be found on the OSHA web site: http://www.osha.gov)

Standard Precautions

In a healthcare setting, one is not always aware of which patients are infected with HIV, HBV, HCV, or other communicable pathogens. Thus, to prevent transmission of pathogens within healthcare settings, two levels of safety precautions have been developed by the CDC: Standard Precautions and Transmission-Based Precautions. Standard Precautions combine the major features of Universal Precautions and Body Substance Isolation Precautions,[f] and are intended to be applied to the care of *all* patients in *all* healthcare settings, regardless of the suspected or confirmed presence of an infectious agent. Transmission-Based Precautions (discussed in a subsequent section), on the other hand, are enforced only for certain specific types of infections.

> Standard Precautions are to be applied to the care of ALL patients in ALL healthcare settings, regardless of the suspected or confirmed presence of an infectious agent.

Implementation of Standard Precautions constitutes the primary strategy for the prevention of healthcare-associated transmission of infectious agents among patients and healthcare personnel. Standard Precautions are based on the principle that all blood, body fluids, secretions, excretions except sweat, non-intact skin, and mucous membranes may contain transmissible infectious agents. Standard Precautions provide infection prevention guidelines regarding hand hygiene; wearing of gloves, gowns, masks, eye protection; respiratory hygiene/cough etiquette; safe injection practices; lumbar puncture; cleaning of patient-care equipment; environmental control (including cleaning and disinfection); handling of soiled linens; handling and disposal of used needles and other sharps; resuscitation devices; and patient placement. Whereas OSHA guidelines are designed to protect healthcare personnel, Standard Precautions will protect *both* healthcare personnel and their patients from becoming infected with HIV, HBV, HCV, and many other pathogens. The sign shown in Figure 12-3 summarizes the most important aspects of Standard Precautions.

> Implementation of Standard Precautions constitutes the primary strategy for the prevention of healthcare-associated transmission of infectious agents among patients and healthcare personnel.

Vaccinations

Because healthcare personnel are at particular risk for several vaccine-preventable infectious diseases, the CDC recommends that they receive the following vaccines:

- Hepatitis B recombinant vaccine
- Influenza vaccine
- Measles live-virus vaccine
- Mumps live-virus vaccine
- Rubella live-virus vaccine
- Varicella-zoster live-virus vaccine

---

[f] Universal Precautions (published in 1985, 1987, and 1988) pertained to blood and body fluids, whereas Body Substance Isolation Precautions (published in 1987) were designed to reduce the risk of transmission of pathogens from moist body substances.

FIGURE 12-3.
Standard Precautions sign. (From McCall RE, Tankersley CM. Phlebotomy Essentials, 4th ed. Philadelphia: Lippincott Williams & Wilkins, 2008. Courtesy of the Brevis Corp., Salt Lake City, UT.)

STANDARD PRECAUTIONS

FOR INFECTION CONTROL

Handwashing
Wash after touching **body fluids**, after **removing gloves**, and between **patient contacts**.

Gloves
Wear **Gloves** before touching **body fluids**, **mucous membranes**, and **nonintact skin**.

Mask & Eye Protection or Face Shield
Protect eyes, nose, mouth during procedures that cause **splashes** or **sprays** of **body fluids**.

Gown
Wear **Gown** during procedures that may cause **splashes** or **sprays** of **body fluids**.

Patient-Care Equipment
Handle soiled equipment so as to prevent personal contamination and transfer to other patients.

Environmental Control
Follow hospital procedures for cleaning beds, equipment, and frequently touched surfaces.

Linen
Handle linen soiled with **body fluids** so as to prevent personal contamination and transfer to other patients.

Occupational Health & Bloodborne Pathogens
Prevent injuries from needles, scalpels, and other sharp devices.
Never recap needles using both hands.
Place sharps in puncture-proof sharps containers.
Use **Resuscitation Devices** as an alternative to mouth-to-mouth resuscitation.

Patient Placement
Use a Private Room for a patient who contaminates the environment.

"**Body Fluids**" include **blood**, **secretions**, and **excretions**.

Form No. **SPR-C**   BREVIS CORP., 3310 S 2700 E, SLC, UT 84109   © 1996 Brevis Corp.

Condensed Version

Hand Hygiene

It cannot be said too often: the most important and most basic technique in preventing and controlling infections and preventing the transmission of pathogens is handwashing. Because contaminated hands are a prime cause of cross-infection (i.e., transmission of pathogens from one patient to another), healthcare personnel caring for hospitalized patients must wash their hands thoroughly between patient contacts (i.e., before and after each patient contact). In addition, hands should be washed between tasks and procedures on the same patient to prevent cross-contamination of different body sites. Hands must be washed after touching blood, body fluids, secretions, excretions, and contaminated items, even when gloves are worn. Hands must be washed immediately after gloves are removed.

A plain (nonantimicrobial) soap may be used for routine handwashing, but an antimicrobial or antiseptic agent should be used in certain circumstances (e.g., before entering an operating room or to control

> The most important and most basic technique in preventing and controlling infections and preventing the transmission of pathogens is handwashing.

HISTORICAL NOTE
The Father of Handwashing

Ignaz Philipp Semmelweis (1818–1865) has been referred to as the "Father of Handwashing," the "Father of Hand Disinfection," and the "Father of Hospital Epidemiology." Semmelweis, a Hungarian physician, was employed in the maternity department of a large Viennese hospital during the 1840s. Many of the women whose babies were delivered in one of the hospital's clinics became ill and died of a disease known as puerperal fever (also known as childbed fever), the cause of which was unknown at the time. (It is now known that puerperal fever is caused by *Streptococcus pyogenes*.) Semmelweis observed that physicians and medical students often went directly from an autopsy room to the obstetrics clinic to assist in the delivery of a baby. Although they washed their hands with soap and water upon entering the clinic, Semmelweis noted that their hands still had a disagreeable odor. He concluded that the puerperal fever that the women later developed was caused by "cadaverous particles" present on the hands of the physicians and students. In May 1847, Semmelweis instituted a policy that stated that "all students or doctors who enter the wards for the purpose of making an examination must wash their hands thoroughly in a solution of chlorinated lime that will be placed in convenient basins near the entrance of the wards." Thereafter, the maternal mortality rate dropped dramatically. This was the first evidence that cleansing contaminated hands with an antiseptic agent reduces HAIs more effectively than handwashing with plain soap and water. It is interesting to note that Oliver Wendell Holmes (1809–1894), an American physician, had concluded some years earlier that puerperal fever was spread by healthcare workers' hands. However, the recommendations Holmes made in his historical essay of 1843, entitled *The Contagiousness of Puerperal Fever*, met with opposition (as did Semmelweis's recommendations) and had little impact on obstetric practices of the time.

HELPFUL HINTS REGARDING HANDWASHING

To make sure that you have washed your hands sufficiently, rub your soapy hands and interlaced fingers together for as long as it takes you to sing the birthday song ("Happy Birthday to You") twice through, or all verses of "Twinkle, Twinkle, Little Star" once. Alternatively, you could use a quick-drying alcohol foam, gel, or lotion. Studies have shown that these convenient products are at least as effective as old-fashioned soap and water. They are quick, they dry in about 15 seconds, and by using them, you eliminate the possibility of someone overhearing you singing off key!

Personal Protective Equipment

There are many components of personal protective equipment (PPE). The most common are listed here.

Gloves. Gloves can protect both patients and healthcare personnel from exposure to infectious materials that may be carried on hands. Healthcare personnel should wear gloves when:

- Anticipating direct contact with blood or body fluids, mucous membranes, nonintact skin, and other potentially infectious materials
- Having direct contact with patients who are colonized or infected with pathogens transmitted by the contact route
- Handling or touching visibly or potentially contaminated patient care equipment and environmental surfaces

Gloves must be changed between tasks and procedures on the same patient whenever there is risk of transferring microorganisms from one body site to another. Always remove gloves promptly after use and before going to another patient. Thoroughly wash your hands immediately after removing gloves; there is always the possibility that the gloves contained small tears in them or that your hands became contaminated while removing the gloves. Figure 12-5 illustrates the proper method of glove removal.

> PPE includes gloves, gowns, masks, eye protection, and respiratory protection.

Isolation Gowns. Isolation gowns are worn in conjunction with gloves and with other PPE when indicated. Gowns are usually the first piece of PPE to be donned. They protect the healthcare worker's arms and exposed body areas and prevent contamination of clothing with blood, body fluids, and other potentially infectious material. When applying Standard Precautions, an isolation gown is worn only if contact with blood or body fluid is anticipated. However, when Contact Precautions are

outbreaks within the hospital). Figure 12-4 contains the step-by-step instructions for effective handwashing. According to the CDC, alcohol-based handrubs that do not require the use of water can be used in place of handwashing when hands are not visibly soiled. The volume of handrub to be used varies from product to product; thus, manufacturer's directions must be followed. Artificial fingernails and rings should not be worn by healthcare personnel who provide direct patient care.

STEP	EXPLANATION/RATIONALE
1. Stand back so that you do not touch the sink.	The sink may be contaminated.
2. Turn on the faucet and wet hands under warm running water.	Water should not be too hot or too cold and hands should be wet before applying soap to minimize drying, chapping, or cracking of hands from frequent handwashing.

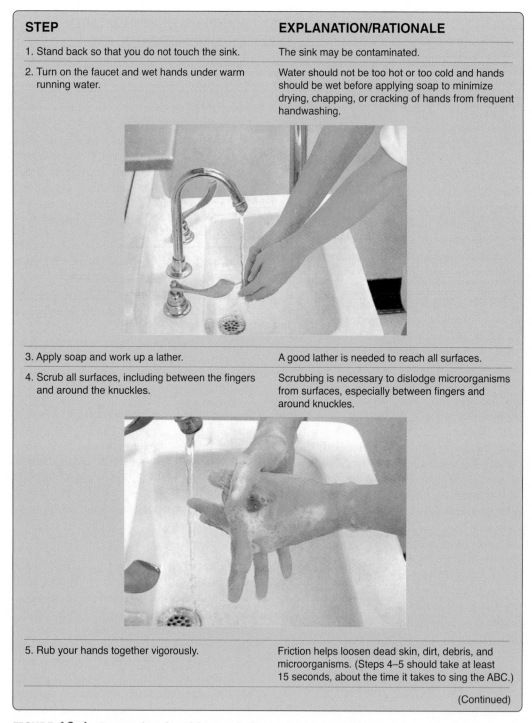

STEP	EXPLANATION/RATIONALE
3. Apply soap and work up a lather.	A good lather is needed to reach all surfaces.
4. Scrub all surfaces, including between the fingers and around the knuckles.	Scrubbing is necessary to dislodge microorganisms from surfaces, especially between fingers and around knuckles.
5. Rub your hands together vigorously.	Friction helps loosen dead skin, dirt, debris, and microorganisms. (Steps 4–5 should take at least 15 seconds, about the time it takes to sing the ABC.)

(Continued)

FIGURE 12-4. Proper handwashing technique. (From McCall RE, Tankersley CM. Phlebotomy Essentials, 4th ed. Philadelphia: Lippincott Williams & Wilkins, 2008.)

STEP	EXPLANATION/RATIONALE
6. Rinse your hands in a downward motion from wrists to fingertips.	Rinsing with the hands downward allows contaminants to be flushed from the hands and fingers into the sink rather than flowing back up the arm or wrist.

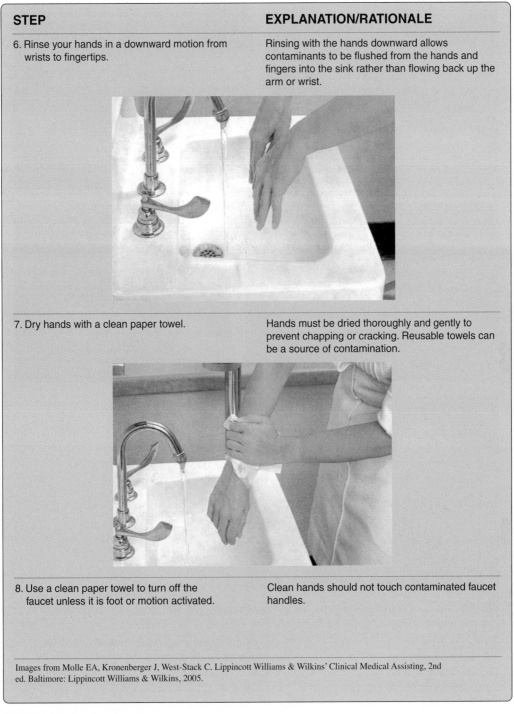

STEP	EXPLANATION/RATIONALE
7. Dry hands with a clean paper towel.	Hands must be dried thoroughly and gently to prevent chapping or cracking. Reusable towels can be a source of contamination.

STEP	EXPLANATION/RATIONALE
8. Use a clean paper towel to turn off the faucet unless it is foot or motion activated.	Clean hands should not touch contaminated faucet handles.

Images from Molle EA, Kronenberger J, West-Stack C. Lippincott Williams & Wilkins' Clinical Medical Assisting, 2nd ed. Baltimore: Lippincott Williams & Wilkins, 2005.

FIGURE 12-4. (*continued*)

FIGURE 12-5. Proper procedure for glove removal. (A) The wrist of one glove is grasped with the opposite gloved hand. **(B)** The glove is pulled inside out, over, and off the hand. **(C)** With the first glove held in the gloved hand, the fingers of the nongloved hand are slipped under the wrist of the remaining glove without touching the exterior surfaces. **(D)** The glove is then pulled inside out over the hand so that the first glove lies within the second glove, with no exterior glove surfaces exposed. **(E)** Contaminated gloves ready to be placed into the proper biohazardous waste receptacle. (From McCall RE, Tankersley CM. Phlebotomy Essentials, 4th ed. Philadelphia: Lippincott Williams & Wilkins, 2008.)

used, donning of both gown and gloves upon room entry is indicated. Isolation gowns should be removed before leaving the patient care area to prevent possible contamination of the environment outside the patient's room. Isolation gowns should be removed in a manner that prevents contamination of clothing or skin. The outer, "contaminated," side of the gown is turned inward and rolled into a bundle, and then discarded into a designated container for waste or linen to contain contamination.

Masks. Masks are used for three primary purposes in healthcare settings:

1. They are worn by healthcare personnel to protect them from contact with infectious material from patients.
2. They are worn by healthcare personnel when engaged in procedures requiring sterile technique to protect patients from exposure to pathogens that may be present in a healthcare worker's mouth or nose.

FIGURE 12-6. The type N95 respirator. See text for details. (From McCall RE, Tankersley CM. Phlebotomy Essentials, 4th ed. Philadelphia: Lippincott Williams & Wilkins, 2008. Courtesy of 3M Occupational Health and Environmental Safety Division, St. Paul, MN.)

3. They are placed on coughing patients to limit potential dissemination of infectious respiratory secretions from the patient to others.

Eye Protection. Types of eye protection include goggles and disposable or nondisposable face shields. Masks may be used in combination with goggles, or a face shield may be used instead of a mask and goggles. Even when Droplet Precautions are not indicated, eye, nose, and mouth protection are necessary when it is likely that there will be a splash or spray of any respiratory secretions or other body fluids. Eye protection and masks are removed after gloves are removed.

Respiratory Protection. Respiratory protection requires the use of a respirator with N95 of higher filtration to prevent inhalation of infectious particles (Fig. 12-6).[g] Do not confuse masks with particulate respirators. Respirators are recommended when working with patients with tuberculosis, SARS, and smallpox, and during the performance of aerosol-generating procedures on patients with avian or pandemic influenza.

Patient-Care Equipment

Organic material (e.g., blood, body fluids, secretions, excretions) must be removed from medical equipment, instruments, and devices prior to high level disinfection and sterilization because residual proteinaceous material reduces the effectiveness of disinfection and sterilization processes. All such equipment and devices must be

handled in a manner that will prevent healthcare workers and the environment with potentially infectious material. Cleaning and disinfection must include computer keyboards and personal digital assistants (PDAs). Whenever possible, the use of dedicated medical equipment, such as stethoscopes, blood pressure cuffs, and electronic thermometers, reduces the potential for transmission. Items such as commodes, intravenous pumps, and ventilators must be thoroughly cleaned and disinfected before use by or on another patient.

Environmental Control

The hospital must have, and employees must comply with, adequate procedures for the routine care, cleaning, and disinfection of environmental surfaces such as bedrails, bedside tables, commodes, doorknobs, sinks, and any other surfaces and equipment in close proximity to patients.

Linens

Textiles such as bedding, towels, and patient gowns that have become soiled with blood, body fluids, secretions, or excretions must be handled, transported, and laundered in a safe manner. Soiled textiles must not be shaken, must not come in contact with the healthcare worker's body or clothing, and must be contained in a laundry bag or designated bin.

Disposal of Sharps

Needlestick injuries and injuries resulting from broken glass and other sharps are the primary manner in which healthcare workers become infected with pathogens such as HIV, HBV, and HCV. Thus, Standard Precautions include guidelines regarding the safe handling of such items. Needles and other sharp devices must be handled in a manner that prevents injury to the user and to others who may encounter the device during or after a procedure. Accidents can be prevented by employing safer techniques (such as by not recapping needles), by disposing of used needles in appropriate sharps disposal containers, and by using safety-engineered sharp devices. Safety devices may be an integral part of the needle (including butterfly needles), the evacuated tube holder, or the syringe.

Listed here are desirable characteristics of needle safety features:

- It is as simple to use as possible, requiring little training to use it effectively.
- It is an integral part of the device, not an accessory.
- It provides a barrier between the hands of the healthcare worker and the needle after its use.
- It allows the worker's hands to remain behind the needle at all times.
- It is in effect before disassembly and remains in effect after disposal to protect users and trash handlers and for environmental safety.

Contaminated needles and other contaminated sharps must not be bent, recapped, or removed, and shearing

[g] N95 respirators are tight-fitting, adjustable masks that are designed to protect against small droplets of respiratory fluids and other airborne particles in addition to all the protection afforded by surgical masks.

or breaking of needles is prohibited. All contaminated needles, lancets, scalpel blades, and other sharps must be disposed of immediately after use, by placing them in special containers known as sharps containers. This is true whether or not the sharp contains a safety feature. Sharps containers are rigid, puncture resistant, leak proof, disposable, and clearly marked with a biohazard label (Fig. 12-7). Sharps containers must be easily accessible to all personnel needing them and must be located in all areas where needles are commonly used, as in areas where blood is drawn, including patient rooms, emergency rooms, ICUs, and surgical suites. When full, sharps containers are properly disposed of as biohazardous waste.

Transmission-Based Precautions

Within a healthcare setting, pathogens are transmitted by three major routes: contact, droplet, and airborne. Transmission-Based Precautions are | **The three types of Transmission-Based Precautions are used *in addition to* Standard Precautions.**

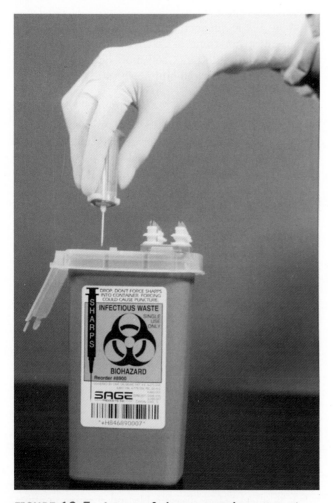

FIGURE 12-7. A type of sharps container. Note the biohazard symbol. (From McCall RE, Tankersley CM. Phlebotomy Essentials, 2nd ed. Philadelphia: Lippincott Williams & Wilkins, 1998. Courtesy of Sage Products, Inc., Crystal Lake, IL.)

used for patients who are known or suspected to be infected or colonized with highly transmissible or epidemiologically important pathogens for which additional safety precautions *beyond* Standard Precautions are required to interrupt transmission within hospitals. There are three types of Transmission-Based Precautions, which may be used either singly or in combination: Contact Precautions, Droplet Precautions, and Airborne Precautions. It is very important to understand that Transmission-Based Precautions are to be used *in addition to* the Standard Precautions already being used. Infectious diseases requiring Transmission-Based Precautions are listed in Table 12-3.

Contact Precautions

Contact transmission is the most important and frequent mode of transmission of HAIs. Contact Precautions are used for patients known or suspected to be infected or colonized with epidemiologically important pathogens that can be transmitted by direct or indirect contact. Examples include multidrug-resistant bacteria, *C. difficile*-associated diseases, respiratory syncytial virus (RSV) infection in children, scabies, impetigo, chickenpox or shingles, and viral hemorrhagic fevers. Contact Precautions are summarized on the sign shown in Figure 12-8. Infectious diseases requiring Contact Precautions are listed in Table 12-3.

| **Contact transmission is the most important and frequent mode of transmission of HAIs.**

Droplet Precautions

Technically, droplet transmission is a form of contact transmission. However, in droplet transmission, the mechanism of transfer is quite different than either direct or indirect contact transmission. Droplets are produced primarily as a result of coughing, sneezing, and talking, as well as during hospital procedures such as suctioning and bronchoscopy. Transmission occurs when droplets (larger than 5 μm in diameter) containing microbes are propelled a short distance through the air and become deposited on another person's conjunctiva, nasal mucosa, or mouth. Because of their size, droplets do not remain suspended in the air. Droplet Precautions must be used for patients known or suspected to be infected with microbes transmitted by droplets that can be generated in the ways previously mentioned. Droplet Precautions are summarized on the sign shown in Figure 12-9. Infectious diseases requiring Droplet Precautions are listed in Table 12-3.

| **Droplet Precautions are used for particles that are larger than 5 μm in diameter.**

Airborne Precautions

Airborne transmission involves either airborne droplet nuclei or dust particles containing a pathogen. Airborne droplet nu-

| **Airborne Precautions are used when particles are 5 μm or less in diameter.**

TABLE 12-3	Infectious Diseases Requiring Transmission-Based Precautions
TYPE OF TRANSMISSION-BASED PRECAUTIONS	**INFECTIOUS DISEASES OR CONDITIONS**[a]
Contact Precautions	Acute viral (hemorrhagic) conjunctivitis; adenovirus pneumonia; any acute respiratory infectious disease in infants and young children; adverse events following vaccinia vaccination; aseptic meningitis in infants and young children; bronchiolitis; chickenpox; *Clostridium difficile* gastroenteritis; congenital rubella in children <1 year of age; cutaneous diphtheria; decubitus ulcer; disseminated shingles in any patient; localized shingles in immunocompromised patients; extrapulmonary tuberculosis with draining lesion; gastroenteritis due to adenovirus, *Campylobacter*, cholera, *Cryptosporidium*; enterohemorrhagic 0157:H7 *E. coli*, giardiasis, norovirus, rotavirus, *Salmonella, Shigella, Vibrio parahemolyticus* or *Yersinia enterocolitica* in diapered or incontinent persons; group A streptococcus infections if skin lesions are present head lice; human metapneumovirus infection; impetigo; infection or colonization with multidrug-resistant organisms; major draining abscesses; major wound infections; monkeypox; poliomyelitis; respiratory parainfluenza virus infection in infants and young children; respiratory syncytial virus infection in infants, young children, and immunocompromised adults; rotavirus gastroenteritis; severe mucocutaneous herpes simplex infections; neonatal herpes simplex infections; scabies; severe acute respiratory syndrome (SARS); smallpox; staphylococcal furunculosis in infants and young children; staphylococcal scalded skin syndrome (Ritter's diseases); major staphylococcal or streptococcal disease of skin, wounds, or burns; type A or type E viral hepatitis in diapered or incontinent patients; viral hemorrhagic fevers due to Lassa, Ebola, Marburg, or Crimean-Congo fever viruses
Droplet Precautions	Adenovirus infection in infants and young children; adenovirus pneumonia; epiglottitis or meningitis caused by *Haemophilus influenzae* type b; group A streptococcus infections (major skin, wound, or burn infections; pharyngitis in infants and young children; scarlet fever in infants and young children; serious invasive disease); influenza; meningitis or pneumonia caused by *Neisseria meningitidis*; mumps; *Mycoplasma* pneumonia; parvovirus B19 skin infection; pertussis (whooping cough); pharyngeal diphtheria; pneumonic plague; rhinovirus infection; rubella (German measles); severe acute respiratory syndrome (SARS); viral hemorrhagic fevers due to Lassa, Ebola, Marburg, or Crimean-Congo fever viruses
Airborne Precautions	Chickenpox, confirmed or suspected pulmonary or laryngeal tuberculosis; extrapulmonary tuberculosis with draining lesions; disseminated shingles in any patient; localized shingles in immunocompromised patients, measles (rubeola); monkeypox; severe acute respiratory syndrome (SARS); smallpox

[a]This is not an all-inclusive list of diseases.

clei are small-particle residues (5 μm or less in diameter) of evaporated droplets containing microbes; because of their small size, they remain suspended in air for long periods. Airborne Precautions are summarized on the sign shown in Figure 12-10. Airborne Precautions apply to patients known or suspected to be infected with epidemiologically important pathogens that can be transmitted by the airborne route. Infectious diseases requiring Airborne Precautions are listed in Table 12-3.

Patient Placement

Whenever possible, single-patient rooms are used for patients who might contaminate the hospital environment or who do not (or cannot be expected to) assist in maintaining appropriate hygiene or environmental control. Single rooms are always indicated for patients placed on Airborne Precautions and are preferred for patients requiring Contact or Droplet Precautions.

Airborne Infection Isolation Rooms

The preferred placement for patients who are infected with pathogens that are spread via airborne droplet nuclei and, therefore, require Airborne Precautions, is in an airborne infection isolation room (AIIR). An AIIR (Fig. 12-11) is a single-patient room that is equipped with special air handling and ventilation systems. AIIRs are under negative pressure to prevent AIIRs are under negative pressure, and air that is evacuated from these rooms passes through HEPA filters.

FIGURE 12-8. Contact Precautions sign. (From McCall RE, Tankersley CM. Phlebotomy Essentials, 4th ed. Philadelphia: Lippincott Williams & Wilkins, 2008. Courtesy of the Brevis Corp., Salt Lake City, UT.)

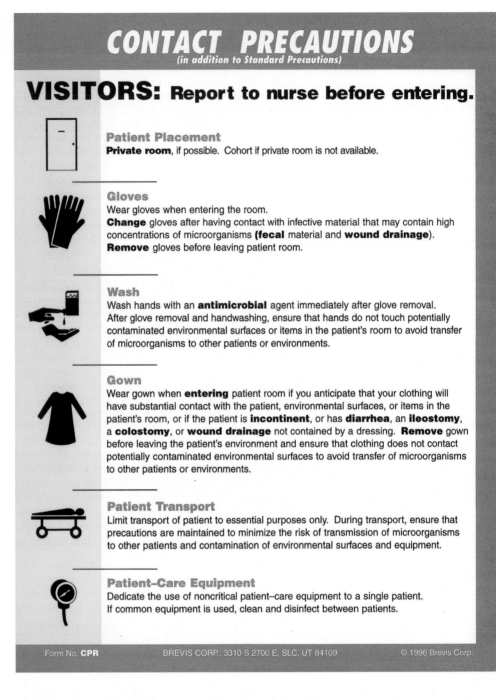

CONTACT PRECAUTIONS
(in addition to Standard Precautions)

VISITORS: Report to nurse before entering.

Patient Placement
Private room, if possible. Cohort if private room is not available.

Gloves
Wear gloves when entering the room.
Change gloves after having contact with infective material that may contain high concentrations of microorganisms **(fecal** material and **wound drainage)**.
Remove gloves before leaving patient room.

Wash
Wash hands with an **antimicrobial** agent immediately after glove removal. After glove removal and handwashing, ensure that hands do not touch potentially contaminated environmental surfaces or items in the patient's room to avoid transfer of microorganisms to other patients or environments.

Gown
Wear gown when **entering** patient room if you anticipate that your clothing will have substantial contact with the patient, environmental surfaces, or items in the patient's room, or if the patient is **incontinent**, or has **diarrhea**, an **ileostomy**, a **colostomy**, or **wound drainage** not contained by a dressing. **Remove** gown before leaving the patient's environment and ensure that clothing does not contact potentially contaminated environmental surfaces to avoid transfer of microorganisms to other patients or environments.

Patient Transport
Limit transport of patient to essential purposes only. During transport, ensure that precautions are maintained to minimize the risk of transmission of microorganisms to other patients and contamination of environmental surfaces and equipment.

Patient–Care Equipment
Dedicate the use of noncritical patient–care equipment to a single patient. If common equipment is used, clean and disinfect between patients.

Form No. **CPR**   BREVIS CORP., 3310 S 2700 E, SLC, UT 84109   © 1996 Brevis Corp.

room air from entering the corridor when the door is opened, and air that is evacuated from such rooms passes through high-efficiency particulate air (HEPA) filters to remove pathogens. Standard and Airborne Precautions are strictly enforced.

Protective Environments

Certain patients are especially vulnerable to infection, particularly to invasive environmental fungal infections. Examples of such patients are patients with severe burns, those who have leukemia, patients who have received a transplant (such as a hematopoietic stem cell transplant), immunosuppressed persons, those receiving radiation treatments, leukopenic patients (those having abnormally low white blood cell counts), and premature infants. These patients can be protected by placing them in a Protective Environment (sometimes referred to as protective isolation or positive pressure isolation). The Protective Environment is a well-sealed single-patient room in which vented air entering the room is passed through HEPA filters. The room is under positive pressure to prevent corridor air from entering when the door is opened (Fig. 12-12). Strategies to minimize dust include scrubbable surfaces rather than upholstery and carpet. Crevices and sprinkler heads are routinely

Protective Environments are rooms that are under positive pressure, and vented air that enters these rooms passes through HEPA filters.

FIGURE 12-9. Droplet Precautions sign. (From McCall RE, Tankersley CM. Phlebotomy Essentials, 4th ed. Philadelphia: Lippincott Williams & Wilkins, 2008. Courtesy of the Brevis Corp., Salt Lake City, UT.)

cleaned. Appropriate Standard and Transmission-Based Precautions are strictly enforced.

Handling Food and Eating Utensils

Contaminated food provides an excellent environment for the growth of pathogens. Most often, human carelessness, especially neglecting the practice of handwashing, is responsible for this contamination. Foodborne pathogens and the diseases they cause are discussed in Chapter 11. Regulations for safe handling of food and eating utensils are not difficult to follow. They include:

- Using high-quality, fresh food
- Properly refrigerating and storing food
- Properly washing, preparing, and cooking food
- Properly disposing of uneaten food
- Thoroughly washing hands and fingernails before handling food and after visiting a restroom
- Properly disposing of nasal and oral secretions in tissues and then thoroughly washing hands and fingernails

FIGURE 12-10. Airborne Precautions sign. (From McCall RE, Tankersley CM. Phlebotomy Essentials, 4th ed. Philadelphia: Lippincott Williams & Wilkins Publishers, 2008. Courtesy of the Brevis Corp., Salt Lake City, UT.)

FIGURE 12-11. Airborne infection isolation room. See text for details.

FIGURE 12-12. Protective Environment. See text for details.

- Covering hair and wearing clean clothes and aprons
- Providing periodic health examinations for kitchen workers
- Prohibiting anyone with a respiratory or gastrointestinal disease from handling food or eating utensils
- Keeping all cutting boards and other surfaces scrupulously clean
- Rinsing and then washing cooking and eating utensils in a dishwasher in which the water temperature is greater than 80°C

According to the CDC, the combination of hot water and detergents used in dishwashers is sufficient to decontaminate dishware and eating utensils; no special precautions are needed.

Handling Fomites

As previously described, fomites are any nonliving or inanimate objects other than food that may harbor and transmit microbes. Examples of fomites in healthcare settings are patients' gowns, bedding, towels, and eating and drinking utensils; and hospital equipment such as bedpans, stethoscopes, latex gloves, electronic thermometers, and electrocardiographic electrodes that become contaminated by pathogens from the respiratory tract, intestinal tract, or the skin of patients. Telephones and computer keyboards in patient-care areas can also serve as fomites. Transmission of pathogens by fomites can be prevented by observing the following rules:

- Use disposable equipment and supplies wherever possible
- Disinfect or sterilize equipment as soon as possible after use
- Use individual equipment for each patient
- Use electronic or glass thermometers fitted with one-time use, disposable covers or use disposable, single-use

thermometers; electronic and glass thermometers must be cleaned or sterilized on a regular basis, following manufacturer's instructions
- Empty bedpans and urinals, wash them in hot water, and store them in a clean cabinet between uses
- Place bed linen and soiled clothing in bags to be sent to the laundry

Medical Waste Disposal

Materials or substances that are harmful to health are referred to as biohazards (short for biologic hazards). They must be identified by a biohazard symbol, which was shown in Figure 12-7. According to OSHA standards, medical wastes must be disposed of properly. These standards include the following:

- Any receptacle used for decomposable solid or liquid waste or refuse must be constructed so that it does not leak and must be maintained in a sanitary condition. This receptacle must be equipped with a solid, tight-fitting cover, unless it can be maintained in a sanitary condition without a cover.
- All sweepings, solid or liquid wastes, refuse, and garbage shall be removed to avoid creating a menace to health and shall be removed as often as necessary to maintain the place of employment in a sanitary condition.
- The medical facility's infection control program must address the handling and disposal of potentially contaminated items.

Disposal of sharps was discussed earlier in the chapter.

Infection Control in Dental Healthcare Settings

In 2003, the CDC published a set of infection control guidelines applicable to dental healthcare settings, entitled *Guidelines for Infection Control in Dental Healthcare Settings*,

2003. Students in dental-related programs, such as dental assistant, dental hygienist, and dental laboratory technician programs should familiarize themselves with these guidelines. Listed here are some of the major considerations addressed in the CDC publication:

- Development of a written infection control program that includes policies, procedures, and guidelines for education and training of dental healthcare personnel, immunizations, exposure prevention and postexposure management, work restriction caused by medical conditions, and maintenance of records, data management, and confidentiality
- Preventing transmission of bloodborne pathogens, including HBV vaccination and preventing exposures to blood and other potentially infectious materials
- Hand hygiene and PPE; Figure 12-13 illustrates the protection afforded by PPE

- Contact dermatitis and latex hypersensitivity
- Sterilization and disinfection of patient-care items
- Environmental infection control, including use of disinfectants, housekeeping services, spills of blood or body substances, and medical waste
- Special considerations, such as dental handpieces, dental radiology, aseptic technique for parenteral medications, oral-surgical procedures, handling of biopsy specimens and extracted teeth, dental laboratory, and patients with tuberculosis

Infection Control Committees and Infection Control Professionals

All healthcare facilities should have some type of formal infection control program in place. Its functions will vary slightly from one type of healthcare facility to another. In a hospital setting, the infection control program is usually under the jurisdiction of the hospital's Infection Control Committee (ICC) or Epidemiology Service. The ICC is composed of representatives from most of the hospital's departments, including medical and surgical services, pathology, nursing, hospital administration, risk management, pharmacy, housekeeping, food services, and central supply. The chairperson is usually an Infection Control Professional (ICP), such as a physician (e.g., an epidemiologist or infectious disease specialist), an infection control nurse, a microbiologist, or some other person knowledgeable about infection control.

> A hospital's infection control program is usually under the jurisdiction of the hospital's ICC or Epidemiology Service.

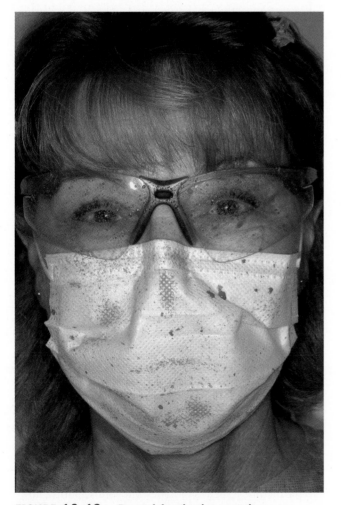

FIGURE 12-13. Dental hygienist wearing appropriate PPE. A red dye was used to simulate a patient's saliva that can spatter onto a hygienist's face, mask, and protective eyewear during a polishing procedure. (From Molinari JA and Harte JA. Cotton's Practical Infection Control in Dentistry, 3rd ed. Philadelphia: Lippincott Williams & Wilkins, 2010.)

SPOTLIGHTING INFECTION CONTROL PROFESSIONALS

Individuals wishing to combine their interest in detective work with a career in medicine might consider a career as an ICP. ICPs include physicians (infectious disease specialists or epidemiologists), nurses, clinical laboratory scientists (medical technologists), and microbiologists. Most ICPs are nurses, many having baccalaureate degrees and some with master of science degrees. In addition to having strong clinical skills, ICPs require knowledge and expertise in such areas as epidemiology, microbiology, infectious disease processes, statistics, and computers. To be effective, they must be part detective, part diplomat, part administrator, and part educator. In addition, ICPs function as role models, patient advocates, and consultants.

Within the hospital, ICPs provide valuable services that minimize the risks of infection and spread of disease, thereby aiding patients, healthcare professionals,

(continues)

and visitors. The ICP is the key person in implementing and facilitating the institution's infection control program. The ICP is often the head of the hospital's ICC and, as such, is responsible for scheduling, organizing, and conducting ICC meetings. At these meetings, medical records are reviewed of all patients suspected of having incurred a hospital-associated infection since the previous meeting. The committee discusses possible or known causes of such infections and ways to prevent them from occurring in the future. The ICP receives timely information from the clinical microbiology laboratory (CML) concerning possible outbreaks of infection within the hospital and is responsible for rapidly organizing a team to investigate these outbreaks. ICPs are also responsible for educating healthcare personnel about infection risk, prevention, and control.

The primary responsibilities of an ICP are as follows:

- Possess knowledge of infectious diseases processes, reservoirs, incubation periods, periods of communicability, and susceptibility of patients
- Conduct surveillance and epidemiologic investigations
- Prevent/control the transmission of pathogens to include strategies for hand hygiene, antisepsis, cleaning, disinfection, sterilization, patient care settings, patient placement, medical waste disposal, and implementation of outbreak control measures
- Manage the facility's infection control program
- Communicate with the public, facility staff, and state and local health departments concerning infection control-related issues
- Evaluate new medical products that could be associated with increased infection risk

The ICC periodically reviews the hospital's infection control program and the incidence of HAIs. It is a policy-making and review body that may take drastic action (e.g., instituting quarantine measures) when epidemiologic circumstances warrant. Other ICC responsibilities include patient surveillance, environmental surveillance, investigation of outbreaks and epidemics, and education of the hospital staff regarding infection control.

Although every department of the hospital endeavors to maintain aseptic conditions, the total environment is constantly bombarded with microbes from outside the hospital. These must be controlled for the protection of the patients. Hospital personnel (usually ICPs) entrusted with this aspect of healthcare diligently and constantly work to maintain the proper environment. In the event of an epidemic, the ICP notifies city, county, and state health authorities so they can assist in ending the epidemic.

Role of the Microbiology Laboratory in Healthcare Epidemiology

Listed here are some of the ways in which CML personnel participate in healthcare epidemiology and infection control:

> A hospital's CML participates in that hospital's infection control program in various ways.

- By monitoring the types and numbers of pathogens isolated from hospitalized patients. In most hospitals, such monitoring is accomplished using computers and appropriate software programs.
- By performing antimicrobial susceptibility testing, detecting emerging resistance patterns, and preparing and distributing periodic cumulative antimicrobial susceptibility summary reports (see information on "pocket charts" in Chapter 9)
- By notifying the appropriate ICP should an unusual pathogen or an unusually high number of isolates of a common pathogen be detected. The ICP will then initiate an investigation of the outbreak.
- By processing environmental samples, including samples from hospital employees that have been collected from within the affected ward(s), with the goal of pinpointing the exact source of the pathogen that is causing the outbreak. Examples of environmental samples include air samples, nasal swabs from healthcare personnel, and swabs of sink drains, whirlpool tubs, respiratory therapy equipment, bed rails, and ventilation grates and ducts.
- By performing biochemical, immunological, and molecular identification and typing procedures to compare various isolates of the same species. *Example*: Assume that there is an epidemic of *Klebsiella pneumoniae* infections on the pediatric ward and that *K. pneumoniae* has been isolated from a certain environmental sample collected on that ward. How do CML personnel determine that the *K. pneumoniae* that has been isolated from the environmental sample is the same strain of *K. pneumoniae* that has been isolated from the patients? Traditionally, the two most commonly used methods have been by biotype and antibiogram. If the two strains produce the same biochemical test results, they are said to have the same biotype. If they produce the same susceptibility and resistance patterns when antimicrobial susceptibility testing is performed, they are said to have the same antibiogram. Having the same biotype and antibiogram is evidence (but not absolute proof) that they are the same strain. Because of the limitations of phenotypic methods (such as biotypes and antibiograms), however, most hospitals are currently using what is known as molecular epidemiology, in which genotypic (as opposed to phenotypic) typing methods are used. Most often, these methods involve genotyping of plasmid or chromosomal DNA. Genotypic methods provide more accurate data than phenotypic methods. If the two iso-

lates of *K. pneumoniae* in the given example have exactly the same genotype (i.e., possess exactly the same genes), they are the same strain; therefore, the source of the epidemic has been found. Action will then be taken to eliminate the source.

CONCLUDING REMARKS

An HAI can add several weeks to a patient's hospital stay and may lead to serious complications and even death. From an economic viewpoint, insurance companies rarely reimburse hospitals and other healthcare facilities for the costs associated with HAIs. Insurance companies take the position that HAIs are the fault of the healthcare facility and, therefore, that the facility should bear any additional patient costs related to such infections. Sadly, cross-infections transmitted by hospital personnel, including physicians, are all too common; this is particularly true when hospitals and clinics are overcrowded and the staff is overworked. However, HAIs can be avoided through proper education and disciplined compliance with infection control practices.

All healthcare workers must fully comprehend the problem of HAIs, must be completely knowledgeable about infection control practices, and must personally do everything in their power to prevent HAIs from occurring.

ON THE CD-ROM
- Terms Introduced in This Chapter
- Review of Key Points
- Insight
  - Learning About Florence Nightingale
  - Healthcare-Associated Zoonoses
  - Donning PPE
  - Removing PPE
- Increase Your Knowledge
- Critical Thinking
- Additional Self-Assessment Exercises

SELF-ASSESSMENT EXERCISES

After studying this chapter, answer the following multiple-choice questions.

1. An HAI is one that:
   a. develops during hospitalization or erupts within 14 days of hospital discharge.
   b. develops while the patient is hospitalized.
   c. is acquired in the community.
   d. the patient has at the time of hospital admission.
2. An example of a fomite would be:
   a. a drinking glass used by a patient.
   b. bandages from an infected wound.
   c. soiled bed linens.
   d. all of the above.

3. Which of the following Gram-positive bacteria is most likely to be the cause of an HAI?
   a. *C. difficile*
   b. *S. aureus*
   c. *Streptococcus pneumoniae*
   d. *S. pyogenes*
4. Which of the following Gram-negative bacteria is least likely to be the cause of an HAI?
   a. a *Klebsiella* species
   b. a *Salmonella* species
   c. *E. coli*
   d. *P. aeruginosa*
5. A Protective Environment would be appropriate for a patient:
   a. infected with MRSA.
   b. with leukopenia.
   c. with pneumonic plague.
   d. with tuberculosis.
6. Which of the following is not part of Standard Precautions?
   a. handwashing between patient contacts
   b. placing a patient in a private room having negative air pressure
   c. properly disposing of needles, scalpels, and other sharps
   d. wearing gloves, masks, eye protection, and gowns when appropriate
7. A patient suspected of having tuberculosis has been admitted to the hospital. Which one of the following is not appropriate?
   a. Droplet Precautions
   b. an AIIR
   c. Standard Precautions
   d. use of a type N95 respirator by healthcare professional who are caring for the patient
8. Which of the following statements about medical asepsis is false?
   a. Disinfection is a medical aseptic technique.
   b. Handwashing is a medical aseptic technique.
   c. Medical asepsis is considered a clean technique.
   d. The goal of medical asepsis is to exclude all microorganisms from an area.
9. Which of the following statements about an AIIR is false?
   a. Air entering the room is passed through HEPA filters.
   b. The room is under negative air pressure.
   c. An AIIR is appropriate for patients with meningococcal meningitis, whooping cough, or influenza.
   d. Transmission-Based Precautions will be necessary.
10. Contact Precautions are required for patients with:
    a. *C. difficile*-associated diseases.
    b. infections caused by multidrug-resistant bacteria.
    c. viral hemorrhagic fevers.
    d. all of the above.

13 DIAGNOSING INFECTIOUS DISEASES

LEARNING OBJECTIVES

AFTER STUDYING THIS CHAPTER, YOU SHOULD BE ABLE TO:

- Discuss the role of healthcare professionals in the collection and transport of clinical specimens
- List the types of clinical specimens that are submitted to the Clinical Microbiology Laboratory for the diagnosis of infectious diseases
- Discuss general precautions that must be observed during the collection and handling of clinical specimens
- Describe the proper procedures for obtaining blood, urine, cerebrospinal fluid, sputum, throat, wound, GC, and fecal specimens for submission to the Clinical Microbiology Laboratory
- State the information that must be included on specimen labels and laboratory test requisitions
- Outline the organization of the Pathology Department and the Clinical Microbiology Laboratory
- Compare and contrast the anatomical and clinical pathology divisions of the Pathology Department
- Identify the various types of personnel that work in anatomical and clinical pathology

INTRODUCTION

The proper diagnosis of an infectious disease requires (a) taking a complete patient history, (b) conducting a thorough physical examination of the patient, (c) carefully evaluating the patient's signs and symptoms, and (d) implementing the proper selection, collection, transport, and processing of appropriate clinical specimens. The latter topics—those involving clinical specimens—are discussed in this chapter. The other topics are beyond the scope of this book.

CLINICAL SPECIMENS

The various types of speci- | The clinical specimens
mens, such as blood, urine, | that are used to
feces, and cerebrospinal fluid, | diagnose infectious
that are collected from patients | diseases must be of the
and used to diagnose or follow | highest possible quality.
the progress of infectious dis-
eases are referred to as *clinical specimens*. The most common types of clinical specimens that are sent to the hospital's microbiology laboratory (hereafter referred to as

TABLE 13-1	Types of Clinical Specimens Submitted to the Clinical Microbiology Laboratory		
TYPE OF SPECIMEN	**TYPE(S) OF INFECTIOUS DISEASE THAT THE SPECIMEN IS USED TO DIAGNOSE**	**TYPE OF SPECIMEN**	**TYPE(S) OF INFECTIOUS DISEASE THAT THE SPECIMEN IS USED TO DIAGNOSE**
Blood	B, F, P, V	"Scotch tape prep"	P
Bone marrow	B	Skin scrapings	F
Bronchial and bronchoalveolar washes	V	Skin snip	P
Cerebrospinal fluid (CSF)	B, F, P, V	Sputum	B, F, P
Cervical and vaginal swabs	B	Synovial (joint) fluid	B
Conjunctival swab or scraping	B, V	Throat swabs	B, V
Feces and rectal swabs	B, P, V	Tissue (biopsy and autopsy) specimens	B, F, P, V
Hair clippings	F	Urethral discharge material	B
Nail (fingernail and toenail) clippings	F	Urine	B, P, V
Nasal swabs	B	Urogenital secretions (e.g., vaginal discharge material, prostatic secretions)	B, P
Pus from a wound or abscess	B	Vesicle fluid or scraping	V

B, bacterial infections; F, fungal infections; P, parasitic infections; V, viral infections.

the Clinical Microbiology Laboratory or CML) are listed in Table 13-1. It is extremely important that these specimens are of the highest possible quality and that they are collected in a manner that does not jeopardize either the patient or the person collecting the specimen.

Role of Healthcare Professionals in the Submission of Clinical Specimens

A close working relationship among the members of the healthcare team is essential for the proper diagnosis of infectious diseases. When a clinician suspects that a patient has a particular infectious disease, appropriate clinical specimens must be obtained and certain diagnostic tests requested. The doctor, nurse, medical technologist, or other qualified healthcare professional must select the appropriate specimen, collect it properly, and then properly transport it to the CML for processing (Fig. 13-1). Laboratory findings must then be conveyed to the attending clinician as quickly as possible to facilitate the prompt diagnosis and

Laboratory professionals make laboratory observations and generate test results which are used by clinicians to diagnose infectious diseases and initiate appropriate therapy.

treatment of the infectious disease. Although laboratory professionals do not themselves make diagnoses, they make laboratory observations and generate test results that assist clinicians to correctly diagnose infectious diseases and initiate appropriate therapy.

Healthcare professionals who collect and transport clinical specimens should exercise extreme caution during the collection and transport of clinical specimens to avoid sticking themselves with needles, cutting themselves with other types of sharps, or coming in contact with any type of specimen. Healthcare personnel who collect clinical specimens must strictly adhere to the safety policies known as Standard Precautions (discussed in detail in Chapter 12). According to the Clinical and Laboratory Standards Institute (CLSI), "All specimens should be collected or transferred into a leakproof primary container with a secure closure. Care should be taken by the person collecting the specimen not to contaminate the outside of the primary container. . . . Within the institution, the primary container should be placed into a second container, which will contain the specimen if the primary container breaks or leaks in transit to the laboratory." (CLSI Document M29-A3, 2005.) Within the laboratory, all specimens are handled carefully,

FIGURE 13-1. Diagrammatic representation of the steps involved in the diagnosis of infectious diseases. (Modified from Winn WC Jr, et al. Koneman's Color Atlas and Textbook of Diagnostic Microbiology. 6th ed. Philadelphia: Lippincott Williams & Wilkins, 2006.)

following Standard Precautions and ultimately disposed of as infectious waste.

Importance of High-Quality Clinical Specimens

Specimens submitted to the CML must be of the highest possible quality. High-quality clinical specimens are required to achieve accurate, *clinically relevant laboratory results*—meaning results that *truly* provide information about the patient's infectious disease. **It has often been stated that the quality of the laboratory work performed in a CML can be only as good as the quality of the specimens it receives.** It is impossible for a CML to obtain and report high-quality test results if the laboratory receives poor quality specimens or the wrong types of specimens.

The three components of specimen quality are (a) proper specimen selection (i.e., the correct type of specimen must be submitted), (b) proper specimen collection, and (c) proper

> High-quality clinical specimens are required to achieve accurate, clinically relevant laboratory results.

> The laboratory must provide written instructions for the proper selection, collection, and transport of clinical specimens.

transport of the specimen to the laboratory. The laboratory must provide written guidelines regarding specimen selection, collection, and transport in the form of a manual. Although the name of the manual varies from one institution to the next, it is referred to in this book as the "Laboratory Policies and Procedures Manual" (Lab P&P Manual). Copies of the Lab P&P Manual must be available to every ward, floor, clinic, and department. Often, it is accessible through the hospital's computer system. **Although the laboratory provides guidelines, it is the person who collects the specimen who is ultimately responsible for its quality.**

It would not be feasible in a book of this size to provide a complete discussion of the proper methods for

---

STUDY AID

Three Components of Specimen Quality

1. Proper selection of the specimen (i.e., to select the appropriate type of specimen for diagnosis of the suspected infectious disease)
2. Proper collection of the specimen
3. Proper transport of the specimen to the laboratory

selecting, collecting, and transporting clinical specimens. Only a few important concepts are discussed here. See "Insight: Specimen Quality and Clinical Relevance" on the CD-ROM for additional details.

When clinical specimens are improperly collected and handled, (a) the etiologic agent (causative agent) may not be found or may be destroyed, (b) overgrowth by indigenous microflora may mask the pathogen, and/or (c) contaminants may interfere with the identification of pathogens and the diagnosis of the patient's infectious disease.

Proper Selection, Collection, and Transport of Clinical Specimens

When collecting clinical specimens for microbiology, these general precautions should be taken:

- The specimen must be properly selected. That is, it must be the appropriate type of specimen for diagnosis of the suspected infectious disease.
- The specimen must be properly and carefully collected. Whenever possible, specimens must be collected in a manner that will eliminate or minimize contamination of the specimen with indigenous microflora.
- The material should be collected from a site where the suspected pathogen is most likely to be found and where the least contamination is likely to occur.
- Whenever possible, specimens should be obtained before antimicrobial therapy has begun. If this is not possible, the laboratory should be informed as to which antimicrobial agent(s) the patient is receiving.
- The acute stage of the disease—when the patient is experiencing the symptoms of the disease—is the appropriate time to collect most specimens. Some viruses, however, are more easily isolated during the prodromal or onset stage of disease.
- Specimen collection should be performed with care and tact to avoid harming the patient, causing discomfort, or causing undue embarrassment. If the patient is to collect the specimen, such as sputum or urine, the patient must be given clear and detailed collection instructions.
- A sufficient quantity of the specimen must be obtained to provide enough material for all required diagnostic tests. The amount of specimen to collect should be specified in the Lab P&P Manual.
- All specimens should be placed or collected into a sterile container to prevent contamination of the specimen by indigenous microflora and airborne microbes. Appropriate types of collection devices and specimen containers should be specified in the Lab P&P Manual.
- Specimens should be protected from heat and cold and promptly delivered to the laboratory so that the results of the analyses will validly represent the number and types of organisms present at the time of collection. If delivery to the laboratory is delayed, some delicate pathogens might die; therefore, certain types of specimens must be rushed to the laboratory immediately after collection. Some types of specimens must be placed on ice during delivery to the laboratory, whereas other specimens should never be refrigerated or placed on ice because of the fragile and sensitive nature of the pathogens. Obligate anaerobes die when exposed to air and therefore must be protected from oxygen during transport to the CML. Any indigenous microflora in the specimen may overgrow, inhibit, or kill pathogens. Specimen transport instructions should be contained in the Lab P&P Manual.
- Specimens must be handled with great care to avoid contamination of the patients, couriers, and healthcare professionals. Specimens must be placed in a sealed plastic bag for immediate and careful transport to the laboratory. Whenever possible, sterile, disposable specimen containers should be used.
- The specimen container must be properly labeled and accompanied by an appropriate laboratory test requisition containing adequate instructions. Labels should contain the patient's name, unique hospital identification number, and hospital room number; requesting clinician's name; culture site; and date and time of collection. Laboratory test requisitions should contain the patient's name, age, sex, and unique hospital identification number; name of the requesting clinician; specific information about the type of specimen and the site from which it was collected; date and time of collection; initials of the person who collected the specimen; and information about any antimicrobial agent(s) that the patient is receiving. The laboratory should always be given sufficient clinical information to aid in performing appropriate analyses. For example, the laboratory test requisition that accompanies a wound specimen should not merely state "wound"; rather, it should state the specific *type* of wound (e.g., burn wound, dog bite wound, surgical site infection, etc.), the anatomical site, and whether it is on the left side or right side, if applicable.
- Ideally, specimens should be collected and delivered to the laboratory as early in the day as possible to give CML professionals sufficient time to process the material, especially when the hospital or clinic does not have 24-hour laboratory service.

Contamination of Clinical Specimens with Indigenous Microflora

As mentioned in Chapter 1, vast numbers of microbes live on and in the human body. Usually, they are collectively referred to as indigenous microflora, although the older term, "normal flora," is sometimes used. Clinical specimens must be collected in a manner that eliminates, or at least reduces, contamination of the specimens with members of the indigenous microflora. Recall that many members of our indigenous microflora are opportunistic pathogens. Thus, when present in specimens, these organisms *might* merely be contaminants, but it is also possible that they are causing an infection.

Types of Clinical Specimens Usually Required to Diagnose Infectious Diseases

Specific techniques for the collection and transport of clinical specimens vary from institution to institution and are contained in the institution's Lab P&P Manual. Only a few of the most important considerations are mentioned here.

Blood

Blood consists of a mixture of cells and fluid (Fig. 13-2). Within the human body, the liquid portion of blood is called plasma; it makes up about 55% of the volume of blood. When a blood specimen is allowed to clot, the liquid portion is called serum. (Thus, serum is plasma that no longer contains clotting factors.) The cells (also referred to as cellular or *formed elements*) make up about 45% of the volume of blood. The various blood cells include red blood cells (RBCs or erythrocytes), white blood cells (WBCs or leukocytes), and platelets (or thrombocytes). The three major categories of WBCs are granulocytes, monocytes, and lymphocytes. Lymphocytes are discussed in detail in Chapter 16. The three types of granulocytes are neutrophils, basophils, and eosinophils.

> Within the body, the liquid portion of blood is called *plasma*, but if a blood specimen is allowed to clot, the liquid portion is called *serum*.

As it circulates throughout the body, blood is usually sterile. However, blood sometimes contains bacteria. The presence of bacteria in the bloodstream (*bacteremia*) may indicate a disease, although temporary or transient bacteremias may occur after oral surgery, tooth extraction, or even aggressive tooth brushing that causes bleeding. Bacteremia may occur during certain stages of many infectious diseases. These diseases include bacterial meningitis, typhoid fever and other salmonella infections, pneumococcal pneumonia, urinary infections, endocarditis, brucellosis, tularemia,

> Bacteremia—the presence of bacteria in the bloodstream—may or may not be a sign of disease. Septicemia, on the other hand, *is* a disease.

plague, anthrax, syphilis, and wound infections caused by beta-hemolytic streptococci, staphylococci, and other invasive bacteria. Bacteremia should not be confused with septicemia. *Septicemia* is a serious disease characterized by chills, fever, prostration, and the presence of bacteria or their toxins in the bloodstream. The most severe types of septicemia are those caused by Gram-negative bacilli, owing to the endotoxin that is released from their cell walls. Endotoxin can induce fever and septic shock, which can be fatal. To diagnose either bacteremia or septicemia, it is recommended that at least three blood cultures be collected during a 24-hour period.

To prevent contamination of the blood specimen with indigenous skin flora, extreme care must be taken to use aseptic technique when collecting blood for culture. The person drawing the blood must wear sterile gloves, and gloves must be changed between patients.

FIGURE 13-2. Composition of whole blood. Following centrifugation, the layer of white blood cells and platelets—referred to as the buffy coat—lies above the red blood cells. (From Cohen BJ. Memmler's The Human Body in Health and Disease, 11th ed. Philadelphia: Lippincott Williams & Wilkins, 2009.)

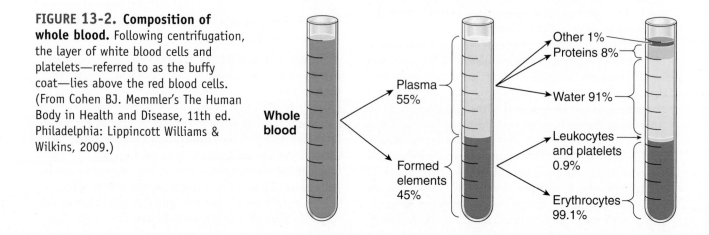

Whole blood

Plasma 55%

Formed elements 45%

Other 1%
Proteins 8%
Water 91%
Leukocytes and platelets 0.9%
Erythrocytes 99.1%

FIGURE 13-3. Proper method of preparing the venipuncture site when obtaining blood for culture. (From McCall RE, Tankersley CM. Phlebotomy Essentials, 4th ed. Philadelphia: Lippincott Williams & Wilkins, 2008.)

Blood for culture is usually obtained from a vein located at the antecubital fossa.[a] After locating a suitable vein, the skin at the site is disinfected with 70% isopropyl alcohol and then with an iodophor. (It should be noted that the protocol for skin disinfection varies from one medical facility to another. For example, some facilities use isopropyl alcohol or tincture of iodine alone; some use povidone-iodine or chlorhexidine alone; some use a combination of ethyl alcohol and povidone-iodine.) When disinfecting the site, a concentric swabbing motion is used, starting at the point at which the needle is to be inserted and working outward from that point (Fig. 13-3). The iodophor is then allowed to dry. A tourniquet is applied and the appropriate amount of blood is withdrawn. It is important not to touch the site after it has been disinfected.

---

[a] The antecubital fossa is located on the inner part of the arm, opposite the bend of the elbow. The major superficial veins in this area are referred to as antecubital veins.

Traditionally, blood has been injected into a pair of blood culture bottles (one aerobic bottle and one anaerobic bottle), but there are many different types of blood culture systems currently available (Fig. 13-4). The rubber tops of blood culture bottles must be disinfected prior to insertion of the needle. Then an appropriate volume of blood is injected; the amount will depend on the type of blood culture being used. Following the venipuncture procedure, the iodophor should be removed from the skin using alcohol. The blood culture bottle(s) should be transported promptly to the laboratory for incubation at 37°C. Blood culture bottles should not be refrigerated.

SPOTLIGHTING PHLEBOTOMISTS

As stated in the American Medical Association's Health Care Careers Directory, 2008–2009 (available at http://www.ama-assn.org), "Phlebotomists collect, transport, handle, and process blood specimens for analysis; identify and select equipment, supplies, and additives used in blood collection; and understand factors that affect specimen collection procedures and test results. Recognizing the importance of specimen collection in the overall patient care system, phlebotomists adhere to infection control and safety policies and procedures. They practice safe blood collection and handling techniques that protect patients

(continues)

FIGURE 13-4. Various types of blood culture systems. (A) BACTEC blood culture bottles (Courtesy of Becton Dickinson, Franklin Lakes, NJ). **(B)** BacT/Alert blood culture supplies (Courtesy of bioMerieux, Durham, NC. Both **[A]** and **[B]** are from McCall RE, Tankersley CM. Phlebotomy Essentials, 4th ed. Philadelphia: Lippincott Williams & Wilkins, 2008.)

from injury, safeguard themselves from accidents, and produce high-quality specimens while demonstrating compassion for the patient. Phlebotomists monitor quality control within predetermined limits while demonstrating professional conduct, stress management, and communication skills with patients, peers, and other healthcare personnel as well as with the public." Information concerning educational requirements and programs, certification, and salary is available at the AMA web site.

Urine

Urine is ordinarily sterile while it is in the urinary bladder. However, during urination, it becomes contaminated by indigenous microflora of the distal urethra (the portion of the urethra farthest from the bladder). Contamination can be reduced by collecting a *clean-catch, midstream urine* (CCMS urine). "Clean-catch" refers to the fact that the area around the external opening of the urethra is cleansed by washing with soap and rinsing with water before urinating. This removes the indigenous microflora that live in the area. "Midstream" refers to the fact that the initial portion of the urine stream is directed into a toilet or bedpan, and then the urine stream is directed into a sterile container. Thus, the microorganisms that live in the distal urethra are flushed out of the urethra by the initial portion of the urine stream, into the toilet or bedpan, rather than into the specimen container. In some circumstances, the clinician may prefer to collect a catheterized specimen or use the suprapubic needle aspiration technique to obtain a sterile sample of urine. In the latter technique, a needle is inserted through the abdominal wall into the urinary bladder, and a syringe is used to withdraw urine from the bladder. To prevent continued bacterial growth, all urine specimens must be processed within 30 minutes of collection, or refrigerated at 4°C until they can be analyzed. Refrigerated urine specimens should be cultured within 24 hours. Failure to refrigerate a urine specimen will cause an inflated colony count (described later), which could lead to an incorrect diagnosis of a urinary tract infection (UTI).

> The ideal specimen for a urine culture is a clean-catch, midstream urine specimen.

CLINICAL PROCEDURE
Collecting a Clean-Catch, MidStream Urine Specimen

Instructions for Female Patients

1. Sit comfortably on the toilet and swing one knee to the side as far as you can.
2. Spread your genital area with one hand and hold it spread open while you wash and rinse the area and collect the specimen.

3. Wash your genital area, using the cleaning materials supplied. Wipe yourself as carefully as you can from front to back, between the folds of skin.
4. After washing, rinse with a water-moistened pad with the same front-to-back motion. Use each pad only once, and then throw it away.
5. Hold the specimen collection cup with your fingers on the outside; do not touch the rim. Pass a small amount of urine into the toilet before passing urine into the cup. Fill the cup approximately half full.
6. Place the lid on the cup carefully and tightly, and give it to the nurse or laboratory assistant.

Instructions for Male Patients

1. Retract the foreskin (if uncircumcised).
2. Wash the glans (the head of the penis), using the cleaning materials supplied.
3. After washing, rinse with a water-moistened pad. Use each pad only once, and then throw it away.
4. Hold the specimen collection cup with your fingers on the outside; do not touch the rim. Pass a small amount of urine into the toilet before passing urine into the cup. Fill the cup approximately half full.
5. Place the lid on the cup carefully and tightly, and give it to the nurse or laboratory assistant.

There are actually three parts to a urine culture: (a) a colony count, (b) isolation and identification of the pathogen, and (c) antimicrobial susceptibility testing. The colony count is a way of estimating the number of viable bacteria that are present in the urine specimen. A calibrated loop is used to perform the colony count. A *calibrated loop* is a bacteriologic loop that has been manufactured so that it contains a precise volume of urine. There are two types of calibrated loops: those calibrated to contain 0.01 mL of fluid, and those calibrated to contain 0.001 mL of fluid. The calibrated loop is dipped into the CCMS urine specimen. Then the volume of urine within the calibrated loop is inoculated over the entire surface of a blood agar plate, which is then incubated overnight at 37°C (Fig. 13-5). After incubation, the colonies are counted and this number is then multiplied by the dilution factor (either 100 or 1,000) to obtain the number of colony-forming units (CFU) per milliliter of urine. (The dilution factor is 100 if a 0.01-mL calibrated loop was used, or 1,000 if a 0.001-mL calibrated loop was used.) **Example:** If the number of colonies is 300 and a 0.001-mL calibrated loop was used, then the colony count is $300 \times 1,000$ or 300,000 (3×10^5) CFU/mL.

A CFU count that is 100,000 (1×10^5) CFU/mL or higher is indicative of a UTI, although high colony counts may also be caused by contamination of the urine specimen with indigenous microflora during

> A complete urine culture consists of a colony count, isolation and identification of the pathogen, and antimicrobial susceptibility testing.

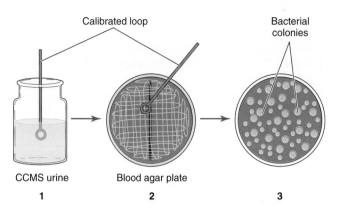

FIGURE 13-5. Obtaining a urine colony count.
(1) A calibrated loop is dipped into a clean-catch, mid-stream (CCMS) urine specimen. **(2)** The volume of urine contained within the calibrated loop is spread over the entire surface of a blood agar plate, which is then incubated overnight at 37°C. **(3)** The colonies are counted after the plate is removed from the incubator. (See text for additional details.)

specimen collection or failure to refrigerate the specimen between collection and transport to the laboratory. The mere presence of bacteria in the urine (*bacteriuria*) is not significant, as urine always becomes contaminated with bacteria during urination (voiding). However, the presence of two or more bacteria per × 1,000 microscopic field of a Gram-stained urine smear is indicative of a UTI with 100,000 or more CFU per milliliter.

Cerebrospinal Fluid

Meningitis, encephalitis, and meningoencephalitis are rapidly fatal diseases that can be caused by various microbes, including bacteria, fungi, protozoa, and viruses. *Meningitis* is inflammation or infection of the membranes (meninges) that surround the brain and spinal column. *Encephalitis* is inflammation or infection of the brain. *Meningoencephalitis* is inflammation or infection of both the brain and the meninges. To diagnose these diseases, *cerebrospinal fluid* (also referred to as spinal fluid or CSF) must be collected into a sterile tube by a lumbar puncture (spinal tap) under surgically aseptic conditions (Fig.13-6). This technically difficult procedure is performed by a physician. CSF specimens must be rushed to the laboratory and must not be refrigerated. Refrigeration might kill any fragile pathogens present in the specimen.

Because of the extremely serious nature of central nervous system (CNS) infections, the CSF will be treated as a STAT (emergency) specimen in the CML, and a workup of the specimen will be initiated immediately. Information obtained as a result of examining a Gram stain of the spinal fluid sediment will be reported by telephone to the clinician immediately; this is what is known as a *preliminary report*. Preliminary reports are laboratory reports that are communicated (usually by telephone) to the requesting clinician before the availability of the final report. Preliminary reports containing

> Cerebrospinal fluid specimens are treated as STAT (emergency) specimens in the CML, where workup of the specimens is initiated immediately upon receipt.

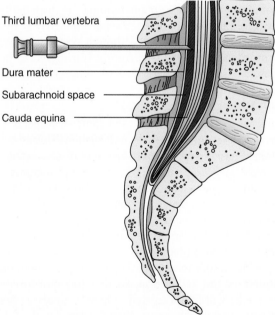

Third lumbar vertebra

Dura mater

Subarachnoid space

Cauda equina

FIGURE 13-6. Technique of lumbar puncture. (Taylor C, et al. Fundamentals of Nursing, 2nd ed. Philadelphia: JB Lippincott, 1993.)

CSF Gram stain observations frequently enable clinicians to make diagnoses and initiate therapy, and often save patients' lives.

Sputum

Sputum is pus that accumulates deep within the lungs of a patient with pneumonia, tuberculosis, or other lower respiratory infection. Laboratory workup of a good quality sputum specimen can provide important information about a patient's lower respiratory infection. Unfortunately, many of the sputum specimens that are submitted to the CML are actually saliva. A laboratory workup of a patient's saliva will not provide clinically relevant information about the patient's lower respiratory infection and will be a waste of time, effort, and money. This situation can be avoided if someone (most often, a nurse) takes a moment to explain to the patient what is required. (e.g., "The next time you cough up some of that thick, greenish material from your lungs, Mr. Smith, please spit it into this container.") If proper mouth hygiene is maintained, the sputum will not be severely contaminated with oral flora. If tuberculosis is suspected, extreme care in collecting and handling the specimen should be exercised because one could easily be infected with the pathogens. Usually, sputum specimens may be refrigerated for several hours without loss of the pathogens.

> Laboratory workup of a good quality sputum specimen can provide important information about a patient's lower respiratory infection, whereas workup of a patient's saliva cannot.

The clinician may wish to obtain a better quality specimen by bronchial aspiration through a bronchoscope or by a process known as transtracheal aspiration. Needle biopsy of the lungs may be necessary for diagnosis of *Pneumocystis jiroveci* pneumonia (as in patients with acquired immunodeficiency syndrome [AIDS] and for certain other pathogens). Although once classified as a protozoan, *P. jiroveci* is currently considered to be a fungus.

Throat Swabs

Routine throat swabs are collected to determine whether a patient has strep throat (*Streptococcus pyogenes* pharyngitis). If any other pathogen (e.g., *Neisseria gonorrhoeae* or *Corynebacterium diphtheriae*) is suspected by the clinician to be causing the patient's pharyngitis, a specific culture for that pathogen must be noted on the laboratory test requisition, so that the appropriate culture media will be inoculated. There is an art to the proper collection of a throat swab, as described in the following box.

> If a clinician suspects a pathogen other than *S. pyogenes* to be causing a patient's pharyngitis, that information must be included on the laboratory test requisition.

CLINICAL PROCEDURE
Proper Technique for Obtaining a Throat Swab Specimen

1. Using a tongue depressor to hold the patient's tongue down, observe the back of the throat and tonsillar area for localized areas of inflammation (redness) and exudate.
2. Remove a Dacron or calcium alginate swab from its packet.
3. Under direct observation, carefully but firmly rub the swab over any areas of inflammation or exudate or over the tonsils and posterior pharynx. Do not touch the cheeks, teeth, or gums with the swab as you withdraw it from the mouth.
4. Insert the swab back into its packet and crush the transport medium vial in the transport container.
5. Transport the swab to the laboratory as soon as possible. If transport will be delayed beyond 1 hour, refrigerate the swab.

Wound Specimens

Whenever possible, a wound specimen should be an aspirate (i.e., pus that has been collected using a small needle and syringe assembly), rather than a swab specimen. Specimens collected by swab are frequently contaminated with indigenous skin microflora and often dry out before they can be processed in the CML. The person collecting the specimen should always indicate the type of wound infection (e.g., dog bite, surgical site, or burn wound infection) on the laboratory test requisition and the anatomical site from which the specimen was obtained. This provides valuable information that will enable CML personnel to inoculate appropriate types of media and be on the lookout for specific organisms. For example, *Pasteurella multocida* is frequently isolated from dog bite wound infections, but this Gram-negative bacillus is rarely encountered in other types of specimens. Merely stating "wound" on the laboratory test requisition is insufficient.

> The laboratory test requisition that accompanies a wound specimen must indicate the type of wound and its anatomical location.

GC Cultures

The initials GC represent an abbreviation for *gonococci*, a term referring to *N. gonorrhoeae*. As mentioned earlier, *N. gonorrhoeae* is a fastidious bacterium that is microaerophilic and capnophilic. Only Dacron, calcium alginate, or nontoxic cotton swabs should be used to collect GC specimens. Ordinary cotton swabs contain fatty acids, which can be

> When attempting to culture *Neisseria gonorrhoeae*, one should remember that it is a fastidious, microaerophilic, and capnophilic organism.

FIGURE 13-7. Transgrow bottles used in gonococcal cultures. (Courtesy of Dr. A. Schroeter and the CDC.)

toxic to *N. gonorrhoeae*. When attempting to diagnose gonorrhea, swabs (vaginal, cervical, urethral, throat, and rectal) should be inoculated immediately onto Thayer-Martin or Martin-Lewis medium and incubated in a carbon dioxide (CO_2) environment. Alternatively, they should be inoculated into a tube or bottle (e.g., Transgrow) that contains an appropriate culture medium and an atmosphere containing 5% to 10% CO_2 (Fig. 13-7). To prevent loss of the CO_2, the bottle should be held in an upright position while inoculating. Otherwise, the CO_2 spills out and is displaced by room air. These cultures should be incubated at 37°C overnight and then shipped to a microbiology laboratory for positive identification of *N. gonorrhoeae*. If it is necessary to transport a swab specimen, the swab should be placed into a transport medium for shipment. Never refrigerate GC swabs because the low temperature might kill the *N. gonorrhoeae*.

Fecal Specimens

Ideally, fecal specimens (stool specimens) should be collected at the laboratory and processed immediately to prevent a decrease in temperature, which allows the pH to drop, causing the death of many *Shigella* and *Salmonella* species. Alternatively, the specimen may be placed in a container with a preservative that maintains a pH of 7.0.

Because the colon is anaerobic, fecal bacteria are obligate, aerotolerant, and facultative anaerobes. However, fecal specimens are cultured anaerobically only when *Clostridium difficile*-associated disease is suspected or to diagnose clostridial food poisoning. In gastrointestinal infections, the pathogens

> In gastrointestinal infections, the pathogens frequently overwhelm the indigenous intestinal microflora, so that they are the predominant organisms seen in smears and cultures.

frequently overwhelm the indigenous intestinal microflora, so that they are the predominant organisms seen in smears and cultures. A combination of direct microscopic examination, culture, biochemical tests, and immunologic tests may be performed to identify Gram-negative and Gram-positive bacteria (e.g., enteropathogenic *Escherichia coli*, *Salmonella* spp., *Shigella* spp., *Clostridium perfringens*, *C. difficile*, *Vibrio cholerae*, *Campylobacter* spp., and *Staphylococcus* spp.), fungi (*Candida*), intestinal protozoa (*Giardia*, *Entamoeba*), and intestinal helminths.

THE PATHOLOGY DEPARTMENT ("THE LAB")

The clinical specimens just described are submitted to the CML. Within a hospital setting, the CML is an integral part of the Pathology Department

> Within a hospital, the CML is an integral part of the Pathology Department.

(which is frequently referred to simply as "the lab"). Because virtually all healthcare personnel will interact in some way(s) with the Pathology Department, they should understand how it is organized and the types of laboratory tests that are performed there.

The Pathology Department is under the direction of a *pathologist* (a physician who has had extensive, specialized training in *pathology*—the study of the structural and functional manifestations of disease). As shown in Figure 13-8, the Pathology Department consists of two major divisions: Anatomical Pathology and Clinical Pathology.

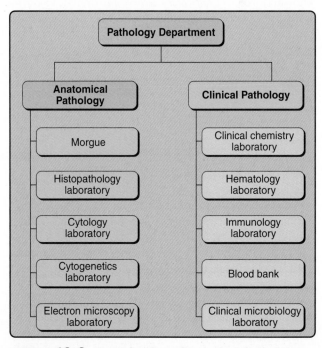

FIGURE 13-8. Organization of a typical Pathology Department.

Anatomical Pathology

Most pathologists work in Anatomical Pathology, where they perform autopsies in the morgue and examine diseased organs, stained tissue sections, and cytology specimens. Other healthcare professionals employed in Anatomical Pathology include cytogenetic technologists, cytotechnologists, histologic technicians, histotechnologists, and pathologist's assistants.

In addition to the morgue, Anatomical Pathology houses the Histopathology Laboratory, the Cytology Laboratory, and the Cytogenetics Laboratory. In some Pathology Departments, the Electron Microscopy Laboratory is also located in Anatomical Pathology.

Clinical Pathology

In addition to the CML, Clinical Pathology consists of several other laboratories: the Clinical Chemistry Laboratory (or Clinical Chemistry/Urinalysis Laboratory), the Hematology Laboratory (or Hematology/Coagulation Laboratory), the Blood Bank (or Immunohematology Laboratory), and the Immunology Laboratory (described in Chapter 16). In smaller hospitals, immunodiagnostic procedures are performed in the Immunology Section (or Serology Section) of the CML.

> The CML is located in the Clinical Pathology division of the Pathology Department.

Personnel working in Clinical Pathology include pathologists; specialized scientists such as chemists and microbiologists, who have graduate degrees in their specialty areas; **clinical laboratory scientists** (also known as *medical technologists* or MTs), who have 4-year baccalaureate degrees; and **clinical laboratory technicians** (also known as *medical laboratory technicians* or MLTs), who have 2-year associate degrees.

SPOTLIGHTING MEDICAL LABORATORY PROFESSIONALS

Medical laboratory professionals are important members of the highly skilled medical team who work together to collect clinical data and diagnose diseases. Medical laboratory professionals include pathologists, clinical laboratory scientists (CLSs; also known as medical technologists, MTs), clinical laboratory technicians (CLTs; also known as medical laboratory technicians, MLTs), histologic technicians, cytotechnologists, blood bank technologists, phlebotomy technicians, pathologist assistants, and cytogeneticists. Practice settings for these professionals include hospital laboratories; clinics; nursing homes; city, state, and federal public health facilities (e.g., the Centers for Disease Control and Prevention [CDC]); molecular diagnostic and biotechnology laboratories; research laboratories; educational institutions; and commercial companies (e.g., pharmaceutical companies and food service industries).

Clinical laboratory scientists (CLSs or MTs) and clinical laboratory technicians (CLTs or MLTs) work in all areas of the clinical laboratory, including blood bank, chemistry, hematology, immunology, urinalysis, and microbiology. They perform a wide variety of laboratory tests used in the detection, diagnosis, and treatment of many diseases. CLSs have many responsibilities and are held accountable for accurate and reliable test results.

Education and training in Clinical Laboratory Science not only prepare the individual for a rewarding career in the profession, but also serve as a foundation for jobs in other fields (e.g., medicine, medical research, forensics, biotechnology). Individuals interested in pursuing a career in Clinical Laboratory Science should have a strong background in the high school and college sciences (i.e., biology and chemistry), as well as math and computer science.

There are two levels of Clinical Laboratory Science training available. The minimum formal education requirements for a CLT are a 2-year associate degree and completion of an accredited CLT program. CLTs perform routine tests in all areas of the laboratory under the supervision of a CLS. The CLS requires a 4-year baccalaureate degree and clinical experience in an accredited Clinical Laboratory Science program. CLSs are able to correlate results with disease states, establish and monitor quality control, and operate complex electronic equipment and computers. CLSs must be able to work in stressful situations and they must be reliable, self-sufficient, precise, and thorough. Clinical education programs for CLSs may be located in hospitals or university settings and include instruction in microbiology, chemistry, hematology, immunology, blood banking, virology, phlebotomy, urinalysis, management, and education. To ensure competency, graduates of both CLS and CLT clinical education programs must be certified by one or both of the two national credentialing agencies: the American Society for Clinical Pathology (ASCP), or the National Credentialing Agency (NCA). Additional information concerning these professions, including educational programs, certification, and salaries can be found at the following web sites:

- American Medical Association (http://www.ama-assn.org)
- American Society for Clinical Laboratory Science (http://www.ascls.org)
- American Society for Clinical Pathology (http://www.ascp.org)
- National Accrediting Agency for Clinical Laboratory Sciences (http://www.naacls.org)
- National Credentialing Agency (http://www.nca-info.org)

THE CLINICAL MICROBIOLOGY LABORATORY

Organization

Depending on the size of the hospital, the CML may be under the direction of a pathologist, a microbiologist (having either a master or doctor of clinical microbiology degree), or, in smaller hospitals, a medical technologist who has had many years of experience working in microbiology. Most of the actual bench work that is performed in the CML is performed by CLSs and CLTs.

As shown in Figure 13-9, the CML is divided into various sections, which, to a large degree, correspond to the various categories of microbes. With the exception of the Immunology Section, the responsibilities of the specific sections of the CML are described in this chapter. Procedures performed in the Immunology Section are described in Chapter 16.

Responsibilities

The primary mission of the CML is to assist clinicians in the diagnosis and treatment of infectious diseases. To accomplish this mission, the four major, day-to-day responsibilities of the CML are to:

1. Process the various clinical specimens that are submitted to the CML (described later)
2. Isolate pathogens from those specimens
3. Identify (speciate) the pathogens
4. Perform antimicrobial susceptibility testing when appropriate to do so

The exact steps in the processing of clinical specimens vary from one specimen type to another and also depend on the specific section of the CML to which the specimen is submitted. In general, processing includes the following steps:

- Examining the specimen macroscopically and recording pertinent observations (e.g., cloudiness or the presence of blood, mucus, or an unusual odor)
- Examining the specimen microscopically and recording pertinent observations (e.g., the presence of white blood cells or microorganisms)
- Inoculating the specimen to appropriate culture media in an attempt to isolate the pathogen(s) from the specimen and get them growing in pure culture in the laboratory

The four major responsibilities of the CML are to (a) process clinical specimens, (b) isolate pathogens, (c) identify (speciate) pathogens, and (d) perform antimicrobial susceptibility testing when appropriate to do so.

In general, the processing of clinical specimens in the CML includes (a) examining the specimen macroscopically, (b) examining the specimen microscopically, and (c) inoculating the specimen to appropriate culture media.

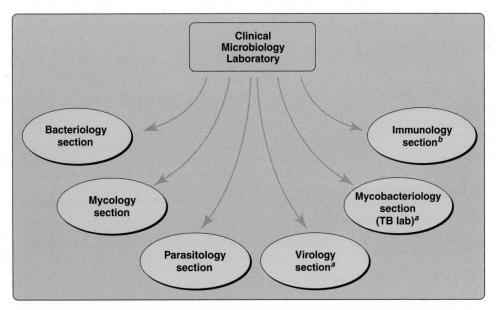

FIGURE 13-9. Organization of a typical Clinical Microbiology Laboratory.
[a]Virology and Mycobacteriology Sections are usually found only in larger hospitals and medical centers. Lacking these sections, most of the smaller hospitals would instead send virology and mycobacteriology specimens to a reference laboratory. [b]Only smaller hospitals would have Immunology Sections, where some immunodiagnostic procedures would be performed. Larger hospitals and medical centers would have an Immunology Laboratory, which would perform a much wider variety of immunologic procedures and would operate independently of the CML.

SOMETHING TO THINK ABOUT

Although the results of some laboratory procedures (such as certain of the automated procedures performed in the Chemistry Section) are often available within hours after arrival of the specimens in the laboratory, such is usually *not* the case with CML procedures. CML procedures frequently require a pure culture of the suspected pathogen, which often takes a minimum of 24 hours to obtain. Once a pure culture is available, an additional 24 hours or more are often required to obtain a species identification and antimicrobial susceptibility test results. **Therefore, individuals who submit specimens to the CML should expect a 1- or 2-day delay between submission of the specimens and receipt of CML results.** Fortunately, certain of the newer techniques (such as molecular and immunodiagnostic procedures) do provide same day results.

The CML is sometimes called on to assume an additional responsibility, namely the processing of environmental samples (i.e., samples collected from within the hospital environment). Such samples are processed by the CML whenever there is an outbreak or epidemic within the hospital, in an attempt to locate the source of the pathogen involved. Environmental samples include those collected from appropriate hospital sites (e.g., floors, sink drains, showerheads, whirlpool baths, respiratory therapy equipment) and employees (e.g., nasal swabs, material from open wounds).

> A less frequent responsibility of the CML is to process environmental samples whenever there is an outbreak or epidemic within the hospital.

Frequently, CML personnel are the first people to recognize that an outbreak is occurring within the hospital. For example, CML personnel might note an unusually high number of isolates of a particular pathogen from specimens submitted from a particular ward. The CML would notify the Hospital Infection Control Committee (described in Chapter 12) of the unusually high number of isolates, and the committee would then be responsible for collecting appropriate environmental samples and submitting them to the CML for processing.

Isolation and Identification (Speciation) of Pathogens

In an effort to isolate bacteria (including mycobacteria) and fungi (yeasts and moulds) from clinical specimens, the specimens are inoculated into liquid culture media or onto solid culture media. The goal is to get any pathogens that are present

> To isolate bacteria and fungi from clinical specimens, specimens are inoculated into liquid culture media or onto solid culture media.

in the specimen growing in pure culture (by themselves), and in large number, so that there will be a sufficient quantity of the organism to inoculate appropriate identification and antimicrobial susceptibility testing systems. Specific types of media were discussed in Chapter 8. The manner in which pathogens are identified depends on the particular section of the CML to which that the specimen was submitted. (Note: As previously mentioned, throughout this book, the term "to identify an organism" means to learn the organism's name; i.e., to speciate it.)

Bacteriology Section

The overall responsibility of the Bacteriology Section of the CML is to assist clinicians in the diagnosis of bacterial diseases. In the Bacteriology Section, various types of clinical specimens are processed, bacterial pathogens are isolated from the specimens, tests are performed to identify the bacterial pathogens, and antimicrobial susceptibility testing is performed whenever it is appropriate to do so (Fig. 13-10). Once they are isolated from clinical specimens,

> The overall responsibility of the Bacteriology Section of the CML is to assist clinicians in the diagnosis of bacterial diseases.

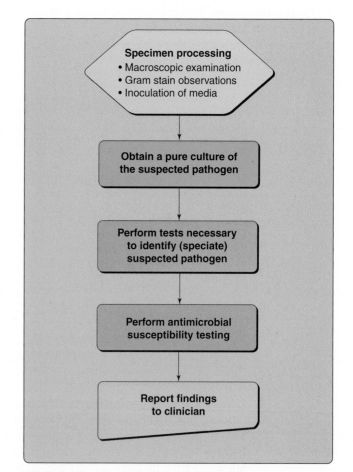

FIGURE 13-10. Flowchart illustrating the sequence of events that occur within the Bacteriology Section of the Clinical Microbiology Laboratory.

FIGURE 13-11. Clinical Microbiology Laboratory professionals are very much like detectives and crime scene investigators. They gather "clues" about a pathogen until they have enough information to identify (speciate) the culprit.

bacterial pathogens are identified by gathering clues (phenotypic characteristics). Thus, CML professionals are very much like detectives and crime scene investigators (Fig. 13-11), gathering "clues" about a pathogen until they are have sufficient clues to identify it.

The various phenotypic characteristics (clues) useful in identifying bacteria include the following:

> CML professionals gather "clues" (phenotypic characteristics) about a pathogen until they have sufficient information to identify (speciate) it.

- Gram reaction (i.e., Gram-positive or Gram-negative)
- Cell shape (e.g., cocci, bacilli, curved, spiral-shaped, filamentous, branching)
- Morphologic arrangement of cells (e.g., pairs, tetrads, chains, clusters)
- Growth or no growth on various types of plated media
- Colony morphology (e.g., color, general shape, elevation, margin)
- Presence or absence of a capsule
- Motility
- Number and location of flagella
- Ability to sporulate
- Location of spores (terminal or subterminal)
- Presence or absence of various enzymes (e.g., catalase, coagulase, oxidase, urease)
- Ability to catabolize various carbohydrates and amino acids (miniaturized biochemical test systems—"minisystems"—are often used for this purpose; see Fig. 13-12)
- Ability to reduce nitrate
- Ability to produce indole from tryptophan
- Atmospheric requirements
- Type of hemolysis produced (Fig. 13-13)

Mycology Section

The overall responsibility of the Mycology Section of the CML is to assist clinicians in the diagnosis of fungal infections (mycoses). In the Mycology Section, various types of clinical specimens are processed, fungal

> The overall responsibility of the Mycology Section of the CML is to assist clinicians in the diagnosis of fungal infections (mycoses).

FIGURE 13-12. An example of a minisystem (API-20E). These three API 20E strips were inoculated with suspensions of three different members of the family Enterobacteriaceae. After 18 to 20 hours of incubation, the colors in the compartments are interpreted as either positive or negative results. Based on the positive and negative reactions, a seven-digit biotype number is calculated. In most cases, the number is specific for a particular bacterial species. (From Winn WC Jr, et al. Koneman's Color Atlas and Textbook of Diagnostic Microbiology, 6th ed. Philadelphia: Lippincott Williams & Wilkins, 2006.)

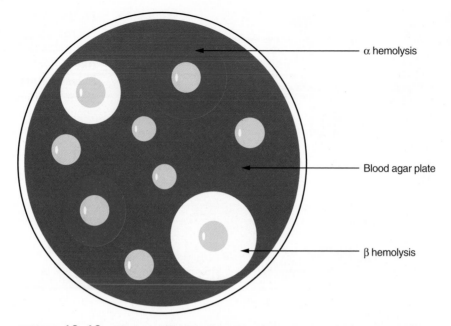

FIGURE 13-13. Diagram illustrating the three types of hemolysis that can be observed on a blood agar plate. Alpha-hemolysis is a green zone around the bacterial colony. Alpha-hemolytic bacteria produce an enzyme that causes a partial breakdown of hemoglobin in the red blood cells in the medium, resulting in a green color. Beta-hemolysis is a clear zone around the bacterial colony. Beta-hemolytic bacteria produce an enzyme that completely destroys (lyses) the red blood cells, thus producing a clear zone. Gamma-hemolysis is no hemolysis at all (neither a green nor a clear zone around the bacterial colony). Gamma-hemolytic bacteria (also referred to as nonhemolytic bacteria) produce neither of these enzymes and, therefore, cause no change in the red blood cells.

pathogens are isolated, and tests are performed to identify the fungal pathogens. In general, the specimens processed in the Mycology Section are the same types of specimens that are processed in the Bacteriology Section. However, three types are specimens are much more commonly submitted to the Mycology Section than to the Bacteriology Section: hair clippings, nail clippings, and skin scrapings.

A potassium hydroxide preparation (KOH prep) is performed on hair clippings, nail clippings, and skin scrapings. (See CD-ROM Appendix 4 for details of the KOH preparation.) The KOH acts as a clearing agent by dissolving keratin in the specimens. This enables the technologist to see into the specimens when they are examined microscopically, and to determine whether any fungal elements (e.g., yeasts or hyphae) are present in the specimen (Fig. 13-14).

Specimens will also be inoculated onto Sabouraud dextrose agar, a selective medium for fungi. Bacteria do not grow on this medium because of the low pH (pH 5.6), but most fungi grow quite well.

When isolated from clinical specimens, yeasts are identified by using various biochemical tests, primarily by their ability to catabolize various carbohydrates. Moulds are identified using a combination of rate of growth and macroscopic and microscopic observations, *not* by performing biochemical tests. Macroscopic observations are things that you can learn about the mycelium by looking at it with the naked eye—like color, texture, and topography (see Figs. 13-15 and 13-16).

To examine a mould microscopically, a tease mount is prepared. A drop of stain is placed on a glass microscope slide. A small piece of the mycelium is placed into the drop. Teasing needles (also known as dissecting needles) are used to gently pull (tease) the piece of mycelium apart, enabling the CML professional to see various identifying characteristics of the mould. A glass coverslip is added, and the tease mount preparation is examined under the microscope. The stain that is used in the tease mount is lactophenol cotton blue (LPCB), containing lactic acid, phenol, and cotton blue. The lactic acid preserves morphol-

When isolated from clinical specimens, yeasts are identified using various biochemical tests, primarily based on their ability to catabolize various carbohydrates.

When isolated from clinical specimens, moulds are identified using a combination of rate of growth and macroscopic and microscopic observations.

FIGURE 13-14. Fungal hyphae (arrows) in a KOH preparation of skin scrapings from a patient with tinea corporis. (Schaechter M, et al., eds.). Mechanisms of Microbial Disease, 3rd ed. Philadelphia, Lippincott Williams & Wilkins, 1999.)

ogy. The phenol kills the organisms, so they will not be infectious. The cotton blue stains the mycelial structures blue.

When the tease mount preparation is examined microscopically, the first thing to determine is whether

FIGURE 13-15. A colony (mycelium) of an Aspergillus species. Moulds in the genus Aspergillus can cause sinusitis, lower respiratory infections, and infections of the eyes, heart, kidneys, skin, and other organs, most commonly in immunosuppressed patients. (From Winn WC Jr, et al. Koneman's Color Atlas and Textbook of Diagnostic Microbiology, 6th ed. Philadelphia: Lippincott Williams & Wilkins, 2006.)

FIGURE 13-16. Colonies (mycelia) of a Penicillium species. Although penicillin is derived from Penicillium, various species in this genus can also cause lung, liver, and skin infections in immunosuppressed patients. (From Winn WC Jr, et al. Koneman's Color Atlas and Textbook of Diagnostic Microbiology, 6th ed. Philadelphia: Lippincott Williams & Wilkins, 2006.)

the mould has septate or aseptate hyphae (described in Chapter 5). Next, the technologist will look for spores and the structures on or within which the spores are produced. The appearance of these structures further enables the technologist to identify the mould (refer back to Fig. 5-6 in Chapter 5).

Susceptibility testing of fungi is not currently performed in most CMLs; however, because of the ever-growing problem of drug resistance in fungi, it is likely that such testing will become routine in the near future.

Parasitology Section

The overall responsibility of the Parasitology Section of the CML is to assist clinicians in the diagnosis of parasitic diseases—specifically, infections caused by endoparasites (parasites that live within the body), such as parasitic protozoa and helminths (parasitic worms). In general, parasitic infections are diagnosed by observing and recognizing various parasite life cycle stages (e.g., trophozoites and cysts of protozoa; microfilariae, eggs, and larvae of helminths) in clinical specimens. Parasites are identified primarily by the characteristic appearance (e.g., size, shape, internal details) of the various life cycle stages that are seen in clinical specimens. Sometimes, whole worms or segments of worms are observed in fecal specimens. Parasites are described in detail in Chapter 21.

Virology Section

The overall responsibility of the Virology Section of the CML is to assist clinicians in the diagnosis of viral diseases. Many viral diseases are diagnosed using immunodiagnostic procedures (described in Chapter 16). Other techniques used to identify viral pathogens are:

> The overall responsibility of the Virology Section of the CML is to assist clinicians in the diagnosis of viral diseases.

- Observation of intracytoplasmic or intranuclear viral inclusion bodies in specimens by cytologic or histologic examination
- Observation of viruses in specimens using electron microscopy
- Molecular techniques such as nucleic acid probes and polymerase chain reaction assays (described on the CD-ROM)
- Virus isolation by use of cell cultures; viruses are identified primarily by the type(s) of cell lines that they are able to infect and the physical changes (called cytopathic effect or CPE) that they cause in the infected cells (Fig. 13-17.)

FIGURE 13-17. Cytopathic effect (CPE).
(A) Normal appearance of human diploid fibroblasts.
(B) The appearance of the same cells, 48 hours after being inoculated with herpes simplex type 2 virus.
(From Engleberg NC, et al. Schaechter's Mechanisms of Microbial Disease, 4th ed. Philadelphia: Lippincott Williams & Wilkins, 2007.)

Mycobacteriology Section

The primary responsibility of the Mycobacteriology Section (or "TB Lab," as it is often called) of the CML is to assist clinicians in the diagnosis of tuberculosis. In the Mycobacteriology Section, various types of specimens (primarily sputum specimens) are processed, acid-fast staining is performed, mycobacteria are isolated and identified, and susceptibility testing is performed. *Mycobacterium* spp. are identified using a combination of growth characteristics (e.g., growth rate, colony pigmentation, photoreactivity, and morphology) and various biochemical tests. *Mycobacterium tuberculosis*, the primary cause of human tuberculosis, is a very slow-growing organism. Fortunately, the acid-fast stain (described in Chapter 4) enables rapid presumptive diagnosis of tuberculosis.

> The primary responsibility of the Mycobacteriology Section ("TB Lab") of the CML is to assist clinicians in the diagnosis of tuberculosis.

Additional information pertaining to the CML, including molecular diagnostic procedures, antimicrobial susceptibility testing, quality assurance and quality control in the CML, and safety in the CML, can be found in CD-ROM Appendix 3: "Responsibilities of the Clinical Microbiology Laboratory."

> **ON THE CD-ROM**
> - Terms Introduced in This Chapter
> - Review of Key Points
> - Insight
>   - Specimen Quality and Clinical Relevance
> - Increase Your Knowledge
> - Critical Thinking
> - Additional Self-Assessment Exercises

SELF-ASSESSMENT EXERCISES

After studying this chapter, answer the following multiple-choice questions.

1. Assuming that a clean-catch, midstream urine was processed in the CML, which of the following colony counts is (are) indicative of a urinary tract infection?
   a. 10,000 CFU/mL
   b. 100,000 CFU/mL
   c. >100,000 CFU/mL
   d. both b and c
2. Which of the following statements about blood is false?
   a. As it circulates throughout the human body, blood is usually sterile.
   b. Following centrifugation, the layer of leukocytes and platelets is referred to as the buffy coat.
   c. Bacteremia and septicemia are synonyms.
   d. Plasma constitutes about 55% of whole blood.

3. Which of the following statements about cerebrospinal fluid (CSF) specimens is false?
   a. They are collected only by clinicians.
   b. They are treated as STAT (emergency) specimens in the laboratory.
   c. They should always be refrigerated.
   d. They should be rushed to the laboratory after collection.

4. All clinical specimens submitted to the CML must be:
   a. properly and carefully collected.
   b. properly labeled.
   c. properly transported to the laboratory.
   d. all of the above

5. Which of the following is *not* one of the three parts of a urine culture?
   a. isolation and identification of the pathogen
   b. performing a colony count
   c. performing a microscopic observation of the urine specimen
   d. performing antimicrobial susceptibility testing

6. Which of the following matches is false?
   a. CPE . . . Virology Section
   b. KOH preparation . . . Mycology Section
   c. Tease mount . . . Bacteriology Section
   d. Type of hemolysis . . . Bacteriology Section

7. Who is primarily responsible for the quality of specimens submitted to the CML?
   a. microbiologist who is in charge of the CML
   b. pathologist who is in charge of "the lab"
   c. person who collects the specimen
   d. person who transports the specimen to the CML

8. Which of the following is *not* one of the four major day-to-day responsibilities of the CML?
   a. identify (speciate) pathogens
   b. isolate pathogens from clinical specimens
   c. perform antimicrobial susceptibility testing when appropriate
   d. process environmental samples

9. Which of the following sections is *least* likely to be found in the CML of a small hospital?
   a. Bacteriology Section
   b. Mycology Section
   c. Parasitology Section
   d. Virology Section

10. In the Mycology Section of the CML, moulds are identified by _____.
   a. biochemical test results
   b. macroscopic observations
   c. microscopic observations
   d. a combination of b and c

14 PATHOGENESIS OF INFECTIOUS DISEASES

LEARNING OBJECTIVES

AFTER STUDYING THIS CHAPTER, YOU SHOULD BE ABLE TO:

- Cite four reasons why an individual might not develop an infectious disease after exposure to a pathogen
- Discuss the four periods or phases in the course of an infectious disease
- Differentiate between localized and systemic infections
- Explain how acute diseases differ from subacute and chronic diseases
- Differentiate between "symptoms" of a disease and "signs" of a disease and cite several examples of each
- Cite several examples of latent infections
- Differentiate between primary and secondary infections
- List six steps in the pathogenesis of an infectious disease
- Define virulence and virulence factors
- List three bacterial structures that serve as virulence factors
- List six bacterial exoenzymes that serve as virulence factors
- Differentiate between endotoxins and exotoxins
- List six bacterial exotoxins and the diseases they cause

- Describe three mechanisms by which pathogens escape the immune response

INTRODUCTION

By definition, microbes are too small to be seen with the unaided eye. How is it possible for such tiny organisms and infectious particles to cause disease in plants and animals, which are gigantic in comparison to microbes? This chapter will attempt to answer that question, with emphasis on disease in humans.

The prefix *path-* comes from the Greek word "pathos," meaning disease. Examples of words containing this prefix are *pathogen* (a microbe capable of causing disease), *pathology* (the study of the structural and functional manifestations of disease), *pathologist* (a physician who has specialized in pathology), *pathogenicity* (the ability to cause disease), and *pathogenesis* (the steps or mechanisms involved in the development of a disease).

Words containing the prefix "path-" or "patho-" pertain to disease.

INFECTION VERSUS INFECTIOUS DISEASE

As discussed previously in this book, an infectious disease is a disease caused by a microbe, and the microbes that cause infectious diseases are collectively | In general usage, the terms *infection* and *infectious disease* are synonyms. |

referred to as pathogens. The word *infection* tends to be confusing because the term is used in different ways. Most commonly, infection is used as a synonym for infectious disease. For example, saying that "the patient has an ear infection" is the same thing as saying that "the patient has an infectious disease of the ear." Because this is how the word infection is used by physicians, nurses, other healthcare professionals, the mass media, and most other people, this is how infection is used in this book.

Many microbiologists, however, reserve use of the word infection to mean colonization by a pathogen (i.e., when a pathogen lands on or enters a person's body and establishes residence there, then the person is infected with that pathogen). That pathogen may or may not go on to cause disease in the person. In other words, it is possible for a person to be infected with a certain pathogen, but *not* have the infectious disease caused by that pathogen (recall the discussion of carriers in Chapter 11).

WHY INFECTION DOES NOT ALWAYS OCCUR

Many people who are exposed to pathogens do not get sick. Listed here are some possible explanations: | Many factors influence whether or not exposure to a pathogen results in disease, including a person's immune, nutritional, and overall health status. |

- The microbe may land at an anatomic site where it is unable to multiply. For example, when a respiratory pathogen lands on the skin, it may be unable to grow there because the skin lacks the necessary warmth, moisture, and nutrients required for growth of that particular microbe. Additionally, the low pH and presence of fatty acids make the skin a hostile environment for certain organisms.
- Many pathogens must attach to specific receptor sites (described later) before they are able to multiply and cause damage. If they land at a site where such receptors are absent, they are unable to cause disease.
- Antibacterial factors that destroy or inhibit the growth of bacteria (e.g., the lysozyme that is present in tears, saliva, and perspiration) may be present at the site where a pathogen lands.
- The indigenous microflora of that site (e.g., mouth, vagina, intestine) may inhibit growth of the foreign microbe by occupying space and using up available nutrients. This is a type of *microbial antagonism*, in which one microbe or group of microbes wards off another.
- The indigenous microflora at the site may produce antibacterial factors (proteins called **bacteriocins**) that destroy the newly arrived pathogen. This is also a type of microbial antagonism.
- The individual's nutritional and overall health status often influences the outcome of the pathogen–host encounter. A person who is in good health, with no underlying medical problems, would be less likely to become infected than a person who is malnourished or in poor health.
- The person may be immune to that particular pathogen, perhaps as a result of prior infection with that pathogen or having been vaccinated against that pathogen. Immunity and vaccination are discussed in Chapter 16.
- Phagocytic white blood cells (phagocytes) present in the blood and other tissues may engulf and destroy the pathogen before it has an opportunity to multiply, invade, and cause disease. Phagocytosis is discussed in Chapter 15.

FOUR PERIODS OR PHASES IN THE COURSE OF AN INFECTIOUS DISEASE

Once a pathogen has gained entrance to the body, the course of an infectious disease has four periods or phases (Fig. 14-1): | The four periods or phases of an infectious disease are the (a) incubation period, (b) prodromal period, (c) period of illness, and (d) convalescent period. |

1. **The incubation period** is the time that elapses between arrival of the pathogen and the onset of symptoms. The length of the incubation period is influenced by many factors, including the overall health and nutritional status of the host, the immune status of the host (i.e., whether the host is immunocompetent or immunosuppressed), the virulence of the pathogen, and the number of pathogens that enter the body.
2. **The prodromal period** is the time during which the patient feels "out of sorts" but is not yet experiencing actual symptoms of the disease. Patients may feel like they are "coming down with something" but are not yet sure what it is.
3. **The period of illness** is the time during which the patient experiences the typical symptoms associated with that particular disease (e.g., sore throat, headache, sinus congestion). Communicable diseases are most easily transmitted during this third period.
4. **The convalescent period** is the time during which the patient recovers. For certain infectious diseases, especially viral respiratory diseases, the convalescent period can be quite long. Although the patient may recover from the illness itself, permanent damage may be

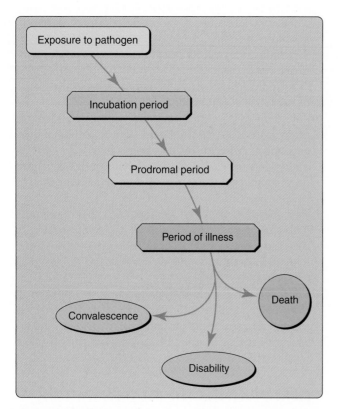

FIGURE 14-1. Periods in the course of an infectious disease.

caused by destruction of tissues in the affected area. For example, brain damage may follow encephalitis or meningitis, paralysis may follow poliomyelitis, and deafness may follow ear infections.

LOCALIZED VERSUS SYSTEMIC INFECTIONS

Once an infectious process is initiated, the disease may remain localized to one site or it may spread. Pimples, boils, and abscesses are examples of **localized infections**. If the pathogens are not contained at the original site of infection, they may be carried to other parts of the body by way of lymph, blood, or, in some cases, phagocytes. When the infection has spread throughout the body, it is referred to as either a **systemic infection** or a *generalized infection*. For example, the bacterium that causes tuberculosis—*Mycobacterium tuberculosis*—may spread to many internal organs, a condition known as miliary (disseminated) tuberculosis.

> An infection may remain localized or it may spread, becoming a systemic or generalized infection.

ACUTE, SUBACUTE, AND CHRONIC DISEASES

A disease may be described as being acute, subacute, or chronic. An **acute disease** has a rapid onset, usually followed by a relatively rapid recovery; measles, mumps, and influenza are examples. A **chronic disease** has an insidious (slow) onset and lasts a long time; examples are tuberculosis, leprosy (Hansen disease), and syphilis. Sometimes, a disease having a sudden onset can develop into a long-lasting disease. Some diseases, such as bacterial endocarditis, come on more suddenly than a chronic disease, but less suddenly than an acute disease; they are referred to as **subacute diseases**. An example of a subacute disease is subacute bacterial endocarditis, often referred to merely as SBE.

> A disease may be acute, subacute, or chronic, depending on the length of its incubation period and duration.

SYMPTOMS OF A DISEASE VERSUS SIGNS OF A DISEASE

A **symptom of a disease** is defined as some evidence of a disease that is experienced or perceived by the patient; something that is subjective. Examples of symptoms include any type of ache or pain, a ringing in the ears (tinnitus), blurred vision, nausea, dizziness, itching, and chills. Diseases, including infectious diseases, may be either symptomatic or asymptomatic. A **symptomatic disease** (or clinical disease) is a disease in which the patient is experiencing symptoms. An **asymptomatic disease** (or subclinical disease) is a disease that the patient is unaware of because he or she is not experiencing any symptoms.

> Symptoms of a disease are subjective, in that they are perceived by the patient.

In its early stages, gonorrhea (caused by the bacterium, *Neisseria gonorrhoeae*) is usually symptomatic in male patients (who develop a urethral discharge and experience pain while urinating), but asymptomatic in female patients. Only after several months, during which the organism may have caused extensive damage to her reproductive organs, is pain experienced by the infected woman. In trichomoniasis (caused by the protozoan, *Trichomonas vaginalis*), the situation is reversed. Infected women are usually symptomatic (experiencing vaginitis), whereas infected men are usually asymptomatic. These two sexually transmitted diseases are especially difficult to control because people are often unaware that they are infected and unknowingly transmit the pathogens to others during sexual activities.

A **sign of a disease** is defined as some type of objective evidence of a disease. For example, while palpating a patient, a physician might discover a lump or an enlarged liver (hepatomegaly) or spleen (splenomegaly). Other signs of disease include abnormal heart or breath sounds, blood pressure, pulse rate, and laboratory results as well as abnormalities that appear on radiographs, ultrasound studies, or computed tomography (CT) scans.

> Signs of a disease are objective findings, such as laboratory test results, which are not perceived by the patient.

LATENT INFECTIONS

An infectious disease may go from being symptomatic to asymptomatic and then, some time later, go back to being symptomatic. Such diseases are referred to as **latent infections**, from the Greek word "latens," meaning to lie hidden. Herpes virus infections, such as cold sores (fever blisters), genital herpes infections, and shingles, are examples of latent infections. Cold sores occur intermittently, but the patient continues to harbor the herpes virus between cold sore episodes (Fig. 14-2). The virus remains dormant within cells of the nervous system until some type of stress acts as a trigger. The stressful trigger may be a fever, sunburn, extreme cold, or emotional stress. A person who had chickenpox as a child may harbor the virus throughout his or her lifetime and then, later in life, as the immune system weakens, that person may develop shingles. Shingles, a painful infection of the nerves, is considered a latent manifestation of chickenpox.

> A latent disease is a disease that is lying dormant, not currently manifesting itself.

If not successfully treated, syphilis progresses through primary, secondary, latent, and tertiary stages (Fig. 14-3). During the primary stage, the patient has an open lesion called a chancre, which contains the spirochete *Treponema pallidum* (Fig. 14-4). Four to six weeks after the spirochete enters the bloodstream, the chancre disappears, and the symptoms of the secondary stage arise, including rash, fever, and mucous membrane lesions. These symptoms disappear within weeks to 12 months, and the disease enters a latent stage, which may last for weeks to years (sometimes for a lifetime). During the latent stage, the patient has few or no symptoms. In tertiary syphilis, the spirochetes cause destruction of the organs in which they have been

> If not successfully treated, syphilis can progress through several stages, including a latent stage.

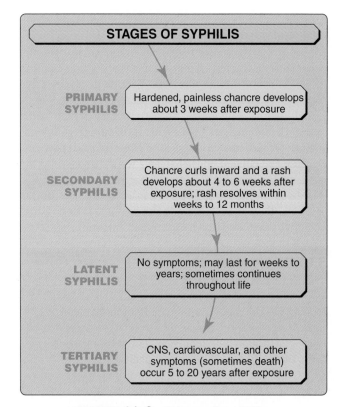

STAGES OF SYPHILIS

PRIMARY SYPHILIS — Hardened, painless chancre develops about 3 weeks after exposure

SECONDARY SYPHILIS — Chancre curls inward and a rash develops about 4 to 6 weeks after exposure; rash resolves within weeks to 12 months

LATENT SYPHILIS — No symptoms; may last for weeks to years; sometimes continues throughout life

TERTIARY SYPHILIS — CNS, cardiovascular, and other symptoms (sometimes death) occur 5 to 20 years after exposure

FIGURE 14-3. Stages of syphilis.

hiding—the brain, heart, and bone tissue—sometimes leading to death.

PRIMARY VERSUS SECONDARY INFECTIONS

One infectious disease may commonly follow another, in which case the first disease is referred to as a **primary infection** and the second disease is referred to as a **secondary infection**. For example, serious

> A primary infection caused by one pathogen can be followed by a secondary infection caused by a different pathogen.

FIGURE 14-2. Cold sore caused by herpes simplex virus. (Courtesy of Dr. Hermann and the Centers for Disease Control and Prevention [CDC].)

FIGURE 14-4. Syphilis chancre on penile shaft. (Courtesy of Dr. Gavin Hart, Dr. NJ Fiumara, and the CDC.)

cases of bacterial pneumonia frequently follow relatively mild viral respiratory infections. During the primary infection, the virus causes damage to the ciliated epithelial cells that line the respiratory tract. The function of these cells is to move foreign materials up and out of the respiratory tract and into the throat where they can be swallowed. While coughing, the patient may inhale some saliva, containing an opportunistic bacterial pathogen, such as *Streptococcus pneumoniae* or *Haemophilus influenzae*. Because the ciliated epithelial cells were damaged by the virus, they are unable to clear the bacteria from the lungs. The bacteria then multiply and cause pneumonia. In this example, the viral infection is the primary infection and bacterial pneumonia is the secondary infection.

STEPS IN THE PATHOGENESIS OF INFECTIOUS DISEASES

In general, the pathogenesis of infectious diseases often follows the following sequence (Fig. 14-5):

> An infection may follow the sequence of entry, attachment, multiplication, invasion, evasion of host defenses, and damage to host tissues.

1. **Entry** of the pathogen into the body. Portals of entry include penetration of skin or mucous membranes by the pathogen, inoculation of the pathogen into bodily tissues by an arthropod, inhalation (into the respiratory tract), ingestion (into the gastrointestinal tract), introduction of the pathogen into the genitourinary tract, or introduction of the pathogen directly into the blood (e.g., through blood transfusion or the use of shared needles by intravenous drug abusers).
2. **Attachment** of the pathogen to some tissue(s) within the body.
3. **Multiplication** of the pathogen. The pathogen may multiply in one location of the body, resulting in a localized infection (e.g., abscess), or it may multiply throughout the body (a systemic infection).
4. **Invasion or spread** of the pathogen.
5. **Evasion of host defenses.**
6. **Damage to host tissue(s).** The damage may be so extensive as to cause the death of the patient.

It is important to understand that not all infectious diseases involve *all* these steps. For example, once ingested, some exotoxin-producing intestinal pathogens are capable of causing disease without adhering to the intestinal wall or invading tissue.

VIRULENCE

The terms *virulent* and **virulence** tend to be confusing because they are used in several different ways. Sometimes virulent is used as a synonym for

> Virulent strains of a microbe are capable of causing disease, whereas avirulent strains are not.

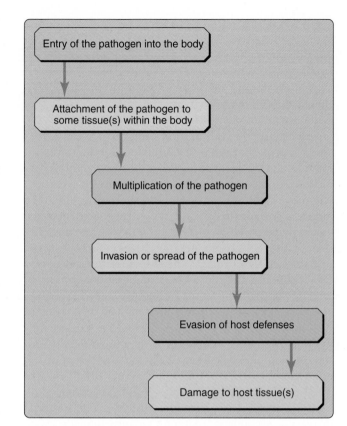

FIGURE 14-5. Steps in the pathogenesis of infectious diseases. Not all infectious diseases involve *all* of the steps shown. For example, once ingested, some exotoxin-producing intestinal pathogens are capable of causing disease without adhering to the intestinal wall or invading tissue.

pathogenic. For example, there may be virulent (pathogenic) strains and *avirulent* (nonpathogenic) strains of a particular species. The **virulent strains** are capable of causing disease, whereas the **avirulent strains** are not. For example, toxigenic strains of the bacterium, *Corynebacterium diphtheriae*, (i.e., strains that produce diphtheria toxin) are virulent, whereas nontoxigenic strains are not. Encapsulated strains of the bacterium, *S. pneumoniae*, can cause disease, but nonencapsulated strains of *S. pneumoniae* cannot. As will be discussed in a subsequent section, piliated strains of certain pathogens are able to cause disease, whereas nonpiliated strains are not; thus, the piliated strains are virulent, but the nonpiliated strains are avirulent.

Sometimes virulence is used to express a measure or degree of pathogenicity. Although all pathogens cause disease, some are more virulent than others

> Some strains of a given pathogen can be more virulent than other strains.

(i.e., they are better able to cause disease). In bacterial diarrhea, for example, it only takes about 10 *Shigella* cells to cause shigellosis, but it takes between 100 and 1,000 *Salmonella* cells to cause salmonellosis. Thus, *Shigella* is considered to be more virulent than *Salmonella*. In some cases, certain strains of a particular species are more virulent than others. For example, the "flesh-eating" strains of the bacterium, *Streptococcus pyogenes*, are more virulent than other strains of *S. pyogenes* because they produce certain necrotizing enzymes that are not produced by the other strains. Similarly, only certain strains of *S. pyogenes* produce **erythrogenic toxin** (the cause of scarlet fever); these strains are considered more virulent than the strains of *S. pyogenes* that do not produce erythrogenic toxin. Strains of the bacterium, *Staphylococcus aureus*, that produce toxic shock syndrome toxin-1 (TSST-1) are considered more virulent than strains of *S. aureus* that do not produce this toxin.

Sometimes virulence is used in reference to the severity of the infectious diseases that are caused by the pathogens. Used in this manner, one pathogen is more virulent than another if it causes a more serious disease.

VIRULENCE FACTORS

The physical attributes or properties of pathogens that enable them to escape various host defense mechanisms and cause disease are called **virulence factors**. Virulence factors are phenotypic characteristics that, like all phenotypic characteristics, are dictated by the organism's genotype. Toxins are obvious virulence factors,

> Virulence factors are phenotypic characteristics that enable microbes to be virulent (to cause disease).

but other virulence factors are not so obvious. Some virulence factors are shown in Figure 14-6.

Attachment

Perhaps you have noticed that certain pathogens infect dogs but not humans, whereas others infect humans but not dogs. Perhaps you have wondered why certain pathogens cause respiratory infections whereas others cause gastrointestinal infections. Part of the explanation has to do with the type or types of cells to which the pathogen is able to attach. To cause disease, some pathogens must be able to anchor themselves to cells after they have gained access to the body.

Receptors and Adhesins

The general terms *receptor* and *integrin* are used to describe the molecule on the surface of a host cell that a particular pathogen is able to recognize and attach to (Fig 14-7). Often, these receptors are glycoprotein molecules. A particular pathogen can only attach to cells bearing the appropriate receptor. Thus, certain viruses cause respiratory infections because they are able to recognize and attach to certain receptors that are present on cells that line the respiratory tract. Because those particular receptors are not present on cells lining the gastrointestinal tract, the virus is unable to cause

> Molecules on a host cell's surface that pathogens are able to recognize and attach to are called *receptors* or *integrins*.

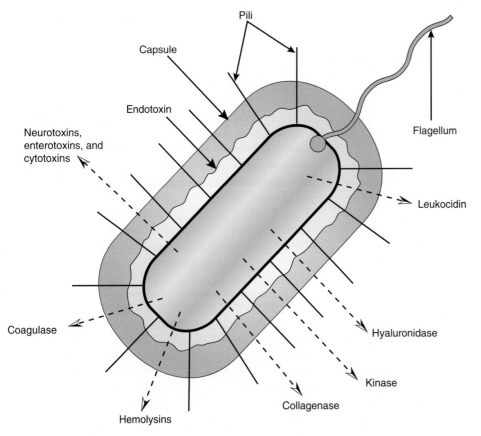

FIGURE 14-6. Virulence factors. See text for details.

Pili

Capsule

Endotoxin

Neurotoxins, enterotoxins, and cytotoxins

Coagulase

Hemolysins

Collagenase

Kinase

Hyaluronidase

Leukocidin

Flagellum

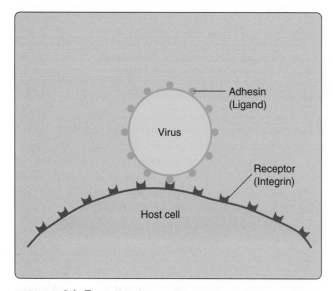

FIGURE 14-7. Adhesins and receptors. See text for details.

gastrointestinal infections. Similarly, certain viruses cause infections in dogs, but not in humans, because dog cells possess a receptor that human cells lack.

S. pyogenes cells have an adhesin (called protein F) on their surfaces that enables this pathogen to adhere to a protein—fibronectin—that is found on many host cell surfaces. Human immunodeficiency virus (HIV; the virus that causes acquired immunodeficiency syndrome [AIDS]) is able to attach to cells bearing a surface receptor called CD4. Such cells are known as CD4$^+$ cells. A category of lymphocytes called T-helper cells (the primary target cells for HIV) are examples of CD4$^+$ cells.

The general terms *adhesin* and *ligand* are used to describe the molecule on the surface of a pathogen that is able to recognize and bind to a particular receptor (Fig. 14-7). For example, the adhesin on the envelope of HIV that recognizes and binds to the CD4 receptor is a glycoprotein molecule designated gp120. (Entry of HIV into a host cell is a rather complex event, requiring several adhesins and several co-receptors.) Because adhesins enable pathogens to attach to host cells, they are considered virulence factors. In some cases, antibodies directed against such adhesins prevent the pathogen from attaching and, thus, prevent infection by that pathogen. (As will be discussed in Chapter 16, antibodies are proteins that our immune systems produce to protect us from pathogens and infectious diseases.)

> Molecules on a pathogen's surface that recognize and attach to receptors on a host cell's surface are called *adhesins* or *ligands.*

Bacterial Fimbriae (Pili)

Bacterial fimbriae (pili) are long, thin, hairlike, flexible projections composed primarily of an array of proteins called pilin (refer back to Fig. 3-13). Fimbriae are considered to be virulence factors because they enable

bacteria to attach to surfaces, including various tissues within the human body. Fimbriated (piliated) strains of *N. gonorrhoeae* are able to anchor themselves to the inner walls of the urethra and cause urethritis. Should nonfimbriated (nonpiliated) strains of *N. gonorrhoeae* gain access to the urethra, they are flushed out by urination and are thus unable to cause urethritis. Therefore, with respect to urethritis, fimbriated strains of *N. gonorrhoeae* are virulent and nonfimbriated strains are avirulent.

> Bacterial fimbriae (pili) are virulence factors, in that they enable fimbriated (piliated) bacteria to adhere to cells and tissues within the human body.

Similarly, fimbriated strains of *Escherichia coli* that gain access to the urinary bladder are able to anchor themselves to the inner walls of the bladder and cause cystitis; thus, with respect to cystitis, fimbriated strains of *E. coli* are virulent. Should nonfimbriated strains of *E. coli* gain access to the urinary bladder, they are flushed out by urination and are unable to cause cystitis; thus, nonfimbriated strains are avirulent.

The fimbriae of group A, beta-hemolytic streptococci (*S. pyogenes*) contain molecules of M-protein. M-protein serves as a virulence factor in two ways: (a) it enables the bacteria to adhere to pharyngeal cells; and (b) it protects the cells from being phagocytized by white blood cells (i.e., the M-protein serves an antiphagocytic function).

Other bacterial pathogens possessing fimbriae are *Vibrio cholerae*, *Salmonella* spp., *Shigella* spp., *Pseudomonas aeruginosa*, and *Neisseria meningitidis*. Because bacterial fimbriae enable bacteria to colonize surfaces, they are sometimes referred to as colonization factors.

Obligate Intracellular Pathogens

Certain pathogens, such as Gram-negative bacteria in the genera *Rickettsia* and *Chlamydia* must live within host cells to survive and multiply; they are referred to as **obligate intracellular pathogens** (or obligate intracellular parasites). Rickettsias invade and live within endothelial cells and vascular smooth muscle cells. Rickettsias are capable of synthesizing proteins, nucleic acids, and adenosine triphosphate (ATP), but are thought to require an intracellular environment because they possess an unusual membrane transport system; they are said to have leaky membranes.

> Rickettsias and chlamydias are obligate intracellular pathogens.

The different species and serotypes of chlamydias invade different types of cells, including conjunctival epithelial cells and cells of the respiratory and genital tracts. Although chlamydias produce ATP molecules, they preferentially use ATP molecules produced by host cells; this has earned them the title of "energy parasites." In the laboratory, obligate intracellular pathogens are propagated using cell cultures, laboratory animals, or embryonated chicken eggs.

Ehrlichia spp. and *Anaplasma phagocytophilum* are Gram-negative bacteria that closely resemble *Rickettsia* spp. They are **intraleukocytic pathogens**. *Ehrlichia* spp. live within monocytes, causing a disease known as human monocytic ehrlichiosis (HME). *A. phagocytophilum* lives within granulocytes, causing a condition known as human anaplasmosis (formerly called human granulocytic ehrlichiosis or HGE). Certain sporozoan protozoa, such as the *Plasmodium* spp. that cause human malaria and the *Babesia* spp. that cause human babesiosis, are **intraerythrocytic pathogens** (i.e., they live within erythrocytes).

> *Ehrlichia* and *Anaplasma* spp. are intraleukocytic pathogens, whereas *Plasmodium* and *Babesia* spp. are intraerythrocytic pathogens.

Facultative Intracellular Pathogens

Some pathogens, referred to as **facultative intracellular pathogens** (or facultative intracellular parasites), are capable of both an intracellular and extracellular existence. Many facultative intracellular pathogens that can be grown in the laboratory on artificial culture media are also able to survive *within* phagocytes. How facultative intracellular pathogens are able to survive within phagocytes is discussed in the next section. Phagocytosis is discussed in greater detail in Chapter 15.

> Pathogens that can live both within and outside of host cells are called facultative intracellular pathogens.

Intracellular Survival Mechanisms

As will be discussed in Chapter 15, phagocytes play an important role in our defenses against pathogens. The two most important categories of phagocytes in the human body (referred to as "professional phagocytes") are macrophages and neutrophils. Once phagocytized, most pathogens are destroyed within the phagocytes by hydrolytic enzymes (e.g., lysozyme, proteases, lipases,

> The two most important categories of phagocytes in the human body—referred to as "professional phagocytes"—are macrophages and neutrophils.

DNase, RNase, myeloperoxidase), hydrogen peroxide, superoxide anions, and other mechanisms. However, certain pathogens are able to survive and multiply within phagocytes after being ingested (Table 14-1).

Some pathogens (such as the bacterium, *M. tuberculosis*) have a cell wall composition that resists digestion. Mycobacterial cell walls contain waxes, and it is thought that these waxes protect the organisms from digestion. Other pathogens (like the protozoan, *Toxoplasma gondii*) prevent the fusion of lysosomes (vesicles that contain digestive enzymes) with the phagocytic vacuole (phagosome). Other pathogens, such as the bacterium, *Rickettsia rickettsii*, produce phospholipases that destroy the phagosome membrane, thus preventing lysosome-phagosome fusion. Other pathogens (such as the bacteria, *Brucella abortus*, *Francisella tularensis*, *Legionella pneumophila*, *Listeria monocytogenes*, *Salmonella* spp., and

> Many bacteria, including *M. tuberculosis*, are facultative intracellular pathogens.

STUDY AID
The Word Facultative
Wherever the word *facultative* appears in this book, it implies a choice. For example, the term *facultative anaerobe* was introduced in Chapter 4. Such an organism can live either in the presence or absence of oxygen; it has a choice! In this chapter, the term *facultative intracellular pathogen* is introduced. Such an organism can live either extracellularly or intracellularly (within host cells); it has a choice! The term *facultative parasite* will be introduced in Chapter 21. Such an organism can live either a free-living or parasitic existence; it has a choice!

TABLE 14-1	Pathogens that Routinely Multiply within Macrophages	
CATEGORY OF PATHOGENS	**EXAMPLES**	**DISEASE(S)**
Viruses	Herpes viruses	Genital herpes, herpes labialis (cold sores or fever blisters)
	HIV	AIDS
	Rubeola virus	Measles
	Poxviruses	Smallpox, monkeypox
Rickettsias	*Rickettsia rickettsii*	Rocky Mountain spotted fever
	Rickettsia prowazeki	Epidemic (louseborne) typhus
Other bacteria	*Brucella* spp.	Brucellosis
	Legionella pneumophila	Legionellosis
	Listeria monocytogenes	Listeriosis
	Mycobacterium leprae	Hansen disease (leprosy)
	Mycobacterium tuberculosis	Tuberculosis
Protozoa	*Leishmania* spp.	Leishmaniasis
	Toxoplasma gondii	Toxoplasmosis
	Trypanosoma cruzi	Chagas' disease (American trypanosomiasis)
Fungi	*Cryptococcus neoformans*	Cryptococcosis

Yersinia pestis) are able to survive by means of mechanisms that are not yet understood.

Capsules

Bacterial capsules (refer back to Fig. 3-10) are considered to be virulence factors because they serve an antiphagocytic function (i.e., they protect encapsulated bacteria from being phagocytized by phagocytic white blood cells). Phagocytes are unable to attach to encapsulated bacteria because they lack surface receptors for the polysaccharide material of which the capsule is made. If they cannot adhere to the bacteria, they cannot ingest them. Because encapsulated bacteria that gain access to the bloodstream or tissues are protected from phagocytosis, they are able to multiply, invade, and cause disease. Nonencapsulated bacteria, on the other hand, are phagocytized and killed. Encapsulated bacteria include *S. pneumoniae*, *Klebsiella pneumoniae*, *H. influenzae*, and *N. meningitidis*. The capsule of the yeast, *Cryptococcus neoformans*, is also considered to be a virulence factor (refer back to Fig. 5-8).

> Bacterial capsules serve an antiphagocytic function (i.e., they protect encapsulated bacteria from being phagocytized).

Flagella

Bacterial *flagella* are considered virulence factors because flagella enable flagellated (motile) bacteria to invade aqueous areas of the body that nonflagellated (nonmotile) bacteria are unable to reach. Perhaps flagella also enable bacteria to avoid phagocytosis—it is more difficult for phagocytes to catch a moving target.

> Flagella are considered to be virulence factors because they enable flagellated bacteria to invade areas of the body that nonflagellated bacteria cannot reach.

Exoenzymes

Although pili, capsules, and flagella are considered virulence factors, they really do not explain how bacteria and other pathogens actually *cause* disease. **The major mechanisms by which pathogens cause disease are certain exoenzymes or toxins that they produce.** Some pathogens (e.g., certain strains of *S. pyogenes*) produce *both* exoenzymes and toxins.

> The most important virulence factors are certain exoenzymes and toxins that pathogens produce.

Some pathogens release enzymes (called **exoenzymes**) that enable them to evade host defense mechanisms, invade, or cause damage to body tissues.[a] These exoenzymes include necrotizing enzymes, coagulase, kinases, hyaluronidase, collagenase, hemolysins, and lecithinase.

Necrotizing Enzymes

Many pathogens produce exoenzymes that destroy tissues; these are collectively referred to as necrotizing enzymes. Notorious examples are the flesh-eating strains of *S. pyogenes*, which produce proteases and other enzymes that cause very rapid destruction of soft tissue, leading to a disease called necrotizing fasciitis (Fig. 14-8). The various *Clostridium* species that cause gas gangrene (myonecrosis) produce a variety of necrotizing enzymes, including proteases and lipases.

> Necrotizing enzymes are exoenzymes that cause destruction of cells and tissues.

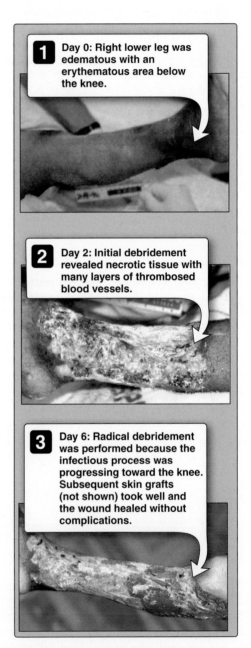

FIGURE 14-8. Necrotizing fasciitis. (From Harvey RA, et al. Lippincott's Illustrated Reviews: Microbiology, 2nd ed. Philadelphia: Lippincott Williams & Wilkins, 2007.)

---

[a] Enzymes that are produced within cells and remain within those cells to catalyze intracellular reactions are called endoenzymes.

Coagulase

An important identifying feature of *S. aureus* in the laboratory is its ability to produce a protein called **coagulase**. Coagulase binds to prothrombin, forming a complex called staphylothrombin. The protease activity of thrombin is activated in this complex, causing the conversion of fibrinogen to fibrin. In the body, coagulase may enable *S. aureus* to clot plasma and thereby to form a sticky coat of fibrin around themselves for protection from phagocytes, antibodies, and other host defense mechanisms.

> Coagulase is a virulence factor that causes clotting.

Kinases

Kinases (also known as fibrinolysins) have the opposite effect of coagulase. Sometimes the host will cause a fibrin clot to form around pathogens in an attempt to wall them off and prevent them from invading deeper into body tissues. Kinases are enzymes that lyse (dissolve) clots; therefore, pathogens that produce kinases are able to escape from clots. **Streptokinase** is the name of a kinase produced by streptococci, and **staphylokinase** is the name of a kinase produced by staphylococci. Streptokinase has been used to treat patients with coronary thrombosis. Because *S. aureus* produces both coagulase and staphylokinase, not only can *S. aureus* cause the formation of clots, but it can also dissolve them.

> Kinases are exoenzymes that dissolve clots.

Hyaluronidase

The "spreading factor," as **hyaluronidase** is sometimes called, enables pathogens to spread through connective tissue by breaking down **hyaluronic acid**, the polysaccharide "cement" that holds tissue cells together. Hyaluronidase is secreted by several pathogenic species of *Staphylococcus*, *Streptococcus*, and *Clostridium*.

> Hyaluronidase and collagenase are virulence factors that dissolve hyaluronic acid and collagen, respectively, enabling pathogens to invade deeper into tissues.

Collagenase

The enzyme **collagenase**, produced by certain pathogens, breaks down collagen (the supportive protein found in tendons, cartilage, and bones). This enables the pathogens to invade tissues. *Clostridium perfringens*, a major cause of gas gangrene, spreads deeply within the body by secreting both collagenase and hyaluronidase.

Hemolysins

Hemolysins are enzymes that cause damage to the host's red blood cells (erythrocytes). Not only does the lysis (bursting or destruction) of red blood cells harm the host, but it also provides the pathogens with a source of iron. In the

> Hemolysins are enzymes that damage red blood cells.

laboratory, the effect an organism has on the red blood cells in blood agar enables differentiation between alpha-hemolytic (α-hemolytic) and beta-hemolytic (β-hemolytic) bacteria. The hemolysins produced by α-hemolytic bacteria cause a partial breakdown of hemoglobin in the red blood cells, resulting in a green zone around the colonies of α-hemolytic bacteria. The hemolysins produced by β-hemolytic bacteria cause complete lysis of the red blood cells, resulting in a clear zone around the colonies of β-hemolytic bacteria (refer back to Fig. 13-13). Hemolysins are produced by many pathogenic bacteria, but the type of hemolysis produced by an organism is of most importance when attempting to speciate a *Streptococcus* in the laboratory. Some *Streptococcus* spp. are α-hemolytic, some are β-hemolytic, and some are γ-hemolytic (nonhemolytic).

Lecithinase

C. perfringens, the major cause of gas gangrene, is able to rapidly destroy extensive areas of tissue, especially muscle tissue. One of the enzymes produced by *C. perfringens*, called **lecithinase**, breaks down phospholipids that are collectively referred to as **lecithin**. This enzyme is destructive to cell membranes of red blood cells and other tissues.

> Lecithinase is an exoenzyme that causes destruction of host cell membranes.

Toxins

The ability of pathogens to damage host tissues and cause disease may depend on the production and release of various types of poisonous substances, referred to as toxins. The two major categories of toxins are endotoxins and exotoxins. **Endotoxins**, which are integral parts of the cell walls of Gram-negative bacteria, can cause a number of adverse physiologic effects. **Exotoxins**, on the other hand, are toxins that are produced within cells and then released from the cells.

> The two major categories of toxins are endotoxins and exotoxins.

Endotoxin

Septicemia (often referred to as *sepsis*) is a very serious disease consisting of chills, fever, prostration (extreme exhaustion), and the presence of bacteria or their toxins in the bloodstream. Septicemia caused by Gram-negative bacteria, sometimes referred to as Gram-negative sepsis, is an especially serious type of septicemia. The cell walls of Gram-negative bacteria contain lipopolysaccharide (LPS), the lipid portion of which is called lipid-A or endotoxin. Endotoxin can cause serious, adverse, physiologic effects such as fever and shock. Substances that cause fever are known as **pyrogens**.

> Endotoxin is a component of the cell walls of Gram-negative bacteria.

Shock is a life-threatening condition resulting from very low blood pressure and an inadequate blood supply to body tissues and organs, especially the kidneys and brain. The type of shock that results from Gram-negative sepsis is known as **septic shock**. Symptoms include reduced mental alertness, confusion, rapid breathing, chills, fever, and warm, flushed skin. As shock worsens, several organs begin to fail, including the kidneys, lungs, and heart. Blood clots may form within blood vessels. More than 500,000 cases of sepsis occur annually in the United States; approximately half of these are caused by Gram-negative bacteria. There is a 30% to 35% mortality rate associated with Gram-negative sepsis.

Exotoxins

Exotoxins are poisonous proteins that are secreted by a variety of pathogens; they are often named for the target organs that they affect. Examples include neurotoxins, enterotoxins, cytotoxins, exfoliative toxin, erythrogenic toxin, and diphtheria toxin.

> Exotoxins are poisonous proteins that are secreted by a variety of pathogens.

The most potent exotoxins are **neurotoxins**, which affect the central nervous system. The neurotoxins produced by *Clostridium tetani* and *Clostridium botulinum*—tetanospasmin and botulinal toxin—cause tetanus and botulism, respectively. Tetanospasmin

> Neurotoxins are exotoxins that adversely affect the central nervous system.

affects control of nerve transmission, leading to a spastic, rigid type of paralysis in which the patient's muscles are contracted (Fig. 14-9). Botulinal toxin also blocks nerve impulses but by a different mechanism, leading to a generalized, flaccid type of paralysis in which the patient's muscles are relaxed. Both diseases are often fatal. See this book's CD-ROM for "A Closer Look at Botulinal Toxin."

Other types of exotoxins, called **enterotoxins**, are toxins that affect the gastrointestinal tract, often causing diarrhea and sometimes vomiting. Examples of bacterial pathogens that produce enterotoxins are *Bacillus cereus*, certain serotypes of *E. coli, Clostridium difficile, C. perfringens, Salmonella* spp., *Shigella* spp., *V. cholerae*, and some strains of *S. aureus*. In addition to releasing an enterotoxin (called toxin A), *C. difficile* also produces a cytotoxin (called toxin B) that damages the lining of the colon, leading to a condition known as pseudomembranous colitis.

> Enterotoxins are exotoxins that adversely affect the gastrointestinal tract.

Symptoms of toxic shock syndrome are caused by exotoxins secreted by certain strains of *S. aureus* and, less commonly, *S. pyogenes*. Staphylococcal TSST-1 primarily affects the integrity of capillary walls. **Exfoliative toxin** (or epidermolytic toxin) of *S. aureus* causes the epidermal layers of skin to slough away, leading to a disease known

FIGURE 14-9. Tetanus patient displaying the bodily posture known as opisthotonos. This condition of abnormal posturing involves rigidity and severe arching of the back, with the head thrown backward. If a patient displaying opisthotonos was placed on their back, only the back of their head and their heels would touch the supporting surface. (Courtesy of the CDC.)

as scalded skin syndrome. *S. aureus* also produces a variety of toxins that destroy cell membranes.

Erythrogenic toxin, produced by some strains of *S. pyogenes*, causes scarlet fever. **Leukocidins** are toxins that destroy white blood cells (leukocytes). Thus, leukocidins (which are produced by some staphylococci, streptococci, and clostridia) cause destruction of the very cells that the body sends to the site of infection to ingest and destroy pathogens.

> Erythrogenic toxin, produced by some strains of *S. pyogenes*, causes scarlet fever.

Diphtheria toxin, produced by toxigenic strains of *C. diphtheriae*, inhibits protein synthesis. It kills mucosal epithelial cells and phagocytes and adversely affects the heart and nervous system. The toxin is actually coded for by a bacteriophage gene. Thus, only *C. diphtheriae* cells that are "infected" with that particular bacteriophage are able to produce diphtheria toxin. Other exotoxins that inhibit protein synthesis are *Pseudomonas aeruginosa* exotoxin A, Shiga toxin (produced by *Shigella* spp.), and the Shiga-like toxins produced by certain serotypes of *E. coli*.

> Diphtheria toxin is produced by some strains of *C. diphtheriae*, referred to as toxigenic strains.

Table 14-2 contains a recap of bacterial virulence factors described so far.

Mechanisms by which Pathogens Escape Immune Responses

Immunology, the study of the immune system, is discussed in detail in Chapter 16. A primary role of the immune system is to recognize and destroy pathogens that invade our bodies. However, there are many ways in which pathogens avoid being destroyed by immune responses. Several mechanisms will be mentioned here; others are beyond the scope of this book.

Antigenic Variation

As discussed in Chapter 16, antigens are foreign molecules that evoke an immune response—often stimulating the immune system to produce antibodies. Some pathogens are able to periodically change their surface antigens, a phenomenon known as **antigenic variation**. About the time that the host has produced antibodies in response to the pathogen's surface antigens, those antigens are shed and new ones appear in their place. This renders the antibodies worthless, because they have nothing to adhere to. Examples of pathogens capable of antigenic variation are influenza viruses, HIV, *Borrelia recurrentis* (the causative agent of relapsing fever), *N. gonorrhoeae*,

> Some pathogens periodically change their surface antigens, a phenomenon known as antigenic variation.

TABLE 14-2	Recap of Bacterial Virulence Factors
VIRULENCE FACTOR	**COMMENTS**
Bacterial structures:	
Flagella	Enable bacteria to gain access to anatomic areas that nonmotile bacteria cannot reach; may enable bacteria to "escape" from phagocytes
Capsules	Serve an antiphagocytic function
Pili	Enable bacteria to attach to surfaces
Enzymes:	
Coagulase	Enables bacteria to produce clots within which to "hide"
Kinases	Enable bacteria to dissolve clots
Hyaluronidase	Dissolves hyaluronic acid, enabling bacteria to penetrate deeper into tissues
Lecithinase	Destroys cell membranes
Necrotizing enzymes	Cause massive destruction of tissues
Toxins:	
Endotoxin	Released from the cell walls of Gram-negative bacteria; causes fever and septic shock
Exotoxins	Produced within the cell, but then released from the cell
Neurotoxins	Cause damage to the central nervous system; tetanospasmin and botulinal toxin are examples
Enterotoxins	Cause gastrointestinal disease
Clostridium difficile toxin B	The cytotoxin that causes pseudomembranous colitis
Staphylococcus aureus TSST-1	The toxin that causes most cases of toxic shock syndrome
Exfoliative toxin	Produced by some strains of *S. aureus*; causes scalded skin syndrome
Erythrogenic toxin	Produced by some strains of *Streptococcus pyogenes*; causes scarlet fever
Diphtheria toxin	Produced by toxigenic strains of *Corynebacterium diphtheriae*; causes diphtheria
Leukocidins	Cause the destruction of leukocytes

and the trypanosomes that cause African trypanoso-miasis. Trypanosomes can keep up their antigenic va-riation for 20 years, never presenting the same surface antigens twice.

Camouflage and Molecular Mimicry

Adult schistosomes (trematodes that cause schistosomiasis) are able to conceal their foreign na-ture by coating themselves with host proteins—a sort of camou-flage. In molecular mimicry, the pathogen's surface antigens closely resemble host antigens and are therefore not recognized as being foreign. Although there is little evidence to prove that molecular mimicry leads to a subdued immune response against the pathogens, it is known that the hyaluronic acid capsule of streptococci is almost identical to the hyaluronic acid com-ponent of human connective tissue. It is also interesting that in mycoplasmal pneumonia, antibodies produced by the host against antigens of *Mycoplasma pneumoniae* can cause damage to the host's heart, lung, brain, and red blood cells.

> In molecular mimicry, pathogens cover their surface antigens with host proteins, so the pathogens will not be recognized as being foreign.

Destruction of Antibodies

Several bacterial pathogens, including *H. influenzae*, *N. gonorrhoeae*, and streptococci, produce an enzyme (IgA protease) that destroys IgA antibodies. Thus, these pathogens are capable of destroying some of the antibod-ies that the host's immune system has produced in an attempt to destroy them.

ON THE CD-ROM
- Terms Introduced in This Chapter
- Review of Key Points
- Increase Your Knowledge
- Critical Thinking
- Additional Self-Assessment Exercises

SELF-ASSESSMENT EXERCISES

After studying this chapter, answer the following multiple-choice questions.

1. Which of the following virulence factors enable(s) bacteria to attach to tissues?
   a. capsules
   b. endotoxin
   c. flagella
   d. pili

2. Neurotoxins are produced by:
   a. *Clostridium botulinum* and *Clostridium tetani*.
   b. *Clostridium difficile* and *Clostridium perfringens*.
   c. *Pseudomonas aeruginosa* and *Mycobacterium tuber-culosis*.
   d. *Staphylococcus aureus* and *Streptococcus pyogenes*.

3. Which of the following pathogens produce entero-toxins?
   a. *Bacillus cereus* and certain serotypes of *Escherichia coli*
   b. *C. difficile* and *C. perfringens*
   c. *Salmonella* spp. and *Shigella* spp.
   d. all of the above

4. A bloodstream infection with _____ could re-sult in the release of endotoxin into the bloodstream.
   a. *C. difficile* or *C. perfringens*
   b. *Neisseria gonorrhoeae* or *E. coli*
   c. *S. aureus* or *M. tuberculosis*
   d. *S. aureus* or *S. pyogenes*

5. Communicable diseases are most easily transmitted during the:
   a. incubation period.
   b. period of convalescence.
   c. period of illness.
   d. prodromal period.

6. Enterotoxins affect cells in the:
   a. central nervous system.
   b. gastrointestinal tract.
   c. genitourinary tract.
   d. respiratory tract.

7. Which of the following bacteria is *least* likely to be the cause of septic shock?
   a. *E. coli*
   b. *Haemophilus influenzae*
   c. *Mycoplasma pneumoniae*
   d. *Neisseria meningitidis*

8. Which of the following produces both a cytotoxin *and* an enterotoxin?
   a. *C. botulinum*
   b. *C. difficile*
   c. *C. tetani*
   d. *Corynebacterium diphtheriae*

9. Which of the following virulence factors enable(s) bacteria to avoid phagocytosis by white blood cells?
   a. capsule
   b. cell membrane
   c. cell wall
   d. pili

10. Which of the following can cause toxic shock syndrome?
    a. *C. difficile* and *C. perfringens*
    b. *M. pneumoniae* and *M. tuberculosis*
    c. *N. gonorrhoeae* and *E. coli*
    d. *S. aureus* and *S. pyogenes*

NONSPECIFIC HOST DEFENSE MECHANISMS

15

LEARNING OBJECTIVES

AFTER STUDYING THIS CHAPTER, YOU SHOULD BE ABLE TO:

- Define the following terms: host defense mechanisms, antibody, antigen, lysozyme, microbial antagonism, colicin, bacteriocins, superinfection, pyrogen, interferon, complement cascade, complement, opsonization, inflammation, vasodilation, phagocytosis, and chemotaxis
- Briefly describe the three lines of defense used by the body to combat pathogens and give one example of each
- Explain what is meant by "nonspecific host defense mechanisms" and how they differ from "specific host defense mechanisms"
- Identify three ways by which the digestive system is protected from pathogens
- Describe how interferons function as host defense mechanisms
- Name three cellular and chemical responses to microbial invasion
- Describe the major benefits of complement activation
- List the four main signs and symptoms associated with inflammation
- Discuss the four primary purposes of the inflammatory response
- Describe the four steps in phagocytosis

- Identify the three major categories of leukocytes and the three categories of granulocytes
- State four ways in which pathogens escape destruction by phagocytes
- Categorize the disorders and conditions that affect the body's nonspecific host mechanisms

INTRODUCTION

In Chapter 14, you discovered the ways in which pathogens cause infectious diseases. In this chapter and the next, you will learn how our bodies combat pathogens in an attempt to prevent the infectious diseases that they cause.

Humans and animals have survived on Earth for hundreds of thousands of years because they have many built-in or naturally occurring mechanisms of defense against pathogens and the infectious diseases that they cause. The ability of any animal to resist these invaders and recover from disease is attributable to many complex interacting functions within the body.

Host defense mechanisms—ways in which the body protects itself from pathogens—can be thought of as an army consisting of three lines of defense (Fig. 15-1). If the enemy (the pathogen) breaks through the first line of

FIGURE 15-1. Lines of defense. Host defense mechanisms—ways in which the body protects itself from pathogens—can be thought of as an entrenched army consisting of three lines of defense. (See text for details.)

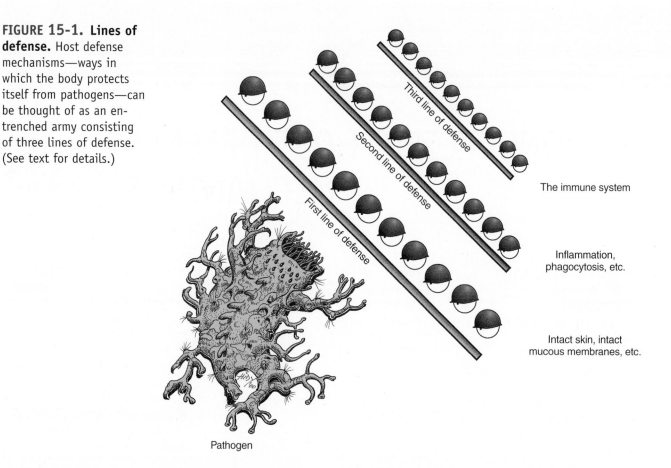

First line of defense

Second line of defense

Third line of defense

The immune system

Inflammation, phagocytosis, etc.

Intact skin, intact mucous membranes, etc.

Pathogen

defense, it will encounter and, hopefully, be stopped by the second line of defense. If the enemy manages to break through and escape the first two lines of defense, there is a third line of defense ready to attack it.

The first two lines of defense are nonspecific; these are ways in which the body attempts to destroy *all* types of substances that are foreign to it, including pathogens. The third line of defense, the immune response, is very specific. In the third line of defense (or *specific host defense mechanisms*), special proteins called *antibodies* are usually produced in the body in response to the presence of foreign substances. These foreign substances are called **antigens** because they stimulate the production of specific antibodies; they are "**anti**body-**gen**erating" substances. The antibodies that are produced are very specific, in that they usually can only recognize and attach to the antigen that stimulated their production. Immune responses are discussed in greater detail in Chapter 16. The various categories of host defense mechanisms are summarized in Figure 15-2.[a]

> The first two lines of defense are nonspecific, in the sense that they are directed against *any* foreign substances that enter our bodies. The third line of defense, on the other hand, is very specific.

---

[a] Some immunologists consider both the second and third lines of defense as parts of the immune system. They refer to the second line of defense as *innate immune responses* (those not requiring immunologic memory) and the third line of defense as *acquired immune responses*.

NONSPECIFIC HOST DEFENSE MECHANISMS

Nonspecific host defense mechanisms are general and serve to protect the body against many harmful substances. One of the nonspecific host defenses is the innate, or inborn, resistance observed among some species of animals and some persons who have a natural resistance to certain diseases. Innate or inherited characteristics make these people and animals more resistant to some diseases

FIGURE 15-2. Categories of host defense mechanisms.

than to others. The exact factors that produce this innate resistance are not well understood, but are probably related to chemical, physiologic, and temperature differences between the species as well as the general state of physical and emotional health of the person and environmental factors that affect certain races, but not others.

Although we are usually unaware of it, our bodies are constantly in the process of defending us against microbial invaders. We encounter pathogens and potential pathogens many times per day, every day of our lives. Usually, our bodies successfully ward off or destroy the invading microbes. Nonspecific host defense mechanisms discussed in this chapter include mechanical and physical barriers to invasion, chemical factors, microbial antagonism by our indigenous microflora, fever, the inflammatory response (inflammation), and phagocytic white blood cells (phagocytes).

FIRST LINE OF DEFENSE

Skin and Mucous Membranes as Physical Barriers

The intact, unbroken skin that covers our bodies represents a nonspecific host defense mechanism, in that it serves as a physical or mechanical barrier to pathogens. Very few pathogens are able to penetrate intact skin. Although certain helminth infections (e.g., hookworm infection, schistosomiasis) are acquired by penetration of the skin by parasites, it is unlikely that many, if any, bacteria are capable of penetrating intact skin. In most cases, it is only when the skin is cut, abraded (scratched), or burned that pathogens gain entrance or when they are injected through the skin (e.g., by arthropods or the sharing of needles by intravenous drug abusers). Even the tiniest of cuts (a paper cut, for example) can serve as a portal of entry for pathogens.

Although they are composed of only a single layer of cells, mucous membranes also serve as a physical or mechanical barrier to pathogens. Most pathogens can only pass through when these membranes are cut or scratched. As is true for skin, even the tiniest of cuts can serve as portals of entry for pathogens. The sticky mucus that is produced by goblet cells within the mucous membranes serves to entrap invaders; thus, it is considered part of the first line of defense.

Intact skin and mucous membranes serve as nonspecific host defense mechanisms by serving as physical or mechanical barriers to pathogens.

Cellular and Chemical Factors

Not only does skin provide a physical barrier, but there are several additional factors that account for the skin's ability to resist pathogens. The dryness of most areas of skin

The dryness, acidity, and temperature of the skin inhibit colonization and growth of pathogens; perspiration flushes them away.

inhibits colonization by many pathogens. Also, the acidity (pH ~5.0) and temperature (<37°C) of the skin inhibit the growth of pathogens. The oily sebum that is produced by sebaceous glands in the skin contains fatty acids, which are toxic to some pathogens. Perspiration serves as a nonspecific host defense mechanism by flushing organisms from pores and the surface of the skin. Perspiration also contains the enzyme, *lysozyme*, which degrades peptidoglycan in bacterial cell walls (especially Gram-positive bacteria). Even the sloughing off of dead skin cells removes potential pathogens from the skin.

In addition to being sticky, the mucus produced at mucous membranes contains a variety of substances (e.g., lysozyme, lactoferrin, lactoperoxidase) that can kill bacteria or inhibit their growth. As previously mentioned, lysozyme destroys bacterial cell walls by degrading peptidoglycan. *Lactoferrin* is a protein that binds iron, a mineral that is required by all pathogens. Because they are unable to compete with lactoferrin for free iron, the pathogens are deprived of this essential nutrient. *Lactoperoxidase* is an enzyme that produces superoxide radicals, highly reactive forms of oxygen, which are toxic to bacteria.

Sticky mucous serves as a nonspecific host defense mechanism by trapping pathogens. It also contains toxic substances, such as lysozyme, lactoferrin, and lactoperoxidase.

Because mucosal cells are among the most rapidly dividing cells in the body, they are constantly being produced and released from mucous membranes. Bacteria that are adhering to the cells are often expelled along with the cells to which they are attached.

The respiratory system would be particularly accessible to invaders that could ride in on dust or other particles inhaled with each breath were it not for the hair, mucous membranes, and irregular chambers of the nose that serve to trap much of the inhaled debris. Also, the cilia (mucociliary covering) present on epithelial cells of the posterior nasal membranes, nasal sinuses, bronchi, and trachea sweep the trapped dust and microbes upward toward the throat, where they are swallowed or expelled by sneezing and coughing. Damage to these ciliated epithelial cells (e.g., damage caused by smoking, other pollutants, bacterial or viral respiratory infections) can increase a person's susceptibility to bacterial respiratory infections. Phagocytes in the mucous membranes may also be involved in this mucociliary clearance mechanism.

The mucociliary covering on epithelial cells in the respiratory tract move trapped dust and microbes upward toward the throat, where they are swallowed or expelled.

Lysozyme and other enzymes that lyse or destroy bacteria are present in nasal secretions, saliva, and tears. Even the swallowing of saliva can be thought of as a nonspecific host defense mechanism, because thousands of bacteria are removed from the oral cavity every time we swallow. Humans swallow approximately 1 L of saliva per day.

To a certain extent, the following factors protect the gastrointestinal (GI) tract from bacterial colonization and are therefore considered to be non-specific host defense mechanisms:

> Pathogens entering the GI tract are often killed by digestive enzymes or the acidity or alkalinity of different anatomical regions.

- Digestive enzymes
- Acidity of the stomach (approximately pH 1.5)
- Alkalinity of the intestines

Bile, which is secreted from the liver into the small intestine, lowers the surface tension and causes chemical changes in bacterial cell walls and membranes that make bacteria easier to digest. As a result of the combination of stomach acid, bile salts, and the rapid flow of its contents, the small intestine is relatively free of bacteria. Many invading microorganisms are trapped in the sticky, mucous lining of the digestive tract, where they may be destroyed by bactericidal enzymes and phagocytes. Peristalsis and the expulsion of feces serve to remove bacteria from the intestine. Bacteria make up about 50% of feces.

> Peristalsis and urination serve to remove pathogens from the GI tract and urinary tract, respectively.

The urinary tract is usually sterile in healthy persons, with the exception of indigenous microorganisms that colonize the distal urethra (that part of the urethra furthest from the urinary bladder). Microorganisms are continually flushed from the urethra by frequent urination and expulsion of mucus secretions. Many urinary bladder infections result from infrequent urination, including the failure to urinate after intercourse. Conditions that obstruct urine flow (e.g., benign prostatic hyperplasia [BPH]) also increase the chances of developing cystitis. The low pH of vaginal fluid usually inhibits colonization of the vagina by pathogens. However, women who are taking certain oral contraceptives are particularly susceptible to some infections because the contraceptives increase the pH of the vagina.

> The acidity of vaginal fluid usually inhibits colonization of the vagina by pathogens.

Microbial Antagonism

As mentioned in Chapter 10, when resident microbes of the indigenous microflora prevent colonization by new arrivals to a particular anatomical site, it is known as *microbial antagonism.* This is another example of a

> When indigenous microflora prevent the establishment of arriving pathogens, it is known as microbial antagonism.

nonspecific host defense mechanism. The inhibitory capability of the indigenous microflora has been attributed to the following factors:

- Competition for colonization sites
- Competition for nutrients
- Production of substances that kill other bacteria

It is thought that the indigenous microflora of the skin, oral cavity, upper respiratory tract, and colon play a major role as a nonspecific host defense mechanism by preventing pathogens and potential pathogens from colonizing these sites. The effectiveness of microbial antagonism is frequently decreased after prolonged administration of broad-spectrum antibiotics. The antibiotics reduce or eliminate certain members of the indigenous microflora (e.g., the vaginal and gastrointestinal flora), leading to overgrowth by bacteria or fungi that are resistant to the antibiotic(s) being administered. This overgrowth or "population explosion" of organisms is called a *superinfection*. A superinfection of *Candida albicans* in the vagina may lead to the condition known as yeast vaginitis. A superinfection of *Clostridium difficile* in the colon may lead to *C. difficile*–associated diseases known as antibiotic-associated diarrhea (AAD) and pseudomembranous colitis (PMC).

> A decrease in the number of indigenous microflora at a particular anatomical site can lead to an overgrowth of pathogens or opportunistic pathogens present at the site; this is referred to as a *superinfection.*

Some bacteria produce proteins that kill other bacteria; collectively, these antibacterial substances are known as *bacteriocins*. An example is *colicin*, which is produced by certain strains of *Escherichia coli*. Similar antibacterial substances are produced by some strains of *Pseudomonas* and *Bacillus* species as well as by certain other bacteria. Bacteriocins have a narrower range of activity than do antibiotics, but they are more potent than antibiotics.

> Colicin and other bacteriocins are proteins produced by some bacteria to kill other bacteria.

SECOND LINE OF DEFENSE

Pathogens able to penetrate the first line of defense are usually destroyed by nonspecific cellular and chemical responses, collectively referred to as the second line of defense. A complex sequence of events develops involving production of fever, production of interferons, activation of the complement system, inflammation, chemotaxis, and phagocytosis. Each of these responses is discussed in this chapter.

> Transferrin, fever, interferons, the complement system, inflammation, and phagocytosis are all part of the second line of defense.

Transferrin

Transferrin, a glycoprotein synthesized in the liver, has a high affinity for iron. Its normal function is to store and deliver iron to host cells. Like lactoferrin (mentioned earlier), transferrin serves as a nonspecific host defense mechanism by sequestering iron and depriving pathogens of this essential nutrient. Studies have shown that transferrin levels in the blood increase dramatically in response to systemic bacterial infections.

> Transferrin serves as a host defense mechanism by depriving pathogens of iron.

Fever

Normal body temperature fluctuates between 36.2°C and 37.5°C (97.2°F and 99.5°F), with an average of about 37°C (98.6°F). A body temperature greater than 37.8°C (100°F) is generally considered to be a fever. Substances that stimulate the production of fever are called *pyrogens* or *pyrogenic substances*. Pyrogens may originate either outside or inside the body. Those from outside the body include pathogens and various pyrogenic substances that they produce or release (e.g., endotoxin). Interleukin 1 (IL-1) is an example of a pyrogen that is produced within the body (i.e., it is an endogenous pyrogen). The resulting increased body temperature (fever) is considered to be a nonspecific host defense mechanism.

> Substances that stimulate the production of fever are called pyrogens or pyrogenic substances.

Fever augments the host's defenses in the following ways:

- By stimulating white blood cells (leukocytes) to deploy and destroy invaders
- By reducing available free plasma iron, which limits the growth of pathogens that require iron for replication and synthesis of toxins
- By inducing the production of IL-1, which causes the proliferation, maturation, and activation of lymphocytes in the immunologic response

Elevated body temperatures also slow down the rate of growth of certain pathogens and can even kill some especially fastidious pathogens.

> A fever can slow down the rate of growth of certain pathogens and can even kill some especially fastidious ones.

The following scenario illustrates one way in which fever develops during an infectious disease:

1. A patient has septicemia caused by Gram-negative bacteria (referred to as *Gram-negative sepsis*). Recall from Chapter 13 that septicemia is a serious disease characterized by chills, fever, prostration, and the presence of bacteria or their toxins in the bloodstream.

2. The bacteria release endotoxin into the patient's bloodstream. (Endotoxin is part of the cell wall structure of Gram-negative bacteria; it is the lipid component of lipopolysaccharide.)
3. Phagocytes ingest (phagocytize) the endotoxin.
4. The ingested endotoxin stimulates the phagocytes to produce IL-1, an endogenous pyrogen. IL-1 is produced primarily by macrophages.
5. IL-1 stimulates the hypothalamus (a part of the brain referred to as the body's thermostat) to produce prostaglandins.
6. Once metabolized, the prostaglandins cause the hypothalamic thermostat to be set at a higher level.
7. The increased thermostatic reading sends out signals to the nerves surrounding peripheral blood vessels. This causes the vessels to contract, thus conserving heat.
8. The increased body heat, resulting from vasoconstriction, continues until the temperature of the blood supplying the hypothalamus matches the elevated thermostat reading. The thermostat can be reset to the normal body temperature when the concentration of endogenous pyrogen decreases.

There are, of course, detrimental aspects of fever—especially prolonged high fevers. These include increased heart rate, increased metabolic rate, increased caloric demand, and mild to severe dehydration.

Interferons

Interferons are small, antiviral proteins produced by virus-infected cells. They are called interferons because they "interfere" with viral replication. The three known types of interferon, referred to as alpha (α), beta (β), and gamma (γ) interferons, are induced by different stimuli, including viruses, tumors, bacteria, and other foreign cells. The different types of interferons are produced by different type of cells. α-Interferon is produced by B lymphocytes (B cells), monocytes, and macrophages; β-interferon, by fibroblasts and other virus-infected cells; and γ-interferon, by activated T lymphocytes (T cells) and natural killer cells (NK cells).

> Interferons are small, antiviral proteins produced by virus-infected cells. They interfere with viral replication.

The interferons produced by a virus-infected cell are unable to save that cell from destruction, but once they are released from that cell, they attach to the membranes of surrounding cells and prevent viral replication from occurring in those cells. Thus, the spread of the infection is inhibited, allowing other body defenses to fight the disease more effectively. In this way, many viral diseases (e.g., colds, influenza, and measles) are limited in duration. Similarly, the acute phase of herpes simplex cold sores is of limited duration. The herpesvirus then enters a latent phase and hides in nerve ganglion cells where it is protected until the person's defenses are down; the cycle of disease and latency is repeated over and over.

Interferons are not virus-specific, meaning that they are effective against a variety of viruses, not just the particular type of virus that stimulated their production. Interferons are species-specific, however, meaning that they are effective only in the species of animal that produced them. Thus, rabbit interferons are only effective in rabbits and could not be used to treat viral infections in humans. Human interferons are industrially produced by genetically engineered bacteria (bacteria into which human interferon genes have been inserted) and are used experimentally to treat certain viral infections (e.g., warts, herpes simplex, hepatitis B and C) and cancers (e.g., leukemias, lymphomas, Kaposi sarcoma in patients with acquired immune deficiency syndrome or acquired immunodeficiency syndrome [AIDS]). In addition to interfering with viral multiplication, interferons also activate certain lymphocytes (NK cells) to kill virus-infected cells. NK cells are discussed in Chapter 16.

> Interferons are not virus-specific, but they are host-specific.

In addition to the beneficial aspects of the interferons that are produced in response to certain viral infections, they actually cause the nonspecific flulike symptoms (malaise, myalgia, chills, fever) that are associated with many viral infections.

The Complement System

Complement is not a single entity, but rather a group of approximately 30 different proteins (including nine proteins designated as C1 through C9) that are found in normal blood plasma. These proteins make up what is called "the complement system"—so named because it is complementary to the action of the immune system. The proteins of the complement system, sometimes collectively referred to as complement components, interact with each other in a stepwise manner, known as the **complement cascade**. A discussion of the somewhat complex steps in the complement cascade is beyond the scope of this book. What is of primary importance is that activation of the complement system is considered a nonspecific host defense mechanism; it assists in the destruction of many different pathogens.

> The proteins of the complement system (collectively referred to as complement components) interact with each other in a stepwise manner, known as the complement cascade—a nonspecific host defense mechanism that assists in the destruction of many different pathogens.

The major consequences of complement activation are listed here:

- Initiation and amplification of inflammation
- Attraction of phagocytes to sites where they are needed (chemotaxis; to be discussed later)
- Activation of leukocytes
- Lysis of bacteria and other foreign cells
- Increased phagocytosis by phagocytic cells (opsonization)

See this book's CD-ROM for "A Closer Look at the Complement System."

Opsonization is a process by which phagocytosis is facilitated by the deposition of **opsonins**, such as antibodies or certain complement fragments, onto the surface of particles or cells. In some cases, phagocytes are unable to ingest certain particles or cells (e.g., encapsulated bacteria) until opsonization occurs. One of the products formed during the complement cascade, called C3b, is an opsonin. It is deposited on the surface of microorganisms. Neutrophils and macrophages possess surface molecules (receptors) that can recognize and bind to C3b.

> Opsonization is a process by which phagocytosis is facilitated by the deposition of opsonins (e.g., antibodies or certain complement fragments) onto the surface of particles or cells.

Complement fragments C3a, C4a, and C5a cause mast cells to degranulate and release histamine, leading to increased vascular permeability and smooth muscle contraction. (Mast cells are discussed in Chapter 16.) C5a also acts as a chemoattractant (chemotactic agent) for neutrophils and macrophages. Chemoattractants are discussed later in the chapter.

There are a variety of hereditary complement deficiencies that interfere with activities of the complement system. Some of these inherited deficiencies are associated with defects in activation of the classical pathway.[b] A deficiency of C3 leads to a defect in activation of both the classical and alternative pathways. Defects of properdin factors impair activation of the alternative pathway. Any of these defects leads to increased susceptibility to pyogenic (pus-producing) staphylococcal and streptococcal infections.

Acute-Phase Proteins

Plasma levels of molecules collectively referred to as *acute-phase proteins* increase rapidly in response to infection, inflammation, and tissue injury. They serve as host defense mechanisms by enhancing resistance to infection and promoting the repair of damaged tissue. Acute-phase proteins include C-reactive protein (which is used as a laboratory marker for, or indication of, inflammation), serum amyloid A protein, protease inhibitors, and coagulation proteins.

Cytokines

Cytokines are chemical mediators that are released from many different types of cells in the human body. They enable cells to communicate with each other. They act as chemical messengers both within the immune system (discussed in Chapter 16) and

> Cytokines are chemical mediators that are released from many different types of cells in the human body. They act as chemical messengers, enabling cells to communicate with each other.

---

[b] As explained on the CD-ROM, the complement system can be activated by any of three pathways: the classical (or classic) pathway, the alternative pathway, and the lectin pathway.

between the immune system and other systems of the body. A cell is able to "sense" the presence of a cytokine if it possesses appropriate surface receptors that can recognize the cytokine. The cytokine mediates (causes) some type of response in a cell that is able to sense its presence. Some cytokines are chemoattractants (to be discussed later), recruiting phagocytes to locations where they are needed. Others, like interferons (previously discussed), have a direct role in host defense.

Inflammation

The body normally responds to any local injury, irritation, microbial invasion, or bacterial toxin by a complex series of events collectively referred to as **inflammation** or the *inflammatory response* (Fig. 15-3). The

> The three major events in acute inflammation are vasodilation, increased permeability of the capillaries, and escape of leukocytes from the capillaries.

three major events in acute inflammation are:

- An increase in the diameter of capillaries (**vasodilation**), which increases blood flow to the site
- Increased permeability of the capillaries, allowing the escape of plasma and plasma proteins
- Escape of leukocytes from the capillaries and their accumulation at the site of injury

The primary purposes of the inflammatory response (Fig. 15-4) are to:

- Localize an infection
- Prevent the spread of microbial invaders
- Neutralize any toxins being produced at the site
- Aid in the repair of damaged tissue

> The primary purposes of the inflammatory response are to localize an infection, prevent the spread of microbial invaders, neutralize toxins, and aid in the repair of damaged tissue.

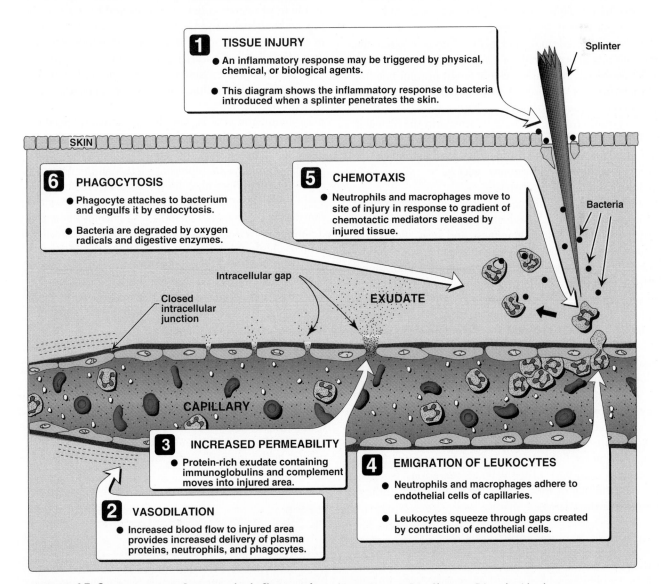

FIGURE 15-3. Sequence of events in inflammation. (From Harvey RA, Champe RA, eds. Lippincott Illustrated Reviews: Microbiology. Philadelphia: Lippincott Williams & Wilkins, 2001.)

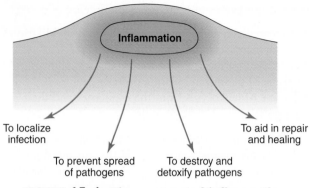

To localize infection

To prevent spread of pathogens

To destroy and detoxify pathogens

To aid in repair and healing

FIGURE 15-4. The purposes of inflammation.

During the inflammatory process, many nonspecific host defense mechanisms come into play. These interrelated physiologic reactions result in the four cardinal (main) signs and symptoms of inflammation: redness, heat, swelling (**edema**), and pain.[c] There is often pus formation, and occasionally a loss of function of the damaged area (e.g., an inflamed elbow might prevent bending of the arm).

> The four cardinal or main signs and symptoms of inflammation are redness, heat, swelling (edema), and pain.

A complex series of physiologic events occurs immediately after the initial damage to the tissue. One of the initial events is vasodilation at the site of injury, mediated by vasoactive agents (e.g., histamine and prostaglandins) released from damaged cells. Vasodilation allows more blood to flow to the site, bringing redness and heat. Additional heat results from increased metabolic activities in the tissue cells at the site. Vasodilation causes the endothelial cells that line the capillaries to stretch and separate, resulting in increased permeability. Plasma escapes from the capillaries into the surrounding area, causing the site to become **edematous** (swollen). Sometimes the swelling is severe enough to interfere with the bending of a particular joint (e.g., knuckle, elbow, knee, ankle), leading to a loss of function.

> Vasodilation—an increase in the diameter of capillaries—leads to redness, heat, and edema.

A variety of chemotactic agents (to be discussed later) are produced at the site of inflammation, leading to an influx of phagocytes. The pain or tenderness that accompanies inflammation may result from actual damage of the nerve fibers because of the injury, irritation by microbial toxins or other cellular secretions (such as prostaglandins), or increased pressure on nerve endings because of the edema.

The accumulation of fluid, cells, and cellular debris at the inflammation site is referred to as an **inflammatory** *exudate*. If the exudate is thick and greenish yellow, containing many live and dead leukocytes, it is known as a **purulent exudate** or *pus*. However, in many inflammatory responses, such as arthritis or pancreatitis, there is no exudate and are no invading microorganisms. When **pyogenic microbes** (pus-producing microbes), such as staphylococci and streptococci, are present, additional pus is produced as a result of the killing effect of bacterial toxins on phagocytes and tissue cells. Although most pus is greenish yellow, the exudate is often bluish green in infections caused by *Pseudomonas aeruginosa*. This is caused by the bluish green pigment (called *pyocyanin*) produced by this organism.

> A purulent inflammatory exudate is often referred to as pus.

When the inflammatory response is over and the body has won the battle, phagocytes clean up the area and help to restore order. The cells and tissues can then repair the damage and begin to function normally again in a homeostatic (equilibrated) state, although some permanent damage and scarring may result.

The lymphatic system—including lymph (the fluid component of the lymphatic system), lymphatic vessels, lymph nodes, and lymphatic organs (tonsils, spleen, and thymus gland)—also plays an important role in defending the body against invaders. The primary functions of this system include draining and circulating intercellular fluids from the tissues and transporting digested fats from the digestive system to the blood. Also, macrophages, B cells, and T cells in the lymph nodes serve to filter the lymph by removing foreign matter and microbes, and by producing antibodies and other factors to aid in the destruction and detoxification of any invading microbes.

> The primary functions of the lymphatic system include draining and circulating intercellular fluids from tissues, transporting digested fats from the digestive system to the blood, removing foreign matter and microbes from the lymph, and producing antibodies and other factors to aid in the destruction and detoxification of any invading microbes.

The body continually wages war against damage, injury, malfunction, and microbial invasion. The outcome of each battle depends on the person's age, hormonal balance, genetic resistance, and overall state of physical and mental health, as well as the virulence of the pathogens involved.

---

[c] In his written work, *De Medicina* (*On Medicine*), Aulus Cornelius Celsus, a Roman encyclopedist who lived and died before the time of Christ, described the cardinal signs of inflammation using the Latin terms *rubor* (redness), *calor* (warmth), *dolor* (pain), and *tumor* (swelling). These Latin terms are sometimes taught in Physiology courses.

STUDY AID
Beware of Similar Sounding Terms
Pyrogenic substances (pyrogens) are fever-producing substances. Pyogenic means pus-producing; thus, pyogenic microbes are pus-producing microbes.

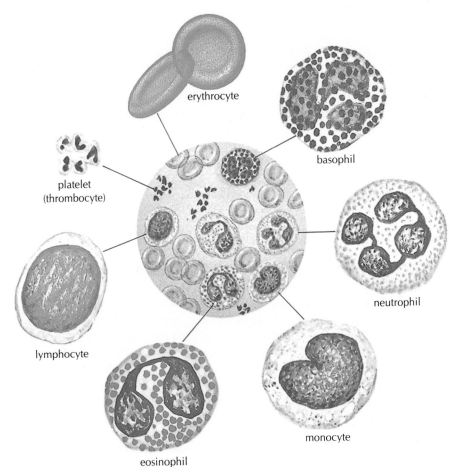

FIGURE 15-5. Cellular elements of the blood, as seen in a Wright's-stained peripheral blood smear. Wright's stain contains two dyes: eosin (a reddish orange acidic dye, which stains basic substances) and methylene blue (a dark blue dye, which stains acidic substances). Eosinophil granules stain reddish orange because their contents are basic and, therefore, attract the acidic dye. Basophil granules stain dark blue because their contents are acidic and, therefore, attract the basic dye. The contents of neutrophil granules are neutral (neither basic nor acidic) and, therefore attract neither the acidic dye nor the basic dye. (From McCall RE, Tankersley CM. Phlebotomy Essentials, 2nd ed. Philadelphia: Lippincott-Raven Publishers, 1998.)

Labels on figure: erythrocyte, basophil, platelet (thrombocyte), neutrophil, lymphocyte, monocyte, eosinophil

Phagocytosis

The cellular elements of blood are shown in Figure 15-5. Recall from Chapter 13 that the three major categories of leukocytes found in blood are monocytes, lymphocytes, and granulocytes. The three types of granulocytes are neutrophils, eosinophils, and basophils.

The three major categories of leukocytes found in blood are monocytes, lymphocytes, and granulocytes.

Phagocytic white blood cells are called **phagocytes**, and the process by which phagocytes surround and engulf (ingest) foreign material is called **phagocytosis**. The two most important groups of phagocytes in the human body are macrophages and neutrophils; they are some-

The two most important groups of phagocytes in the human body—sometimes referred to as "professional phagocytes"—are macrophages and neutrophils.

times called "professional phagocytes," because phagocytosis is their major function.[d] Macrophages serve as a "clean-up crew" to rid the body of unwanted and often harmful substances, such as dead cells, unused cellular secretions, debris, and microorganisms.

Granulocytes are named for the prominent cytoplasmic granules that they possess. Phagocytic granulocytes include **neutrophils** and **eosinophils**. Neutrophils (also known as polymorphonuclear cells, polys, and PMNs) are much more efficient at phagocytosis than eosinophils. An abnormally high number of eosinophils in the peripheral

Granulocytes include basophils, eosinophils, and neutrophils.

STUDY AID
Cellular Elements of Blood
Erythrocytes (red blood cells)
Thrombocytes (platelets)
Leukocytes (white blood cells)
   Granulocytes
      Basophils
      Eosinophils
      Neutrophils
   Monocytes/Macrophages
   Lymphocytes
      B cells
      T cells
         Helper T cells (T_H cells)
         Cytotoxic T cells (T_C cells)
      Natural killer cells (NK cells)

---

[d] Macrophages and neutrophils are not the only body cells capable of phagocytosis, but they are the most important phagocytic cells.

bloodstream is known as **eosinophilia**. Examples of conditions that cause eosinophilia are allergies and helminth infections. A third type of granulocyte, **basophils**, are also involved in allergic and inflammatory reactions, although they are not phagocytes. Basophil granules contain histamine and other chemical mediators. Basophils are further discussed in Chapter 16.

Macrophages develop from a type of leukocyte called **monocytes** during the inflammatory response to infections. Those that leave the bloodstream and migrate to infected areas are called **wandering macrophages**. **Fixed macrophages** (also known as *histocytes* or *histiocytes*) remain within tissues and organs and serve to trap foreign debris. Macrophages are extremely efficient phagocytes. They are found in tissues of the **reticuloendothelial system** (RES). This nonspecific defensive system includes cells in the liver (Kupffer cells), spleen, lymph nodes, and bone marrow as well as the lungs (alveolar or dust cells), blood vessels, intestines, and brain (microglia). The principal function of the entire RES is the engulfment and removal of foreign and useless particles, living or dead, such as excess cellular secretions, dead and dying leukocytes, erythrocytes, and tissue cells as well as foreign debris and microorganisms that gain entrance to the body.

> Wandering macrophages leave the bloodstream and migrate to sites of infection and other areas where they are needed. Fixed macrophages remain within tissues and organs.

The four steps in phagocytosis are chemotaxis, attachment, ingestion, and digestion. They are discussed next and are summarized in Table 15-1.

Chemotaxis

Phagocytosis begins when phagocytes move to the site where they are needed. This directed migration is called **chemotaxis** and is the result of

> The directed migration of phagocytes is called chemotaxis. It is caused by chemicals referred to as chemotactic agents.

chemical attractants referred to as **chemotactic agents** (also called chemotactic factors, chemotactic substances, and chemoattractants). Chemotactic agents that are produced by various cells of the human body are called **chemokines**.[e] Chemotactic agents are produced during the complement cascade and inflammation. The phagocytes move along a concentration gradient, meaning that they move from areas of low concentrations of chemotactic agents to the area of highest concentration. The area of highest concentration is the site where the chemotactic agents are being produced or released—often the site of inflammation. Thus, the phagocytes are attracted to the site where they are needed. Different types of chemotactic agents attract different types of leukocytes; some attract monocytes, others neutrophils, and still others eosinophils.

Attachment

The next step in phagocytosis is attachment of the phagocyte to the object (e.g., a yeast or bacterial cell) to be ingested. Phagocytes can only ingest objects to which they can attach.

> In opsonization, a particle becomes coated with opsonins—either complement fragments or antibodies.

As previously mentioned, opsonization is sometimes necessary to enable phagocytes to attach to certain particles (e.g., encapsulated bacteria). In opsonization, the particle becomes coated with opsonins (either complement fragments or antibodies). Because the phagocyte possesses surface molecules (receptors) for complement fragments and antibodies, the phagocyte can now attach to the particle (Fig. 15-6).

Ingestion

The phagocyte then surrounds the object with pseudopodia, which fuse together, and the object is ingested (is phagocytized or phagocytosed) (Fig. 15-7). Phagocytosis is one type of endocytosis, the process of ingesting material from outside a cell. Within the cytoplasm of the phagocyte, the object is contained within a membrane-bound vesicle called a **phagosome**.

> During ingestion, the particle becomes surrounded by a membrane. The membrane-bound vesicle is called a phagosome.

Digestion

The phagosome next fuses with a nearby lysosome to form a digestive vacuole (**phagolysosome**), within which killing and digestion occur (Fig. 15-8). Recall from Chapter 3 that

> The fusion of a lysosome and a phagosome results in a phagolysosome, within which the ingested particle is digested.

TABLE 15-1	Four Steps in Phagocytosis
STEP	**BRIEF DESCRIPTION**
1. Chemotaxis	Phagocytes are attracted by chemotactic agents to the site where they are needed
2. Attachment	A phagocyte attaches to an object
3. Ingestion	Pseudopodia surround the object, and it is taken into the cell
4. Digestion	The object is broken down and dissolved by digestive enzymes and other mechanisms

---

[e] Various types of cells within the human body, including cells of the immune system, communicate with each other. They do so by means of chemical messages—proteins known as cytokines. If the cytokines are chemotactic agents, attracting leukocytes to areas where they are needed, they are referred to as chemokines.

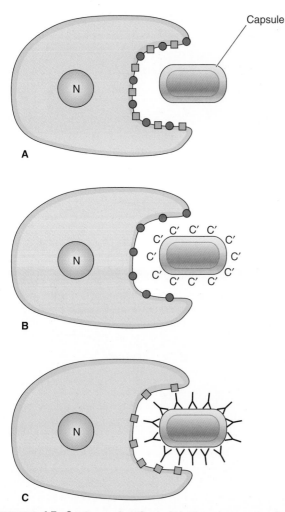

FIGURE 15-6. Opsonization. (A) The phagocyte shown here is unable to attach to the encapsulated bacterium because there are no molecules (receptors) on the surface of the phagocyte that can recognize or attach to the polysaccharide capsule. **(B)** Complement fragments (represented by the symbol C′) have been deposited onto the surface of the capsule. (In this example, the opsonins are complement fragments.) Now the phagocyte can attach to the bacterium because there are receptors (represented by ●) on the phagocyte's surface that can recognize and bind to complement fragments. **(C)** Antibodies (the Y-shaped molecules) have attached to the capsule. (In this example, the opsonins are antibodies.) Now the phagocyte can attach to the bacterium because there are receptors (represented by ■) on the phagocyte's surface that can recognize and bind to the Fc region of antibody molecules. (See text for additional details.) *N*, nucleus.

lysosomes are membrane-bound vesicles containing digestive enzymes. Digestive enzymes found within lysosomes include lysozyme, β-lysin, lipases, proteases, peptidases, DNAses, and RNAses, which degrade carbohydrates, lipids, proteins, and nucleic acids.

Other mechanisms also participate in the destruction of phagocytized microorganisms. In neutrophils, for example, a membrane-bound enzyme called nicotinamide adenine dinucleotide phosphate (NADPH) oxidase reduces oxygen to very destructive products such as superoxide anions, hydroxyl radicals, hydrogen peroxide, and singlet oxygen. These highly reactive reduction products assist in the destruction of the ingested microbes. Another killing mechanism involves the enzyme myeloperoxidase. After lysosome fusion, myeloperoxidase is released, which in the presence of hydrogen peroxide and chloride ion, produces a potent microbicidal agent called hypochlorous acid.

Figures 15-9 and 15-10 depict *Giardia lamblia* trophozoites being phagocytized by rat leukocytes. *G. lamblia* (also known as *Giardia intestinalis*) is a flagellated protozoan parasite that causes a diarrheal disease known as giardiasis. These photomicrographs and electron micrographs were taken during a laboratory research project involving opsonization of *Giardia* trophozoites.

Mechanisms by which Pathogens Escape Destruction by Phagocytes

During the initial phases of infection, capsules serve an antiphagocytic function, protecting encapsulated bacteria from being phagocytized. Some **Some bacteria and protozoa are able to survive within phagocytes.** bacteria produce an exoenzyme (referred to as a toxin by some scientists) called *leukocidin*, which kills phagocytes. As mentioned in Chapter 14, not all bacteria engulfed by phagocytes are destroyed within phagolysosomes. For example, waxes in the cell wall of *Mycobacterium tuberculosis* protect the organism from digestion. The bacteria are even able to multiply within the phagocytes and are transported within them to other parts of the body. Other pathogens that are able to survive within phagocytes include bacteria such as *Rickettsia rickettsii*, *Legionella pneumophila*, *Brucella abortus*, *Coxiella burnetii*, *Listeria monocytogenes*, and *Salmonella* spp., as well as protozoan parasites such as *Toxoplasma gondii*, *Trypanosoma cruzi*, and *Leishmania* spp. The mechanism by which each pathogen evades digestion by lysosomal enzymes differs from one pathogen to another; in some cases, the mechanism is not yet understood. These pathogens may remain dormant within phagocytes for months or years before they escape to cause disease. Thus, these types of virulent pathogens usually win the battle with phagocytes. Unless antibodies or complement fragments are present to aid in the destruction of these pathogens, the infection may progress unchecked.

Ehrlichia and *Anaplasma* spp., closely related to rickettsias, are obligate, intracellular, Gram-negative bacteria that live within leukocytes (i.e., they are *intraleukocytic pathogens*). **_Ehrlichia_ and _Anaplasma_ spp. are intraleukocytic bacteria, able to live and multiply within leukocytes.** These organisms cause two endemic, tickborne diseases in the United States. *Ehrlichia* spp. cause human monocytic

FIGURE 15-7. The ingestion phase of phagocytosis. (A) A phagocyte has attached to a bacterial cell. **(B)** Pseudopodia extend around the bacterial cell. **(C)** The pseudopodia meet and fuse together. **(D)** The bacterial cell, surrounded by a membrane, is now inside the phagocyte. The membrane-bound structure, containing the ingested bacterial cell, is called a phagosome. *N*, nucleus.

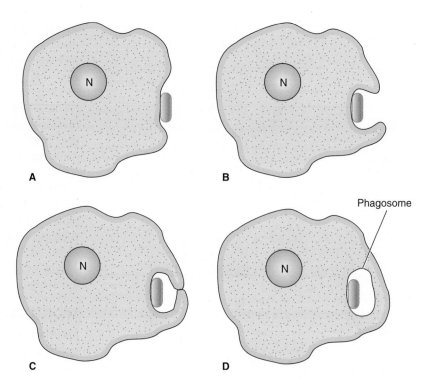

FIGURE 15-8. The digestion phase of phagocytosis. (A) A lysosome, containing digestive enzymes, approaches a phagosome. **(B)** The lysosome membrane fuses with the phagosome membrane. **(C)** The lysosome and phagosome become a single membrane-bound vesicle, known as a phagolysosome. The phagolysosome contains the ingested bacterial cell plus digestive enzymes. **(D)** The bacterial cell is digested within the phagolysosome. *N*, nucleus.

FIGURE 15-9. Photomicrograph of rat leukocytes, some of which contain phagocytized *Giardia* trophozoites. The phagocytosis occurred under experimental conditions in a research laboratory. (Provided by S. Koester and P. Engelkirk.)

ehrlichiosis (HME), a condition in which the bacteria infect monocytic phagocytes. *Anaplasma* spp. cause human anaplasmosis (or human granulocytic ehrlichiosis [HE], as it is sometimes called), a condition in which the bacteria infect granulocytes. The bacteria are somehow able to prevent the fusion of lysosomes with phagosomes.

Disorders and Conditions that Adversely Affect Phagocytic and Inflammatory Processes

Leukopenia

Some patients have an abnormally low number of circulating leukocytes—a condition known as **leukopenia**. (Although the terms *leukopenia* and *neutropenia* are often used synonymously, they are not

> Leukopenia—an abnormally low number of circulating leukocytes. Neutropenia—an abnormally low number of circulating neutrophils.

really synonyms. Technically, neutropenia is an abnormally low number of circulating neutrophils; neutropenia = neutrophilic leukopenia.) Leukopenia may result from bone marrow injury as a result of ionizing radiation or drugs, nutritional deficiencies, or congenital stem cell defects.

Disorders and Conditions Affecting Leukocyte Motility and Chemotaxis

The inability of leukocytes to migrate in response to chemotactic agents may be related to a defect in the production of actin, a structural protein associated with motility. Some drugs (e.g., corticosteroids) can also inhibit the chemotactic activity of leukocytes. Decreased neutrophil chemotaxis also occurs in the inherited childhood disease known as Chediak-Higashi syndrome (CHS). In addition, the PMNs of individuals with CHS contain abnormal lysosomes that do not readily fuse with phagosomes, resulting in decreased bactericidal activity. CHS is characterized by symptoms such as albinism, central nervous system abnormalities, and recurrent bacterial infections.

FIGURE 15-10. Scanning electron micrographs (A,B) illustrating the phagocytosis of *Giardia* trophozoites (G) by rat leukocytes (L). The phagocytosis occurred under experimental conditions in a research laboratory. (Provided by S. Erlandsen and P. Engelkirk.)

TABLE 15-2	Additional Factors that Can Impair Host Defense Mechanisms
FACTOR	**COMMENTS**
Nutritional status	Malnutrition is accompanied by decreased resistance to infections
Increased iron levels	High concentrations of iron make it easier for bacteria to satisfy their iron requirements; high concentrations of iron reduce the chemotactic and phagocytic activities of phagocytes; increased iron levels may result from a variety of conditions or habits
Stress	People living under stressful conditions are more susceptible to infections than people living under less stressful conditions
Age	Newborn infants lack a fully developed immune system; the efficiency of the immune system and other host defenses declines after age 50
Cancer and cancer chemotherapy	Cancer chemotherapeutic agents kill healthy cells and malignant ones
AIDS	Destruction of the AIDS patient's helper T cells (T_H cells) decreases the patient's ability to produce antibodies to certain pathogens (discussed in Chapter 16)
Drugs	Steroids and alcohol, for example
Various genetic defects	B-cell and T-cell deficiencies, for example

Disorders and Conditions Affecting Intracellular Killing by Phagocytes

The phagocytes of some individuals are capable of ingesting bacteria, but are incapable of killing certain species. This is usually the result of deficiencies in myeloperoxidase or an inability to generate superoxide anion, hydrogen peroxide, or hypochlorite. Chronic granulomatous disease (CGD) is an often fatal genetic disorder that is characterized by repeated bacterial infections. The PMNs of individuals with CGD can ingest bacteria but cannot kill certain species. In one form of CGD, the person's PMNs are unable to produce hydrogen peroxide. In another hereditary disorder, the individual's PMNs completely lack myeloperoxidase. Their PMNs do possess other microbicidal mechanisms, however, so these individuals usually do not experience recurrent infections.

Additional Factors

Table 15-2 lists some additional factors that can impair host defense mechanisms.

ON THE CD-ROM
- Terms Introduced in This Chapter
- Review of Key Points
- Increase Your Knowledge
- Critical Thinking
- Additional Self-Assessment Exercises

SELF-ASSESSMENT EXERCISES

After studying this chapter, answer the following multiple-choice questions.

1. Host defense mechanisms—ways in which the body protects itself from pathogens—can be thought of as an army consisting of how many lines of defense?
   a. two
   b. three
   c. four
   d. five

2. Which of the following is *not* part of the body's first line of defense?
   a. fever
   b. intact skin
   c. mucus
   d. pH of the stomach contents

3. Each of the following is considered a part of the body's second line of defense except:
   a. fever.
   b. inflammation.
   c. interferons.
   d. lysozyme.

4. Which of the following is *not* a consequence of activation of the complement system?
   a. attraction and activation of leukocytes
   b. increased phagocytosis by phagocytic cells (opsonization)
   c. lysis of bacteria and other foreign cells
   d. repair of damaged tissue

5. Each of the following is a primary purpose of the inflammatory response except:
    a. to localize the infection.
    b. to neutralize any toxins being produced at the site.
    c. to prevent the spread of microbial invaders.
    d. to stimulate the production of opsonins.
6. Which of the following cells is a granulocyte?
    a. eosinophil
    b. lymphocyte
    c. macrophage
    d. monocyte
7. All the following would be considered an aspect of microbial antagonism except:
    a. competition for nutrients.
    b. competition for space.
    c. production of bacteriocins.
    d. production of lysozyme.
8. Which of the following function as opsonins?
    a. antibodies
    b. antigens
    c. complement fragments
    d. both a and c
9. Which of the following statements about interferons is false?
    a. Interferons are virus-specific.
    b. Interferons have been used to treat hepatitis C and certain types of cancer.
    c. Interferons produced by a virus-infected cell will not save that cell from destruction.
    d. Interferons produced by virus-infected rabbit cells cannot be used to treat viral diseases in humans.
10. Which of the following is *not* one of the four cardinal signs or symptoms of inflammation?
    a. edema
    b. heat
    c. loss of function
    d. redness

16 SPECIFIC HOST DEFENSE MECHANISMS: AN INTRODUCTION TO IMMUNOLOGY

CHAPTER OUTLINE

LEARNING OBJECTIVES

AFTER STUDYING THIS CHAPTER, YOU SHOULD BE ABLE TO:

- Define the following terms: immunology, immunity, antigenic determinant, immunoglobulins, primary response, secondary response, agammaglobulinemia, hypogammaglobulinemia, T cell, B cell, plasma cell, and immunosuppression
- Differentiate between humoral and cell-mediated immunity (CMI)
- Distinguish between active acquired immunity and passive acquired immunity
- Distinguish between natural active acquired immunity and artificial active acquired immunity and cite an example of each
- Distinguish between natural passive acquired immunity and artificial passive acquired immunity and cite an example of each
- Outline the steps involved in the processing of T-independent antigens and T-dependent antigens
- Identify the two primary functions of the immune system
- Construct a diagram of a monomeric antibody molecule

- Identify and describe the five immunoglobulin classes (isotypes)
- List the types of cells that are killed by natural killer (NK) cells
- Name the four types of hypersensitivity reactions
- Outline the steps involved in allergic reactions, starting with the initial sensitization to an allergen and ending with the typical symptoms of an allergic reaction
- Cite six examples of allergens
- List five possible explanations for a positive tuberculosis (TB) skin test

INTRODUCTION

Immunology is the scientific study of the immune system and immune responses. Scientists who study various aspects of the immune system are called immunologists.

The immune system is considered to be a specific host defense mechanism and the third line of defense.

The immune system is considered to be the third line of defense. It is considered a *specific* host defense mechanism because it springs into action to defend against a specific pathogen (or other foreign object) that has gained entrance to the body.

Immune responses involve complex interactions among many different types of body cells and cellular secretions. Only certain basic fundamentals of immunology and immune responses are presented in this chapter. Topics briefly discussed here include active and passive acquired immunity to infectious agents, vaccines, antigens and antibodies, processes involved in antibody production, cell-mediated immune responses, allergies and other types of hypersensitivity reactions, autoimmune diseases, immunosuppression, and immunodiagnostic procedures (IDPs).

THE KEY TO UNDERSTANDING IMMUNOLOGY

An understanding of immunology boils down to an understanding of two terms: *antigens* and *antibodies*. For the moment, think of antigens as molecules (usually proteins) that stimulate a person's immune system to produce antibodies. Think of antibodies as protein molecules that a person's immune system produces in response to antigens. Later in the chapter, antigens and antibodies will be discussed in more detail. As you study this chapter, keep in mind that if you understand antigens and antibodies, you are well on your way to understanding immunology.

> Antigens are molecules that stimulate the immune system to produce antibodies. Antibodies are proteins produced by the immune system in response to antigens.

PRIMARY FUNCTIONS OF THE IMMUNE SYSTEM

According to accepted doctrine, the primary functions of the immune system are to:

- Differentiate between "self" and "nonself" (something foreign), and
- Destroy that which is nonself.[a]

> The primary functions of the immune system are to differentiate between "self" and "nonself" (something foreign), and destroy that which is nonself.

MAJOR ARMS OF THE IMMUNE SYSTEM

There are two major arms of the immune system: humoral immunity and CMI (Fig. 16-1).

Humoral immunity always involves the production of antibodies in response to antigens. After their production, these humoral (circulating) antibodies remain in blood plasma, lymph, and other body secretions where they protect against the specific pathogens that stimulated their production. Thus, in humoral immunity, a person is immune to a particular pathogen because of the presence of specific protective antibodies that are effective against that pathogen. Because

> Antibodies play a major role in humoral immunity, but play only a minor role, if any, in CMI.

---

[a] An Alternative Viewpoint. For more than 50 years, immunologists have relied on the self/nonself theory of immunity, which states that the immune system reacts to, or "does battle with," nonself (foreign molecules), but does not react to self (molecules that are part of the human body). However, there are certain immunologic events that are seemingly at odds with this theory. Recently, an alternative model of immunity has been proposed, called the Danger Model. This model "suggests that the immune system is more concerned with [tissue] damage than with foreignness, and is called into action by [danger or] alarm signals [emitted] from injured tissues, rather than by the recognition of nonself....When distressed, [the tissues] stimulate immunity, and...they may also determine the [specific type] of [immune] response." The immune response "is tailored to the tissue in which the response occurs, rather than being tailored by the targeted pathogen." Thus, "immunity is controlled by an internal conversation between tissues and the cells of the immune system." (From Matzinger P. The danger model: a renewed sense of self. Science 2002;296:301–305.)

FIGURE 16-1. The two major arms of the immune system.

humoral immunity is mediated by antibodies, it is also known as *antibody-mediated immunity* (AMI).

The second major arm of the immune system—**CMI**—involves various cell types, with antibodies only playing a minor role, if any. These immune responses are referred to as cell-mediated immune responses; they are briefly discussed later in this chapter.

> CMI involves various cell types, with antibodies only playing a minor role, if any.

IMMUNITY

A significant result of immune responses is to make a person resistant to certain infectious diseases. When one is resistant to a certain disease, one is said to be immune. The condition of being immune is usually referred to as **immunity**. Humans are immune to certain infectious diseases simply because they are humans. For example, humans are not infected with some of the pathogens that infect their pets. One explanation for this is that human cells do not possess the appropriate cell surface receptors for some of the pathogens that cause diseases of pets. Other reasons for this natural or innate resistance are far more complex and, in some cases, not fully understood, and will not be addressed here.

STUDY AID
Different Uses of the Term Resistant
As you have learned in previous chapters, bacteria can become resistant to certain antibiotics, meaning that they are no longer killed by those antibiotics. Such bacteria are said to be drug resistant. Humans do not become resistant to antibiotics. Humans can become resistant (immune) to certain infectious diseases, however, in ways that are discussed in this chapter.

What will be discussed in this section are the various types of immunities that humans acquire as life progresses, from conception onward—these types of immunity are collectively referred to as *acquired immunity*. Such immunity is often the result of the presence of protective antibodies that are directed against various pathogens.

Acquired Immunity

Immunity that results from the active production or receipt of protective antibodies during one's lifetime is called **acquired immunity**. If the antibodies are actually produced within the person's body, the immunity is called **active acquired immunity**; such protection is usually long lasting. In **passive acquired immunity**, the person receives antibodies that were produced by another person or by more than one person, or, in some cases, by an animal; such protection is usually only temporary. In either case, active or passive, the immunity may result from either a natural or an artificial event. The four categories of acquired immunity are summarized in Table 16-1.

> Immunity that results from the active production or receipt of protective antibodies during one's lifetime is called acquired immunity.

Active Acquired Immunity

There are two types of active acquired immunity:

> Acquired immunity may be the result of a natural or artificial event.

1. Natural (or naturally occurring) active acquired immunity, which, as the name implies, occurs naturally.
2. Artificial (or artificially occurring) active acquired immunity, which does not occur naturally; rather, it is artificially induced.

TABLE 16-1	Types of Acquired Immunity
ACTIVE ACQUIRED IMMUNITY	
Natural active acquired immunity	Immunity that is acquired in response to the entry of a live pathogen into the body (i.e., in response to an actual infection)
Artificial active acquired immunity	Immunity that is acquired in response to vaccines
PASSIVE ACQUIRED IMMUNITY	
Natural passive acquired immunity	Immunity that is acquired by a fetus when it receives maternal antibodies in utero or by an infant when it receives maternal antibodies contained in colostrum
Artificial passive acquired immunity	Immunity that is acquired when a person receives antibodies contained in antisera or gamma globulin

People who have had a specific infection usually have developed some resistance to reinfection by the causative pathogen because of the presence of antibodies and stimulated lymphocytes. This is called **natural active acquired immunity**. Symptoms of the disease may or may not be present when these antibodies are formed. Such resistance to reinfection may be permanent, lasting for a person's entire lifetime, or it may only be temporary. Antibodies that protect us from infection or reinfection are called **protective antibodies**. Sometimes, there is no immunity to reinfection after recovery from certain infectious diseases, even though antibodies are produced against the pathogens that cause these diseases. This is because the antibodies that are produced are *not* protective antibodies.

> Antibodies that protect us from infection or reinfection are called protective antibodies.

Artificial active acquired immunity is the second type of active acquired immunity. This type of immunity results when a person receives a vaccine. The administration of a vaccine (Fig. 16-2) stimulates a person's immune system to produce specific protective antibodies—antibodies that will protect the person should he or she become colonized with that particular pathogen in the future. Vaccines are discussed more fully in the following section.

> Immunity that results from receipt of a vaccine is called artificial active immunity.

Vaccines. The mere mention of the names of certain infectious diseases struck fear into the hearts of our ancestors. Today, thanks to childhood vaccines, residents of the United States rarely hear of those diseases, let alone live in fear of them. The Centers for Disease Control and Prevention (CDC) has stated that "Immunizations are one of the great public health success stories of the 20th century, having made once-common diseases such as diphtheria, measles, mumps, and pertussis diseases of the past. Vaccines are now available to protect children and adults against 15 life-threatening or debilitating diseases." (http://www.cdc.gov/vaccines)

FIGURE 16-2. Child receiving a vaccine. (Courtesy of Judy Schmidt, James Gathany, and the CDC.)

HISTORICAL NOTE

Vaccination

Since the time of the ancient Greeks, it has been observed that people who have recovered from certain infectious diseases, such as plague, smallpox, and yellow fever, rarely contract the same diseases again. The use of vaccines to prevent diseases may date as far back as the 11th century, when the Chinese used a powder prepared from dried smallpox scabs to immunize people, either by introducing the powder into a person's skin or by having the person inhale the powder. This method of preventing smallpox— using actual smallpox scabs—was known as the *Chinese method*. One of those immunized in this manner was Edward Jenner, a British physician. Some years later, Jenner investigated the widespread belief that milkmaids, who usually had clear, unblemished skin, never developed smallpox. He hypothesized that having had cowpox (a much milder disease than smallpox and one that leaves no scars) protected the milkmaids from getting smallpox. Jenner prepared a smallpox vaccine, using material obtained from cowpox lesions. People injected with Jenner's vaccine were protected from smallpox. The words "vaccine" and "vaccination" come from *vacca*, the Latin word for cow. Because Jenner was the first person to publish (in 1798) the successful results of vaccination, he is generally given credit for originating the concept. During the late 19th century, Louis Pasteur developed successful vaccines to prevent cholera in chickens, anthrax in sheep and cattle, and rabies in dogs and humans. It was actually Pasteur who first used the terms *vaccine* and *vaccination*.

A **vaccine** is defined as material that can artificially induce immunity to an infectious disease, usually after injection or, in some cases, ingestion of the material (e.g., oral polio vaccine). A person is deliberately exposed to a harmless version of a pathogen (or toxin), which will stimulate that person's immune system to produce protective antibodies and memory cells (described later in the chapter), but will not cause disease in that person. In this manner, the person's immune system is primed to mount a strong protective response should the actual pathogen (or toxin) be encountered in the future.

> Vaccination deliberately exposes a person to a harmless version of a pathogen (or toxin), to stimulate that person's immune system to produce protective antibodies and memory cells.

An ideal vaccine is one that:

• Contains enough antigenic determinants to stimulate the immune system to produce protective antibodies (i.e., antibodies that will protect individuals from infection by the pathogen)

- Contains antigenic determinants from all the strains of the pathogen that cause that disease (e.g., the three strains of virus that cause polio); such vaccines are referred to as multivalent or polyvalent vaccines
- Has few (preferably, no) side effects
- Does not cause disease in the vaccinated person

Types of Vaccines. Various materials are used in vaccines (Table 16-2). Most vaccines are made from living or dead (inactivated) pathogens or from certain toxins they produce. The use of such vaccines illustrates a very important and practical application of the principles of microbiology and immunology. In general, vaccines made from living organisms are most effective, but they must be prepared from harmless organisms that are antigenically closely related to the pathogens or from weakened (attenuated) pathogens that have been genetically changed so that they are no longer pathogenic.

> Some vaccines contain weakened (attenuated) pathogens, whereas others contain dead (inactivated) pathogens.

As microbiologists made further studies of the characteristics of vaccines, they found that it was practical to vaccinate against several diseases by combining specific vaccines in a single injection. Thus, the diphtheria-tetanus-pertussis (DTP) vaccine contains toxoids to prevent diphtheria and tetanus and antigenic portions of killed bacteria (*Bordetella pertussis*) to prevent whooping cough (pertussis). Another example is the measles-mumps-rubella (MMR) vaccine.

According to the CDC, American children should receive the following vaccines between birth and entry into school:

- Hepatitis B (Hep B) vaccine
- Rotavirus vaccine
- Diphtheria toxoid-tetanus toxoid-acellular pertussis (DTaP) vaccine
- *Haemophilus influenzae* type b (Hib) conjugate vaccine
- Inactivated poliovirus vaccine
- MMR vaccine
- Varicella (chickenpox) vaccine
- Influenza vaccine
- Pneumococcal vaccine (recommended for children in certain high-risk groups)
- Hepatitis A vaccine (recommended for children in certain high-risk groups)
- Meningococcal vaccine (recommended for children in certain high-risk groups)
  (Reference: http://www.cdc.gov/vaccines)

Many additional vaccines are available for use when needed. They include vaccines for protection against anthrax, cholera, genital warts, Lyme disease, rabies, smallpox, tuberculosis, typhoid fever, and yellow fever. A successful vaccine for colds has not been developed, because so many different types of viruses cause colds. Maintaining a successful vaccine for influenza is difficult because influenza viruses frequently change their surface antigens—a phenomenon known as **antigenic variation**.

SOMETHING TO THINK ABOUT

"In some surprising ways, we are in danger of becoming the victims of our own success. As our collective memory of infectious diseases like whooping cough and polio fades, the rare complications from vaccination loom large. Because of concerns about such complications, some parents are choosing not to have their children appropriately immunized. This poses a significant threat to the public health, because the microbes that cause the diseases are still very much with us. With the appearance of a large number of susceptible people again, we can expect to see the return of diseases we thought conquered."

(From Needham C, et al. *Intimate Strangers: Unseen Life on Earth.* Washington, DC: ASM Press, 2000.) The quote is as true today as when it was published.

How Vaccines Work. Vaccines stimulate the recipient's immune system to produce protective antibodies. The protective antibodies and/or memory cells produced in response to the vaccine then remain in the recipient's body to "do battle with" a particular pathogen, should that pathogen enter the recipient's body at some time in the future.

For example, when a person receives tetanus toxoid (an altered form of the toxin, tetanospasmin), protective antibodies referred to as antitoxins are produced. The antitoxins remain in the person's body. Should *Clostridium tetani* enter the person's body at some time in the future, and start to produce tetanospasmin, the antitoxins are there to attach to and neutralize the toxin.

Some vaccines stimulate the body to produce protective antibodies that are directed against surface antigens. When the pathogen enters the person's body, the antibodies attach to the surface antigens. This prevents the pathogen from adhering to host cells. In the case of viruses, if they are unable to attach, they are unable to enter the cell and are thus unable to multiply and cause cell destruction. Antibodies produced in response to molecules on the surface of bacterial pili would adhere to the pili, preventing the bacteria from attaching to tissues and, thus, preventing the bacteria from causing disease.

In some cases, protective antibodies attached to pathogens' surface antigens act as opsonins (discussed in Chapter 15), enabling phagocytes to attach to the pathogens. Once attached to a pathogen, the phagocyte can ingest and digest it. In other cases, attachment of protective antibodies to surface antigens activates the complement cascade, with the end result being lysis of the pathogen.

TABLE 16-2	Types of Available Vaccines

TYPE OF VACCINE	EXAMPLES
Attenuated vaccines. The process of weakening pathogens is called attenuation, and the vaccines are referred to as *attenuated vaccines*. Most live vaccines are avirulent (nonpathogenic) mutant strains of pathogens that have been derived from the virulent (pathogenic) organisms; this is accomplished by growing them for many generations under various conditions or by exposing them to mutagenic chemicals or radiation. Attenuated vaccines should not be administered to immunsuppressed individuals, because even weakened pathogens could cause disease in these persons.	**Attenuated viral vaccines:** adenovirus, chicken pox (varicella), measles (rubeola), mumps, German measles (rubella), polio (oral Sabin vaccine), rotavirus, smallpox, yellow fever **Attenuated bacterial vaccines:** BCG (for protection against tuberculosis), cholera, tularemia, typhoid fever (oral vaccine)
Inactivated vaccines. Vaccines made from pathogens that have been killed by heat or chemicals—called *inactivated vaccines*—can be produced faster and more easily, but they are less effective than live vaccines. This is because the antigens on the dead cells are usually less effective and produce a shorter period of immunity.	**Inactivated viruses or viral antigens:** hepatitis A, influenza, Japanese encephalitis, other (EEE, WEE, Russian) encephalitis vaccines, polio (subcutaneous Salk vaccine), rabies **Inactivated bacterial vaccines:** anthrax, typhoid fever (subcutaneous vaccine), Q fever
Subunit vaccines. A *subunit vaccine* (or *acellular vaccine*) is one that uses antigenic (antibody-stimulating) portions of a pathogen, rather than using the whole pathogen. For example, a vaccine containing pili of *Neisseria gonorrhoeae* could theoretically stimulate the body to produce antibodies that would attach to *N. gonorrhoeae* pili, thus preventing the bacteria from adhering to cells. If *N. gonorrhoe* cannot adhere to cells that line the urethra, they cannot cause urethritis. The material that is used to protect healthcare workers and others from hepatitis caused by hepatitis B virus (HBV) is being produced by genetically engineered yeasts. The genes that code for hepatitis B surface protein were introduced into yeast cells, which then produced large quantities of that protein. The proteins are then injected into people. Antibodies against the protein are produced in their bodies, and these antibodies serve to protect the people from HBV hepatitis.	Hepatitis B, Lyme disease, whooping cough
Conjugate vaccines. Successful conjugate vaccines have been made by conjugating bacterial capsular antigens (which by themselves are not very antigenic) to molecules that stimulate the immune system to produce antibodies against the less antigenic capsular antigens.	Hib (for protection against *Haemophilus influenzae* type b), meningococcal meningitis (*Neisseria meningitidis* serogroup C), pneumococcal pneumonia
Toxoid vaccines. A **toxoid** is an exotoxin that has been inactivated (made nontoxic) by heat or chemicals. Toxoids can be injected safely to stimulate the production of antibodies that are capable of neutralizing the exotoxins of pathogens, such as those that cause tetanus, botulism, and diphtheria. Antibodies that neutralize toxins are called **antitoxins**, and a serum containing such antitoxins is referred to as an **antiserum**.	Diphtheria, tetanus. Commercial antisera containing antitoxins are used to treat diseases such as tetanus and botulism. Such antisera are also used in certain types of laboratory tests, known as immunodiagnostic procedures.
DNA vaccines. Currently, *DNA vaccines* or *gene vaccines* are only experimental. A particular gene from a pathogen is inserted into plasmids, and the plasmids are then injected into skin or muscle tissue. Inside host cells, the genes direct the synthesis of a particular microbial protein (antigen). Once the cells start churning out copies of the protein, the body then produces antibodies directed against the protein, and these antibodies protect the person from infection with the pathogen.	Laboratory animals have been successfully protected using this technique, and reports of the induction of cellular immune responses in humans to a malarial parasite antigen, using DNA vaccines, have been published.
Autogenous vaccines. An *autogenous vaccine* is one that has been prepared from bacteria isolated from a localized infection, such as a staphylococcal boil. The pathogens are killed and then injected into the same person to induce production of more antibodies.	

Passive Acquired Immunity

Passive acquired immunity differs from active acquired immunity, in that antibodies formed in one person are transferred to another to protect the latter from infection. Thus, in passive acquired immunity, a person receives antibodies, rather than producing them. Because the person receiving the antibodies did not actively produce them, the immunity is temporary, lasting only about 3 to 6 weeks. The antibodies of passive acquired immunity may be transferred naturally or artificially.

> In passive acquired immunity, a person *receives* antibodies, rather than producing them. This can occur naturally or in an artificial manner.

In **natural passive acquired immunity**, small antibodies (like immunoglobulin G [IgG], which is described later in this chapter) present in the mother's blood cross the placenta to reach the fetus while it is in the uterus (in utero). Also, colostrum, the thin, milky fluid secreted by mammary glands a few days before and after delivery, contains maternal antibodies to protect the infant during the first months of life.

> A fetus receiving maternal antibodies in utero and an infant receiving maternal antibodies in colostrum are examples of natural passive acquired immunity.

Artificial passive acquired immunity is accomplished by transferring antibodies from an immune person to a susceptible person. After a patient has been exposed to a disease, the length of the incubation period usually does not allow sufficient time for postexposure vaccination to be an effective preventive measure. This is because a span of about 2 weeks is needed before sufficient antibodies are formed to protect the exposed person. To provide temporary protection in these situations, the patient is given human gamma globulin or "pooled" immune serum globulin (ISG); that is, antibodies taken from the blood of many immune people. In this manner, the patient receives some antibodies to all of the diseases to which the donors are immune. The ISG may be given to provide temporary protection against measles, mumps, polio, diphtheria, and hepatitis in people, especially infants, who are not immune and have been exposed to these diseases.

> Receiving a shot of gamma globulin is an example of artificial passive acquired immunity.

Hyperimmune serum globulin (or specific immune globulin) has been prepared from the serum of persons with high antibody levels (titer) against certain diseases. For example, hepatitis B immune globulin (HBIG) is given to protect those who have been, or are apt to be, exposed to hepatitis B virus; tetanus immune globulin (TIG) is used to prevent tetanus in nonimmunized patients with deep, dirty wounds; and rabies immune globulin (RIG) may be given to prevent rabies after a person is bitten by a rabid animal. Other examples include chickenpox immune globulin, measles immune globulin, pertussis immune globulin, poliomyelitis immune globulin, and zoster immune globulin. In potentially lethal cases of botulism, antitoxin antibodies are used to neutralize the toxic effects of the botulinal toxin. Remember that passive acquired immunity is always temporary because the antibodies are not actively produced by the B cells of the protected person.

CELLS OF THE IMMUNE SYSTEM

As stated earlier, the immune system involves very complex interactions among many different types of cells and cellular secretions. The major cell types that participate in immune responses are:

- T lymphocytes (T cells)
- B lymphocytes (B cells)
- NK cells (a category of lymphocytes)
- Macrophages

The cells involved in immune responses originate in bone marrow, from which most blood cells develop. Three lines of lymphocytes—B lymphocytes (B cells), T lymphocytes (T cells), and NK cells—are derived from lymphoid stem cells of bone marrow.

There are two major categories of T cells: helper T cells and cytotoxic T cells. Helper T cells are also known as T-helper cells, T_H cells, and CD4$^+$ cells. The term CD4$^+$ cells refers to the fact that these cells possess on their surface an antigen designated as CD4. The primary function of helper T cells is secretion of cytokines. T_H1 cells and T_H2 cells are subcategories of helper T cells. Cytokines secreted by T_H1 cells (referred to as type 1 cytokines) support cell-mediated immune responses (described later in the chapter), involving macrophages, cytotoxic T cells, and NK cells. Cytokines secreted by T_H2 cells (referred to as type 2 cytokines) support humoral immune responses (described later in the chapter) by inducing B-cell activation and differentiation of activated B cells into plasma cells.

> The two major types of T cells are helper T cells and cytotoxic T cells.

Cytotoxic T cells are also known as T cytotoxic cells, T_C cells, and CD8$^+$ cells. The term CD8$^+$ cells refers to the fact that these cells possess on their surface an antigen designated as CD8. The primary function of cytotoxic T cells is to destroy virally infected host cells, foreign cells, and tumor cells.

STUDY AID
Sorting Out the -Kines
Various types of cells within the human body, including cells of the immune system, communicate with each other. They do so by means of chemical messages—proteins known as **cytokines**. If the cytokines are chemotactic agents, attracting leukocytes to areas where they are needed, they are referred to as **chemokines**.

WHERE DO IMMUNE RESPONSES OCCUR?

Although it encompasses the whole body, the lymphatic system is the site and source of most immune activity. Immune responses to antigens in the blood are usually initiated in the

> Immune responses occur at many body sites, including the spleen, lymph nodes, tonsils, and adenoids.

spleen, whereas responses to microbes and other antigens in tissues are generated in lymph nodes located near the affected area. Antigens entering the body through mucosal surfaces (e.g., after inhalation or ingestion) activate immune responses in mucosa-associated lymphoid tissues. For example, immune responses to intranasal and inhaled antigens occur in the tonsils and adenoids. Ingested antigens enter specialized epithelial cells called microfold or M cells, which then transport the antigens to Peyer's patches in the intestinal mucosa, where the immune responses are initiated. All of the various types of cells (macrophages, B cells, T cells, etc.) that collaborate to produce immune responses are present at these sites (spleen, lymph nodes, tonsils, adenoids, Peyer's patches).

HUMORAL IMMUNITY

In **humoral immunity**, special glycoproteins (molecules composed of carbohydrate and protein) called antibodies are produced by B cells in response to antigens. In many cases, these antibodies are capable of recognizing, binding to, and inactivating or destroying specific pathogens.

A Closer Look at Antigens

Most **antigens** are foreign organic substances that are large enough to stimulate the production of antibodies; in other

> Antigens stimulate the immune system to produce antibodies.

words, an antigen generates antibody production—it is an *anti*body-*gen*erating substance. Substances capable of stimulating the production of antibodies are said to be **antigenic**. Antigens may be proteins of more than 10,000 daltons[b] (d) molecular weight, polysaccharides larger than 60,000 d, large molecules of DNA or RNA, or any combination of biochemical molecules (e.g., glycoproteins, lipoproteins, and nucleoproteins) that are cellular components of either microorganisms or macroorganisms (e.g., helminths). Foreign proteins are the best antigens.

A bacterial cell has many molecules on its surface capable of stimulating the production of antibodies; these individual molecules or antigenic sites are known as **antigenic determinants** (or *epitopes*). A bacterial cell could be

described as a mosaic of antigenic determinants. The important point is that, in most cases, antigens must be *foreign* materials that the human body does not recognize as *self* antigens. Certainly, all invading microbes fall into this category.

> Individual molecules that stimulate the production of antibodies are referred to as antigenic determinants or epitopes.

Some small molecules called **haptens** may act as antigens only if they are coupled with a large carrier molecule such as a protein. Then the antibodies formed against the antigenic determinant(s) of the hapten may combine with the hapten molecules when they are not coupled with the carrier protein. As an example, penicillin and other low–molecular-weight chemical molecules may act as haptens, causing some people to become allergic (or hypersensitive) to them.

Processing of Antigens in the Body

For antibodies to be produced within the body, a complex series of events must occur, some of which are not completely understood. It is known that macrophages, T cells, and B cells often are involved in a cooperative effort. (The processing of antigens within the body is actually far more complex than the abbreviated explanation that follows.)

T-dependent antigens. The majority of antigens are referred to as *T-dependent antigens*, because T cells (specifically, T_H cells) are involved in their processing. In other words, processing of these antigens is *dependent* on T cells. The processing of T-dependent antigens also involves macrophages and B cells.

> The processing of T-dependent antigens requires the participation of helper T cells, as well as macrophages and B cells.

T-independent antigens. Other antigens are known as *T-independent antigens*, the processing of which requires only B cells. In other words, the processing occurs independently of T cells (see Fig. 16-3). T-inde-

> Helper T cells are not involved in the processing of T-independent antigens; only B cells are required.

pendent antigens are large polymeric molecules (usually polysaccharides) containing repeating antigenic determinants; examples include the lipopolysaccharide (LPS) found in the cell walls of Gram-negative bacteria, bacterial flagella, and bacterial capsules.

Table 16-3 summarizes the processing of T-independent and T-dependent antigens. Note that the processing of either category of antigen—

> The cells that secrete antibodies are called plasma cells; they are derived from B cells.

T-independent or T-dependent—results in B cells developing into **plasma cells** that are capable of secreting antibodies.

---

[b] The term dalton is a unit of mass equal to 1/12 the mass of a carbon-12 (^{12}C) atom. A dalton is equal to 1 in the atomic mass scale. Daltons are used to express molecular weight.

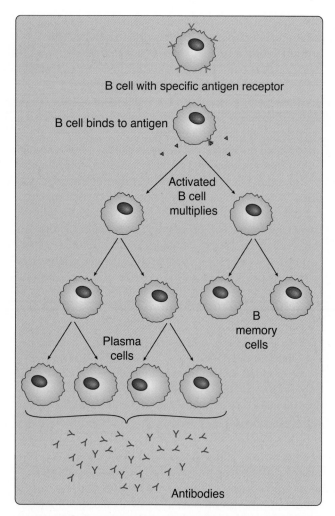

FIGURE 16-3. Processing of T-independent antigens.
See Table 16-3 for details. (From Cohen BJ. Memmler's The Human Body in Health and Disease, 11th ed. Philadelphia: Lippincott Williams & Wilkins, 2009.)

are given to protect against certain pathogens that one might encounter throughout life, such as the bacterium, *C. tetani* (the cause of tetanus). In addition to memory B cells, memory T cells also contribute to immunologic memory.

A Closer Look at Antibodies

Humoral immunity (or AMI) involves the production of antibodies, as opposed to CMI (discussed later in this chapter), which does not involve antibody production. *Antibodies* are proteins produced by lymphocytes in response to the presence of an antigen. (As previously described, the antibody-producing cells are a specific type of lymphocyte called B lymphocytes [or B cells], which usually work in coordination with T lymphocytes [T cells] and macrophages.) A bacterial cell has numerous antigenic determinants on its cell membrane, cell wall, capsule, and flagella that stimulate the production of many different antibodies. Usually, an antibody is specific in that it will recognize and bind to only the antigenic determinant that stimulated its production. **Example:** Antibodies produced against molecules located on bacterial pili can only recognize and bind to those particular molecules. Occasionally however, an antibody will bind to an antigenic determinant that is similar, but not identical, in structure to the antigenic determinant that stimulated its production; in this case, it is referred to as a cross-reacting antibody.

> Antibodies are usually very specific, binding only with the antigenic determinant that stimulated their production.

All antibodies are in a category of proteins called **immunoglobulins**—globular glycoproteins in the blood that participate in immune reactions. The term *antibodies* is used to refer to immunoglobulins with particular specificity for an antigen. In addition to being found in blood, immunoglobulins are found in lymph, tears, saliva, and colostrum

> An antibody is an immunoglobulin having particular specificity for an antigen.

The initial immune response to a particular antigen is called the **primary response**. In the primary response to an antigen, it takes about 10 to 14 days for antibodies to be produced. When the antigen is used up, the number of antibodies in the blood declines as the plasma cells die. Other antigen-stimulated B cells become memory cells, which are small lymphocytes that can be stimulated to rapidly produce large quantities of antibodies when later exposed to the same antigens. This increased production of antibodies after the second exposure to the antigen (e.g., a booster shot) is called the **secondary response**, *anamnestic response*, or *memory response*. A second booster shot of antigen many months later causes the antibody concentration to exceed the level of the secondary response. This is the reason why booster shots

> The initial response to an antigen is called the primary response, whereas a subsequent response to the same antigen is referred to as the secondary, anamnestic, or memory response.

TABLE 16-3	Mechanisms by which T-Dependent and T-Independent Antigens Are Processed by the Immune System

T-INDEPENDENT ANTIGEN	T-DEPENDENT ANTIGEN
Processing of T-independent antigens is initiated when an appropriate B cell makes physical contact with the free antigenic determinant (i.e., an antigenic determinant not bound to a major histocompatibility complex [MHC] molecule[a]).	After invasion of the body, an antigen (e.g., a bacterial cell) is ingested and digested by a macrophage.
↓	↓
The activated B cell next undergoes extensive cell division, producing a clone of identical B cells.	Within the macrophage, antigenic determinants of the bacterial cell (referred to as antigenic peptides or APs) attach to molecules called major histocompatibility complex (MHC) molecules.
↓	↓
Some of the members of the newly formed clone mature into antibody-producing plasma cells, whereas others become memory cells (Fig. 16-3).	The combined AP-MHC molecules are then displayed on the surface of the macrophage; at this point, the macrophage is referred to as an **antigen-presenting cell** (APC).
	↓
	A T_H cell attaches to one of the AP-MHC molecules, divides, and "sends out" (secretes) chemical signals (cytokines). (Note that T_H cells assist in the production of antibodies, but do not manufacture antibodies themselves.)
	↓
	When the chemical signals reach a B cell that is capable of recognizing that particular signal, the activated B cell divides, producing a clone of identical B cells.
	↓
	Some of the members of the newly formed clone mature into antibody-producing plasma cells. Antibodies are expelled rapidly for several days until the plasma cell dies. Each plasma cell makes only one type of antibody; one that will bind with the antigenic determinant that activated the B cell and stimulated production of that antibody. Members of the clone that do not become plasma cells, and some of the activated T cells, remain in the body as memory cells, able to respond very quickly should the antigen enter the body again at a later date.

[a]Major histocompatibility complex (MHC) molecules are cell surface molecules that play roles in antigen presentation and rejection of foreign tissue transplants.

(Fig. 16-4). Antibodies found in the blood are called humoral or circulating antibodies. As previously mentioned, antibodies that provide protection against infectious diseases are called protective antibodies.

The amount and type of antibodies produced by a given antigenic stimulation depend on the nature of the antigen, the site of antigenic stimulus, the amount of antigen, and the number of times the person is exposed to the antigen. After the initial exposure to an antigen (such as a vaccine), there is a delayed primary response in the production of antibodies. During this lag phase, the antigen is processed by cells of the immune system.

Antibody Structure

As previously mentioned, antibodies belong to a category of glycoproteins called immunoglobulins. All antibodies are immunoglobulins, but not all immunoglobulins are antibodies. (However, to avoid any confusion, the terms are used synonymously in this book.) Antibodies are produced by plasma cells in response to stimulation of B cells by foreign antigens.

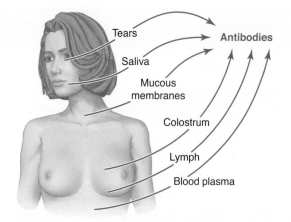

FIGURE 16-4. Body fluids and sites where antibodies are found.

The basic structure of an immunoglobulin molecule resembles the letter Y (Fig. 16-5). It consists of two identical light polypeptide chains (located at the top of the Y), two identical heavy polypeptide chains, two antigen-binding sites (located at the top of the Y), and an F_C region (located at the base of the Y). In this basic form, the molecule is referred to as a **monomer**. The light chains, which contain fewer amino acids than the heavy chains, are shorter and lighter in weight than the heavy chains. The chains are connected to each other

> A monomer resembles the letter Y. It consists of two heavy chains, two light chains, two antigen-binding sites, and an F_C region.

by disulfide (—S—S—) bonds. The monomer is bivalent in the sense that it has two sites (called *antigen-binding sites*) that can bind specifically to the antigenic determinant that stimulated production of that antibody.[c] The amino acid sequence within the variable regions of heavy and light chains enables the antibody molecule to bind to a particular antigenic determinant. The F_C region enables the molecule to bind to cells (e.g., neutrophils, macrophages, basophils, mast cells) that possess surface receptors able to recognize various sites on the F_C region.

Studies of the gamma globulin component of human blood have revealed that five classes (or *isotypes*) of immunoglobulins exist, designated IgA, IgD, IgE, IgG, and IgM. (Ig stands for immunoglobulin). IgA and IgG have subclasses. The amino acid sequence within the constant regions of heavy and light chains varies from one immunoglobulin class to another. Information about the various classes of immunoglobulins is presented in Table 16-4 and Figure 16-6.

> The five immunoglobulin classes are IgA, IgD, IgE, IgG, and IgM.

Antigen–Antibody Complexes

When an antibody combines with an antigen, an **antigen–antibody complex** (or Ag–Ab complex, or *immune complex*) is formed. Antigen–antibody complexes are capable of activating the complement cascade (by the classical pathway), resulting in, among other effects, the activation of leukocytes, lysis of bacterial cells, and increased phagocytosis as a result of opsonization. Thus, acute extracellular bacterial infections are controlled almost entirely by AMI. There is also a "dark side" to immune complexes, which will be discussed in a later section ("Type III Hypersensitivity Reactions").

> The combination of an antibody and an antigen is called an antigen–antibody complex, Ag–Ab complex, or immune complex.

How Antibodies Protect Us from Pathogens and Infectious Diseases

As previously mentioned, once they are produced, antibodies are very specific. Usually, a given antibody can only recognize and bind to the antigenic determinant that stimulated its production. Table 16-5 illustrates several of the ways in which antigen–antibody interactions protect us from pathogens and infectious diseases. Several examples are given here:

Example 1. A pathogen has entered a person's body and has started producing a toxin. That person's immune system responds by producing antibodies against the toxin; such antibodies are called **antitoxins**. Once produced,

FIGURE 16-5. Basic structure of a monomeric immunoglobulin molecule.

---

[c] It is important to note that the two antigen-binding sites can attach only to copies of the antigenic determinant that stimulated production of that antibody.

TABLE 16-4	Immunoglobulin Classes		
IG CLASS	**MOLECULAR WEIGHT (IN DALTONS)**	**% OF TOTAL IG IN SERUM (APPROXIMATE)**	**FUNCTIONS**
IgA	160,000 to 385,000; can exist as a monomer or as a dimer (two monomers held together by a short protein chain called a J-chain ["J" for joining])	10 to 20	The predominant immunoglobulin class in saliva, tears, seminal fluid, colostrum, breast milk, and mucous secretions of the nose, lungs, and gastrointestinal tract. In secretions, IgA is primarily present as secretory IgA (sIgA), a dimer that contains an additional protein called the secretory component. The secretory component apparently facilitates the transport of sIgA into secretions and may serve to protect the IgA molecule from enzymatic damage within the gastrointestinal tract. Protects external openings and mucous membranes from the attachment, colonization, and invasion of pathogens. IgA in colostrum and breast milk helps protect nursing newborns. In the intestine, IgA attaches to viruses, bacteria, and protozoal parasites, such as *Entamoeba histolytica*, and prevents the pathogens from adhering to mucosal surfaces, thus preventing invasion.
IgD	180,000 to 184,000 (a monomer)	<1	Found in large quantities on the surface of B cells. Its function is unknown, but it is possible that the IgD molecules on the B cell's surface serve as antigen receptors and determine which specific antigen that particular B cell is able to respond to.
IgE	188,000 to 200,000 (a monomer)	<1	In atopic individuals, IgE is produced in response to allergens. Found on the surfaces of basophils and mast cells. Plays a major role in allergic responses. (Basophils are granulocytes that circulate in the blood. Mast cells are morphologically very similar to basophils, but they are found in tissues—especially tissues that surround the eyes, nose, respiratory tract, and gastrointestinal tract.)
IgG	146,000 to 170,000 (a monomer; the lightest of the immunoglobulins)	70 to 85 (the most abundant immunoglobulin type in serum)	The only class of immunoglobulin that can cross the placenta. Maternal IgG antibodies that cross the placenta help protect the newborn during its first months of life. Antigen-bound IgG can bind to and activate complement, a process known as "complement fixation." IgG molecules can bind to a wide range of cellular receptors to promote phagocytosis and antibody-dependent cytotoxicity. As a result of memory cells, high levels of IgG are produced very rapidly (within 1 to 3 days) during the secondary response to antigens (described earlier). IgG antibodies are long-lived, sometimes persisting for the lifetime of the individual.
IgM	900,000 to 970,000 (a pentamer, consisting of five monomers held together by a J-chain; the largest of the immunoglobulins)	10	Because a pentamer has 10 antigen-binding sites, IgM can potentially bind to 10 identical antigenic determinants. Theoretically, an IgM molecule could bind to 10 separate virus particles, thus preventing the viruses from attaching to target cells. IgM antibodies are the first antibodies formed in the primary response to antigens (including pathogens), although IgG antibodies later become the most prevalent class. IgM antibodies are relatively short-lived, remaining in the bloodstream for only a few months. Because of its large size, IgM does not cross the placenta. Provides protection in the earliest stages of infection. Bactericidal to Gram-negative bacteria. IgM is the most efficient complement-fixing (complement-binding) immunoglobulin.

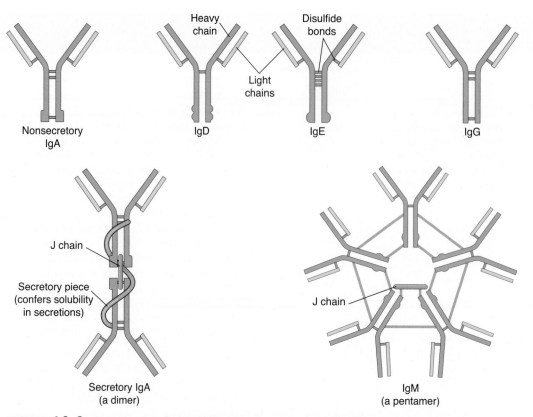

FIGURE 16-6. Structures of the different classes of antibodies. IgG, IgD, IgE, and nonsecretory IgA are monomers. Secretory IgA is a dimer (composed of two monomers), and IgM is a pentamer (composed of five monomers). J chains ("J" for joining) are short protein chains that bind monomers together. The secretory piece (or component) protects IgA molecules from proteolytic (protein-splitting) enzymes and facilitates transport of IgA molecules through membranes.

the antitoxins recognize, bind to, and neutralize the toxin molecules, so that they can no longer cause harm (i.e., they are no longer toxic).

Example 2. Recall from Chapter 14 that viruses can only bind to host cells that bear the appropriate receptor on their surface. The molecule on the virus that recognizes and binds to the receptor is called an adhesin. A person has received a vaccine containing an attenuated virus (a virus that is no longer infectious). The vaccine stimulates that person's immune system to produce antibodies against the adhesin molecules. At some later date, should that same virus enter the person's body, those antibodies will adhere to the adhesin molecules, making it impossible for the virus to bind to host cells. If the virus is unable to bind to the appropriate host cell, it is unable to enter the cell, and the person is protected from infection with that virus.

Example 3. A person is infected with a piliated bacterium. (Recall that pili enable bacteria to attach to host cells, which, with certain bacterial pathogens, is necessary for the bacteria to cause disease.) That person's immune system responds by producing antibodies against

the pili. The antibodies bind to the pili, making it impossible for the bacterial cells to bind to tissue. If the bacteria are unable to attach to tissue, they are unable to cause disease.

Example 4. A person is infected with an encapsulated bacterium. (Recall that bacterial capsules serve an antiphagocytic function, meaning that phagocytic white blood cells are unable to phagocytize encapsulated bacteria. The reason for this is that the phagocytes have no receptors on their surface that recognize the polysaccharide molecules. If the phagocyte is unable to attach to the encapsulated bacterium, it is unable to phagocytize it.) That person's immune system responds by producing antibodies against the capsular polysaccharide molecules. The antibodies attach to the capsule. This makes it possible for the phagocytes to bind to the encapsulated bacteria. Why? Because the phagocytes have receptors on their surface that can recognize and bind to antibody molecules.

> Among other functions, antibodies can neutralize toxins, prevent attachment of pathogens to host cells, and promote phagocytosis.

TABLE 16-5	Antigen–Antibody Interactions and Their Effects	
INTERACTION		**EFFECTS**
Prevention of attachment	Antibody / Virus	A pathogen coated with antibody is prevented from attaching to a cell.
Clumping of antigen	Foreign cell / Antibody	Antibodies link antigens together, forming a cluster that phagocytes can ingest.
Neutralization of toxins	Toxin / Antibody	Antibodies bind to toxin molecules to prevent them from damaging cells.
Help with phagocytosis	Foreign cell / Antibody / Phagocyte	Phagocytes can attach more easily to antigens that are coated with antibody.
Activation of complement	Complement / Antibody / Foreign cell	When complement attaches to antibody on a cell surface, a series of reactions begins that activates complement to destroy cells.
Activation of NK cells	Nk cell / Antibody / Foreign cell	NK cells respond to antibody adhering to a cell surface and attack the cell.

(Courtesy of Cohen BJ. Memmler's The Human Body in Health and Disease, 11th ed. Philadelphia: Lippincott Williams & Wilkins, 2009.)

Monoclonal Antibodies

Purified antibodies that are directed against specific antigens have been produced in laboratories by an innovative technique in which a single plasma cell that produces only one specific type of antibody is fused with a rapidly dividing tumor cell. The new long-lived, antibody-producing cell is called a **hybridoma**. These hybridomas are capable of producing large amounts of specific antibodies called **monoclonal antibodies**. The first monoclonal antibodies were produced in 1975; since then, many uses have been found for them. They are commonly used in **IDPs**—immunologic procedures used in laboratories to diagnose diseases. The first diagnostic kit containing monoclonal antibodies was

Monoclonal antibodies are produced by long-lived cells called hybridomas.

approved for use in the United States in 1981. Many other monoclonal antibody-based IDPs have been developed during the past 30 years. Monoclonal antibodies are also being evaluated for possible use in fighting diseases, killing tumor cells, boosting the immune system, and preventing organ rejection

CELL-MEDIATED IMMUNITY

Antibodies are unable to enter cells, including cells containing intracellular pathogens. Fortunately, there is an arm of the immune system capable of controlling chronic infections by intracellular pathogens (e.g.,

Cell-mediated immune responses involve many types of cells and cytokines; antibodies are rarely, if ever, involved.

bacteria, protozoa, fungi, viruses). It is called CMI—a complex system of interactions among many types of cells and cellular secretions (cytokines). (Only a brief overview of CMI can be provided here.) Included among the various cells that participate in CMI are macrophages, T_H cells, T_C cells, NK cells, and granulocytes. Although CMI does not involve the production of antibodies, antibodies produced during humoral immunity can play a minor role in some cell-mediated responses.

A typical cell-mediated cytotoxic response would involve the following steps:

Step 1. A macrophage engulfs and partially digests a pathogen. Fragments (antigenic determinants) of the pathogen are then displayed on the surface of the macrophage (i.e., the macrophage acts as an antigen-presenting cell).

Step 2. A T_H cell binds to one of the antigenic determinants being displayed on the macrophage surface. The T_H cell produces cytokines, which reach an effector cell of the immune system (e.g., a T_C cell or NK cell).

Step 3. The effector cell binds to a target cell (i.e., a pathogen-infected host cell displaying the same antigenic determinant on its surface).

Step 4. Vesicular contents of the effector cell are discharged. These include perforin and other proteins and enzymes, which literally punch holes in the target cell membrane. Other cytokines released by effector cells are tumor necrosis factor (TNF) and NK cytotoxic factor.

Step 5. Toxins produced by the effector cells enter the target cell, causing disruption of DNA and organelles. The target cell dies.

Both humoral and cell-mediated immune responses play a role in the body's defense against viral infections. In cytolytic viral infections (e.g., herpes infections), the viruses can be neutralized and destroyed by antibodies and the complement system when they move in body fluids from a lysed cell to an intact cell. When the virus is established within body cells, the cell-mediated immune response can destroy the virus-infected cells, preventing viral multiplication. If the virus is not completely destroyed, however, it may become latent in nerve ganglion cells, as in herpes infections (e.g., shingles).

T_C cells and NK cells kill infected host cells when pathogens are established inside the cells. Thus, infected liver cells are destroyed in hepatitis infections during the body's battle against the disease. The acquired immunodeficiency syndrome (AIDS) virus (human immunodeficiency virus [HIV]) that targets T_H cells is particularly destructive because it destroys the very cells that would have helped fight the infection. The lack of T_H cells impairs both humoral and CMI, making AIDS patients very susceptible to many opportunistic infections and malignancies.

Natural Killer Cells

NK cells are in a subpopulation of lymphocytes called large granular lymphocytes. Although they morphologically resemble lymphocytes, NK cells lack typical T- or B-cell surface markers. They also differ from T and B cells in other ways. For example, they do not proliferate in response to antigen and appear not to be involved in antigen-specific recognition. As the name implies, NK cells kill target cells, including foreign cells, host cells infected with viruses or bacteria, and tumor cells. Although NK cell activity is not dependent on antibodies, NK cells have receptors on their surface for the F_C region of IgG antibodies. These receptors enable the cells to attach to and kill antibody-coated target cells; this is known as antibody-dependent cellular cytotoxicity. Once attached to an antibody-coated target cell, the NK cell inserts a molecule called perforin into the cell membrane of the target cell, creating an opening (pore), through which cytotoxic granules called granzymes are injected. Although firm evidence is lacking for an immune surveillance system within our bodies that monitors for and destroys malignant cells, NK cells may participate in such a system.

> Cytotoxic T cells and NK cells kill foreign cells, host cells infected with viruses or bacteria, and tumor cells.

HYPERSENSITIVITY AND HYPERSENSITIVITY REACTIONS

The term *hypersensitivity* refers to an overly sensitive or overly reactive immune system. In such situations, the immune system, in an attempt to protect the person, causes irritation or damage to certain cells and tissues in the body.

> Hypersensitivity can be thought of as an overly sensitive immune system.

There are several different types of **hypersensitivity reactions**. Some types involve antibodies, whereas others do not. All types depend on the presence of antigen and T cells that are sensitized to that antigen. Hypersensitivity reactions are divided into two general categories—immediate-type and delayed-type—depending on the nature of the immune reaction and the time required for an observable reaction to occur (Table 16-6). **Immediate-type hypersensitivity reactions** occur from within a few minutes to 24 hours after contact with a particular antigen. There are three categories of immediate-type hypersensitivity reactions, referred to as type I, type II, and type III hypersensitivity reactions. A **delayed-type hypersensitivity reaction** usually takes more than

> Immediate-type hypersensitivity reactions occur within 24 hours of exposure to an antigen, whereas delayed-type hypersensitivity reactions take longer than 24 hours to manifest themselves.

TABLE 16-6	Types of Hypersensitivity Reactions	
IMMEDIATE-TYPE HYPERSENSITIVITY REACTIONS (OCCUR FROM WITHIN A FEW MINUTES TO 24 HOURS AFTER CONTACT WITH A PARTICULAR ANTIGEN)		
Type I hypersensitivity reactions	Anaphylactic reactions (allergic reactions)	
Type II hypersensitivity reactions	Cytotoxic reactions (involve damage to or death of body cells)	
Type III hypersensitivity reactions	Immune complex reactions (damage to tissues and organs is initiated by antigen–antibody complexes)	
DELAYED-TYPE HYPERSENSITIVITY (DTH) REACTIONS (USUALLY TAKE 24 TO 48 HOURS OR LONGER TO MANIFEST THEMSELVES)		
Type IV hypersensitivity reactions	Also known as cell-mediated reactions; antibodies play only a minor role, if any; an example is a positive TB skin test	

FIGURE 16-7. Factors in the development of type I hypersensitivity (allergies).

to the surface of basophils and mast cells by their F_C regions. The type and severity of an allergic reaction depend on a combination of factors, including the nature of the antigen, the amount of antigen entering the body, the route by which it enters, the length of time between exposures to the antigen, the person's ability to produce IgE antibodies, and the site of IgE attachment (Fig. 16-7).

People who are prone to allergies are described as being atopic. They produce IgE antibodies when they are exposed to allergens (antigens that cause allergic reactions).

The allergic reaction results from the presence of IgE antibodies bound to basophils in the blood or to mast cells[d] in connective tissues—IgE antibodies that were produced in response to the person's first exposure to the allergen. When the allergen binds to cell-bound IgE during a subsequent exposure to the allergen, the sensitized cells respond by degranulation—the discharge

Following their production, IgE antibodies bind to the surface of basophils and mast cells. Degranulation of the basophils and mast cells occurs when allergen binds to these IgE antibodies.

24 hours to manifest itself. Delayed-typed hypersensitivity reactions are also known as type IV hypersensitivity reactions and cell-mediated reactions.

Type I Hypersensitivity Reactions

Type I hypersensitivity reactions (also known as *anaphylactic reactions*) include classic allergic responses such as hay fever symptoms, asthma, hives, and gastrointestinal symptoms that result from food allergies; allergic responses to insect stings and drugs; and anaphylactic shock. These reactions all involve IgE antibodies and the release of chemical mediators (especially histamine) from mast cells and basophils.

Classic allergic responses like hay fever and food allergies are examples of type I hypersensitivity reactions, which are immediate-type hypersensitivity reactions.

The Allergic Response

Type I immediate hypersensitivity is probably the most commonly observed type of hypersensitivity, because more than half the American population is allergic to something. People who are prone to allergies (**atopic persons**) produce IgE (sometimes called reagin) antibodies when they are exposed to **allergens** (antigens that cause allergic reactions). The IgE molecules bind

[d] Mast cells can be thought of as basophils that reside in tissues other than blood. They are most plentiful in the tissues that surround the eyes, respiratory tract, and gastrointestinal tract.

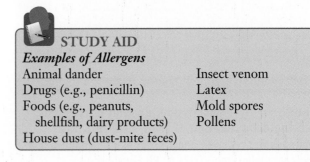

STUDY AID
Examples of Allergens

Animal dander	Insect venom
Drugs (e.g., penicillin)	Latex
Foods (e.g., peanuts, shellfish, dairy products)	Mold spores
House dust (dust-mite feces)	Pollens

FIGURE 16-8. Events that occur in type I hypersensitivity reactions. (From Harvey RA, Champe PA, eds. Lippincott Illustrated Reviews: Microbiology. Philadelphia: Lippincott Williams & Wilkins, 2001.)

and outpouring of granules and their irritating and damaging contents (chemical mediators) (Figs. 16-8 through 16-10). These mediators of the allergic responses include histamine, prostaglandins, serotonin, bradykinin, slow-reacting substance of anaphylaxis (SRS-A), leukotrienes, and chemicals that attract eosinophils (eosinophilotactic agents).

Localized Anaphylaxis

Type I hypersensitivity reactions (**anaphylactic reactions**) may be localized or systemic. Localized reactions usually involve mast cell degranulation, whereas systemic reactions usually involve basophil degranulation. Hay fever, asthma, and hives are examples of localized anaphylaxis. The symptoms depend on how the allergen enters the body and the sites of IgE attachment. If the allergen (e.g., pollens, dust, fungal spores) is inhaled and deposits on the mucous membranes of the respiratory tract, the IgE antibodies that are produced attach to mast cells in that area. Subsequent exposure to those inhaled allergens allows them to bind to the attached IgE, causing mast cell degranulation. The released histamine initiates the classic symptoms of hay fever. Antihistamines function by binding to and thus blocking the sites where histamine binds. However, antihistamines are not as effective in treating asthma, because the mediators of this lower respiratory allergy include chemical mediators in addition to histamine. Allergens (e.g., food and drugs) entering through the digestive tract can also

> Type I hypersensitivity reactions (anaphylactic reactions) may either be localized or systemic. Systemic reactions tend to be more severe than localized reactions.

FIGURE 16-9. Transmission electron micrograph showing degranulation of a rat mast cell. The degranulation occurred under experimental conditions in a research laboratory. (TEM by PG Engelkirk.)

FIGURE 16-10. Transmission electron micrograph showing phagocytosis of rat mast cell granules by a rat eosinophil. The phagocytosis occurred under experimental conditions in a research laboratory. (TEM by PG Engelkirk.)

sensitize the host, and subsequent exposure may result in the symptoms of food allergies (hives, vomiting, and diarrhea).

Systemic Anaphylaxis

Systemic **anaphylaxis** results from the release of chemical mediators from basophils in the bloodstream. It occurs throughout the body and thus tends to be a more serious condition than localized anaphylaxis. It may lead to a severe, potentially fatal condition known as **anaphylactic shock**. Most often, the allergens involved in systemic anaphylaxis are drugs or insect venom to which the host has been sensitized. Penicillin is an example of a hapten—a substance that must first bind to a host blood protein (a carrier protein) before IgE antibodies are produced. The IgE antibodies then bind to circulating basophils. Subsequent injections of penicillin into the sensitized host may cause degranulation of the basophils and release of large amounts of histamine and other chemical mediators into the circulatory system.

> Systemic anaphylactic reactions can lead to anaphylactic shock, which, if not treated quickly and properly, can lead to death.

The shock reaction usually occurs immediately (within 20 minutes) after reexposure to the allergen. The first symptoms are flushing of the skin with itching, headache, facial swelling, and difficulty breathing; this is followed by falling blood pressure, nausea, vomiting, abdominal cramps, and urination (caused by smooth muscle contractions). In many cases, acute respiratory distress, unconsciousness, and death may follow shortly. Swift treatment with epinephrine (adrenaline) and antihistamine usually stops the reaction.

Healthcare professionals must take particular care to ask patients whether they have any allergies or sensitivities before administering drugs. In particular, those people with allergies to penicillin and other drugs and to insect stings should wear MedicAlert jewelry, so that they do not receive improper treatment during a medical crisis.

Latex Allergy

Healthcare workers frequently come in contact with latex by wearing latex gloves and using other products containing latex. The National Institute for Occupational Safety and Health (NIOSH) has stated that "for some workers, exposures to latex may result in skin rashes; hives; flushing; itching; nasal, eye, or sinus symptoms; and (rarely) shock" (http://www.cdc.gov/niosh/latexalt.html). "Reports . . . indicate that from 1% to 6% of the general population and about 8% to 12% of regularly exposed healthcare workers are sensitized to latex." Latex can trigger any of the following three types of reactions:

- **Irritant contact dermatitis.** This is the most common reaction to latex products. The affected individual experiences dry, itchy, irritated areas on the skin, usu-

ally the hands. This is not a true allergy because the immune system is not involved.
- **Allergic contact dermatitis.** This results from exposure to chemicals added to latex during harvesting, processing, or manufacturing. These chemicals can cause skin reactions similar to those caused by poison ivy. This is a type of delayed hypersensitivity or type IV allergy.
- **Latex allergy.** This is an immediate type hypersensitivity that can be a more serious reaction to latex than irritant contact dermatitis or allergic contact dermatitis. Certain products in latex may cause sensitization. Subsequent exposure to latex can then trigger mild to severe reactions. Mild reactions include skin redness, hives, or itching. More severe reactions include respiratory symptoms (runny nose, sneezing), itchy eyes, scratchy throat, and asthma. Rarely, shock may occur. Latex allergy is a systemic type I, IgE-mediated reaction.

Latex allergy can be diagnosed using antibody-detection procedures and skin testing. Once an individual becomes allergic to latex, special precautions are needed to prevent exposures. Certain medications may reduce the allergy symptoms, but complete latex avoidance, although quite difficult, is the most effective approach. Many healthcare facilities maintain latex-safe areas for affected patients and workers. Additional information about the diagnosis and treatment of latex allergy can be found at the NIOSH web site.

> Many healthcare workers develop latex allergy, necessitating measures to avoid contact with latex-containing products.

Allergy Skin Testing and Allergy Shots

Anaphylactic reactions can be prevented by avoiding known allergens. In some cases, skin tests (scratch tests or intradermal injections of allergens) are used to identify the offending allergens. A skin test is considered positive if **cutaneous anaphylaxis** (i.e., swelling and redness at the scratch or injection site) occurs; this is often referred to as a "wheal and flare" reaction.

> A positive skin test result is swelling and redness (wheal and flare) at the site that the allergen was introduced into the skin.

Once the offending allergen is identified, immunotherapy may be accomplished by injecting small doses of allergen, repeatedly, several days apart. In hyposensitization, circulating IgG antibodies are produced rather than IgE antibodies. In theory, when the patient is later exposed in a natural manner to the allergen, the circulating IgG antibodies should bind with the allergen and block its attachment to the basophil- or mast cell-bound IgE. Such circulating IgG molecules, produced in response to allergy

> Allergy shots result in the production of IgG-blocking antibodies, which prevent the allergen from attaching to basophil- or mast cell-bound IgE.

shots, are called **blocking antibodies**. Immunotherapy has been used in patients allergic to plant allergens, insect venoms, cat dander, and fire ant venom.

Type II Hypersensitivity Reactions

Type II hypersensitivity reactions are cytotoxic reactions, meaning that body cells are destroyed during these reactions. Type II hypersensitivity reactions include the cytotoxic reactions that occur in incompatible blood transfusions, Rh incompatibility reactions, and myasthenia gravis; all of these reactions involve IgG or IgM antibodies and complement. A typical type II hypersensitivity reaction might follow this sequence:

> Type II hypersensitivity reactions are cytotoxic reactions.

Step 1. A particular drug binds to the surface of a body cell.
Step 2. Antidrug antibodies then bind to the drug.
Step 3. This initiates complement activation on the cell surface.
Step 4. The complement cascade leads to lysis of the body cell.

Type III Hypersensitivity Reactions

Recall that immune complexes are the result of binding of an antibody with the antigen that stimulated its production. Earlier in the chapter, it was stated that immune complexes have a "dark side." The dark side is that immune complexes can result in *type III hypersensitivity reactions* (also known as immune complex reactions). Examples of type III hypersensitivity reactions are serum sickness

> Type III hypersensitivity reactions are immune complex reactions.

FIGURE 16-11. Mantoux skin test. This test is performed by injecting 0.1 mL of tuberculin or PPD intradermally and observing the results 48 to 72 hours later. If the person has been exposed to mycobacteria in the past, redness and swelling will occur at the injection site; this constitutes a positive TB skin test result. The diameter of induration (the palpable raised hardened area)—not the area of redness—is measured and the results are interpreted using standardized criteria. (Courtesy of Gabrielle Benenson, Greg Knobloch, and the CDC.)

and certain autoimmune diseases (e.g., systemic lupus erythematosus [SLE] and rheumatoid arthritis). These reactions involve IgG or IgM antibodies, complement, and neutrophils. Serum sickness is a cross-reacting antibody immune reaction in which antibodies formed to globular proteins in horse serum may also bind with similar proteins in the patient's blood. The formation of these immune complexes (antigen + antibody + complement) causes the symptoms of hives, fever, kidney malfunction, and joint lesions of serum sickness. Horse serum containing antitoxins is used to treat botulism. About 10% of patients receiving this antiserum develop serum sickness.

Certain complications (sequelae) of untreated or inadequately treated strep throat and other *Streptococcus pyogenes* infections are the result of type III hypersensitivity reactions. IgG and IgM antibodies produced in response to *S. pyogenes* infection may bind with streptococcal antigens (e.g., M-protein). The resultant immune complexes become deposited in heart tissue, joints, or the glomeruli of the kidney. This causes inflammation at the site, leading to scarring, and, in some cases, abnormalities in or loss of function. Deposition of immune complexes in heart tissue leads to rheumatic heart, in joints leads to arthritis, and in kidneys leads to glomerulonephritis.

> Immune complications of *Streptococcus pyogenes* infections include rheumatic heart, arthritis, and glomerulonephritis.

Type IV Hypersensitivity Reactions

Type IV hypersensitivity reactions are referred to as *delayed-type hypersensitivity* (DTH) or cell-mediated immune reactions, and are part of CMI. (Recall that the two major arms of the immune system are humoral immunity and CMI.) Type IV hypersensitivity reactions are called DTH reactions because they are usually observed 24 to 48 hours or longer after exposure or contact. They occur in tuberculin and fungal skin tests, contact dermatitis, and transplantation rejection. DTH is the prime mode of defense against *intracellular* bacteria and fungi. DTH involves various cell types, including macrophages, cytotoxic T cells, and NK cells, but antibodies do not play a major role.

> Type IV hypersensitivity reactions are also known as delayed-type hypersensitivity reactions or cell-mediated immune reactions. They typically take 24 to 48 hours to manifest themselves.

A classic example of a DTH reaction is a positive TB skin test (also called the Mantoux skin test).[e] Either tuberculin or purified protein derivative (PPD), protein extracts prepared from *Mycobacterium tuberculosis* cultures, is injected intradermally into a person (Fig. 16-11). If an "immunologic memory" of the *M. tuberculosis* proteins exists in the person's body, a DTH reaction will

---

[e] The Mantoux skin test is named after Charles Mantoux, the French physician who introduced this test in 1908.

occur, producing the typical swelling and redness (wheal and flare) associated with a positive test result.

The following events occur to produce the positive reaction:

Step 1. Within 2 to 3 hours after injection of the PPD, there is an influx of polymorphonuclear cells (PMNs) into the site.

Step 2. This is followed by an influx of lymphocytes and macrophages while the PMNs disperse.

Step 3. Within 12 to 18 hours, the area becomes red (*erythematous*) and swollen (*edematous*).

Step 4. The *erythema* (redness) and *edema* (swelling) reach maximum intensity between 24 and 48 hours.

Step 5. With time, as the swelling and redness disappear, the lymphocytes and macrophages disperse.

A positive TB skin test result does not necessarily mean that a person has tuberculosis, although that is one possibility. Actually, a positive TB skin test result may indicate any of five possibilities:

> A positive TB skin test indicates that an individual has been exposed to mycobacterial antigens. That individual may or may not have active tuberculosis.

1. The person has active tuberculosis (in which case, a chest radiograph will show the disease, the person will probably be coughing, and the person's sputum will contain acid-fast bacilli).

2. The person had tuberculosis at some time in the past and recovered (in this case, the person should remember having had tuberculosis or the person's medical records will contain this information).

3. The person was infected with *M. tuberculosis* at some time in the past, but the organisms were killed by that person's host defense mechanisms (even though this person currently harbors no live *M. tuberculosis* cells, he or she will receive a 6-month course of isoniazid, because there is no way to differentiate possibility 3 from possibility 4).

4. The person currently harbors live *M. tuberculosis* organisms but does not actually have tuberculosis (in this case, a 6-month course of isoniazid will be initiated in an attempt to kill any *M. tuberculosis* cells in the person's body).

5. The person had received Bacillus Calmette-Guérin (BCG) vaccine at some time in the past (the person should remember having received BCG vaccine or he or she is from a country where BCG vaccine is routinely administered).

Many countries (excluding the United States) routinely immunize their citizens against tuberculosis using BCG vaccine. "BCG" stands for "bacillus Calmette-Guérin," a vaccine prepared from an attenuated strain of *Mycobacterium bovis*.[f] Although this vaccine is only about 50% effective in preventing tuberculosis, it does cause recipients to have positive TB skin test results for variable periods after immunization.

A reaction that is similar to the positive TB skin test occurs in contact dermatitis (contact hypersensitivity), after contact with certain metals, the catechols of poison ivy, cosmetics, and topical medications. The rejection of transplanted tissues containing foreign histologic (tissue) antigens appears to occur in a similar manner, except that cytokines and antibodies cause the rejection of the transplant.

AUTOIMMUNE DISEASES

An **autoimmune disease** results when a person's immune system no longer recognizes certain body tissues as self and attempts to destroy those tissues as if they were nonself or foreign. This may occur with

> An autoimmune disease results when a person's immune system attacks that person's body tissues as if they were nonself or foreign.

certain tissues that are not exposed to the immune system during fetal development, so that they are not recognized as self. Such tissues may include the lens of the eye, the brain and spinal cord, and sperm. Subsequent exposure to this tissue (by surgery or injury) may allow antibodies (IgG or IgM) to be formed, which together with complement could cause destruction of these tissues, resulting in blindness, allergic encephalitis, or sterility. It is believed that certain drugs and viruses may alter the antigens on host cells, thus inducing the formation of autoantibodies or sensitized T cells to react against these altered tissue cells.

There are more than 80 recognized autoimmune diseases. It has been estimated that more than 10 million people in the United States suffer from these diseases.

Autoimmune diseases can be classified as organ-specific and non–organ-specific. Examples of organ-specific autoimmune diseases are Hashimoto's thyroiditis, Graves disease, and primary myxoedema thyrotoxicosis (all three of which affect the thyroid); pernicious anemia affects the gastric mucosa; Addison's disease affects the adrenal glands; and insulin-dependent diabetes mellitus, also known as type 1 diabetes, affects the pancreas. Non–organ-specific autoimmune diseases involve the skin, kidneys, joints, and muscles; examples include myasthenia gravis (affects muscle), dermatomyositis (affects skin), SLE (affects kidneys, lungs, skin, and brain), scleroderma (affects skin, lungs, kidneys, and the gastrointestinal tract), and rheumatoid arthritis (affects joints). Autoimmune diseases are the result of types II, III, or IV hypersensitivity reactions. For example, myasthenia gravis is the result of type II hypersensitivity, whereas rheumatoid arthritis and SLE are the result of type III hypersensitivity.

IMMUNOSUPPRESSION

If a person's immune system is functioning properly, that person is said to be an **immunocompetent person**. If a

---

[f] BCG vaccine is named for Albert Calmette and Camille Guérin, French bacteriologists who developed this vaccine. The vaccine was first tested in 1921.

person's immune system is not functioning properly, that person is said to be **immunosuppressed**, *immunodepressed*, or *immunocompromised*. The most common cause of immune deficiency worldwide is malnutrition. In addition, there are acquired and inherited immunodeficiencies.

> If a person's immune system is not functioning properly, that person is said to be immunosuppressed, immunodepressed, or immunocompromised.

Acquired immunodeficiencies may be caused by drugs (e.g., cancer chemotherapeutic agents and drugs given to transplant

> Immunodeficiencies may either be inherited or acquired.

patients), irradiation, or certain infectious diseases (e.g., HIV infection). HIV infection leads to a decrease in T_H cells, which in turn prevents the production of antibodies against T-dependent antigens and, consequently, results in an inability to fight off certain pathogens. These pathogens overwhelm the patient's host defenses, eventually causing death. Persons with AIDS usually die of various devastating infectious diseases, including viral, bacterial, fungal, and parasitic diseases. Immune responsiveness and the ability to produce antibodies also decline as the normal body ages, perhaps the result of a declining ability of T cells to regulate the immune response. This, in turn, results in greater susceptibility of the elderly to serious infectious diseases.

Inherited immunodeficiency diseases can be the result of deficiencies in antibody production, complement activity, phagocytic function, or NK cell function. Several inherited immunodeficiency diseases have already been mentioned: chronic granulomatous disease, and Chediak-Higashi syndrome. Others include severe combined immune deficiency (SCID), DiGeorge syndrome, and Wiskott-Aldrich syndrome. SCID patients have deficiencies of B cells or T cells or both, resulting in severe recurrent infections.

In DiGeorge syndrome, there is a congenital absence of the thymus and parathyroid glands; patients suffer frequent infections and delayed development. Wiskott-Aldrich syndrome patients have deficiencies in B cells, T cells, monocytes, and platelets; effects on the patient include bleeding, recurrent infections, and eczema. Bone marrow transplantation and gene therapy may be valuable in treating certain immunodeficiency diseases.

It is hoped that the increased knowledge of genetics that is being gained as a result of the Human Genome Project will lead to an increased understanding of these diseases and various new methods by which they may be treated.

Some people are born lacking the ability to produce protective antibodies. Because they are unable to produce antibodies, they have no gamma globulins in their blood. This abnormality is called **agammaglobulinemia**. These persons are very susceptible to infections by even the least virulent microorganisms in their environment. One treatment for agammaglobulinemia that is often successful

consists of a bone marrow transplant, which involves the transfer of precursor white blood cells from a closely related person. Some of these cells become lymphocytes. These lymphocytes may be implanted in the lymph nodes and become immunocompetent (i.e., capable of being stimulated by antigens to produce antibodies).

> A person lacking the ability to produce antibodies is said to have agammaglobulinemia, whereas a person who produces too few antibodies is said to have hypogammaglobulinemia.

Persons who produce an insufficient amount of antibodies are said to have **hypogammaglobulinemia**. Their resistance to infection is lower than normal, so they usually do not recover from infectious diseases as readily as most other persons. One type, called Bruton's hypogammaglobulinemia, is a hereditary disease in which the numbers of circulating B cells are profoundly low or totally absent.

THE IMMUNOLOGY LABORATORY

As mentioned in Chapter 13, immunologic procedures may be performed in an Immunology Laboratory that is separate from the Clinical Microbiology Laboratory (CML), or within the Immunology Section of the CML, depending on the size of the medical facility. Immunologic procedures include tests to diagnose infectious diseases and immune system disorders, determine tissue compatibility for organ and tissue transplants, and detect and measure various serum components (immunochemical procedures). Only a few of these procedures are discussed here.

Immunodiagnostic Procedures

Historically, the amount of time it takes to get laboratory results has been the most common criticism of the CML. Sometimes days or even weeks are necessary to isolate pathogens from clinical specimens, to get them growing in pure culture and large numbers, and to perform the tests necessary to identify them. With certain infectious diseases, it is impossible to isolate the pathogens, either because they are obligate intracellular pathogens or are extremely fastidious.

One solution to these problems has been the development of IDPs—laboratory procedures that help to diagnose infectious diseases by detecting either antigens or antibodies in clinical specimens. The results

> Immunodiagnostic procedures are laboratory procedures that use principles of immunology to diagnose diseases.

of such procedures are often available on the same day that the clinical specimen is collected from the patient. IDPs performed on serum specimens are sometimes referred to as **serologic procedures**.

Some IDPs are designed to detect antigens, whereas others detect antibodies (Fig. 16-12). Detection of

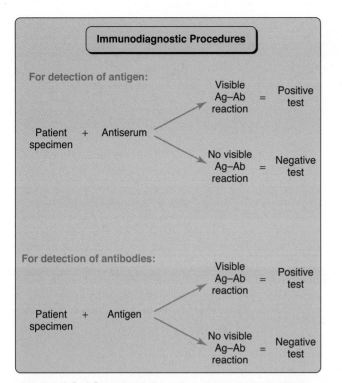

FIGURE 16-12. Principles of antigen and antibody detection procedures. Depending on the type of immunodiagnostic procedure being performed, the visible antigen–antibody (Ag–Ab) reaction might be agglutination (clumping) of cells or latex particles, formation of a precipitin line or band, fluorescence, or production of a color (as in enzyme immunoassays).

antigens in a clinical specimen is an indication that a particular pathogen is present in the patient, thus providing direct evidence that the patient is infected with that pathogen. Detection of antibodies directed against a particular pathogen is indirect evidence of infection with that pathogen. Actually, there are three possible explanations for the presence of antibodies to a particular pathogen:

Detecting antibodies to a particular pathogen in a clinical specimen may represent present infection, past infection, or prior vaccination against that pathogen

• Present infection (i.e., the person is currently infected with the pathogen).
• Past infection (i.e., the person was infected with the pathogen in the past, and antibodies are still present in the person's body).
• Vaccination (i.e., the antibodies are the result of the person having been vaccinated against that particular pathogen at some time in the past; for example, a person's serum may contain antibodies against influenza viruses because the person received a flu shot last year).

Because several explanations are possible for the presence of antibodies in a clinical specimen, the presence of

antigens provides the best proof of current infection. Unfortunately, antigen detection procedures are not available for many infectious diseases. Another problem with antibody detection procedures is that it takes a person approximately 10 to 14 days to produce detectible antibodies; thus, even if the person is infected with a particular pathogen, antibodies will not be detectible for about 2 weeks.

Two ways to increase the value of antibody detection procedures to diagnose present infection are (a) to specifically test for IgM antibodies and (b) to use paired sera. Because IgM antibodies are the first antibodies to be produced during the initial exposure to an antigen

The value of antibody detection procedures can be improved by specific detection of IgM antibodies or via the use of paired sera (i.e., acute and convalescent sera).

(the primary response) and are relatively short-lived, the presence of IgM antibodies directed against a particular pathogen is evidence that the pathogen is currently infecting the individual. To test paired sera, one serum specimen (called the *acute serum*) is collected during the acute stage of the disease and another (called the *convalescent serum*) is collected 2 weeks later. A significant rise in antibody titer (concentration) between the acute and convalescent sera is evidence that the patient was actively producing antibodies against that pathogen during the 2-week period and, therefore, that pathogen is the cause of the patient's current infection. The use of paired sera is useful for epidemiologic purposes (e.g., to determine the prevalent strain of influenza virus during a seasonal flu epidemic).

Laboratories purchase the reagents used to detect either antigens or antibodies from commercial companies. The reagent used to detect antigens contains antibodies and is called an antiserum. An antiserum is usually prepared by inoculating a laboratory animal with the pathogen (usually dead pathogens are used), and then collecting blood from the animal several weeks later. The blood is allowed to clot, and the serum is drawn off. The reagent used to detect antibodies contains antigens. This is usually a suspension of the dead pathogen.

The reagent used to detect antigens contains antibodies and is called an antiserum. The reagent used to detect antibodies contains antigens.

A variety of different laboratory tests have been designed so that a visible reaction will be observed if an antigen–antibody reaction takes place. Such tests, which include agglutination (involving the clumping of particles such as red blood cells or latex beads), precipitin procedures (involving the production of a precipitate), immunofluorescence procedures, and enzyme-linked immunosorbent

Tests used to determine that an antigen–antibody reaction occurred include agglutination, precipitin procedures, immunofluorescence procedures, and enzyme-linked immunosorbent assays.

TABLE 16-7   Immunodiagnostic Procedures for Detection of Antibodies in a Patient's Serum

REACTION IN VITRO	REAGENTS			RESULTS	
	Antigen	Antibody	Other	Positive	Negative
Agglutination	Red blood cells or bacteria	Patient's serum		Clumping	No clumping
Precipitin	Toxins, hormones, proteins	Patient's serum	Agar or solution	Precipitate	No precipitate
Lysis by Complement	Cells, bacteria	Patient's serum	Complement	Lysis	No lysis
Fluorescent Antibody Technique	Pathogen	Patient's serum	Fluorescein-tagged rabbit antihuman antiserum	Fluorescent pathogen	No fluorescence
Capsular Swelling (Quellung Reaction)	Encapsulated bacteria	Patient's serum		Capsule appears to swell	No appearance of swelling
Enzyme-linked assay	Test microbe	Patient's serum	Enzyme-linked antibody +Substrate	Color change	No color change

assays (ELISAs), are represented diagrammatically in Table 16-7. In the Blood Bank, agglutination tests are used to learn a person's blood type, which is determined by the types of antigens that are present on that person's red blood cells.

Antigen Detection Procedures

For detection of antigen, the clinical specimen is mixed with a particular antiserum (see Fig. 16-12). A visible re-action is the result of the formation of antigen–antibody complexes and indicates that the antigen is present in the clinical specimen; in such a case, the test result is consid-ered positive. If the visible reaction is not observed, then the antigen is not present in the specimen and the test result is negative. **Example:** A drop of cerebrospinal fluid (CSF) from a patient with meningitis is mixed with a drop of antiserum containing antibodies against *H. influenzae*. A visible antigen–antibody reaction is evi-dence that the patient's CSF contained *H. influenzae* antigens, and the patient's condition is diagnosed as meningitis caused by *H. influenzae*.

Antibody Detection Procedures

For detection of antibodies, the clinical specimen is mixed with a suspension of a particular antigen (see Fig. 16-12). A visible reaction indicates that antibodies against that pathogen are present in the clinical specimen, and the test result is positive. If the visible reaction is not observed, then antibodies against that pathogen are not present in the specimen and the test result is negative. **Example:** A drop of serum from a patient suspected of having Lyme disease is mixed with a suspension of *Borrelia burgdorferi* (the causative agent of Lyme disease). A visible antigen–antibody reaction is evidence that the patient's serum contained antibodies against *B. burgdorferi*, and the pa-tient's condition is diagnosed as Lyme disease.

The radioallergosorbent test (RAST) is used to detect and measure circulating IgE antibodies produced against allergens that individuals inhale, ingest, or otherwise come in contact with. RAST is used in place of or as an adjunct to intradermal skin testing (traditional allergy testing) to determine the allergen(s) to which a person is allergic.

Skin Testing as a Diagnostic Tool

Skin testing is another type of IDP, but one that is per-formed in vivo (in the patient) rather than in vitro (in the laboratory). In skin testing, antigens are injected within or beneath the skin (intradermally or subcutaneously, respectively). An example of a commonly used skin test is the TB skin test (previously described). Skin testing is also used to determine the allergens to which an atopic individual is allergic.

Procedures Used in the Diagnosis of Immunodeficiency Disorders

In addition to IDPs, tests are performed in the Immunology Laboratory that enable the assessment of a patient's immune status and evaluation of immunodefi-ciency disorders. These include tests to diagnose B-cell deficiency states (humoral immunodeficiencies), cell-me-diated immunodeficiencies, combined humoral and cell-mediated immunodeficiencies, phagocytic deficiency states, and complement deficiencies.

ON THE CD-ROM
- Terms Introduced in This Chapter
- Review of Key Points
- Increase Your Knowledge
- Critical Thinking
- Additional Self-Assessment Exercises

SELF-ASSESSMENT EXERCISES

After studying this chapter, answer the following multiple-choice questions.

1. Of the following, which is the *least* likely to be involved in CMI?
   a. antibodies
   b. cytokines
   c. macrophages
   d. T cells
2. Antibodies are secreted by:
   a. basophils.
   b. macrophages.
   c. plasma cells.
   d. T cells.
3. Humoral immunity involves all the following except:
   a. antibodies.
   b. antigens.
   c. NK cells.
   d. plasma cells.
4. Immunity that develops as a result of an actual infec-tion is called:
   a. artificial active acquired immunity.
   b. artificial passive acquired immunity.
   c. natural active acquired immunity.
   d. natural passive acquired immunity.
5. Artificial passive acquired immunity would result from:
   a. having the measles.
   b. ingesting colostrum.
   c. receiving a gamma globulin injection.
   d. receiving a vaccine.
6. The vaccines that are used to protect people from diphtheria and tetanus are:
   a. antitoxins.
   b. attenuated vaccines.
   c. inactivated vaccines.
   d. toxoids.

7. Natural passive acquired immunity would result from:
   a. having the measles.
   b. ingesting colostrum.
   c. receiving a gamma globulin injection.
   d. receiving a vaccine.

8. Which of the following statements about IgM is *false*?
   a. IgM contains a J chain.
   b. IgM has a total of 10 antigen-binding sites.
   c. IgM is a pentamer.
   d. IgM is a long-lived molecule.

9. Which of the following could be an effect of type III hypersensitivity?
   a. glomerulonephritis
   b. rheumatoid arthritis
   c. SLE
   d. all of the above

10. Most likely, immunology got its start in 1890 when these scientists discovered antibodies while developing a diphtheria antitoxin.
    a. Edward Jenner and Louis Pasteur
    b. Elie Metchnikoff and Robert Koch
    c. Emil Behring and Kitasato Shibasaburo
    d. Jonas Salk and Albert Sabin

OVERVIEW OF INFECTIOUS DISEASES

17

LEARNING OBJECTIVES

AFTER STUDYING THIS CHAPTER, YOU SHOULD BE ABLE TO:

- Define the terms and abbreviations introduced in this chapter
- Categorize various infectious diseases by body system (e.g., cystitis is an infection of the urinary bladder, which is part of the genitourinary [GU] system; myelitis is an infection of the brain and spinal cord)

INTRODUCTION

Human diseases fall into many different categories, including:

- Degenerative diseases
- Immune disorders
- Infectious diseases
- Metabolic disorders
- Neoplasms (cancers and other types of tumors)
- Nutritional disorders
- Psychiatric disorders

Of these disease categories, only infectious diseases are caused by microbes.[a] Recall from Chapter 1 that

pathogens actually cause two general categories of diseases: microbial intoxications and infectious diseases. **Microbial intoxications**, which follow ingestion of a toxin produced outside the body (in vitro) by a

> Infectious diseases are diseases that are caused by pathogens, following colonization of some body site by the pathogen.

pathogen, are discussed in CD-ROM Appendix 1. **Infectious diseases (or infections)**, on the other hand, follow colonization of some body site by a pathogen. This chapter provides an overview of the major infectious diseases of humans. Chapters 18 through 21 provide detailed information about specific infectious diseases.

This chapter is divided into sections that describe infectious diseases of various anatomical sites, including skin, ears, eyes, respiratory system, the oral region, gastrointestinal (GI) tract, GU system, circulatory system, and central nervous system (CNS). Although a particular

> Some infectious diseases affect more than one anatomical site, and some pathogens move from one body site to another during the course of a disease.

disease may be described within one particular section of this chapter (e.g., in the section describing infectious diseases of the respiratory system), readers should keep in mind that some infectious diseases involve several body systems simultaneously, and that the pathogen(s) causing a

---

[a] Some types of cancer are also known to be caused by viruses, but these are not discussed in this book.

What to Learn?

After studying Chapter 17, students should be able to define the terms and abbreviations introduced in this chapter and categorize various infectious diseases by body system (e.g., that myocarditis is an inflammation of the muscular walls of the heart—the myocardium; that encephalitis is an inflammation of the brain).

particular infection may move from one body site to another during the course of that disease.

INFECTIOUS DISEASES OF THE SKIN

As mentioned in Chapter 15, intact skin is a type of nonspecific host defense mechanism, serving as a physical barrier (Fig. 17-1). It is part of the body's first line of defense. Very few pathogens can penetrate intact skin. The indigenous microflora of the skin, a low pH, and the presence of chemical substances like lysozyme and sebum also serve to prevent colonization of the skin by pathogens. Nonetheless, skin infections do occur. Listed here are some terms relating to skin and infectious diseases of the skin:

- **Epidermis.** The superficial portion of the skin.
- **Dermis.** The inner layer of skin, containing blood and lymphatic vessels, nerves, and nerve endings, glands, and hair follicles.
- **Dermatitis.** Inflammation of the skin.
- **Sebaceous glands.** Glands in the dermis that usually open into hair follicles and secrete an oily substance known as **sebum**.
- **Folliculitis.** Inflammation of a hair follicle, the sac that contains a hair shaft.
- **Sty (or stye).** Inflammation of a sebaceous gland that opens into a follicle of an eyelash.
- **Furuncle.** A localized pyogenic (pus-producing) infection of the skin, usually resulting from folliculitis; also known as a **boil**.
- **Carbuncle.** A deep-seated pyogenic infection of the skin, usually arising from a coalescence of furuncles.
- **Macule.** A surface lesion that is neither raised nor depressed, such as the lesions of measles.

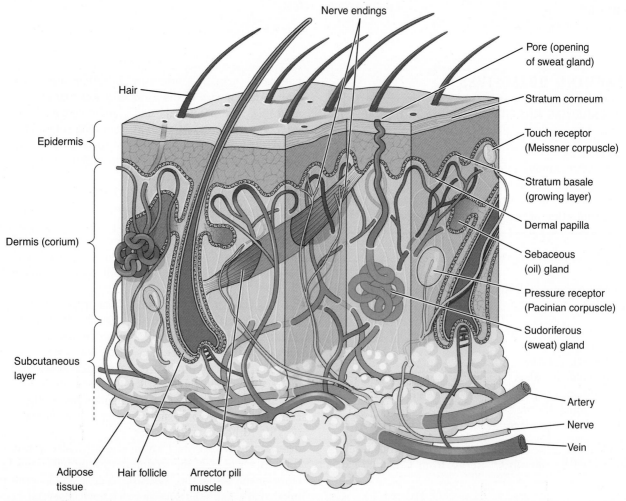

FIGURE 17-1. Cross section of the skin. (From Cohen BJ. Memmler's The Human Body in Health and Disease, 11th ed. Philadelphia: Lippincott Williams & Wilkins, 2009.)

- **Papule.** A surface lesion that is firm and raised, such as the lesions of chickenpox.
- **Vesicle.** A blister or small fluid-filled sac, such as is seen in chickenpox and shingles.
- **Pustule.** A pus-filled surface lesion.

A Macule

B Papule

C Vesicle

D Pustule

FIGURE 17-2. Types of surface lesions. (A) Macules, **(B)** Papules, **(C)** Vesicles, **(D)** Pustules. (From Cohen BJ. Memmler's The Human Body in Health and Disease, 11th ed. Philadelphia: Lippincott Williams & Wilkins, 2009.)

Various types of surface lesions are shown in Figure 17-2.

INFECTIOUS DISEASES OF THE EARS

The anatomy of the ear is shown in Figure 17-3. There are three pathways for pathogens to enter the ear: (a) through the eustachian (auditory) tube, from the throat and nasopharynx; (b) from the external ear; and (c) via the blood or lymph. Usually, bacteria are trapped in the middle ear when a bacterial infection in the throat and nasopharynx causes the eustachian tube to close. The result is an anaerobic condition in the middle ear, allowing obligate and facultative anaerobes to proliferate and cause pressure on the tympanic membrane (eardrum). Swollen lymphoid (adenoid) tissues, viral infections, and allergies may also close the eustachian tube, especially in young children. Infection of the middle ear is known as **otitis media**, whereas infection of the outer ear canal is known as **otitis externa**.

> Infection of the middle ear is known as otitis media, whereas infection of the outer ear canal is known as otitis externa.

INFECTIOUS DISEASES OF THE EYES

The anatomy of the eye is shown in Figure 17-4. Terms relating to the eye and infectious diseases of the eye include the following:

- **Conjunctiva.** The thin, tough lining that covers the inner wall of the eyelid and the sclera (the white of the eye).
- **Conjunctivitis.** An infection or inflammation of the conjunctiva.
- **Keratitis.** An infection or inflammation of the cornea—the domed covering over the iris and lens.
- **Keratoconjunctivitis.** An infection that involves both the cornea and conjunctiva.

INFECTIOUS DISEASES OF THE RESPIRATORY SYSTEM

For practical purposes, the discussion of the respiratory system is divided into the upper respiratory tract (URT) and the lower respiratory tract (LRT). The URT includes the paranasal sinuses, nasopharynx, oropharynx, epiglottis, and larynx ("voice box"). The LRT includes the trachea ("windpipe"), bronchial tubes, and alveoli of the lungs. The respiratory system is depicted in Figure 17-5.

Indigenous microflora of the URT may cause opportunistic infections of the respiratory system. Infectious diseases of the URT (e.g., colds

> Lower respiratory tract infections are the most common cause of death from infectious diseases.

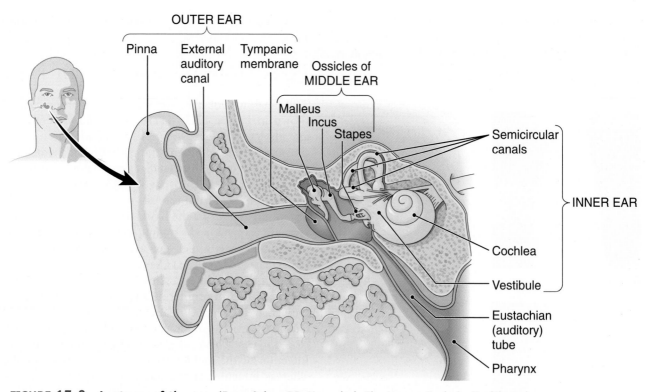

FIGURE 17-3. Anatomy of the ear. (From Cohen BJ. Memmler's The Human Body in Health and Disease, 11th ed. Philadelphia: Lippincott Williams & Wilkins, 2009.)

and sore throats) are more common than infectious diseases of the LRT. They may predispose the patient to more serious infections, such as sinusitis, otitis media, bronchitis, and pneumonia. LRT infections are the most common cause of death from infectious diseases.

Terms relating to infectious diseases of the respiratory system include the following:

• **Bronchitis.** Inflammation of the mucous membrane lining of the bronchial tubes; most commonly caused by respiratory viruses.

FIGURE 17-4. Anatomy of the eye. (From Cohen BJ. Memmler's The Human Body in Health and Disease, 11th ed. Philadelphia: Lippincott Williams & Wilkins, 2009.)

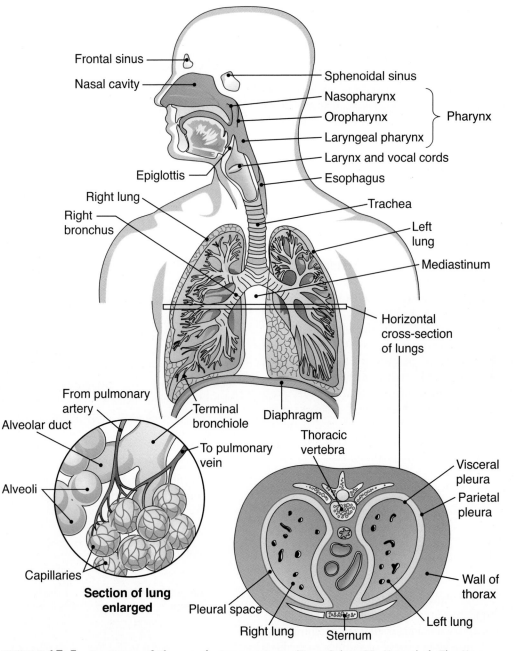

FIGURE 17-5. Anatomy of the respiratory system. (From Cohen BJ. Memmler's The Human Body in Health and Disease, 11th ed. Philadelphia: Lippincott Williams & Wilkins, 2009.)

- **Bronchopneumonia.** Combination of bronchitis and pneumonia.
- **Epiglottitis.** Inflammation of the epiglottis (the mouth of the windpipe); may cause respiratory obstruction, especially in children; frequently caused by *Haemophilus influenzae* type b (Hib).
- **Laryngitis.** Inflammation of the mucous membrane of the larynx (voice box).
- **Pharyngitis.** Inflammation of the mucous membrane and underlying tissue of the pharynx; commonly referred to as **sore throat**. "Strep throat" is pharyngitis caused

Even though *S. pyogenes* is the most "publicized" cause of pharyngitis, viruses cause most cases of pharyngitis.

by *Streptococcus pyogenes*. Even though *S. pyogenes* is the most "publicized" cause of pharyngitis, most cases of pharyngitis are caused by viruses.
- **Pneumonia.** Inflammation of one or both lungs. Alveolar sacs become filled with exudate, inflammatory cells, and fibrin. Most cases of pneumonia are caused by bacteria or viruses, but pneumonia can also be caused by fungi and protozoa.
- **Sinusitis.** Inflammation of the lining of one or more of the paranasal sinuses. The most common causes are the bacteria, *Streptococcus pneumoniae* and *H. influenzae*. Less common causes are the bacteria, *S. pyogenes*, *Moraxella catarrhalis*, and *Staphylococcus aureus*.

Typical versus Atypical Pneumonia

Patients with **typical pneumonia** experience chest pain, dyspnea (shortness of breath), fever, chills, and a productive cough (one that produces purulent sputum). Less common symptoms include anorexia, headache, nausea, diarrhea, and vomiting. X-ray abnormalities are proportional to the physical symptoms. Common causes of typical pneumonia are the bacteria, *S. pneumoniae*, *H. influenzae*, and *S. aureus*, and viruses such as influenza virus types A and B, parainfluenza viruses, and respiratory syncytial virus (RSV). Other causes are *Legionella pneumophila*, *Mycoplasma pneumoniae*, *Chlamydophila pneumoniae*, and other Gram-negative bacilli. **Atypical pneumonia** has a more insidious (slower) onset than typical pneumonia. Patients present with headache, fever, cough with little sputum, and myalgia. X-ray abnormalities are usually greater than the physical symptoms would predict. Common causes of atypical pneumonia are the bacteria, *M. pneumoniae*, *C. pneumoniae*, and *L. pneumophila*, and viruses such as influenza viruses, RSV, and adenoviruses. Other causes are *Chlamydophila psittaci* (a bacterium), *Pneumocystis jiroveci* (a fungus), varicella-zoster virus, and parainfluenza viruses. Note that some pathogens can produce either typical or atypical pneumonia.

SPOTLIGHTING RESPIRATORY THERAPISTS

As stated in the American Medical Association's (AMA) Health Care Careers Directory for 2008–2009 (available at http://www.ama-assn.org), "Respiratory therapists work in a wide variety of settings to evaluate, treat, and manage patients of all ages with respiratory illnesses and cardiopulmonary disorders. Entry-level respiratory therapists perform general respiratory care procedures. They may assume clinical responsibility for specified respiratory care modalities involving the application of therapeutic techniques under the supervision of an advanced-level therapist and/or a physician. The advanced-level respiratory therapist participates in clinical decision-making and patient education, develops and implements respiratory care plans, applies patient-driven protocols, utilizes evidence-based clinical practice guidelines, and participates in health promotion, disease prevention, and disease management. The advanced-level respiratory therapist may be required to exercise considerable independent judgment, under the supervision of a physician, in the respiratory care of patients." Information concerning educational requirements and programs, certification, and salary can be found on the AMA web site.

INFECTIOUS DISEASES OF THE ORAL REGION

As discussed in Chapter 10, the oral cavity (mouth) is a complex ecosystem suitable for growth and interrelationships of many types of microorganisms (Fig. 17-6). Although the actual indigenous microflora of the mouth varies greatly from one person to the next, studies have shown that it includes about 300 identified species of bacteria, both aerobes and anaerobes. Many additional, as yet unclassified bacteria also live there. Some members of the oral microflora are beneficial in that they produce secretions that are antagonistic to other bacteria. Although several bacterial species, such as *Streptococcus* (*Streptococcus salivarius*, *Streptococcus mitis*, *Streptococcus sanguis*, and *Streptococcus mutans*) and *Actinomyces* spp., often interact to protect the oral surfaces, in other circumstances, they are involved in oral disease.

> Most infections of the oral cavity are caused by members of the indigenous oral microflora, sometimes one member acting independently and other times several members acting together.

In the healthy mouth, saliva secreted by salivary glands helps control the growth of opportunistic oral flora. Saliva

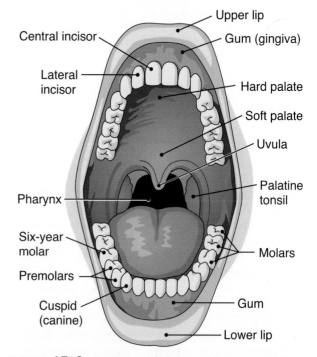

FIGURE 17-6. Anatomy of the mouth. (From Cohen BJ. Memmler's The Human Body in Health and Disease, 11th ed. Philadelphia: Lippincott Williams & Wilkins, 2009.)

contains enzymes (including lysozyme), immunoglobulins (IgA), and buffers to control the near-neutral pH and continually flushes microbes and food particles through the mouth. Other antimicrobial secretions and phagocytes are found in the mucus that coats the oral surfaces. The hard, complex, calcium tooth enamel, bathed in protective saliva, usually resists damage by oral microbes. However, if the ecological balance is upset or is not properly maintained, oral disease may result. The following terms relate to infectious diseases of the oral cavity:

- **Dental caries**. Tooth decay or cavities. Dental caries start when the external surface (the enamel) of a tooth is dissolved by organic acids produced by masses of microorganisms attached to the tooth (dental plaque). This is followed by enzymatic destruction of the protein matrix, cavitation, and bacterial invasion. The most common cause of tooth decay is *S. mutans*, which produces lactic acid as an end product in the fermentation of glucose.
- **Gingivitis**. Inflammation of the gingiva (gums).
- **Periodontitis**. Inflammation of the periodontium (tissues that surround and support the teeth, including the gingiva and supporting bone); in severe cases, teeth loosen and fall out.

Oral infections result from a combination of the unique microbial population, reduced host defenses, improper diet, and poor dental hygiene. These diseases are the consequence of at least four microbial activities, including (a) formation of dextran (a polysaccharide) from sugars by streptococci, (b) acid production by lactic acid–producing bacteria, (c) deposition of calculus by *Actinomyces*, and (d) secretion of inflammatory substances (endotoxin) by *Bacteroides* species. This combination of circumstances damages the teeth, soft tissues (gingiva), alveolar bone, and the periodontal fibers that attach teeth to bone. Oral diseases such as gingivitis, periodontitis, and trench mouth are collectively known as **periodontal diseases**.

Periodontal diseases can be prevented by maintaining good health, proper oral hygiene (tooth brushing, using tartar-control toothpaste, and flossing), an adequate diet without sugars, and regular fluoride treatments to help control the microbial population and to prevent damaging bacterial interactions. Severe gingivitis and periodontitis require professional care by a specially trained dentist called a periodontist. Using techniques known as scaling and planing, periodontists remove tartar that has accumulated on tooth surfaces up to one fifth of an inch below the gum line—areas where tooth brushing and flossing cannot reach. After dental surgery, periodontists often prescribe a chlorhexidine mouth rinse as a temporary substitute for brushing and flossing.

INFECTIOUS DISEASES OF THE GASTROINTESTINAL TRACT

The GI tract consists of a long tube with many expanded areas designed for digestion of food, absorption of nutrients, and elimination of undigested materials (Fig. 17-7). Transient and resident microbes continuously enter and leave the GI tract. Most of the microorganisms ingested with food are destroyed in the stomach and duodenum by the low pH (gastric contents have a pH of approximately 1.5) and are inhibited from growing in the lower intestines by the resident microflora (microbial antagonism). They are then flushed from the colon during defecation, along with large numbers of indigenous microbes. The indigenous microflora of the GI tract were discussed in Chapter 10. Terms relating to infectious diseases of the GI tract include the following:

- **Colitis**. Inflammation of the colon (the large intestine).
- **Diarrhea**. An abnormally frequent discharge of semisolid or fluid fecal matter. Some laboratory workers define diarrheal specimens as "stool specimens that conform to the shape of the container."
- **Dysentery**. Frequent watery stools, accompanied by abdominal pain, fever, and dehydration. The stool specimens may contain blood or mucus.
- **Enteritis**. Inflammation of the intestines, usually referring to the small intestine.
- **Gastritis**. Inflammation of the mucosal lining of the stomach.
- **Gastroenteritis**. Inflammation of the mucosal linings of the stomach and intestines.
- **Hepatitis**. Inflammation of the liver; usually the result of viral infection, but can be caused by toxic agents.

Diarrhea is a symptom in a wide variety of conditions and diseases. It can be caused by certain foods or drugs, or it may be the result of an infectious disease. If diarrhea results from an infectious disease, the pathogen may be a virus, a bacterium, a protozoan, or a helminth. Dysentery may also be caused by various pathogens, including bacteria (e.g., *Shigella* spp. cause bacillary dysentery) and protozoa (e.g., amebiasis and balantidiasis, which are described in Chapter 21).

INFECTIOUS DISEASES OF THE GENITOURINARY SYSTEM

The GU or urogenital system consists of the urinary tract and the genital tract. Infectious diseases of the urinary tract are described first.

FIGURE 17-7. Anatomy of the gastrointestinal tract. (From Cohen BJ. Memmler's The Human Body in Health and Disease, 11th ed. Philadelphia: Lippincott Williams & Wilkins, 2009.)

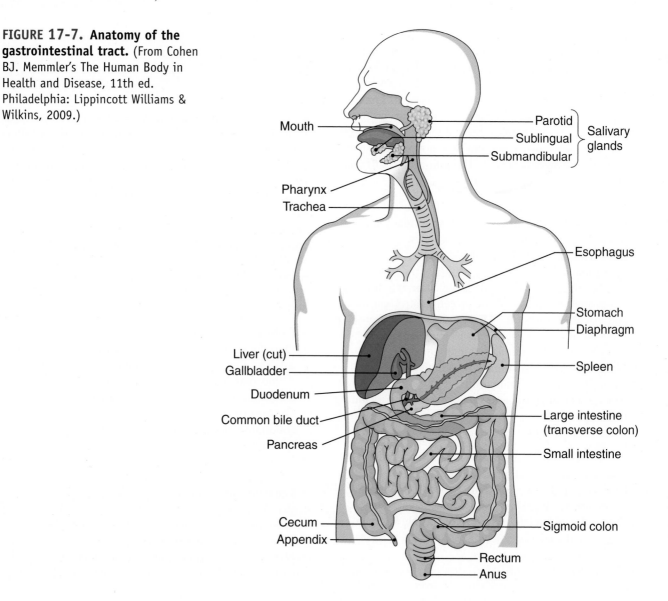

Urinary Tract Infections

For purposes of discussion, urinary tract infections (UTIs) can be divided into upper UTIs and lower UTIs. Upper UTIs include infections of the kidneys (nephritis or **pyelonephritis**) and ureters (ureteritis). Lower UTIs include infections of the urinary bladder (cystitis), the urethra (urethritis), and, in men, the prostate (prostatitis). The anatomy of the urinary tract is shown in Figure 17-8.

UTIs may be caused by any of various microorganisms, introduced by poor personal hygiene, sexual intercourse, the insertion of catheters, and other means. The urinary tract is usually protected from pathogens by the frequent flushing action of urination. The acidity of normal urine also discourages growth of many microorganisms. Indigenous microflora are found at and near the outer opening (meatus) of the urethra of both men and women.

> Urinary tract infections may be caused by any of a variety of microorganisms, introduced by poor personal hygiene, sexual intercourse, the insertion of catheters, and some other means.

Terms relating to infectious diseases of the urinary tract include the following:

- **Cystitis.** Inflammation of the urinary bladder; the most common type of UTI. The most common cause of cystitis is *Escherichia coli*. Other common causes of cystitis are species of *Klebsiella*, *Proteus*, *Enterobacter*, *Pseudomonas*, and *Enterococcus* as well as *Staphylococcus saprophyticus*, *Staphylococcus epidermidis*, and *Candida albicans*.

  > The most common cause of cystitis, nephritis, and pyelonephritis is *E. coli*, whereas the most common cause of urethritis is the bacterium, *C. trachomatis*.

- **Nephritis.** General term referring to inflammation of the kidneys. *Pyelonephritis* is inflammation of the renal parenchyma. *E. coli* is the most common cause of nephritis and pyelonephritis. Most often, nephritis is preceded by cystitis; the bacteria migrate up the ureters, from the urinary bladder to the kidneys. Bacteria may also gain access to the kidneys via the bloodstream.

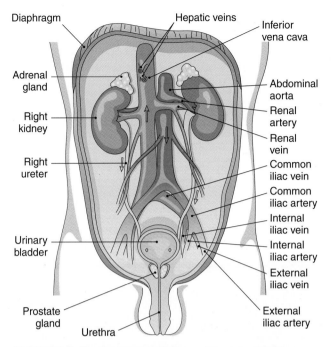

FIGURE 17-8. Anatomy of the urinary tract. (From Cohen BJ. Memmler's The Human Body in Health and Disease, 11th ed. Philadelphia: Lippincott Williams & Wilkins, 2009.)

- **Ureteritis.** Inflammation of one or both ureters. Usually caused by the spreading of infection upward from the urinary bladder or downward from the kidneys.
- **Urethritis.** Inflammation of the urethra. Pathogens are usually transmitted sexually. The most common cause of urethritis is the bacterium, *Chlamydia trachomatis*, but *Neisseria gonorrhoeae*, ureaplasmas, and mycoplasmas can also be the cause. Urethritis that is *not* caused by *N. gonorrhoeae* is often referred to as nonspecific urethritis (NSU) or nongonococcal urethritis (NGU).
- **Prostatitis.** Inflammation of the prostate gland. Most often, prostatitis is not an infectious disease. If it is caused by a pathogen, the pathogen may be a bacterium, a virus, a fungus, or a protozoan.

Infections of the Genital Tract

As previously mentioned, indigenous microflora are found at and near the outer opening of the urethra and within the distal urethra[b] of both men and women. Additionally, the female genital region supports the growth of many other microorganisms. The adult vaginal microflora contains many species of *Lactobacillus*, *Staphylococcus*, *Streptococcus*, *Enterococcus*, *Neisseria*, *Clostridium*, *Actinomyces*, *Prevotella*, diphtheroids, enteric bacilli, and *Candida*. The balance among these microbes depends

> Destruction of some members of the vaginal microflora can lead to an overgrowth (superinfection) of other members.

[b] The distal urethra is that section of the urethra farthest from the urinary bladder.

on the estrogen levels and pH of the site. For example, should something (e.g., antibiotic use) kill the resident lactobacilli, an overgrowth (superinfection) of *C. albicans* can occur, leading to the condition known as yeast vaginitis. Should any of these or other microorganisms invade further into the GU system, various nonspecific infections may occur. The male and female reproductive systems are shown in Figure 17-9.

Genital infections can be caused by a wide variety of microbes. Terms relating to infectious diseases of the genital tract are as follows:

- **Bartholinitis.** Inflammation of the Bartholin's ducts in women.
- **Cervicitis.** Inflammation of the cervix (that part of the uterus that opens into the vagina).
- **Endometritis.** Inflammation of the endometrium (the inner layer of the uterine wall).
- **Epididymitis.** Inflammation of the epididymis (an elongated structure connected to the testis).
- **Pelvic inflammatory disease (PID).** Inflammation of the fallopian tubes; also known as **salpingitis**.
- **Vaginitis.** Inflammation of the vagina. The three most common causes of vaginitis in the United States, each causing about one third of the cases, are *C. albicans* (a yeast), *Trichomonas vaginalis* (a protozoan), and a mixture of bacteria (including bacteria in the genera *Mobiluncus* and *Gardnerella*). When caused by a mixture of bacteria, the infection is referred to as *bacterial vaginosis* (BV). In general, infections that result from the actions of two or more bacteria are called synergistic or polymicrobial infections. A saline wet mount preparation is usually used to diagnose vaginitis (see CD-ROM Appendix 5).

> The three most common causes of vaginitis in the United States are *C. albicans* (a yeast), *T. vaginalis* (a protozoan), and a mixture of bacteria.

- **Vulvovaginitis.** Inflammation of the vulva (the external genitalia of women) and the vagina.

Sexually Transmitted Diseases of the Genital Tract

The term sexually transmitted disease (STD), formerly called venereal disease (VD), includes any of the infections transmitted by sexual activities. It is important to understand that STDs are diseases not only of the genital tract, but can also affect the skin, mucous membranes, blood, lymphatic and digestive systems, and many other body areas. Epidemic STDs include acquired immunodeficiency syndrome (AIDS), chlamydial and herpes infections, gonorrhea, and syphilis. The AIDS virus (human immunodeficiency virus [HIV]) primarily causes damage to helper T cells and thus inhibits antibody production; it is discussed in Chapter 18 in the section entitled "Viral Diseases of the Circulatory System." Diseases

> STDs affect not only the genital tract, but can also involve the skin, mucous membranes, blood, lymphatic and digestive systems, and many other anatomic sites.

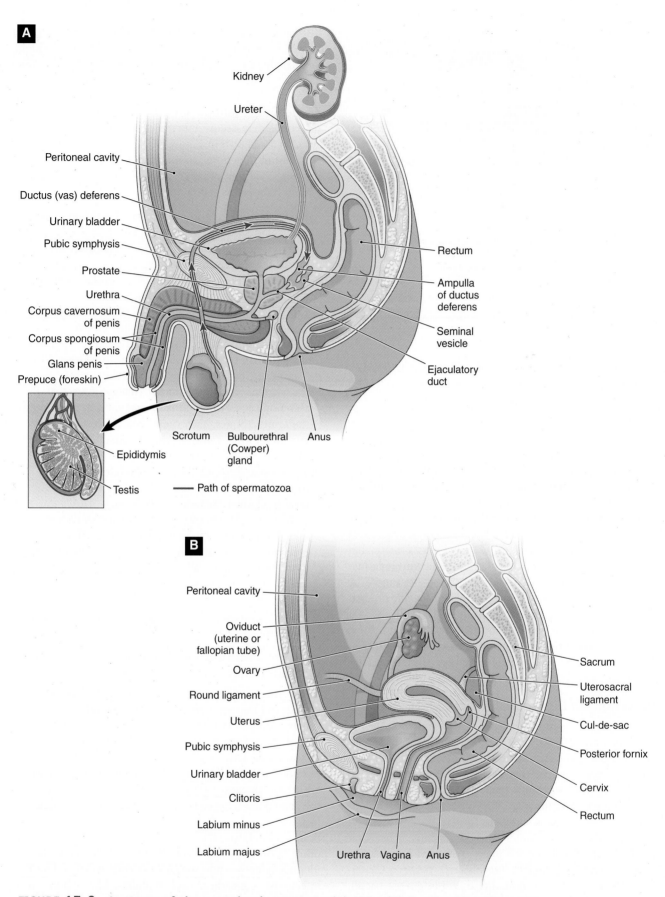

FIGURE 17-9. **Anatomy of the reproductive system. (A)** Male. **(B)** Female. (From Cohen BJ. Memmler's The Human Body in Health and Disease, 11th ed. Philadelphia: Lippincott Williams & Wilkins, 2009.)

such as hepatitis B, amebiasis, and giardiasis can also be transmitted by sexual activities, as can many other diseases.

INFECTIOUS DISEASES OF THE CIRCULATORY SYSTEM

The circulatory system consists of the cardiovascular system and the lymphatic system. The cardiovascular (*cardio* for heart, and *vascular* for the various types of blood vessels) system includes the heart, arteries, capillaries, veins, and blood. Blood is composed of plasma (the liquid portion) plus the various cellular elements. (The cellular elements of blood are discussed in Chapters 13 and 15). Terms relating to infectious diseases of the cardiovascular system are as follows:

• **Endocarditis.** Inflammation of the endocardium—the endothelial membrane that lines the cavities of the heart (Fig. 17-10).

• **Myocarditis.** Inflammation of the myocardium—the muscular walls of the heart.
• **Pericarditis.** Inflammation of the pericardium—the membranous sac around the heart.

SPOTLIGHTING CARDIOVASCULAR TECHNOLOGISTS

As stated in the AMA's Health Care Careers Directory for 2008–2009 (available at http://www .ama-assn.org), "Cardiovascular technologists perform diagnostic examinations and therapeutic interventions of the heart and/or blood vessels at the

(continues)

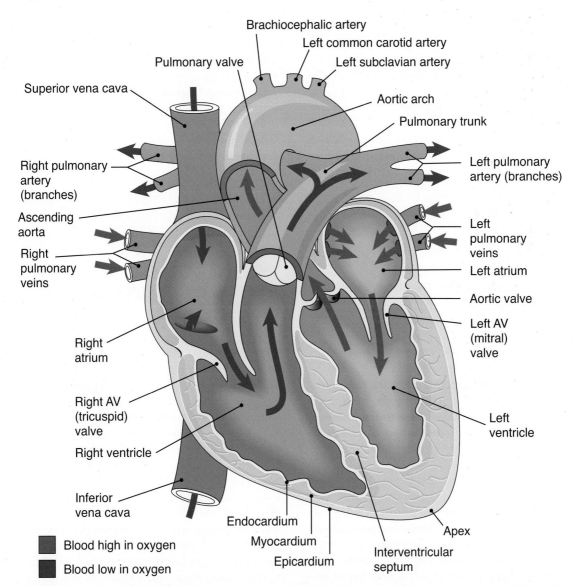

FIGURE 17-10. Anatomy of the heart. (From Cohen BJ. Memmler's The Human Body in Health and Disease, 11th ed. Philadelphia: Lippincott Williams & Wilkins, 2009.)

request or direction of a physician in one or more of the following:

- Invasive cardiovascular laboratories—cardiaccatheterization, blood gas, and electrophysiologylaboratories
- Noninvasive cardiovascular laboratories—echocardiology, exercise stress test, and electrocardiology laboratories
- Noninvasive peripheral vascular studies laboratories—Doppler ultrasound and thermography laboratories

Through subjective sampling and/or recording, the cardiovascular technologist creates as easily definable foundation of data from which a correct anatomic and physiologic diagnosis may be established for each patient."

"The cardiovascular technologist is qualified by specific didactic, laboratory, and clinical technological education to perform various cardiovascular/peripheral vascular diagnostic and therapeutic procedures. The role of the cardiovascular technologist may include but is not limited to:

- Reviewing and/or recoding pertinent patient history and supporting clinical data
- Performing appropriate clinical procedures and obtaining a record of anatomical, pathological, and/or physiological data for interpretation by a physician
- Exercising discretion and judgment in the performance of cardiovascular diagnostic and therapeutic services."

Information concerning educational requirements and programs, certification, and salary can be found on the AMA web site.

Normally, blood is sterile; it contains no resident microflora. The presence of bacteria in the bloodstream is known as **bacteremia**, which can be, but is not always, a sign of disease. **Transient bacteremia** (the temporary presence of bacteria in the blood) often results from dental extractions, wounds, bites, and damage to the intestinal, respiratory, or reproductive tract mucosa. Even aggressive tooth brushing, which causes bleeding of the gums, can lead to transient bacteremia.

However, when pathogenic organisms are capable of resisting or overwhelming the phagocytes and other body defenses—or when an individual is immunosuppressed or is otherwise more susceptible than normal—a systemic disease called *septicemia* may occur. A patient

> The presence of bacteria in a person's bloodstream may or may not be a sign of disease.

> Septicemia is a disease in which the patient experiences chills, fever, and prostration (extreme exhaustion) and has bacteria and/or their toxins in their bloodstream.

with septicemia experiences chills, fever, and prostration (extreme exhaustion) and has bacteria and/or their toxins in the bloodstream.

Although dozens of infectious diseases can be transmitted by donated blood, only the following tests are routinely performed on donor blood in the United States:

- *Treponema pallidum* antigen (*T. pallidum* is the cause of syphilis)
- HIV-1 antibody
- HIV-2 antibody
- HIV p24 antigen
- HTLV-1 antibody (human T-cell lymphotrophic virus type 1 has been associated with several kinds of diseases including demyelinating diseases, leukemia, and lymphoma)
- Hepatitis B surface antigen
- Hepatitis B core antibody
- Hepatitis C antibody

The lymphatic system consists of lymphatic vessels, lymphoid tissue (including lymph nodes, tonsils, thymus, and spleen), and lymph (the liquid that circulates through the lymphatic system). Lymph occasionally picks up microorganisms from the intestine, lungs, and other areas, but these transient organisms are usually quickly engulfed by phagocytic cells in the liver and lymph nodes. The lymphatic system contains many lymphocytes (discussed in Chapter 16). Terms relating to infectious diseases of the lymphatic system include:

- **Lymphadenitis.** Inflamed and swollen lymph nodes.
- **Lymphadenopathy.** Diseased lymph nodes.
- **Lymphangitis.** Inflamed lymphatic vessels.

INFECTIOUS DISEASES OF THE CENTRAL NERVOUS SYSTEM

The nervous system is composed of the CNS and the peripheral nervous system (Fig. 17-11). The CNS consists of the brain, the spinal cord, and the three membranes (or **meninges** [sing., **meninx**]) that cover the brain and spinal cord (Fig. 17-12). The CNS is well protected and remarkably resistant to infection; it is encased in bone, bathed and cushioned in cerebrospinal fluid (CSF), and nourished by capillaries. These capillaries make up the blood-brain barrier, supplying nutrients but not allowing larger particles, such as macromolecules (e.g., antibodies and most antibiotics), cells of the immune system, and microorganisms, to pass from the blood into the brain. The peripheral nervous system consists of nerves that branch from the brain and spinal cord.

There are no indigenous microflora of the nervous system. Microbes gain access to the CNS through trauma (fracture or medical procedure), via the blood and lymph to the CSF, or along the peripheral nerves.

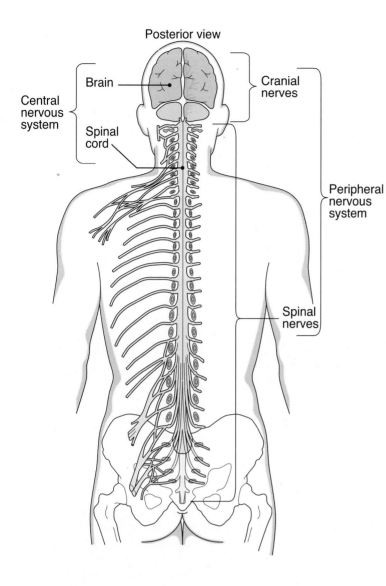

Posterior view

Brain

Central
nervous
system

Spinal
cord

Cranial
nerves

Peripheral
nervous
system

Spinal
nerves

FIGURE 17-11. Anatomy of the central nervous system. (From Cohen BJ. Memmler's The Human Body in Health and Disease, 11th ed. Philadelphia: Lippincott Williams & Wilkins, 2009.)

Terms relating to infectious diseases of the CNS include the following:

- **Encephalitis.** Inflammation of the brain.
- **Encephalomyelitis.** Inflammation of the brain and spinal cord.
- **Meningitis.** Inflammation of the membranes (meninges) that surround the brain and spinal cord.
- **Meningoencephalitis.** Inflammation of the brain and meninges.
- **Myelitis.** Inflammation of the spinal cord.

Infections of the CNS Having Multiple Causes

Meningitis

Meningitis—inflammation of the meninges—can have many causes, including the ingestion of poisons, the ingestion or injection of drugs, a reaction to a vaccine, or a pathogen. If caused by a pathogen, the culprit might be a virus, a bacterium, a fungus, or a protozoan.

Viral meningitis may be caused by a virus that specifically infects the meninges, or may be the result of an immune reaction to a virus that does not specifically infect the brain (e.g., chickenpox, measles, and rubella viruses). Viral meningitis is sometimes referred to as "aseptic meningitis," because in about 50% of the cases, the pathogen cannot be identified. The various types of viruses that cause meningitis include enteroviruses (the major cause in the United States), Coxsackieviruses, echoviruses, mumps virus, **arboviruses** (arthropod-borne viruses), poliovirus, adenoviruses, measles virus, herpes simplex, and varicella virus. Viral meningitis tends to be less serious than bacterial meningitis.

Historically, the three major causes of bacterial meningitis have been *H. influenzae* (the primary cause in children), *Neisseria meningitidis* (the primary cause in

> Meningitis can be caused by the ingestion of poisons, the ingestion or injection of drugs, a reaction to a vaccine, or a pathogen.

> Viral meningitis is sometimes referred to as "aseptic meningitis," because in about 50% of the cases, the pathogen cannot be identified.

FIGURE 17-12. Section of the top of the head showing the meninges and related structures. (From Cohen BJ. Memmler's The Human Body in Health and Disease, 11th ed. Philadelphia: Lippincott Williams & Wilkins, 2009.)

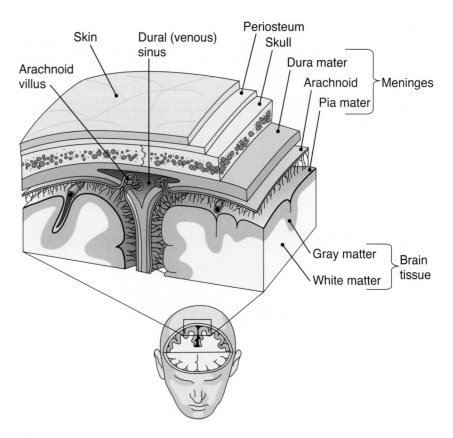

adolescents), and *S. pneumoniae* (the primary cause in the elderly). Vaccination of children with the Hib vaccine[c] has drastically reduced the incidence of *H. influenzae* meningitis in children in the United States. Less common causes of bacterial meningitis are *S. aureus*, *Pseudomonas aeruginosa*, *Salmonella*, and *Klebsiella*.

> Historically, the three major causes of bacterial meningitis have been *H. influenzae*, *Neisseria meningitidis*, and *S. pneumoniae*.

The major causes of bacterial meningitis in neonates are *Streptococcus agalactiae* (Group B, beta-hemolytic streptococci), *E. coli* and other members of the family Enterobacteriaceae, and *Listeria monocytogenes*.

Early symptoms of bacterial meningitis include fever, headache, stiff neck, sore throat, and vomiting. Then neurologic symptoms of dizziness, convulsions, minor paralysis, and coma occur; death may result within a few hours. Meningitis is a medical emergency and steps must be taken immediately to determine the cause. Diagnosis is usually made by a combination of patient symptoms, physical examination, and Gram staining and culture of the CSF.

Free-living amebas that may cause *meningoencephalitis* are in the genera *Naegleria* and *Acanthamoeba*. Other protozoa that may invade the meninges

> Parasites that can cause CNS diseases include free-living amebas and *Toxoplasma* and *Trypanosoma* spp.

are *Toxoplasma* and *Trypanosoma*. Occasionally, fungal pathogens, especially *Cryptococcus neoformans* (an encapsulated yeast), cause meningitis.

Several CNS diseases are caused by toxins. Examples of bacterial neurotoxins are botulinal toxin (the exotoxin that causes botulism) and **tetanospasmin** (the cause of tetanus). Diseases caused by fungal toxins (mycotoxins) include ergot from grain moulds and mushroom poisoning. *Gonyaulax*, an alga found in algal "blooms," produces neurotoxins, which may concentrate in bivalve shell fish and cause paralytic symptoms following ingestion of the

---

STUDY AID

Aseptic Meningitis

The term *aseptic meningitis* implies meningitis that is not caused by a pathogen. Although it is true that some cases of meningitis result from events unrelated to pathogens (e.g., the ingestion of poisons or certain drugs), many cases of aseptic meningitis are actually the result of infections. The term probably originated from meningitis cases where no organisms were recovered on routine bacteriological culture. However, many cases of meningitis are caused by organisms that will not grow on standard bacteriological culture media. Examples of such pathogens are viruses (many different types), fungi, leptospira, and *T. pallidum*. Cases of meningitis caused by these types of organisms are collectively referred to as aseptic meningitis.

---

[c] The *Hib* in Hib vaccine stands for *Haemophilus influenzae* type b, the capsular type of *H. influenzae* that, prior to use of Hib vaccine, was the major cause of meningitis in children.

contaminated shellfish. A variety of other algae also produce neurotoxins (see CD-ROM Appendix 1).

OPPORTUNISTIC INFECTIONS

Recall from Chapter 1 that certain microbes are referred to as "opportunistic pathogens" or "opportunists." These are microbes that usually do not cause disease, but have the potential to cause disease under certain conditions. The term **opportunistic infections** (OIs), refers to infections that normally would not occur in healthy, immunocompetent individuals or would, at most, cause only mild infections. On the other hand, OIs are relatively common in immunosuppressed individuals, and often contribute to their death. Immunosuppressed individuals present an "opportunity" for the pathogens to cause disease.

Listed here are some of the most common OIs:

- **Aspergillosis and other mould infections** (including bread mould infections); can become a systemic infection in immunosuppressed individuals
- **Candidiasis**. A yeast infection of the mouth (thrush), throat, or vagina; can become a systemic infection in immunosuppressed individuals
- **Cytomegalovirus (CMV) infection**. Can cause eye disease that can lead to blindness
- **Herpes simplex virus infections**. The cause of oral herpes (cold sores) and genital herpes, which can occur in immunocompetent individuals, but are more frequent and more severe in immunosuppressed individuals
- **Malaria**. A parasitic infection that occurs in immunocompetent individuals, but is more common and more severe in immunosuppressed individuals
- *Mycobacterium avium* **complex**. A bacterial infection that can cause recurring fevers, problems with digestion, and serious weight loss
- *Pneumocystis* **pneumonia**. A fungal infection that can cause a fatal pneumonia; prior to newer and more aggressive treatments, was once the major killer of AIDS patients
- **Toxoplasmosis ("toxo")**. A protozoal infection of the eyes and brain
- **Tuberculosis (TB)**. A bacterial lower respiratory infection; can cause meningitis; occurs in immunocompetent individuals, but is more common and more severe in immunosuppressed individuals

EMERGING AND REEMERGING INFECTIOUS DISEASES

It was not so very long ago that scientists believed that they had infectious diseases "on the run."[d] They were confident that a combination of surveillance, quarantine, vaccines, antibiotics, and other antimicrobial agents marked the beginning of the end for pathogen-caused diseases. They were wrong.

Not only do "new" (previously unknown) infectious diseases continue to emerge, but other infectious diseases, once thought to be contained or eradicated, continue to reemerge. Causes of emerging diseases include changes in human demographics and behavior; ecological changes such as dams, deforestation, and climate change; increased international travel; increased exposure to exotic animals; misuse of antibiotics and other antimicrobial agents; and breakdown of public health measures. Listed here are some of the infectious diseases that have emerged in the last 30 years:

Avian influenza ("bird flu")
Cryptosporidiosis
E. coli O157 infections (including hemolytic uremic syndrome)
Ebola hemorrhagic fever
Hantavirus pulmonary syndrome (HPS)
Hendra virus infection
HIV infection and AIDS
Human monkeypox
Lassa fever
Legionellosis
Lyme disease
Marburg hemorrhagic fever
Nipah virus encephalitis
Severe acute respiratory syndrome (SARS)
Variant Creutzfeldt-Jakob disease
West Nile virus encephalitis

Causes of reemerging infectious diseases include pathogen mutations and genetic recombinations, acquired drug resistance, decreased compliance with vaccination policies and other breakdowns in public health measures, population shifts, war and civil conflicts, famine, floods, droughts, and bioterrorism. Infectious diseases that have reemerged or shown up in new geographic areas in recent years include cholera, dengue fever, diphtheria, malaria, Rift Valley fever, TB, yellow fever, and infections caused by methicillin-resistant *S. aureus* (MRSA) and other "superbugs."

The journal, *Emerging Infectious Diseases*, published monthly by the Centers for Disease Control and Prevention (CDC), is available at no cost at http://www.cdc.gov/ncidod/EID/index.htm.

---

[d] In the late 1960s, based on progress that had been made reducing the incidence of such infectious diseases as smallpox, polio, and rheumatic fever, the Surgeon General of the United States, William H. Stewart, declared that it was time to close the book on infectious diseases and, to instead, pay closer attention to chronic ailments such as cancer and heart disease.

ON THE CD-ROM
- Terms Introduced in This Chapter
- Review of Key Points
- Increase Your Knowledge
- Additional Self-Assessment Exercises

SELF-ASSESSMENT EXERCISES

After studying this chapter, answer the following multiple-choice questions.

1. Otitis media is an inflammation or infection of the:
   a. ear.
   b. eye.
   c. brain.
   d. urinary bladder.
2. Keratitis is an inflammation or infection of the:
   a. conjunctiva.
   b. cornea.
   c. kidney.
   d. skin.
3. Which of the following is/are the most common cause of pharyngitis?
   a. *Escherichia coli*
   b. *Staphylococcus aureus*
   c. *Streptococcus pyogenes*
   d. viruses
4. Which of the following is the most common cause of tooth decay?
   a. *S. aureus*
   b. *Streptococcus agalactiae*
   c. *Streptococcus mutans*
   d. *S. pyogenes*
5. An infection of the urinary bladder is known as:
   a. cystitis.
   b. pyelonephritis.
   c. ureteritis.
   d. urethritis.
6. The most common cause of cystitis is:
   a. *Candida albicans*.
   b. *E. coli*.
   c. *Staphylococcus epidermidis*.
   d. *Staphylococcus saprophyticus*.
7. The most common cause of urethritis is:
   a. *Chlamydia trachomatis*.
   b. *E. coli*.
   c. *Mycoplasma pneumoniae*.
   d. *S. aureus*.
8. Which of the following terms means swollen lymph glands?
   a. lymphadenitis
   b. lymphadenopathy
   c. lymphangitis
   d. lymphitis
9. Inflammation or infection of the brain is called:
   a. encephalitis.
   b. meningitis.
   c. myelitis.
   d. otitis externa.
10. Which of the following is *not* one of the three most common causes of bacterial meningitis?
    a. *E. coli*
    b. *Haemophilus influenzae*
    c. *Neisseria meningitidis*
    d. *Streptococcus pneumoniae*

VIRAL INFECTIONS   18

LEARNING OBJECTIVES

AFTER STUDYING THIS CHAPTER, YOU SHOULD BE ABLE TO:

- Correlate various viral diseases with body systems (e.g., rhinoviruses with the respiratory system)
- Correlate a particular viral disease with its major characteristics, etiologic agent, reservoir(s), mode(s) of transmission, and diagnostic laboratory procedures
- Name several nationally notifiable viral diseases
- Briefly describe how viruses cause disease
- Describe *Koplik spots* and state the disease with which they are associated
- Characterize the various hepatitis viruses as being either DNA or RNA viruses
- List several viral diseases that are sexually transmitted

INTRODUCTION

It would be impossible in a book this size to describe *all* of the human infectious diseases caused by viruses. Thus, only selected viral diseases are described in this chapter.

Certain of the viral diseases described in this chapter are nationally notifiable infectious diseases, meaning that when a patient is diagnosed with one of these diseases in the United States, the information must be reported to the Centers for Disease Control and Prevention (CDC). As of 2007, there were approximately 21 nationally notifiable viral diseases (see Table 18-1). Most of them are described in this chapter, as are some viral diseases that are not nationally notifiable.

HOW DO VIRUSES CAUSE DISEASE?

Recall from Chapter 4 that viruses can only infect cells bearing appropriate surface receptors (i.e., surface receptors that the virus is able to recognize and bind to). Thus, viruses are specific as to the type of cell(s) that they can infect. For this reason, certain viruses only cause respiratory infections, whereas others only cause gastrointestinal (GI) infections, and so on.

Viruses multiply within host cells, and it is during their escape from those cells—by either cell lysis or budding—that the host cells are destroyed. This cell destruction leads to most of the symptoms of the viral

TABLE 18-1	Nationally Notifiable Viral Diseases

VIRAL DISEASE	NUMBER OF NEW U.S. CASES REPORTED TO THE CDC IN 2007*
AIDS	37,503
Domestic arthropod-borne viral (arboviral) diseases:	
Encephalitis caused by members of the California serogroup	55
Eastern equine encephalitis	4
Powassan virus encephalitis	7
St. Louis encephalitis	9
West Nile virus encephalitis	3,630
Western equine encephalitis	0
Hantavirus pulmonary syndrome	32
Hepatitis A	2,979
Hepatitis B	4,519
Hepatitis C	845
Influenza-associated pediatric mortality	77
Measles	43
Mumps	800
Poliomyelitis	0
Rabies, human	1
Rubella	12
SARS	0
Smallpox	0
Varicella (chickenpox)	40,152
Yellow fever	0

Source: http://www.cdc.gov.
*These figures provide insight as to how frequently these diseases occur in the United States. For updated information, go to the CDC web site; click on "Morbidity & Mortality Weekly Report"; then click on "Notifiable Diseases"; then click on the most recent year that is listed.

STUDY AID

What to Learn?

This chapter contains a large amount of information. Of primary importance will be your ability to later recall the name of the virus that causes a particular viral disease and the manner in which the disease is transmitted. If applicable, you should be able to state the vector that is involved in the transmission of the disease. For example, if your teacher says "dengue fever," you should be able to state the name of the virus that causes the disease (dengue virus), the manner in which dengue fever is transmitted (mosquito bite), and the vector that is involved in the transmission of dengue fever (mosquitoes in the genus *Aedes*).

infection, which vary depending on the location of the infection. Other symptoms are the result of immunological injury (i.e., injury that results from the immune response to the viral pathogen). In the case of the acquired immunodeficiency syndrome (AIDS) virus (human immunodeficiency virus [HIV]), the virus destroys cells of the immune system. This renders the patient unable to ward off various viral, bacterial, fungal, and parasitic pathogens. The AIDS patient's death results from overwhelming infections caused by these pathogens.

VIRAL INFECTIONS OF THE SKIN

Table 18-2 contains information pertaining to viral infections of the skin.

TABLE 18-2 Viral Infections of the Skin

DISEASE	ADDITIONAL INFORMATION
Chickenpox and Shingles. (a) Chickenpox (also known as varicella) is an acute, generalized viral infection, with fever and a skin rash (Fig. 18-1). Vesicles also form in mucous membranes. It is usually a mild, self-limiting disease, but can be severely damaging to a fetus. Serious complications include pneumonia, secondary bacterial infections, hemorrhagic complications, and encephalitis. Reye's (pronounced "rize") syndrome (a severe encephalomyelitis with liver damage) may follow clinical chickenpox if aspirin is given to children younger than 16 years of age. Chickenpox is the leading cause of vaccine-preventable death in the United States. (b) Shingles (also known as herpes zoster) is a reactivation of the varicella virus, often the result of immunosuppression. Shingles involves inflammation of sensory ganglia of cutaneous sensory nerves, producing fluid-filled blisters, pain, and paresthesia (numbness and tingling). Shingles may occur at any age, but is most common after age 50. **Patient Care.** Use Airborne and Contact Precautions for hospitalized patients until their lesions become dry and crusted.	**Pathogen.** Chickenpox and shingles are caused by varicella-zoster virus (VZV); a herpes virus (family Herpesviridae) that is also known as human herpesvirus 3; a DNA virus. **Reservoirs and Mode of Transmission.** Infected humans serve as reservoirs. Transmission is from person to person by direct contact or droplet or airborne spread of vesicle fluid or secretions of the respiratory system of persons with chickenpox. **Laboratory Diagnosis.** Diagnosis is usually made on clinical and epidemiologic grounds. Immunodiagnostic and molecular diagnostic procedures are available, as are cell culture and electron microscopy.
German Measles (Rubella). German measles is a mild, febrile viral disease. A fine, pinkish, flat rash begins 1 or 2 days after the onset of symptoms (Fig. 18-2). The rash starts on the face and neck and spreads to the trunk, arms, and legs. Rubella is a milder disease than hard measles with fewer complications. If acquired during the first trimester of pregnancy, rubella may cause congenital rubella syndrome in the fetus. This can lead to intrauterine death, spontaneous abortion, or congenital malformations of major organ systems. **Patient Care.** Use Droplet Precautions for hospitalized patients until 7 days after the onset of rash.	**Pathogen.** Rubella is caused by rubella virus, an RNA virus in the family Togaviridae. **Reservoirs and Mode of Transmission.** Infected humans serve as reservoirs. Transmission occurs by droplet spread or direct contact with nasopharyngeal secretions of infected people. **Laboratory Diagnosis.** Immunodiagnostic and molecular diagnostic procedures are available for diagnosis of rubella. The virus can be propagated in cell culture.
Measles (Hard Measles, Rubeola). Measles is an acute, highly communicable viral disease with fever, conjunctivitis, cough, photosensitivity (light sensitivity), Koplik spots in the mouth, and red blotchy skin rash (Fig. 18-3). Koplik spots are small red spots, in the center of which can be seen a minute bluish white speck when observed under a strong light (Fig. 18-4). The rash begins on the face between days 3 and 7 and then becomes generalized. Complications include bronchitis, pneumonia, otitis media, and encephalitis. Rarely, autoimmune, subacute, sclerosing panencephalitis (SSPE) may follow a latent period of several years. SSPE is characterized by gradual progressive psychoneurological deterioration, including personality changes, seizures, photosensitivity, ocular abnormalities, and coma. **Patient Care.** Use Airborne Precautions for hospitalized patients until 4 days after the onset of rash.	**Pathogen.** Measles is caused by measles virus (also known as rubeola virus). It is an RNA virus in the family Paramyxoviridae. **Reservoirs and Mode of Transmission.** Infected humans serve as reservoirs. Airborne transmission occurs by droplet spread, direct contact with nasal or throat secretions of infected persons, or with articles freshly soiled with nose and throat secretions. **Laboratory Diagnosis.** Diagnosis of measles is usually made on clinical and epidemiologic grounds. Immunodiagnostic and molecular diagnostic procedures are available, and the virus can be isolated in cell culture.

(continues)

TABLE 18-2   Viral Infections of the Skin (continued)

DISEASE	ADDITIONAL INFORMATION
Monkeypox. Monkeypox is a rare viral disease that causes fever, headache, muscle aches, backache, lymphadenitis, malaise (fatigue), and a rash (Fig. 18-5). A milder disease than smallpox, monkeypox occurs primarily in central and western Africa, although several people in the United States became ill in 2003 after handling infected prairie dogs. Unlike smallpox, monkeypox is rarely fatal. **Patient Care.** Use Airborne and Contact Precautions for hospitalized patients; Airborne Precautions until monkeypox is confirmed and smallpox is excluded; Contact Precautions until lesions become crusted.	**Pathogen.** Monkeypox is caused by monkeypox virus, which is in the same group of viruses (orthopoxviruses) as smallpox virus (variola virus) and the virus used in the smallpox vaccine (vaccinia virus). **Reservoirs and Mode of Transmission.** Infected animals serve as reservoirs. Transmission occurs via animal bite or contact with an infected animal's blood, body fluids, or rash. Person-to-person transmission does occur. **Laboratory Diagnosis.** Monkeypox can be diagnosed by molecular diagnostic procedures, cell culture, electron microscopy, or immunodiagnostic procedures. (see http://www.cdc.gov/ncidod/monkeypox for more information)
Smallpox. Smallpox is a systemic viral infection with fever, malaise, headache, prostration, severe backache, a characteristic skin rash (refer back to Fig. 11-10 in Chapter 11), and occasional abdominal pain and vomiting. The rash is similar to, and must be distinguished from, the rash of chickenpox. Smallpox can become severe, with bleeding into the skin and mucous membranes, followed by death. **Patient Care.** Use Airborne and Contact Precautions for hospitalized patients until all scabs have crusted and separated (3–4 weeks). Use N95 or higher respiratory protection.	**Pathogen.** Smallpox is caused by two strains of variola virus: variola minor (with a fatality rate of <1%), and variola major (with a fatality rate of 20%–40% or higher). Variola virus is a double-stranded DNA virus in the genus Orthopoxvirus, family Poxviridae. Smallpox virus is a potential biological warfare and bioterrorism agent. **Reservoirs and Mode of Transmission.** Before smallpox was eradicated, infected humans were the only source of the virus. There are no known animal or environmental reservoirs. Person-to-person transmission is via the respiratory tract (droplet spread) or skin inoculation. Patients are most contagious before eruption of the rash, by aerosol droplets from oropharyngeal lesions. **Laboratory Diagnosis.** Because of the potential danger of the use of smallpox virus as a bioterrorism agent, physicians must become familiar with the clinical and epidemiologic features of smallpox and how to distinguish smallpox from chickenpox. Laboratory diagnosis is by cell culture, virus neutralization tests, molecular diagnostic procedures, or electron microscopy. These procedures are performed only in biosafety level 4 (BSL-4) facilities.
Warts. Warts consist of many varieties of skin and mucous membrane lesions, including common warts (verrucae vulgaris), venereal warts, and plantar warts. Most are harmless, but some can become cancerous. Venereal or genital warts are discussed in more detail later in the chapter.	**Pathogens.** Warts are caused by at least 70 types of human papillomaviruses (HPV). They are classified in the genus Papillomavirus within the family Papovaviridae. They are DNA viruses. **Reservoirs and Mode of Transmission.** Infected humans serve as reservoirs. Transmission usually occurs by direct contact. Genital warts are sexually transmitted. They are easily spread from one area of the body to another, but most are not very contagious from person to person (genital warts are an exception). **Laboratory Diagnosis.** Diagnosis is made on clinical grounds.

FIGURE 18-1. Chickenpox, with lesions at all stages of development. (From Harvey RA, et al. Lippincott's Illustrated Reviews: Microbiology, 2nd ed. Philadelphia: Lippincott Williams & Wilkins, 2007.)

FIGURE 18-3. Child with measles. (Courtesy of the CDC.)

FIGURE 18-4. Koplik spots. Koplik spots, an early sign of measles, usually appear prior to the onset of skin rash. Koplik spots are irregularly shaped, bright-red spots, often having a bluish white central dot. (From Harvey RA, et al. Lippincott's Illustrated Reviews: Microbiology, 2nd ed. Philadelphia: Lippincott Williams & Wilkins, 2007.)

FIGURE 18-2. Child with rubella. The lesions are not as intensely red as those of measles. (Courtesy of the CDC.)

FIGURE 18-5. Child with monkeypox. (Courtesy of the CDC.)

VIRAL INFECTIONS OF THE EARS

Information about viral and bacterial ear infections can be found in Table 19-3 in Chapter 19.

VIRAL INFECTIONS OF THE EYES

Table 18-3 contains information about viral infections of the eyes.

VIRAL INFECTIONS OF THE RESPIRATORY SYSTEM

Viral Infections of the Upper Respiratory Tract

The Common Cold (Acute Viral Rhinitis, Acute Coryza)

Disease. The common cold is a viral infection of the lining of the nose, sinuses, throat, and large airways. Symptoms include coryza (profuse discharge from nostrils), sneezing, runny eyes, sore throat, chills, and malaise. Additionally, laryngitis, tracheitis, or bronchitis may accompany a cold. Secondary bacterial infections, including sinusitis and otitis media, may follow. The common cold occurs most frequently in fall, winter, and spring. On average, most people have one to six colds annually. It is not a nationally notifiable disease in the United States.

Patient Care. Use Droplet Precautions for hospitalized patients.

Pathogens. Many different viruses cause colds. Rhinoviruses, of which there are more than 100 serotypes, are the major cause in adults. Other cold-causing viruses

TABLE 18-3	Viral Infections of the Eyes
DISEASE	**ADDITIONAL INFORMATION**
Adenoviral Conjunctivitis and Keratoconjunctivitis. These are acute viral diseases of one or both eyes, associated with inflammation of the conjunctiva, edema eyelid and periorbital tissue, pain, photophobia, and blurred vision. The cornea is involved in about 50% of cases, with permanent scarring of the cornea in severe cases. **Patient Care.** Use Contact Precautions for hospitalized patients for the duration of the illness.	**Pathogens.** Adenoviral conjunctitivis and keratoconjunctivitis are caused by various types of adenoviruses. Herpes simplex and varicella-zoster viruses can also cause keratoconjunctivitis. **Reservoirs and Mode of Transmission.** Infected humans serve as reservoirs. Transmission occurs via direct contact with eye secretions or contact with contaminated surfaces, instruments, or solutions. People with viral infections (e.g., cold sores) should wash their hands thoroughly before inserting or removing contact lenses or otherwise touching their eyes. **Laboratory Diagnosis.** Diagnosis is made by cell culture orimmunodiagnostic or molecular diagnostic procedures.
Hemorrhagic Conjunctivitis. This viral disease has a sudden onset, with redness, swelling, and pain in one or both eyes. Small, discrete subconjunctival hemorrhages may enlarge to form confluent subconjunctival hemorrhages. One adenoviral syndrome, called pharyngoconjunctival fever, is characterized by upper respiratory disease, fever, and minor degrees of corneal epithelial inflammation. **Patient Care.** Use Contact Precautions for hospitalized patients for the duration of the illness.	**Pathogens.** Hemorrhagic conjunctivitis is caused by adenoviruses and enteroviruses. **Reservoirs and Mode of Transmission.** Infected humans serve as reservoirs. Transmission occurs by direct or indirect contact with discharge from infected eyes. Adenovirus transmission may be associated with poorly chlorinated swimming pools; this "swimming pool conjunctivitis" can reach epidemic proportions. **Laboratory Diagnosis.** Diagnosis is made by cell culture or immunodiagnostic or molecular diagnostic procedures.

include coronaviruses, parainfluenza viruses, respiratory syncytial virus (RSV), influenza viruses, adenoviruses, and enteroviruses.

Reservoirs and Mode of Transmission. Infected humans serve as reservoirs of infection. Transmission is via respiratory secretions by way of hands and fomites or direct contact with or inhalation of airborne droplets.

Laboratory Diagnosis. Laboratory diagnosis of the common cold usually is not required, but cell-culture techniques can often demonstrate the specific viral pathogen.

Infections of the Lower Respiratory Tract Having Multiple Causes

Information pertaining to infections of the lower respiratory tract having multiple causes can be found in Chapter 19.

Viral Infections of the Lower Respiratory Tract

Table 18-4 contains information pertaining to viral infections of the lower respiratory tract.

VIRAL INFECTIONS OF THE ORAL REGION

Cold Sores (Fever Blisters, Herpes Labialis)

Cold sores are superficial clear vesicles on an erythematous (reddened) base, which may appear on the face or lips (refer back to Fig. 14-2 in Chapter 14). They crust and heal within a few days. Reactivation may be caused by

HISTORICAL NOTE
The World's Worst Influenza Pandemic
The 1918–1919 Spanish flu pandemic (also known as the swine flu pandemic) killed an estimated 20 to 100 million people, worldwide—between 2.5% and 5% of the world population. The pandemic killed between 2% and 20% of those infected compared with a mortality rate of about 0.1% for modern-day flu epidemics. Although most victims of modern-day flu epidemics are very young, very old, and immunosuppressed people, the 1918–1919 pandemic killed primarily healthy young adults. Scientists have recovered the virus (designated A/H1N1) that caused the pandemic from frozen tissue samples, and are currently studying it. They have discovered that the virus kills by causing an overreaction of the body's immune system. This could explain why healthy young adults with strong immune systems were affected to a greater extent than those with weaker immune systems—very young, very old, and immunosuppressed individuals.

trauma, fever (hence the name), physiologic changes, or disease. The infection may be severe and extensive in immunosuppressed individuals. Cold sores are usually caused by herpes simplex virus type 1 (HSV-1), although they can also be caused by herpes simplex virus type 2 (HSV-2). HSV-1 and HSV-2 are also known as human herpesvirus 1 and human herpesvirus 2, respectively. They are DNA viruses in the family Herpesviridae. Either of these viruses may also infect the genital tract, although genital herpes infections are most often caused by HSV-2.

VIRAL INFECTIONS OF THE GASTROINTESTINAL TRACT

Infections of the Gastrointestinal Tract Having Multiple Causes

Diarrhea can have many causes. It may or may not be the result of an infectious disease. When diarrhea is the result of an infectious disease, the pathogen may be a virus, a bacterium, a protozoan, or a helminth. Dysentery (a severe form of diarrhea) may also be caused by various pathogens, including bacteria (e.g., *Shigella* spp. cause bacillary dysentery) and protozoa (e.g., those that cause amebiasis and balantidiasis; see Chapter 21).

Viral Gastroenteritis (Viral Enteritis, Viral Diarrhea)

Disease. Viral gastroenteritis may be an endemic or epidemic illness in infants, children, and adults. Symptoms include nausea, vomiting, diarrhea, abdominal pain, myalgia, headache, malaise, and low-grade fever. Although most often a self-limiting disease lasting 24 to 48 hours, viral gastroenteritis (especially when caused by a rotavirus) can be fatal in an infant or young child. In developing countries, rotavirus infections are responsible for more than 800,000 diarrheal deaths per year. Although viral gastroenteritis is sometimes referred to as "stomach flu" or "24-hour flu," keep in mind that *flu* is an abbreviation of *influenza*, which is a respiratory disease. Viral gastroenteritis is not a nationally notifiable disease in the United States.

Patient Care. Use Standard Precautions for hospitalized patients. Add Contact Precautions for diapered or incontinent patients and for patients with rotavirus infections.

Pathogens. The most common viruses infecting children in their first years of life are enteric adenoviruses, astroviruses, caliciviruses (including noroviruses), and rotaviruses. Those infecting children and adults include norovirus-like viruses and rotaviruses.

Reservoirs and Mode of Transmission. Infected humans are reservoirs of these viruses; contaminated water and shellfish may also be reservoirs. Transmission is most often via the fecal–oral route. Airborne transmission and contact with contaminated fomites may cause epidemics

TABLE 18-4	Viral Infections of the Lower Respiratory Tract

DISEASE	ADDITIONAL INFORMATION
Acute, Febrile, Viral Respiratory Disease. This disease is characterized by fever and one or more of the following systemic reactions: chills, headache, general aching, malaise, anorexia, and sometimes gastrointestinal (GI) disturbances in infants. The disease may include rhinitis, pharyngitis, tonsillitis, laryngitis, bronchitis, pneumonia, conjunctivitis, otitis media, and/or sinusitis. Acute, febrile, viral respiratory diseases are not nationally notifiable diseases in the United States. **Patient Care.** Use Standard Precautions for adult patients; add Contact Precautions for infants and young children for the duration of the illness.	**Pathogen.** Acute, febrile, viral respiratory disease can be caused by one of many viruses, including parainfluenza viruses, respiratory syncytial virus (RSV), adenovirus, rhinoviruses, certain coronaviruses, coxsackieviruses, and echoviruses. RSV is the major viral respiratory tract pathogen of early infancy. RSV may cause pneumonia, croup, bronchitis, otitis media, and death. **Reservoirs and Mode of Transmission.** Infected humans serve as reservoirs. Transmission occurs via direct oral contact or by droplets; indirectly via handkerchiefs, eating utensils, or other fomites; or for some viruses, via the fecal–oral route. **Laboratory Diagnosis.** Diagnosis is made by isolation of the etiologic agent from respiratory secretions, using cell cultures. Immunodiagnostic and molecular diagnostic procedures are available.
Hantavirus Pulmonary Syndrome (HPS). HPS is an acute viral disease characterized by fever, myalgias (muscular pain), GI complaints, cough, difficulty breathing, and hypotension (decreased blood pressure). The Sin Nombre virus—literally, the "virus with no name"—was the cause of the epidemic that occurred in the Four Corners area of the United States in the spring and summer of 1993. Since then, sporadic cases have been reported in many states as well as in South America. **Patient Care.** Use Standard Precautions for hospitalized patients.	**Pathogens.** At least five hantaviruses (Sin Nombre, Bayou, Black Creek Canal, New York-1, Monongahela) have caused HPS in the United States. Other strains have caused HPS in South America. **Reservoirs and Mode of Transmission.** Rodents, including deer mice, pack rats, and chipmunks serve as reservoirs. Transmission occurs via inhalation of aerosolized rodent feces, urine, and saliva. Person-to-person transmission does not occur. **Laboratory Diagnosis.** HPS can be diagnosed by immunodiagnostic and molecular procedures and by cell culture.
Influenza (Flu). Influenza is an acute, viral respiratory infection with fever, chills, headache, aches and pains throughout the body (most pronounced in the back and legs), sore throat, cough, nasal drainage. Influenza sometimes causing bronchitis, pneumonia, and death in severe cases. Nausea, vomiting, and diarrhea may occur, particularly in children. Although the term *stomach flu* is often heard, influenza viruses rarely cause GI symptoms. Stomach flu, also known as the 24-hour flu, is caused by viruses other than influenza viruses. **Patient Care.** Use Droplet Precautions for hospitalized patients, usually for 5 days from onset of symptoms.	**Pathogens.** Influenza is caused by influenza viruses types A, B, and C. They are single-stranded RNA viruses in the family Orthomyxovirus. Influenza A virus cause severe symptoms and is associated with pandemics and severe disease and more localized outbreaks. Influenza C virus usually does not cause epidemics or significant disease. **Reservoirs and Mode of Transmission.** Infected humans are the primary reservoir; pigs and birds also serve as reservoirs. Because pig cells have receptors for both avian and human strains of influenza virus, pigs serve as "mixing bowls," resulting in new strains containing RNA segments from both avian and human strains. It is thought that the 1918 pandemic was caused by an avian influenza virus that jumped directly from birds to humans. Transmission occurs via airborne spread and direct contact. **Laboratory Diagnosis.** Influenza is diagnosed by isolation of influenza virus from pharyngeal or nasal secretions or washings using cell culture techniques, antigen detection, and demonstration of a rise in antibody titer (concentration) between acute and convalescent sera (see Chapter 16), or by molecular diagnostic procedures.

| TABLE 18-4 | Viral Infections of the Lower Respiratory Tract (continued) |

DISEASE	ADDITIONAL INFORMATION
Avian Influenza (Bird Flu). Avian influenza, commonly referred to as bird flu, is primarily a disease of birds, but can cause human disease. In humans, the virus causes a respiratory infection with manifestations ranging from influenza-like symptoms (fever, cough, sore throat, and muscle aches) to eye infections, pneumonia, acute and severe respiratory distress, and other severe and life-threatening complications. **Patient Care.** Use Droplet Precautions for hospitalized patients (see http://www.cdc.gov/flu/avian/professional/infect-control.htm for more information).	**Pathogens.** Bird flu is caused by avian influenza virus type A. The three prominent subtypes of the virus are designated H5, H7, and H9. The strain known as H5N1 is the most virulent strain. **Reservoirs and Mode of Transmission.** Infected wild and domesticated birds serve as reservoirs. Bird-to-human transmission occurs via contact with infected poultry or surfaces that have been contaminated with excretions from infected birds. Person-to-person transmissions are relatively rare. However, influenza viruses commonly mutate, and increased instances of person-to-person transmission are likely to occur in the future. **Laboratory Diagnosis.** Molecular diagnostic procedures or cell culture are the means of diagnosis. **Note:** Additional information about bird flu can be found on the CD-ROM.
Severe Acute Respiratory Syndrome (SARS). SARS is a viral respiratory illness with high fever, chills, headache, a general feeling of discomfort, body aches, and sometimes diarrhea. Most patients develop a dry cough followed by pneumonia. SARS was first reported in Asia in February 2003. Over the next few months, the illness spread to more than 2 dozen countries in Asia, Europe, South America, and North America. During the 2003 outbreak, a total of 8,098 people developed SARS, 774 of whom died. No cases of SARS have been reported since 2004. **Patient Care.** Use Standard, Airborne, Droplet, and Contact Precautions for hospitalized patients for the duration of the illness plus 10 days after resolution of fever. Use N95 or higher respiratory protection and eye protection (see http://www.cdc.gov/ncidod/sars for more information).	**Pathogen.** SARS is caused by SARS-associated coronavirus (SARS-CoV) (Fig.18-6). **Reservoirs and Mode of Transmission.** Infected persons serve as reservoirs. It is possible that an unknown mammalian reservoir exists. Transmission occurs by respiratory droplets or by touching the mouth, nose, or eye after touching a contaminated surface or object. **Laboratory Diagnosis.** Immunodiagnostic or molecular diagnostic procedures or cell culture can be used to diagnose SARS.

FIGURE 18-6. SARS-associated coronavirus virions. Notice the crownlike halo surrounding each virion, which gives rise to the *corona* in *coronavirus*. (Courtesy of Dr. F.A. Murphy and the CDC.)

in hospitals or cruise ships. Foodborne, waterborne, and shellfish transmission have been reported.

Laboratory Diagnosis. Diagnosis is by electron microscopic examination of stool specimens or by immunodiagnostic or molecular procedures.

Viral Hepatitis

Hepatitis, or inflammation of the liver, can have many causes, including alcohol, drugs, and viruses. Viral hepatitis refers to hepatitis caused by any one of about a dozen different viruses, including hepatitis A virus (HAV), hepatitis B virus (HBV), hepatitis C virus (HCV), hepatitis D virus (HDV), hepatitis E virus (HEV), hepatitis G virus (HGV), hepatitis GB virus A (HGBV-A), hepatitis GB virus B (HGBV-B), and hepatitis GB virus C (HGBV-C). Hepatitis can also occur as a result of viral diseases such as infectious mononucleosis, yellow fever, and cytomegalovirus infection. See Table 18-5 for information about viral types, modes of transmission, and

TABLE 18-5	Common Types of Viral Hepatitis		

NAME OF DISEASE	NAME AND TYPE OF VIRUS	MODE OF TRANSMISSION	TYPE OF DISEASE
Type A hepatitis (also known as HAV infection, infectious hepatitis, and epidemic hepatitis)	HAV, a nonenveloped, linear ssRNA virus in the genus Hepatovirus, family Picornaviridae	Fecal–oral transmission; person-to-person; infected food handlers; fecally contaminated foods and water	Abrupt onset; varies in clinical severity from a mild illness lasting 1–2 weeks to a severe, disabling disease lasting several months; no chronic infection
Type B hepatitis (also known as HBV infection and serum hepatitis)	HBV, an enveloped, circular dsDNA virus in the genus Orthohepadnavirus, family Hepadnaviridae; the only DNA virus that causes hepatitis	Sexual or household contact with an infected person; mother-to-infant before or during birth; injected drug use; tattooing; needlesticks and other types of healthcare-associated transmission.	Usually has an insidious (gradual) onset; severity ranges from inapparent cases to fulminating, fatal cases; chronic infections occur; may lead to cirrhosis or hepatocellular carcinoma
Type C hepatitis (also known as HCV infection and non-A, non-B hepatitis)	HCV, an enveloped, linear ssRNA virus in the genus Hepacivirus, family Flaviviridae	Primarily parenterally transmitted (e.g., via blood transfusion); rarely sexually transmitted	Usually an insidious onset; 50%–80% of patients develop a chronic infection; may lead to cirrhosis or hepatocellular carcinoma
Type D hepatitis (also known as delta hepatitis)	HDV or delta virus, an enveloped, circular ssRNA viral satellite (a defective RNA virus) in the genus Deltavirus	Exposure to infected blood and body fluids; contaminated needles; sexual transmission; coinfection with HBV is necessary	Usually has an abrupt onset; may progress to a chronic and severe disease
Type E hepatitis	HEV, a spherical, nonenveloped, ssRNA virus in the genus Calcivirus, family Calciviridae	Fecal–oral transmission; primarily via fecally contaminated drinking water; also from person to person	Similar to type A hepatitis; no evidence of a chronic form
Type G hepatitis	HGV, a linear ssRNA virus in the genus Hepacivirus, family Flaviviridae.	Parenteral	Can cause chronic hepatitis

ds, double-stranded; ss, single-stranded

types of disease. Use Standard Precautions for hospitalized patients; add Contact Precautions for diapered or incontinent patients. Various immunodiagnostic procedures are available for diagnosis of viral hepatitis.

The World Health Organization (WHO) estimates that 350 million people are chronically infected with HBV worldwide, that about 1 million people die each year as a result of HBV infections, and that more than 2 million new acute clinical cases occur annually.

Vaccines are available for HAV and HBV. The HAV vaccine, which contains inactivated virus grown in cell culture, is recommended for people at increased risk of acquiring hepatitis A (including military personnel and others traveling to regions where HAV is endemic, homosexual and bisexual men, and users of illicit drugs). The HBV vaccine is a subunit vaccine, produced by genetically engineered *Saccharomyces cerevisiae* (common baker's yeast). At first, only recommended for persons at high risk of acquiring HBV infection (such as infants born to HBV antigen-positive mothers, household contacts of HBV carriers,

homosexual and bisexual men, and users of illicit drugs), it is now also routinely administered to U.S. children. It is required for healthcare workers exposed to blood.

In addition to vaccination against HBV, healthcare personnel practice Standard Precautions (described in Chapter 12). Hepatitis B immune globulin can be given to unvaccinated people who have been exposed to HBV, perhaps by accidental needlestick injury.

VIRAL INFECTIONS OF THE GENITOURINARY SYSTEM

Information pertaining to viral sexually transmitted diseases (STDs) is contained in Table 18-6.

VIRAL INFECTIONS OF THE CIRCULATORY SYSTEM

Information pertaining to viral infections of the circulatory system is contained in Table 18-7.

TABLE 18-6	Viral Sexually Transmitted Diseases
DISEASE	**ADDITIONAL INFORMATION**
Anogenital Herpes Viral Infections (Genital Herpes). In general, herpes simplex infections are characterized by a localized primary lesion, latency, and a tendency to localized recurrence. In women, the principal sites of primary anogenital herpes virus infection are the cervix and vulva, with recurrent disease affecting the vulva, perineal skin, legs, and buttocks. In men, lesions appear on the penis (Fig. 18-7), and in the anus and rectum of those engaging in anal sex. The initial symptoms are usually itching, tingling, and soreness, followed by a small patch of redness and then a group of small, painful blisters. The blisters break and fuse to form painful, circular sores, which become crusted after a few days. The sores heal in about 10 days but may leave scars. The initial outbreak is more painful, prolonged, and widespread than subsequent outbreaks and may be associated with fever. **Patient Care.** Use Standard Precautions for hospitalized patients; add Contact Precautions for severe disseminated or primary mucocutaneous herpes.	**Pathogens.** Genital herpes is usually caused by HSV-2, but is occasionally caused by HSV-1. **Reservoirs and Mode of Transmission.** Infected humans serve as reservoirs. Transmission occurs via direct sexual contact or oral–genital, oral–anal, or anal–genital contact during presence of lesions. Mother-to-fetus or mother-to-neonate transmission occurs during pregnancy and birth. **Laboratory Diagnosis.** Genital herpes is diagnosed by observation of characteristic cytologic changes in tissue scrapings or biopsy specimens, and the presence of multinucleated giant cells with intranuclear inclusions, and confirmation by immunodiagnostic and molecular diagnostic procedures.
Genital Warts (Genital Papillomatosis, Condyloma Acuminatum). Genital warts start as tiny, soft, moist, pink or red swellings, which grow rapidly and may develop stalks. Their rough surfaces give them the appearance of small cauliflowers. Multiple warts often grow in the same area, most often on the penis in men and the vulva, vaginal wall, cervix, and skin surrounding the vaginal area in women. Genital warts also develop around the anus and in the rectum in men or women who engage in anal sex. These warts can become malignant.	**Pathogens.** Genital warts are caused by HPVs of the Papovaviridae family of DNA viruses (human wart viruses). HPV genotypes 16 and 18 have been associated with cervical cancer. **Reservoirs and Mode of Transmission.** Infected humans serve as reservoirs. Transmission occurs via direct contact, usually sexual; through breaks in skin or mucous membranes; or from mother to neonate during birth. **Laboratory Diagnosis.** Genital warts are usually diagnosed clinically. Molecular diagnostic procedures are available.

FIGURE 18-7. Herpes simplex lesions on a penile shaft. (From Harvey RA, et al. Lippincott's Illustrated Reviews: Microbiology, 2nd ed. Philadelphia: Lippincott Williams & Wilkins, 2007.)

DISEASE

ADDITIONAL INFORMATION

HIV Infection and AIDS. The signs and symptoms of acute HIV infection (i.e., infection with "the AIDS virus") usually occur within several weeks to several months after infection with HIV. Initial symptoms include an acute, self-limited mononucleosis-like illness lasting 1 or 2 weeks. Unfortunately, acute HIV infection is often undiagnosed or misdiagnosed, because anti-HIV antibodies are usually not present in a high enough concentration to be detected during this early phase of infection. Other signs and symptoms of acute HIV infection include fever, rash, headache, lymphadenopathy, pharyngitis, myalgia (muscle pain), arthralgia (joint pain), aseptic meningitis, retro-orbital pain, weight loss, depression, GI distress, night sweats, and oral or genital ulcers. Without appropriate anti-HIV treatment, approximately 90% of HIV-infected individuals ultimately develop AIDS. AIDS is a severe, life-threatening syndrome that represents the late clinical stage of infection with HIV. Invasion and destruction of helper T cells (see Chapter 16) leads to suppression of the patient's immune system (immunosuppression). Secondary infections caused by viruses (e.g., cytomegalovirus, herpes simplex), protozoa (e.g., *Cryptosporidium*, *Toxoplasma*), bacteria (e.g., mycobacteria), and/or fungi (e.g., *Candida*, *Cryptococcus*, *Pneumocystis*) become systemic and cause death. Persons with AIDS die as a result of overwhelming infections caused by a variety of pathogens, often opportunistic pathogens. Kaposi's sarcoma, a previously rare type of cancer, is a frequent complication of AIDS, thought to be caused by a type of herpes virus called human herpesvirus 8. Previously considered to be a universally fatal disease, certain combinations of drugs, referred to as cocktails, are extending the life of some HIV-positive patients. In the absence of effective anti-HIV treatment, the AIDS case–fatality rate is very high—approaching 100%. (Chapter 11 contains information about the current AIDS pandemic.)

Patient Care. Use Standard Precautions for hospitalized patients and appropriate Transmission-Based Precautions for specific infections that occur in AIDS patients.

Pathogens. AIDS is caused by HIV (refer back to Fig. 4-13 in Chapter 4). Two types have been identified: type 1 (HIV-1), which is the most common type, and type 2 (HIV-2). HIV viruses are single-stranded RNA viruses in the family Retroviridae (retroviruses).

Reservoirs and Mode of Transmission. Infected humans serve as reservoirs. Transmission occurs via direct sexual contact (homosexual or heterosexual); sharing of contaminated needles and syringes by intravenous drug abusers; transfusion of contaminated blood and blood products; transplacental transfer from mother to child; breast-feeding by HIV-infected mothers; transplantation of HIV-infected tissues or organs; and needlestick, scalpel, and broken glass injuries. There is no evidence of HIV transmission via biting insects. Most likely, HIV-1 first invades dendritic cells in the genital and oral mucosa. These cells then fuse with CD4+ lymphocytes (helper T cells) and spread to deeper tissues.

Laboratory Diagnosis. Immunodiagnostic procedures are available for detection of antigen and antibodies. Most HIV-infected patients develop detectable antibodies within 1–3 months after infection. However, there may be a more prolonged interval of up to 6 months, or even longer in some cases. The most commonly used screening test is an enzyme-linked immunosorbent assay (ELISA). If the screening test is positive, a confirmatory test such as the Western blot analysis[a] or indirect fluorescent antibody test is usually performed. Antigen detection procedures detect an HIV antigen known as p24. Molecular diagnostic procedures are also available. Quantitative assessment of viral RNA is used to monitor the effectiveness of antiviral therapy.

Infectious Mononucleosis. Infectious mononucleosis (also called "mono" or the "kissing disease") is an acute viral disease that may be asymptomatic or may be characterized by fever, sore throat, lymphadenopathy (especially posterior cervical lymph nodes), **splenomegaly** (enlarged spleen), and fatigue. Infectious mononucleosis is usually a self-limited disease of 1 to several weeks' duration. It is rarely fatal.

Patient Care. Use Standard Precautions for hospitalized patients.

Pathogen. The etiologic agent of infectious mononucleosis is Epstein-Barr virus (EBV), which is also known as human herpesvirus 4. It is a DNA virus in the family Herpesviridae. EBV infects and transforms B cells, although it also infects other types of cells. EBV is known to be **oncogenic** (cancer causing), causing or being associated with lymphomas (e.g., Hodgkin disease and Burkitt lymphoma), carcinomas (e.g., nasopharyngeal carcinoma and gastric carcinoma), and sarcomas, among other cancers.

Reservoirs and Mode of Transmission. Infected humans serve as reservoirs. Transmission occurs from person to person by direct contact with saliva. Kissing facilitates spread among adolescents. EBV can be transmitted via blood transfusion.

Laboratory Diagnosis. Patients with infectious mononucleosis usually present with a lymphocytosis (abnormally high peripheral lymphocyte count), including 10% or more abnormal lymphocyte forms, and abnormalities in liver function tests. Specific diagnosis is usually made by detection of antibodies. Molecular diagnostic procedures are also available. EBV can be cultured from the buffy coat—the layer of white blood cells that appears in centrifuged blood.

TABLE 18-7   Viral Infections of the Circulatory System (continued)

DISEASE	ADDITIONAL INFORMATION
Mumps (Infectious Parotitis). Mumps is an acute viral infection characterized by fever and swelling and tenderness of the salivary glands (Fig. 18-8). Complications can include **orchitis** (inflammation of the testes), **oophoritis** (inflammation of the ovaries), meningitis, encephalitis, deafness, pancreatitis, arthritis, mastitis, nephritis, thyroiditis, and pericarditis. **Patient Care.** Use Droplet Precautions for hospitalized patients until 9 days after onset of swelling.	**Pathogen.** Mumps is caused by mumps virus, an RNA virus in the genus Rubulavirus, family Paramyxoviridae. **Reservoirs and Mode of Transmission.** Infected humans serve as reservoirs. Transmission occurs via droplet spread and direct contact with the saliva of an infected person. **Laboratory Diagnosis.** Diagnosis of mumps is made using immunodiagnostic procedures or cell culture.
Viral Hemorrhagic Diseases. Viral hemorrhagic diseases are extremely serious, acute viral illnesses. Initial symptoms include sudden onset of fever, malaise (a feeling of general discomfort; feeling "out of sorts"), myalgia, and headache, followed by pharyngitis, vomiting, diarrhea, rash, and internal hemorrhaging. Case fatality rates for Marburg virus infection and Ebola virus infection have been 25% and 50%–90%, respectively. All known cases of both diseases occurred in or could be traced back to Africa. **Patient Care.** Exercise Standard, Droplet, and Contact Precautions for hospitalized patients for the duration of the illness. Emphasize (a) use of sharps safety devices and safe work practices, (b) hand hygiene, (c) barrier protection against blood and body fluids, and (d) appropriate waste handling. Use N95 or higher respirators when performing aerosol-generating procedures.	**Pathogens.** Viral hemorrhagic fevers are caused by many different viruses, including dengue virus, yellow fever virus, Crimean-Congo hemorrhagic fever virus, Lassa virus, Ebola virus, and Marburg virus. Ebola virus and Marburg virus are filamentous viruses in the family Filoviridae. Both are extremely large viruses. Ebola virus is about 80 nm in width and up to 1 mm or longer in length. Marburg virus is about 80 nm in width and 790 nm in length. **Reservoirs and Mode of Transmission.** Infected humans serve as reservoirs; infected African green monkeys also serve as reservoirs of Marburg virus. Transmission is from person to person via direct contact with infected blood, secretions, internal organs, or semen, or by needlestick. The risk is highest when the patient is vomiting, having diarrhea, or hemorrhaging. Crimean-Congo hemorrhagic fever is a tickborne disease. Dengue fever and yellow fever are mosquito-borne diseases, transmitted primarily by mosquitoes in the genus *Aedes*. **Laboratory Diagnosis.** Viral hemorrhagic diseases are diagnosed using immunodiagnostic and molecular procedures, cell culture, or electron microscopy. Laboratory studies of viral hemorrhagic fevers represent an extreme biohazard and should be conducted only in BSL-4 containment facilities.

[a]A Western blot analysis is a laboratory procedure in which proteins separated by electrophoresis in polyacrylamide gels are transferred (blotted) onto nitrocellulose or nylon membranes and identified by specific complexing with tagged antibodies.

FIGURE 18-8. Child with mumps. (Courtesy of Barbara Rice, the National Immunization Program, and the CDC.)

 STUDY AID

Viremia

The presence of viruses in the bloodstream is known as **viremia**. The viruses either may be free in the plasma, or attached to or within red blood cells or white blood cells, such as lymphocytes and monocytes. The number of viruses in the bloodstream is referred to as the **viral load**, which may be described as being heavy or light. The degree of viremia varies from one viral disease to another, and often from one stage of a particular viral infection to another.

VIRAL INFECTIONS OF THE CENTRAL NERVOUS SYSTEM

Table 18-8 contains information pertaining to viral infections of the central nervous system (CNS).

RECAP OF MAJOR VIRAL INFECTIONS OF HUMANS

Table 18-10 provides a recap of some major viral infections of humans.

APPROPRIATE THERAPY FOR VIRAL INFECTIONS

Recommendations for the treatment of infectious diseases change frequently. The viral infections described in this chapter must be treated using appropriate antiviral drugs. Sources of updated information include *The Merck Manual* (http://www.merck.com/pubs) and WebMD (http://www.webmd.com). For certain diseases, serum immune globulins (e.g., varicella-zoster immune globulin) are available for treatment. Additional information about antiviral agents can be found in Chapter 9.

TABLE 18-8	Viral Infections of the Central Nervous System
DISEASE	**ADDITIONAL INFORMATION**
Lymphocytic Choriomeningitis. Lymphocytic horiomeningitis is a rodentborne viral disease that presents as aseptic meningitis, encephalitis, or meningoencephalitis. Asymptomatic or mild febrile disease also occurs. Some patients develop fever, malaise, suppressed appetite, muscle aches, headache, nausea, vomiting, sore throat, coughing, joint pain, chest pain, and salivary gland pain. Possible complications of CNS involvement include deafness and temporary or permanent neurological damage. An association between lymphocytic choriomeningitis virus infection and myocarditis has been suggested. **Patient Care.** Use Standard Precautions for hospitalized patients.	**Pathogen.** Lymphocytic choriomeningitis is caused by lymphocytic choriomeningitis virus (LCMV), a member of the family Arenaviridae. **Reservoirs and Mode of Transmission.** Infected rodents, primarily the common house mice serve as reservoirs. Humans become infected following exposure to mouse urine, droppings, saliva, or nesting materials. The virus can enter broken skin; through nose, the eyes, or mouth; or via the bite of an infected rodent. Organ transplantation is a possible means of transmission. Person-to-person transmission does not occur. **Laboratory Diagnosis.** Diagnosis is primarily by immunodiagnostic procedures and cell culture.
Poliomyelitis (Polio, Infantile Paralysis). In most patients, poliomyelitis causes a minor illness with fever, malaise, headache, nausea, and vomiting. In about 1% of patients, the disease progresses to severe muscle pain, stiffness of the neck and back, with or without flaccid paralysis. Major illness is more likely to occur in older children and adults. Although once a major health problem in the United States, vaccines became available in the 1950s. The WHO is attempting to eradicate polio worldwide. **Patient Care.** Use Contact Precautions for hospitalized patients for the duration of illness.	**Pathogens.** Poliomyelitis is caused by polioviruses, RNA viruses in the family Picornaviridae (pico = small, RNA viruses). **Reservoirs and Mode of Transmission.** Infected humans serve as reservoirs. Transmission is from person to person, primarily via the fecal–oral route; also by throat secretions. **Laboratory Diagnosis.** Diagnosis of poliomyelitis is made by isolation of polio virus from stool samples, cerebrospinal fluid (CSF), or oropharyngeal secretions using cell culture techniques or by immunodiagnostic or molecular diagnostic procedures.
Rabies. Rabies is a usually fatal, acute viral encephalomyelitis of mammals, with mental depression, restlessness, headache, fever, malaise, paralysis, salivation, spasms of throat muscles induced by a slight breeze or drinking water, convulsions, and death caused by respiratory failure. The paralysis usually starts in the lower legs and moves upward through the body. Rabies is endemic in every country of the world except Antarctica and in every state except Hawaii. Worldwide, an estimated 35,000–40,000 people die of rabies annually. **Patient Care.** Use Standard Precautions for hospitalized patients.	**Pathogen.** Rabies is caused by rabies virus, a bullet-shaped, enveloped RNA virus in the family Rhabdoviridae. **Reservoirs and Mode of Transmission.** Reservoirs are various wild and domestic mammals, including dogs, foxes, coyotes, wolves, jackals, skunks, raccoons, mongooses, and bats. Transmission is usually via the bite of a rabid animal, which introduces virus-laden saliva. Airborne transmission from bats in caves also occurs. Person-to-person transmission is rare. **Laboratory Diagnosis.** Diagnosis of rabies is made by cell culture, antibody detection in serum or CSF, antigen detection in tissue samples, molecular diagnostic procedures for brain tissue, or observation of Negri bodies in brain or other tissues. Negri bodies are viral RNA-nucleoprotein complexes found in the cytoplasm of virus-infected cells (i.e., they are intracytoplasmic inclusions).

TABLE 18-8   Viral Infections of the Central Nervous System (continued)

DISEASE	ADDITIONAL INFORMATION
Viral Meningitis. Viral meningitis is also known as aseptic meningitis and nonbacterial or abacterial meningitis. It is a relatively common disease but, fortunately, is rarely serious. Acute illness rarely exceeds 10 day's duration. Viral meningitis is characterized by sudden onset of febrile illness with the signs and symptoms of meningeal involvement. CSF findings include the presence of mononuclear white blood cells, increased protein levels, normal glucose levels, and the absence of bacteria. A rash may develop. When caused by an enterovirus, GI and respiratory symptoms may occur. **Patient Care.** Use Standard Precautions for hospitalized patients. Add Contact Precautions for infants and young children.	**Pathogens.** The most common causes of viral meningitis in the United States are enteroviruses. Other causes include coxsackie viruses, arboviruses, measles virus, mumps virus, herpes simplex and varicella-zoster viruses, lymphocytic choriomeningitis virus, and adenoviruses. Leptospirosis (a bacterial disease) can also cause aseptic meningitis. **Reservoirs and Mode of Transmission.** Reservoirs and modes of transmission vary with the specific etiologic agent. **Laboratory Diagnosis.** During the early stages of the disease, the viral pathogen may be isolated from throat washings and stool, and occasionally from CSF and blood. Diagnosis is made by immunodiagnostic or molecular diagnostic procedures or cell culture.
Viral Encephalitis (Arthropod-borne Viral Encephalitis; Table 18-9). Arthropod-borne viral encephalitis is an acute inflammatory viral disease. A patient with this disease may be asymptomatic or have mild fever and headache. Severe infection is also possible, with headache, high fever, stupor, disorientation, coma, tremors, occasional convulsions, spastic paralysis, and death. The term *arboviruses* is sometimes used in reference to viruses that are transmitted by arthropods. **Patient Care.** Exercise Standard Precautions for hospitalized patients. Transmission-Based Precautions may be necessary, depending on the etiologic agent.	**Pathogens.** See Table 18-9. Over the years, St. Louis encephalitis virus has been the most common mosquito-transmitted pathogen in the United States. The situation changed in 2002, when West Nile virus took over the number one spot. **Reservoirs and Mode of Transmission.** See Table 18-9. Person-to-person transmission is rare; possibly by transfusion, organ transplant, breast milk, or transplacentally. **Laboratory Diagnosis.** Many of the viruses that cause encephalitis, including arboviruses, are difficult to isolate from CSF by cell culture. Appropriate containment facilities must be used when attempting to cultivate arboviruses. Viral encephalitis caused by arboviruses is usually diagnosed using immunodiagnostic or molecular diagnostic procedures, or sometimes by electron microscopy. **Note:** Additional information about West Nile virus can be found on the CD-ROM.

TABLE 18-9   Selected Arthropod-borne Viral Encephalitides of the United States

DISEASE	PATHOGEN	RESERVOIRS	VECTORS
Eastern equine encephalitis (EEE)	EEE virus, an RNA virus in the family Togaviridae	Birds, horses	*Aedes, Coquilletidia, Culex,* and *Culiseta* mosquitoes
California encephalitis	California encephalitis virus, an RNA RNA virus in the family Bunyaviridae	Rodents, rabbits	*Aedes* and *Culex* mosquitoes
La Crosse encephalitis	La Crosse encephalitis virus, an RNA virus in the family Bunyaviridae	Chipmunks, squirrels	*Aedes* mosquitoes
St. Louis encephalitis	St. Louis encephalitis virus, an RNA virus in the family Flaviviridae	Birds	*Culex* mosquitoes
West Nile virus encephalitis	West Nile virus, an RNA virus in the family Flaviviridae	Birds, perhaps horses	*Culex* mosquitoes
Western equine encephalitis (WEE)	WEE virus, an RNA virus in the family Togaviridae	Birds, horses	*Aedes* and *Culex* mosquitoes

TABLE 18-10	Recap of Some Major Viral Infections of Humans
DISEASE	**VIRAL PATHOGEN**
AIDS	HIV
Avian influenza (bird flu)	Avian influenza viruses
Chickenpox	Varicella-zoster virus
Cold sores (fever blisters)	HSVs
Genital herpes	HSVs
Hantavirus pulmonary syndrome	Hantaviruses
Infectious mononucleosis	Epstein-Barr virus
Influenza	Influenza viruses
Monkeypox	Monkeypox virus
Mumps	Mumps virus
Poliomyelitis	Polioviruses
Rabies	Rabies virus
Rubella (German measles)	Rubella virus
Rubeola (hard measles)	Rubeola virus
Severe acute respiratory syndrome (SARS)	SARS-associated coronavirus
Smallpox	Variola virus
Swine flu	Swine flu viruses
Viral hepatitis	Various hepatitis viruses
Warts	Papillomaviruses
West Nile virus encephalitis	West Nile virus

ON THE CD-ROM

- Terms Introduced in This Chapter
- Review of Key Points
- Insight:
  - A Closer Look at Bird Flu
  - A Closer Look at Swine Flu
  - A Closer Look at West Nile Virus
- Increase Your Knowledge
- Critical Thinking
- Case Study
- Additional Self-Assessment Exercises

SELF-ASSESSMENT EXERCISES

After studying this chapter, answer the following multiple-choice questions.

1. Which of the following is the cause of smallpox?
   a. vaccinia virus
   b. varicella virus
   c. variola virus
   d. none of the preceding choices

2. Which of the following are considered to be oncogenic?
   a. Epstein-Barr virus and HPVs
   b. HIV and Ebola virus
   c. rubella and rubeola viruses
   d. variola and varicella viruses

3. Laboratory diagnosis of HIV infection is usually made by which of the following?
   a. electron microscopy
   b. growth of HIV in cell culture
   c. growth of HIV in embryonated chicken eggs
   d. immunodiagnostic procedures for the detection of antigen and antibodies

4. Which of the following is also known as infectious hepatitis?
   a. HAV
   b. HBV
   c. HCV
   d. HDV

5. Mosquitoes serve as vectors in all of the following viral diseases, *except*:
   a. dengue fever.
   b. hepatitis.
   c. West Nile virus disease.
   d. yellow fever.

6. Which of the following viruses is/are *not* transmitted sexually?
   a. hantavirus
   b. HSVs
   c. HIV
   d. papillomaviruses

7. Which of the following is a DNA virus?
   a. HAV
   b. HBV
   c. HCV
   d. HDV

8. Which of the following is a type of herpes virus?
   a. Epstein-Barr virus
   b. measles virus
   c. mumps virus
   d. rabies virus

9. Which of the following viral diseases has been acquired in the United States by handling pet prairie dogs?
   a. chickenpox
   b. hantavirus
   c. monkeypox
   d. smallpox

10. The disease known as severe acute respiratory syndrome (SARS) is caused by a type of:
    a. coronavirus.
    b. herpes virus.
    c. papillomavirus.
    d. picornavirus.

BACTERIAL INFECTIONS 19

LEARNING OBJECTIVES

AFTER STUDYING THIS CHAPTER, YOU SHOULD BE ABLE TO:

- Name at least three nationally notifiable bacterial diseases
- Correlate a particular bacterial disease with its major signs and symptoms, etiologic agent, reservoir(s), mode(s) of transmission, and diagnostic laboratory procedures
- Given a particular body site (e.g., the urinary tract), state at least one example of a bacterial disease at that site
- Differentiate between gangrene and gas gangrene
- Correlate a given bacterial sexually transmitted disease (STD) with its etiologic agent
- Name at least three rickettsial or ehrlichial infections of the cardiovascular system
- Name several diseases caused by anaerobic bacteria
- Describe a biofilm and name at least two human diseases thought to be associated with biofilms
- State the general treatment for bacterial infections

INTRODUCTION

It would be impossible in a book this size to describe *all* of the human infectious diseases caused by bacteria. Thus, only selected bacterial diseases are described in this chapter. Although a certain disease may be described within one particular section of this chapter (e.g., in the section describing bacterial diseases of the respiratory system), readers should keep in mind that some bacterial diseases have various clinical manifestations, affecting several body systems simultaneously, and that the pathogens may move from one body site to another. Readers should also keep in mind that, although most of the bacterial diseases described in this chapter are caused by a single bacterial species, many other diseases are thought to be the result of communities of bacteria consisting of more than one species (biofilms; described in Chapter 10 and later in this chapter).

TABLE 19-1	Nationally Notifiable Bacterial Diseases

BACTERIAL DISEASE	NUMBER OF NEW U.S. CASES REPORTED TO THE CDC IN 2007*
Anthrax	1
Botulism	144
Brucellosis	131
Chancroid	23
Chlamydia	1,108,374
Cholera	7
Diphtheria	0
Ehrlichiosis	1,999
Gonorrhea	355,991
Haemophilus influenzae, invasive disease	2,541
Hansen disease (leprosy)	101
Hemolytic uremic syndrome, postdiarrheal	292
Legionellosis	2,716
Listeriosis	808
Lyme disease	27,444
Meningococcal disease	1,077
Pertussis (whooping cough)	10,454
Plague	7
Psittacosis	12
Q fever	171
Salmonellosis	47,995
Shiga toxin-producing *Escherichia coli*	4,847
Shigellosis	19,758
Streptococcal disease, invasive, group A	5,294
Streptococcal toxic-shock syndrome	132
Streptococcus pneumoniae, invasive disease, drug-resistant, all ages	3,329
Syphilis	40,920
Tetanus	28
Toxic-shock syndrome (*Staphylococcus aureus*)	92
Tuberculosis	13,299
Tularemia	137
Typhoid fever	434
Vancomycin-intermediate *S. aureus*	37
Vancomycin-resistant *S. aureus*	2

*These figures provide insight as to how frequently these diseases occur in the United States. For updated information, go to the CDC web site; click on "Morbidity & Mortality Weekly Report"; then click on "Notifiable Diseases"; then click on the most recent year that is listed. Source: http://www.cdc.gov.

that are not nationally notifiable (e.g., *Campylobacter* enteritis).

HOW DO BACTERIA CAUSE DISEASE?

The various bacterial virulence factors, which enable pathogens to cause disease, were described in Chapter 14. Some of them are listed here:

- Adherence and colonization factors
- Factors that prevent activation of complement
- Factors that enable escape from phagocytosis by white blood cells (WBCs)
- Factors that prevent destruction within phagocytes
- Factors that suppress the host immune system (i.e., factors that cause immunosuppression)
- Endotoxin (a component of the cell walls of Gram-negative bacteria)
- Production of exotoxins (e.g., cytotoxins, enterotoxins, neurotoxins)
- Production of necrotic and other types of destructive enzymes

BACTERIAL INFECTIONS OF THE SKIN

Information pertaining to bacterial infections of the skin is contained in Table 19-2.

Certain of the bacterial diseases described in this chapter are nationally notifiable infectious diseases. When a patient is diagnosed with one of these diseases in the United States, the information must be reported to the Centers for Disease Control and Prevention (CDC). As of 2007, there were approximately 34 nationally notifiable bacterial diseases (Table 19-1). Most of them are described in this chapter, as are some bacterial diseases

TABLE 19-2	Bacterial Infections of the Skin
DISEASE	**ADDITIONAL INFORMATION**
Acne. Acne is a common condition in which pores become clogged with dried sebum, flaked skin, and bacteria, which leads to the formation of blackheads and whiteheads (collectively known as acne pimples) and inflamed, infected abscesses. Acne is most common among teenagers.	**Pathogens.** The etiologic agents of acne are *Propionibacterium acnes* and other *Propionibacterium* spp., all of which are anaerobic, Gram-positive bacilli. **Reservoirs and Mode of Transmission.** Infected humans serve as reservoirs, although acne is probably not transmissible. **Laboratory Diagnosis.** Diagnosis is made on clinical grounds.
Anthrax. Anthrax, also known as woolsorter's disease, can affect the skin (cutaneous anthrax), lungs (inhalation or pulmonary anthrax), or gastrointestinal tract (gastrointestinal anthrax), depending on the portal of entry of the etiologic agent. In cutaneous anthrax, depressed blackened lesions called eschars form as a result of a necrotoxin (a toxin that kills cells) (refer back to Fig. 11-9 in Chapter 11). Inhalation and gastrointestinal anthrax are often fatal, but cutaneous anthrax usually is not. Ordinarily, human cases in the United States are quite rare. However, 22 U.S. cases occurred in the fall of 2001 as a result of the mailing of letters that had purposely been contaminated with *Bacillus anthracis* spores. The 22 cases included 11 cases of inhalation anthrax (5 fatal) and 11 cases of cutaneous anthrax (nonfatal).	**Pathogen.** The etiologic agent of anthrax is *B. anthracis*, an encapsulated, spore-forming, Gram-positive bacillus. **Reservoirs and Mode of Transmission.** Reservoirs include anthrax-infected animals, as well as spores that may be present in soil, animal hair, wool, animal skins and hides, and products made from them. Transmission occurs via entry of endospores through breaks in skin, inhalation of spores, or ingestion of bacteria in contaminated meat. Pulmonary anthrax is not transmitted from person to person. **Laboratory Diagnosis.** Anthrax is diagnosed by isolation of *B. anthracis* from blood, lesions, or discharges, and identification using biochemical- or enzyme-based tests. Immunodiagnostic procedures are available.

(continues)

TABLE 19-2   Bacterial Infections of the Skin (continued)

DISEASE	ADDITIONAL INFORMATION
Patient Care. Use Standard Precautions for hospitalized patients. Add Contact Precautions for cutaneous anthrax patients if there is a large amount of uncontained drainage. Use soap and water for handwashing; alcohol does not have sporicidal activity.	
Gas Gangrene (Clostridial Myonecrosis). After *Clostridium* spores enter and germinate in a wound, the vegetative pathogens produce necrotizing exoenzymes and toxins, which destroy muscle and soft tissue, allowing deeper penetration by the organisms. Gases released from the infecting pathogens cause pockets of gas to develop in the infected tissue. Tissue destruction occurs rapidly, often necessitating amputation of the infected anatomic site. In its most severe forms, gas gangrene produces massive tissue destruction, shock, and renal failure. **Patient Care.** Use Standard Precautions for hospitalized patients.	**Pathogens.** Although *Clostridium perfringens* is the most common cause of gas gangrene, other *Clostridium* spp. can also cause this condition. **Reservoirs and Mode of Transmission.** Soil is the primary reservoir. Humans become infected when soil containing clostridial spores enters an open wound. Person-to-person transmission does not occur. **Laboratory Diagnosis.** The presence of Gram-positive and/or Gram-variable bacilli in Gram-stained smears of wound specimens should lead one to suspect gas gangrene. Often, no leukocytes are observed, as they have been killed by toxins produced by the clostridia. Once isolated on culture media, the etiologic agent can be identified using various phenotypic characteristics, including reactions in biochemical- or enzyme-based tests.
Leprosy. Leprosy is today more commonly known as Hansen disease. There are two forms of leprosy: (a) lepromatous leprosy, characterized by numerous nodules in skin and possible involvement of the nasal mucosa and eyes and (b) tuberculoid leprosy, in which relatively few skin lesions occur. Peripheral nerve involvement tends to be severe, with loss of sensation. Hansen disease is named for G.A. Hansen who, in 1873, discovered the bacillus that causes leprosy. Leprosy occurs primarily in warm, wet areas of the tropics and subtropics. The worldwide prevalence of leprosy was estimated to be about 1.5 million cases in 1997. Most U.S. cases involve people who emigrated from developing countries. **Patient Care.** Use Standard Precautions for hospitalized patients.	**Pathogen.** The etiologic agent of leprosy is *Mycobacterium leprae*, an acid-fast bacillus. **Reservoirs and Mode of Transmission.** Infected humans serve as reservoirs; *M. leprae* is present in nasal discharges and is shed from cutaneous lesions. Armadillos in Texas and Louisiana have a naturally occurring disease that is identical to experimental leprosy in those animals, suggesting that transmission from armadillos to humans is possible. The exact mode of transmission has not been clearly established. The organisms may gain entrance through the respiratory system or broken skin. Leprosy does not appear to be easily transmitted from person to person. Prolonged, close contact with an infected individual appears to be necessary. The tuberculoid form of leprosy is not contagious. **Laboratory Diagnosis.** *M. leprae* cannot be grown on artificial culture media. It can be cultured only in laboratory animals, such as nine-banded armadillos or mouse foot pads. Diagnosis is made by demonstration of acid-fast bacilli in skin smears or skin biopsy specimens.
Staphylococcal Skin Infections (Folliculitis, Furuncles, Carbuncles, Abscesses, Impetigo, Impetigo of the Newborn, Scalded Skin Syndrome). Virtually all infected hair follicles, boils (furuncles), carbuncles, and stys involve *Staphylococcus aureus*. The majority of common skin lesions are localized, discrete, and uncomplicated. However, seeding of the bloodstream may lead to pneumonia, lung abscess, osteomyelitis, sepsis, endocarditis, meningitis, or brain abscess. With impetigo, which occurs mainly in children, pus-filled blisters (*pustules*) may appear anywhere on the body. Impetigo of the newborn (impetigo neonatorum) and staphylococcal scalded skin syndrome (SSSS) may occur as epidemics in hospital nurseries.	**Pathogen.** Most staphylococcal infections ("staph infections") are caused by *S. aureus*, a Gram-positive coccus. Impetigo may also be caused by *Streptococcus pyogenes*, which is another Gram-positive coccus. *S. aureus* spreads through skin by producing hyaluronidase (see Chapter 14). SSSS is produced by strains of *S. aureus* that produce exfoliative (or epidermolytic) toxin, which causes the top layer of skin (epidermis) to split from the rest of the skin. **Reservoirs and Mode of Transmission.** Infected humans serve as reservoirs. Persons with a draining lesion or any purulent discharge are the most common sources of epidemic spread. Transmission occurs via direct contact with a person having a purulent lesion or is an

TABLE 19-2	Bacterial Infections of the Skin (continued)
DISEASE	**ADDITIONAL INFORMATION**

Patient Care. Use Standard Precautions for skin, burn, and wound infections if they are minor or limited, and Contact Precautions if they are major. Use Contact Precautions for patients with SSSS. Use Standard Precautions for infections caused by methicillin-resistant *S. aureus* (MRSA); add Contact Precautions if wounds cannot be contained by dressings. Use Contact Precautions for diapered or incontinent children with enterocolitis (staph food poisoning), for the duration of illness.

asymptomatic carrier. In hospitals, staphylococcal infections can be spread by the hands of healthcare workers.

Laboratory Diagnosis. The infecting strain must be isolated on culture media and identified using a variety of phenotypic characteristics, including reactions in biochemical- or enzyme-based tests. Susceptibility testing must be performed because many strains of *S. aureus* are multidrug resistant.
(See Fig. 19-1 and the CD-ROM for additional information regarding diseases caused by *S. aureus*.)

Streptococcal Skin Infections (Impetigo, Scarlet Fever, Erysipelas, Necrotizing Fasciitis). (a) Streptococcal impetigo is usually superficial but may proceed through vesicular, pustular, and encrusted stages. (b) Scarlet fever (scarlatina) includes a widespread, pink-red rash, most obvious on the abdomen, sides of the chest, and in skin folds. Severe cases may be accompanied by high fever, nausea, and vomiting. (c) Erysipelas is an acute cellulitis with fever, constitutional symptoms, and hot, tender, red eruptions (sometimes referred to as St. Anthony's fire). (d) Necrotizing fasciitis is the name of the disease caused by the so-called flesh-eating bacteria. **Fasciitis** is inflammation of the *fascia* (fibrous tissue that envelops the body beneath the skin and also encloses muscles and groups of muscles).

Patient Care. Use Standard Precautions for skin, burn, and wound infections if they are minor or limited, and Contact or Droplet Precautions if they are major. Use Droplet Precautions for infants and young children with strep throat or scarlet fever, and all patients with pneumonia or serious invasive disease. Outbreaks of serious invasive disease have occurred secondary to transmission among patients and healthcare personnel.

Pathogen. These infections are caused by *S. pyogenes*, a Gram-positive coccus, that is also known as group A beta-hemolytic streptococcus, GAS, and "Strep A." Scarlet fever is caused by erythrogenic toxin, produced by some strains of *S. pyogenes*. Scarlet fever can be a complication (sequela) of untreated strep throat (streptococcal pharyngitis).

Reservoirs and Mode of Transmission. Infected humans serve as reservoirs. Transmission occurs from person to person via large respiratory droplets or direct contact with patients or carriers. Transmission rarely occurs by indirect contact through objects.

Laboratory Diagnosis. The infecting strain must be isolated on culture media and identified using various phenotypic characteristics, including biochemical- or enzyme-based tests. Immunodiagnostic procedures are available, some of which are referred to as "rapid strep tests." Currently, susceptibility testing is not routinely performed because *S. pyogenes* has not yet developed resistance to penicillin. Some strains have become resistant to other antimicrobial agents, however.
(See the CD-ROM for "A Closer Look at *Streptococcus pyogenes*.")

STUDY AID
Gangrene versus Gas Gangrene
The term **gangrene** refers to tissue necrosis (death) resulting from local anemia (ischemia). **Ischemia** results from an obstruction, loss, or reduction of blood supply, leading to a lack of oxygen. Gangrene may have nothing whatsoever to do with microorganisms. **Gas gangrene**, on the other hand, is *always* caused by microorganisms—specifically, *Clostridium* spp. The clostridia produce gaseous metabolic byproducts—primarily, hydrogen and nitrogen—that accumulate in the necrotic tissues. Regardless of the cause, gangrenous tissue becomes brownish black and foul smelling.

Wound Infections

When the protective skin barrier is broken as a result of burns, puncture wounds, surgical procedures, or bites, opportunistic indigenous microflora and environmental bacteria can invade and cause local or deep tissue infections. The pathogens may spread via blood or lymph, causing serious systemic infections.

BACTERIAL INFECTIONS OF THE EARS

Information pertaining to viral and bacterial ear infections is contained in Table 19-3.

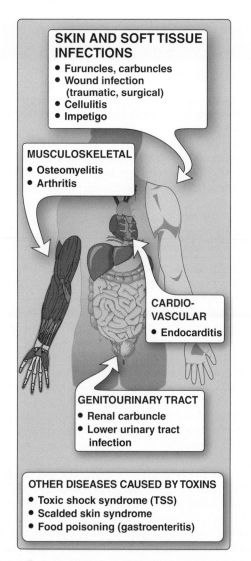

FIGURE 19-1. Diseases caused by *Staphylococcus aureus*. (From Harvey RA, et al. Lippincott's Illustrated Reviews, 2nd ed. Philadelphia: Lippincott Williams & Wilkins, 2007.)

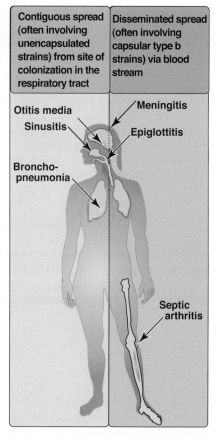

FIGURE 19-2. Infections caused by *Haemophilus influenzae*. (From Harvey RA, et al. Lippincott's Illustrated Reviews, 2nd ed. Philadelphia: Lippincott Williams & Wilkins, 2007.)

TABLE 19-3	Viral and Bacterial Ear Infections
DISEASE	**ADDITIONAL INFORMATION**
Otitis Externa (External Otitis, Ear Canal Infection, Swimmer's Ear). Otitis externa is an infection of the outer ear canal with itching, pain, a malodorous discharge, tenderness, redness, swelling, and impaired hearing. Otitis externa is most common during the summer swimming season; trapped water in the external ear canal can lead to wet, softened skin, which is more easily infected by bacteria or fungi. Otitis externa is referred to as "swimmer's ear" because it often results from swimming in water contaminated with *Pseudomonas aeruginosa*.	**Pathogens.** The usual causes of otitis externa are the bacteria *Escherichia coli*, *P. aeruginosa*, *Proteus vulgaris*, and *Staphylococcus aureus*. Fungi, such as *Aspergillus* spp. are less common causes of otitis externa. **Reservoirs and Mode of Transmission.** Reservoirs include contaminated swimming pool water, sometimes indigenous microflora, or articles inserted into the ear canal for cleaning out debris and wax. **Laboratory Diagnosis.** Material from the infected ear canal should be sent to the microbiology laboratory for culture and susceptibility (C&S). Most strains of *P. aeruginosa* are multidrug resistant.

TABLE 19-3	Viral and Bacterial Ear Infections (continued)
DISEASE	**ADDITIONAL INFORMATION**
Otitis Media (Middle Ear Infection). Otitis media often develops as a complication of the common cold. Manifestations can include persistent and severe earache, temporary hearing loss, pressure in the middle ear, and bulging of the eardrum (tympanic membrane). Nausea, vomiting, diarrhea, and fever may be present in young children. Otitis media may lead to rupture of the eardrum, bloody discharge, and pus. Severe complications, including bone infection, permanent hearing loss, and meningitis, may occur. Otitis media is most common in young children, particularly those between 3 months and 3 years of age.	**Pathogens.** Otitis media may be caused by bacteria or viruses. The three most common bacterial causes are *Streptococcus pneumoniae* (a Gram-positive diplococcus), *Haemophilus influenzae* (a Gram-negative bacillus; see Fig. 19-2), and *Moraxella catarrhalis* (a Gram-negative diplococcus). Less common bacterial causes include *Streptococcus pyogenes* and *S. aureus*. Viral causes include measles virus, parainfluenza virus, and RSV. **Reservoirs and Mode of Transmission.** Otitis medias is probably not communicable. **Laboratory Diagnosis.** If present, a sample of discharge from the ear should be sent to the microbiology laboratory for C&S. β-Lactamase testing should be performed on isolates of *H. influenzae* and *S. pneumoniae*. (See the CD-ROM for "A Closer Look at *Streptococcus pneumoniae*.")

BACTERIAL INFECTIONS OF THE EYES

Table 19-4 contains information pertaining to bacterial infections of the eyes.

BACTERIAL INFECTIONS OF THE RESPIRATORY SYSTEM

Bacterial Infections of the Upper Respiratory Tract

Table 19-5 contains information pertaining to bacterial infections of the upper respiratory tract.

Infections of the Lower Respiratory Tract Having Multiple Causes

Pneumonia

Disease. Pneumonia is an acute nonspecific infection of the small air sacs (alveoli) and tissues of the lung, with fever, productive cough (meaning that sputum is coughed up), acute chest pain, chills, and shortness of breath. It is clinically diagnosed by abnormal chest sounds and chest radiographs. Pneumonia is often a secondary infection that follows a primary viral respiratory infection. About 2 million people have pneumonia in the United States per year. Of those, approximately 40,000 to 70,000 die. In developing countries, pneumonia and dehydration from severe diarrhea are the leading causes of death. Certain specific types of pneumonia (e.g., legionellosis and psittacosis) are nationally notifiable diseases in the United States.

Patient Care. Use Standard Precautions for all hospitalized patients; Droplet and/or Contact Precautions are required in addition to Standard Precautions for pneumonia caused by certain pathogens (e.g., *Burkholderia cepacia*, *Legionella* spp., *Neisseria meningitidis*, *Mycoplasma pneumoniae*, *Streptococcus pyogenes*).

Pathogens. Pneumonia may be caused by Gram-positive or Gram-negative bacteria, mycoplasmas, chlamydias, viruses, fungi, or protozoa. Community-acquired bacterial pneumonia is most frequently caused by *Streptococcus pneumoniae* (pneumococcal pneumonia). *S. pneumoniae* is the most common cause of pneumonia in the world. Other bacterial pathogens include *Haemophilus influenzae*, *Staphylococcus aureus*, *Klebsiella pneumoniae*, and occasionally other Gram-negative bacilli and anaerobic members of the oral flora. Atypical pathogens include *Legionella* (legionellosis), *M. pneumoniae* (mycoplasmal pneumonia; primary atypical pneumonia), and *Chlamydia pneumoniae* (chlamydial pneumonia). Psittacosis (ornithosis; parrot fever), a type of pneumonia caused by *Chlamydia psittaci*, is normally acquired by inhalation of respiratory secretions and desiccated droppings of infected birds (e.g., parrots, parakeets). Fungi such as *Histoplasma capsulatum* (histoplasmosis), *Coccidioides immitis* (coccidioidomycosis), *Candida albicans* (candidiasis), *Cryptococcus neoformans* (cryptococcosis), *Blastomyces* (blastomycosis), *Aspergillus* (aspergillosis; see Fig. 20-4 in Chapter 20), and *Pneumocystis jiroveci* (previously considered to be a protozoan) may be etiologic agents of pneumonia, especially in immunocompromised individuals. Various species of bread moulds can cause

TABLE 19-4	Bacterial Infections of the Eyes

DISEASE	ADDITIONAL INFORMATION
Bacterial Conjunctivitis ("Pinkeye"). Bacterial conjunctivitis involves irritation and reddening of conjunctiva, edema of eyelids, mucopurulent discharge, and sensitivity to light. The disease is highly contagious. **Patient Care.** Use Standard Precautions for hospitalized patients.	**Pathogens.** The most common etiologic agents of pinkeye are *Haemophilus influenzae* subsp. *aegyptius* and *Streptococcus pneumoniae*, although many other bacteria can cause these diseases. **Reservoirs and Mode of Transmission.** Infected humans serve as reservoirs. Human-to-human transmission occurs via contact with eye and respiratory discharges, contaminated fingers, facial tissues, clothing, eye makeup, eye medications, ophthalmic instruments, and contact lens-wetting and lens-cleaning agents. **Laboratory Diagnosis.** Infections of the eye caused by bacteria (including chlamydias) and viruses should be differentiated from allergic manifestations and irritation by microscopic examination of the *exudate* (oozing pus), culture of pathogens, and/or immunodiagnostic procedures.
Chlamydial Conjunctivitis (Inclusion Conjunctivitis, Paratrachoma). In neonates, acute chlamydial conjunctivitis with mucopurulent discharge may result in mild scarring of conjunctivae and cornea. It may be concurrent with chlamydial nasopharyngitis or pneumonia. In adults, chlamydial conjunctivitis may be concurrent with nongonococcal urethritis or cervicitis. **Patient Care.** Use Standard Precautions for hospitalized patients.	**Pathogens.** The etiologic agents of chlamydial conjunctivitis are certain serotypes (serovars[a]) of *Chlamydia trachomatis*, a Gram-negative bacterium and obligate intracellular pathogen. **Reservoirs and Mode of Transmission.** Infected humans serve as reservoirs. Transmission occurs via contact with genital discharges of infected people, contaminated fingers to eye, infection in newborns via an infected birth canal, or non-chlorinated swimming pools ("swimming pool conjunctivitis"). **Laboratory Diagnosis.** Chlamydias do not grow on artificial media. Diagnosis is made by cell culture and/or immunodiagnostic procedures.
Trachoma (Chlamydia Keratoconjunctivitis). Trachoma is a highly contagious, acute, or chronic conjunctival inflammation, resulting in scarring of cornea and conjunctiva, deformation of eyelids, and blindness. Trachoma is most common in poverty-stricken areas of the hot, dry Mediterranean countries and the Far East. It is the leading cause of blindness in the world. Trachoma occurs only rarely in the United States. **Patient Care.** Use Standard Precautions for hospitalized patients.	**Pathogens.** Trachoma is caused by certain serotypes (serovars) of *C. trachomatis*. **Reservoirs and Mode of Transmission.** Infected humans serve as reservoirs. Transmission occurs via direct contact with infectious ocular or nasal secretions or contaminated articles. The disease is also spread by flies serving as mechanical vectors. **Laboratory Diagnosis.** Trachoma is diagnosed by microscopic observation of intracellular chlamydial elementary bodies in epithelial cells of Giemsa-stained conjunctival scrapings or by an immunofluorescence procedure. Alternatively, the chlamydias can be isolated from specimens using cell culture techniques.
Gonococcal Conjunctivitis (Gonorrheal Ophthalmia Neonatorum). Gonococcal conjunctivitis is associated with an acute redness and swelling of conjunctiva and purulent discharge (Fig. 19-3). Corneal ulcers, perforation, and blindness may occur if the disease is untreated. **Patient Care.** Use Standard Precautions for hospitalized patients.	**Pathogen.** Gonococcal conjunctivitis is caused by *Neisseria gonorrhoeae*, a kidney bean–shaped, Gram-negative diplococcus. *N. gonorrhoeae* is also known as gonococcus (pl., gonococci) or GC. **Reservoirs and Mode of Transmission.** Infected humans—specifically, infected maternal birth canals—serve as reservoirs. Transmission occurs via contact with the infected birth canal during delivery. Adult infection can result from finger-to-eye contact with infectious genital secretions. **Laboratory Diagnosis.** Gonococcal conjunctivitis is diagnosed by microscopic observation of Gram-negative diplococci in smears of purulent material and isolation of *N. gonorrhoeae* on appropriate culture media (e.g., chocolate agar or modified chocolate agar, such as Thayer-Martin agar, Martin-Lewis agar, or Transgrow).

[a]The terms serotypes and serovars are synonyms. Serovars of a particular species differ from each other primarily as a result of differences in surface antigens. Sometimes, different serovars of a particular species cause different diseases.

FIGURE 19-3. Gonococcal ophthalmia neonatorum.
(Courtesy of J. Pledger and the CDC.)

TABLE 19-5	Bacterial Infections of the Upper Respiratory Tract

DISEASE	ADDITIONAL INFORMATION
Diphtheria. Diphtheria is a potentially serious upper respiratory tract disease. This acute, contagious bacterial disease primarily involves the tonsils, pharynx, larynx, and nose, and occasionally involves other mucous membranes, skin, conjunctivae, and the vagina. The characteristic lesion is a tough, asymmetrical, adherent gray-white membrane in the throat, with surrounding inflammation. Sore throat, swollen and tender cervical lymph nodes, tonsillitis, and swelling of the neck are common. The membrane may cause airway obstruction. There is also a cutaneous form of diphtheria, which is more common in the tropics. At one time, diphtheria was a major killer of children in the United States. However, as a result of widespread vaccination with diphtheria toxoid (an altered form of diphtheria toxin), diphtheria rarely occurs in the United States. Unfortunately, diphtheria continues to be a major killer of children in developing countries, where epidemics occur. **Patient Care.** Use Droplet Precautions for hospitalized patients with pharyngeal diphtheria and Contact Precautions for hospitalized patients with cutaneous diphtheria.	**Pathogen.** Diphtheria is caused by toxigenic (toxin-producing) strains of *Corynebacterium diphtheriae*, pleomorphic, Gram-positive bacilli that form characteristic V-, L-, and Y-shaped arrangements of bacilli. Only strains infected with a particular corynebacteriophage are toxigenic; the exotoxin (diphtheria toxin) is coded for by a bacteriophage gene. **Reservoirs and Mode of Transmission.** Infected humans serve as reservoirs. Transmission occurs via airborne droplets, direct contact, and contaminated fomites. **Laboratory Diagnosis.** A nasopharyngeal swab and a throat swab, preferably containing a sample of the membrane, should be sent to the microbiology laboratory for culture. Special media called Loeffler serum medium and cystine-tellurite or Tinsdale medium are used for culture and identification of *C. diphtheriae*. Toxigenicity can be determined using laboratory animals (rabbits or guinea pigs).
Streptococcal Pharyngitis (Strep Throat). Strep throat is an acute bacterial infection of the throat with soreness, chills, fever, headache, a beefy red throat, white patches of pus on pharyngeal epithelium, enlarged tonsils, and enlarged and tender cervical lymph nodes. The infection may spread to the middle ear, sinuses, or the organs of hearing. Untreated strep throat can lead to complications (sequelae) such as scarlet fever (caused by erythrogenic toxin), rheumatic fever, and glomerulonephritis. The latter two conditions result from the deposition of immune complexes beneath heart and kidney tissue, respectively. Some strains produce a pyrogenic exotoxin that causes toxic shock syndrome and some strains (the so-called flesh-eating bacteria) can cause necrotizing fasciitis (refer back to Fig. 14-8 in Chapter 14). More than 200,000 cases occur annually in the United States, mostly among children, 3–15 years of age. **Patient Care.** Use Droplet Precautions for hospitalized infants and young children and Standard Precautions for others.	**Pathogen.** Strep throat is caused by *Streptococcus pyogenes*, a beta-hemolytic, catalase-negative, Gram-positive coccus in chains. It is also known as group A streptococcus, GAS, or Strep A. **Reservoirs and Mode of Transmission.** Infected humans serve as reservoirs. Transmission occurs human to human by direct contact, usually hands; aerosol droplets; secretions from patients and nasal carriers; and contaminated dust, lint, or handkerchiefs; contaminated milk and milk products have been associated with foodborne outbreaks of streptococcal pharyngitis. **Laboratory Diagnosis.** The sole purpose of a *routine* throat culture is to determine if a patient does or does not have strep throat. If beta-hemolytic streptococci are isolated, they are tested to determine if they are group A streptococci. Rapid strep tests (based on detection of antigen) can be performed on throat swabs, but if the test is negative, a more traditional test (such as a throat culture and bacitracin susceptibility) should be performed.

pneumonia in immunosuppressed patients; a condition known as **mucormycosis (zygomycosis)**. Viral pneumonia may be caused by adenoviruses, respiratory syncytial virus (RSV), parainfluenza viruses, cytomegalovirus, measles virus, chickenpox virus, and other viruses. Healthcare-associated bacterial pneumonia is most often caused by Gram-negative bacilli, especially *Klebsiella*, *Enterobacter*, *Serratia*, and *Acinetobacter* spp. *Pseudomonas aeruginosa* and *S. aureus* are also frequent causes of healthcare-associated pneumonias. Pneumonia is the most common fatal infection acquired in hospitals.

Reservoirs and Mode of Transmission. In most cases, infected humans; other reservoirs include infected psittacine birds (parrots and parakeets) in psittacosis, soil, and bird droppings in histoplasmosis and cryptococcosis. Depending on the pathogen involved, transmission is by droplet inhalation, direct oral contact, contact with contaminated hands and fomites, or inhalation of yeasts and fungal spores.

Laboratory Diagnosis. A good quality sputum specimen (coughed up from the patient's lungs) must be sent to the microbiology laboratory for culture and sensitivity (C&S). It must be sputum—*not* saliva. A laboratory workup of saliva will not provide clinically relevant information. Laboratory personnel can differentiate between saliva and sputum by preparing and examining a Gram-stained smear of the specimen. Sputum will contain numerous WBCs and few epithelial cells, whereas saliva will contain few (if any) WBCs and numerous epithelial cells.

Bacterial Infections of the Lower Respiratory Tract

Information pertaining to bacterial infections of the lower respiratory tract is contained in Table 19-6.

BACTERIAL INFECTIONS OF THE ORAL REGION

The anaerobic environment produced by oxidation–reduction reactions of the oral flora organisms allows certain genera of anaerobic bacteria (e.g., *Bacteroides*, *Porphyromonas*, *Fusobacterium*, *Prevotella*, *Actinomyces*, and *Treponema* spp.) to become involved in the production of oral diseases. The coating that forms on unclean teeth, called **dental plaque**, is a coaggregation of bacteria and their products. Many of these microorganisms produce a slime layer or glycocalyx that enables them to attach firmly and cause damage to the tooth enamel. Certain carbohydrates, especially sucrose, are metabolized by streptococci (especially *Streptococcus mutans*), lactobacilli, and *Actinomyces* spp., producing lactic acid, which rapidly dissolves the tooth enamel. When plaque remains on teeth for more than 72 hours, it hardens into

tartar or calculus, which cannot be completely removed by brushing and flossing.

Acute Necrotizing Ulcerative Gingivitis

Acute necrotizing ulcerative gingivitis (ANUG) is also called **Vincent's angina** and **trench mouth**.

Disease. The term "trench mouth" originated in World War I, where soldiers developed the infection while fighting in trenches. It is usually the result of a combination of poor oral hygiene, physical or emotional stress, and poor diet. It involves painful, bleeding gums and tonsils, erosion of gum tissue, and swollen lymph nodes beneath the jaw. It causes extremely bad breath.

Patient Care. Use Standard Precautions for hospitalized patients.

Pathogens. Trench mouth is a synergistic infection involving two or more species of anaerobic bacteria of the indigenous oral microflora. The most commonly involved bacteria are *Fusobacterium nucleatum* (an anaerobic, Gram-negative bacillus) and *Treponema vincentii* (a spirochete). Other commonly involved anaerobic Gram-negative bacilli are *Bacteroides* spp., *Prevotella intermedius*, and *Prevotella melaninogenica*.

Prevention and Control. As is true for other periodontal diseases, trench mouth can be prevented by good oral hygiene. Trench mouth is thought to be noncontagious.

TABLE 19-6	Bacterial Infections of the Lower Respiratory Tract

DISEASE	ADDITIONAL INFORMATION
Legionellosis (Legionnaires' Disease, Pontiac Fever). Legionellosis is an acute bacterial pneumonia with anorexia, malaise, myalgia, headache, high fever, chills, and dry cough, followed by a productive cough, shortness of breath, diarrhea, and pleural and abdominal pain. There is about a 40% fatality rate. Pontiac fever, an influenza-like, less severe form of legionellosis, is not associated with pneumonia or death. Legionellosis was first recognized as a disease following an outbreak in a Philadelphia hotel in 1976, but evidence exists that prior epidemics and deaths were caused by *Legionella* spp. Epidemics continue to occur, often associated with hotels, cruise ships, hospitals, and supermarkets. Legionellosis usually affects elderly persons; people with preexisting respiratory disease, diabetes mellitus, renal disease, or malignancy; people who are immuno-compromised; or people who smoke or drink heavily. **Patient Care.** Use Standard Precautions for hospitalized patients.	**Pathogen.** The primary etiologic agent of legionellosis is *Legionella pneumophila*, a poorly staining, Gram-negative bacillus. Other *Legionella* spp. and organisms within related genera can also cause the disease. As of 2003, 40 species of *Legionella* were known. **Reservoirs and Mode of Transmission.** Reservoirs include environmental water sources, such as ponds, lakes, and creeks; hot-water and air-conditioning systems, cooling towers, and evaporative condensers; whirlpool spas, hot tubs, shower heads, humidifiers, tap water, and water distillation systems; decorative fountains; and perhaps dust. Transmission has occurred as a result of aerosols of *Legionella* spp. that have been produced by vegetable misting devices in supermarkets. Legionellosis is not transmitted from person to person. **Laboratory Diagnosis.** Sputum and blood specimens should be sent to the microbiology laboratory for C&S. *Legionella* spp. stain poorly and require cysteine and other nutrients to grow. The recommended culture medium is buffered charcoal yeast extract agar. Immunodiagnostic procedures are available, such as antigen detection in urine.
Mycoplasmal Pneumonia (Primary Atypical Pneumonia). Mycoplasmal pneumonia has a gradual onset with headache, malaise, dry cough, sore throat, and less often, chest discomfort. The amount of sputum the patient produces is scant at first, but may increase as the disease progresses. Illness may last from a few days to a month or more. Mycoplasmal pneumonia is most common in people 5–35 years of age. Pneumonias produced by mycoplasmas and chlamydias are the most common types of atypical pneumonias (i.e., pneumonias usually caused by organisms other than those that are the typical causes of pneumonia). **Patient Care.** Use Droplet Precautions for hospitalized patients for the duration of illness.	**Pathogen.** The etiologic agent of mycoplasmal pneumonia is *Mycoplasma pneumoniae*, a tiny, Gram-negative bacterium, lacking cell walls. **Reservoirs and Mode of Transmission.** Infected humans serve as reservoirs. Transmission occurs via droplet inhalation or direct contact with an infected person, or articles contaminated with nasal secretions or sputum from an ill, coughing patient. **Laboratory Diagnosis.** Mycoplasmal pneumonia is diagnosed by demonstration of a rise in antibody titer between acute and convalescent sera. On artificial media, *M. pneumoniae* produces tiny "fried egg" colonies, having a dense central area and a less-dense periphery.
Tuberculosis (TB). Tuberculosis is an acute or chronic mycobacterial infection of the lower respiratory tract with malaise, fever, night sweats, weight loss, and productive cough. Shortness of breath, chest pain, hemoptysis (coughing up blood), and hoarseness may occur in advanced stages. Widespread tuberculosis, known as military tuberculosis, involves many lesions throughout the body. (See Chapter 11 for additional information regarding the current TB pandemic.) **Patient Care.** Use Airborne Precautions for hospitalized patients with pulmonary or laryngeal disease. Use Standard Precautions for patients with extrapulmonary or meningeal TB and no draining lesions. If the patient has draining lesions, add Airborne and Contact Precautions.	**Pathogens.** Tuberculosis may be caused by any of the species in the *Mycobacterium tuberculosis* complex, but it is most often caused by *M. tuberculosis* (a slow-growing, acid-fast, Gram-positive to Gram-variable bacillus). *M. tuberculosis* is sometimes referred to as the tubercle bacillus. **Reservoirs and Mode of Transmission.** Infected humans are the primary reservoirs; rarely, primates, cattle, and other infected mammals can serve as reservoirs. Transmission occurs via airborne droplets produced by infected people during coughing, sneezing, and even talking or singing; usually following prolonged direct contact with infected individuals. Bovine tuberculosis may result from exposure to infected cattle or ingestion of unpasteurized, contaminated milk or other dairy products.

(continues)

TABLE 19-6	Bacterial Infections of the Lower Respiratory Tract (continued)
DISEASE	**ADDITIONAL INFORMATION**
	Laboratory Diagnosis. Demonstration of acid-fast bacilli (AFB) in sputum specimens provides a rapid, presumptive diagnosis of tuberculosis. Isolation of *M. tuberculosis* on Löwenstein-Jensen or Middlebrook culture media takes about 3–6 weeks because of the organism's long generation time (about 18–24 hours). A variety of more rapid techniques are available for isolation and identification of *M. tuberculosis*, including automated and semiautomated instruments, molecular diagnostic procedures, and gas–liquid chromatography. Susceptibility testing should be performed as soon as possible, because many strains of *M. tuberculosis* are multidrug resistant. Infected patients show a positive delayed hypersensitivity skin test (the Mantoux purified protein derivative [PPD] tuberculin skin test), and pulmonary tubercles may be seen on chest radiographs. Recall from Chapter 16 that a positive TB skin test result may indicate any of five possibilities, including past infection, present infection, or receipt of Bacillus Calmette-Guérin (BCG) vaccine.
Whooping Cough (Pertussis). Whooping cough is a highly contagious, acute bacterial childhood (usually) infection. The first stage (the prodromal or catarrhal stage) of the disease involves mild, coldlike symptoms. The second stage (the paroxysmal stage) produces severe, uncontrollable coughing fits. The coughing often ends in a prolonged, high-pitched, deeply indrawn breath (the "whoop," from which whooping cough gets its name). The coughing fits produce a clear, tenacious mucus and vomiting. They may be so severe as to cause lung rupture, bleeding in the eyes and brain, broken ribs, rectal prolapse, or hernia. The third stage (the recovery or convalescent stage) usually begins within 4 weeks of onset. Parapertussis is a similar but milder disease. **Patient Care.** Use Droplet Precautions for hospitalized patients until 5 days after initiation of effective therapy.	**Pathogen.** Pertussis is caused by *Bordetella pertussis*, a small, encapsulated, nonmotile, Gram-negative coccobacillus that produces endotoxin and exotoxins. Parapertussis is caused by *Bordetella parapertussis*. A related organism, *Bordetella bronchiseptica*, causes respiratory infections in animals, including kennel cough in dogs. **Reservoirs and Mode of Transmission.** Infected humans serve as reservoirs. Transmission occurs via droplets produced by coughing. **Laboratory Diagnosis.** Nasopharyngeal aspirates or swabs should be sent to the microbiology laboratory. Special media, such as Bordet-Gengou agar (a potato-based medium) or Regan-Lowe agar (a charcoal/horse blood medium), are used to isolate *B. pertussis*. Molecular diagnostic and immunodiagnostic procedures are also available.

BACTERIAL INFECTIONS OF THE GASTROINTESTINAL TRACT

Table 19-7 contains information pertaining to bacterial infections of the gastrointestinal (GI) tract.

Enterovirulent *Escherichia coli*

E. coli is a Gram-negative bacillus that is found in the GI tract of all humans. The strains and serotypes of *E. coli* that are part of the indigenous microflora of the GI tract are opportunistic pathogens. They usually cause no harm while in the GI tract, but have the potential to cause serious infections if they gain access to the bloodstream, the urinary bladder, or a wound. *E. coli* is the major cause of septicemia, urinary tract infections (UTIs), and healthcare-associated infections.

There are other strains and serotypes of *E. coli* in nature that are not indigenous microflora of the human colon and always cause disease when they are ingested. Collectively, these strains and serotypes are referred to as enterovirulent *E. coli*. Information pertaining to two general types, the enterohemorrhagic *E. coli* and the enterotoxigenic *E. coli*, is contained in Table 19-8 (p. 338).

Bacterial Foodborne Intoxications (Foodborne Infections, Food Poisoning)

The term "food poisoning" is broad and may include diseases resulting from the ingestion of chemical contaminants as well as bacteria or bacterial toxins, phycotoxins, mycotoxins, viruses, or protozoa. Technically, diseases resulting from the ingestion of toxin-producing microorganisms are called **infectious diseases**, whereas diseases

TABLE 19-7   Bacterial Infections of the Gastrointestinal Tract

DISEASE	ADDITIONAL INFORMATION
Bacterial Gastritis and Gastric Ulcers. Infection with *Helicobacter pylori* can cause chronic bacterial gastritis and duodenal ulcers. Gastritis is suspected when a person has upper abdominal pain with nausea or heartburn. People with duodenal ulcers may experience gnawing, burning, aching, mild-to-moderate pain just below the breastbone, an empty feeling, and hunger. The pain usually occurs when the stomach is empty. Drinking milk, eating, or taking antacids generally relieves the pain, but it usually returns 2 or 3 hours later. Gastric ulcers and gastric adenocarcinoma are also epidemiologically associated with *H. pylori* infection. Gastric ulcers can cause swelling of the tissues leading into the small intestine, which prevents food from easily passing out of the stomach. This, in turn, can cause pain, bloating, nausea, or vomiting after eating. Gastric ulcers and duodenal ulcers are types of peptic ulcers. Complications of peptic ulcers include penetration, perforation, bleeding, and obstruction. **Patient Care.** Use Standard Precautions for hospitalized patients.	**Pathogen.** *H. pylori* is a curved, microaerophilic, capnophilic, Gram-negative bacillus that is found on the mucus-secreting epithelial cells of the stomach. No other bacteria are known to grow in the extremely acidic stomach. **Reservoirs and Mode of Transmission.** Infected humans serve as reservoirs. Transmission probably occurs via ingestion; presumed to be either oral–oral or fecal–oral transmission. **Laboratory Diagnosis.** Diagnostic techniques include staining and culturing of gastric and duodenal biopsy specimens, the urea breath test, the NH_4 excretion test, molecular diagnostic procedures, and immunodiagnostic procedures. In the urea breath test, the patient ingests radioactively labeled urea and his or her breath is analyzed 60 minutes later for radioactively labeled CO_2. The enzyme urease, produced by *H. pylori*, splits the urea into ammonia and CO_2; hence, the presence of radioactively labeled CO_2 indicates the presence of *H. pylori*. In the NH_4 excretion test, the patient consumes urea containing radioactively labeled nitrogen. The ammonia produced in the stomach by *H. pylori* is absorbed into the blood, excreted in the urine, and the amount of radioactively labeled NH_4 in the urine is measured.
***Campylobacter* Enteritis.** Campylobacter enteritis is an acute bacterial enteric disease, ranging from asymptomatic to severe, with diarrhea, nausea, vomiting, fever, malaise, and abdominal pain. The disease is usually self-limiting, lasting 2–5 days. Stools may contain gross or occult (hidden) blood, mucus, and WBCs. *Campylobacter* spp. are the major cause of bacterial diarrhea in the United States. **Patient Care.** Use Standard Precautions for hospitalized patients. Add Contact Precautions for diapered or incontinent patients.	**Pathogens.** The etiologic agents of *Campylobacter* enteritis are *Campylobacter jejuni* and, less commonly, *Campylobacter coli*. *Campylobacter* spp. are curved, S-shaped, or spiral-shaped Gram-negative bacilli, often having a "gull-wing" morphology (a pair of curved bacilli) following cell division. They are microaerophilic and capnophilic, with an optimal growth temperature of 42°C. **Reservoirs and Mode of Transmission.** Reservoirs are animals, including poultry, cattle, sheep, swine, rodents, birds, kittens, puppies, and other pets. Most raw poultry is contaminated with *C. jejuni*, thus necessitating proper methods of cleaning and disinfecting in the kitchen. Transmission occurs via ingestion of contaminated food (e.g., chicken, pork), raw milk, or water; contact with infected pets or farm animals; or contaminated cutting boards. **Laboratory Diagnosis.** Diagnosis depends on the recovery of *Campylobacter* spp. from stool specimens, using selective medium (Campy blood agar, which contains several antimicrobial agents to suppress growth of other bacteria), a Campy gas mixture (5% O_2, 10% CO_2, 85% N_2), and 42°C incubation.
Cholera. Cholera is an acute, bacterial diarrheal disease with profuse watery stools, occasional vomiting, and rapid dehydration. If untreated, circulatory collapse, renal failure, and death may occur. More than 50% of untreated people with severe cholera die. Cholera occurs worldwide, with periodic epidemics and pandemics. A cholera pandemic that started in Peru in 1991 produced more than 950,000 cases and had been reported in 21 countries in the Western Hemisphere by 1994. Most U.S. cases involve the ingestion of raw or undercooked seafood (e.g., oysters) from the coastal waters of Louisiana and Texas.	**Pathogens.** The etiologic agents of cholera are certain biotypes of *Vibrio cholerae* serogroup 01. These are curved (comma-shaped) Gram-negative bacilli that secrete an *enterotoxin* (a toxin that adversely affects cells in the intestinal tract) called *choleragen*. Other *Vibrio* spp. (*Vibrio parahemolyticus*, *Vibrio vulnificus*) also cause diarrheal diseases. Vibrios are halophilic (salt-loving) and thus are found in marine environments.

(continues)

TABLE 19-7   Bacterial Infections of the Gastrointestinal Tract (continued)

DISEASE	ADDITIONAL INFORMATION
Patient Care. Use Standard Precautions for hospitalized patients. Add Contact Precautions for diapered or incontinent patients.	**Reservoirs and Mode of Transmission.** Reservoirs include infected humans and aquatic reservoirs (copepods and other zooplankton). Transmission occurs via the fecal–oral route, contact with feces or vomitus of infected people, ingestion of fecally contaminated water or foods (especially raw or undercooked shellfish and other seafood), or mechanical transmission by flies. **Laboratory Diagnosis.** Rectal swabs or stool specimens should be inoculated onto thiosulfate-citrate-bile-sucrose (TCBS) agar; different *Vibrio* spp. produce different reactions on this medium. Biochemical tests are used to identify the various species. Biotyping is accomplished using commercially available antisera.
Salmonellosis. Salmonellosis is gastroenteritis with sudden onset of headache, abdominal pain, diarrhea, nausea, and sometimes vomiting. Dehydration may be severe. Salmonellosis may develop into septicemia or localized infection in any tissue of the body. **Patient Care.** Use Standard Precautions for hospitalized patients. Add Contact Precautions for diapered or incontinent patients.	**Pathogens.** GI salmonellosis is caused by members of the family Enterobacteriaceae currently named *Salmonella enterica* (of which there are more than 2,000 serotypes or serovars). These Gram-negative bacilli invade intestinal cells, release endotoxin, and produce cytotoxins and enterotoxins. About 200 of the *S. enterica* serotypes cause GI salmonellosis in the United States. The most commonly reported serotypes are *S. enterica* subsp. *enterica* serovar *typhimurium* (also known as *Salmonella typhimurium*) and *S. enterica* subsp. *enterica* serovar *enteritidis* (also known as *Salmonella enteritidis*). **Reservoirs and Mode of Transmission.** Reservoirs include a wide range of wild and domestic animals, such as poultry, swine, cattle, rodents, reptiles (e.g., pet iguanas and turtles), pet chicks, dogs, and cats. Infected humans (e.g., patients, carriers) are also reservoirs. Transmission occurs via ingestion of contaminated food (e.g., eggs, unpasteurized milk, meat, poultry, raw fruits and vegetables), fecal–oral transmission from person to person, food handlers, or contaminated water supplies. **Laboratory Diagnosis.** Stool specimens should be submitted to the microbiology laboratory for C&S. *Salmonella* spp. are nonlactose fermenters and thus produce colorless colonies on MacConkey agar. Biochemical tests are used for identification, and commercially available antisera are used for serotyping.
Typhoid Fever (Enteric Fever). Typhoid fever is a systemic bacterial disease with fever, severe headache, malaise, anorexia, a rash on the trunk in about 25% of patients, nonproductive cough, and constipation. Bacteremia; pneumonia; gallbladder, liver, and bone infection; endocarditis; meningitis, and other complications may occur. About 10% of untreated patients die. Worldwide, an estimated 17 million cases occur per year with approximately 600,000 deaths. **Patient Care.** Use Standard Precautions for hospitalized patients. Add Contact Precautions for diapered or incontinent patients.	**Pathogen.** Typhoid fever is caused by *Salmonella typhi* (also known as the typhoid bacillus), a Gram-negative bacillus that releases endotoxin and produces exotoxins. A similar, but less severe infection is caused by *Salmonella paratyphi*. **Reservoirs and Mode of Transmission.** Infected humans serve as reservoirs for typhoid and paratyphoid; rarely, domestic animals for paratyphoid. Some people become carriers following infection, shedding the pathogens in their feces or urine. (Refer to Chapter 11 for the "Typhoid Mary" story.) Transmission occurs via the fecal–oral route; food or water contaminated by feces or urine of patients or carriers; oysters harvested from fecally contaminated waters; fecally contaminated fruits and raw vegetables; or from feces to food by mechanical transmission by flies.

TABLE 19-7   Bacterial Infections of the Gastrointestinal Tract (conti

DISEASE	ADDITIONAL INFORM
	Laboratory Diagnos by isolation of *S.* marrow, followe Immunodiagno
Shigellosis (Bacillary Dysentery). Shigellosis is an acute bacterial infection of the lining of the small and large intestine, producing diarrhea (as many as 20 bowel movements a day) with blood, mucus, and pus. Other symptoms include nausea, vomiting, cramps, and fever. Sometimes *toxemia* (toxins in the blood) and convulsions (in children) occur. Other serious complications, such as hemolytic uremic syndrome, may occur. Worldwide, shigellosis is estimated to cause approximately 600,000 deaths per year, with about two thirds of the cases and most of the deaths occurring in children younger than 10 years of age. **Patient Care.** Use Standard Precautions for hospitalized patients. Add Contact Precautions for diapered or incontinent patients.	**Pathogens.** The etiologic a *dysenteriae, Shigella flexneri, S* *Shigella soneii.* They are nonmotile Gra that are members of the Enterobacteriaceae plasmid is associated with toxin production and virulence. Relatively few (10–100) organisms are required to cause disease. **Reservoirs and Mode of Transmission.** Infected humans serve as reservoirs. People become infected by direct or indirect fecal–oral transmission from patients or carriers; fecally contaminated hands and fingernails; or fecally contaminated food, milk, and drinking water. Flies can mechanically transfer organisms from latrines to food. **Laboratory Diagnosis.** Leukocytes will be present in stool specimens. Fresh fecal or rectal swabs should be immediately inoculated into Gram-negative (GN) enrichment broth and onto a solid medium (such as MacConkey, xylose lysine deoxycholate [XLD], or Hektoen enteric [HE] agar). *Shigella* spp. produce colorless colonies on MacConkey agar because they are nonlactose fermenters. Isolates are identified by biochemical and immunodiagnostic procedures.
***Clostridium difficile*–Associated Diseases.** *C. difficile* is the major cause of conditions known as antibiotic-associated diarrhea (AAD) and pseudomembranous colitis (PMC), which frequently occur in patients following antibiotic therapy. It does not seem to matter for what condition the patient was receiving antibiotics, which antibiotics the patient was receiving, the dosage, or the route of administration. Antibiotics that have a profound effect on colonic flora, such as cephalosporins, ampicillin, amoxicillin, and clindamycin, are the drugs most frequently implicated. **Patient Care.** Use Contact Precautions for the duration of illness. Use soap and water for handwashing. The alcohol in waterless antiseptic hand rubs lacks sporicidal activity.	**Pathogen.** *C. difficile* (often referred to simply as "C. dif") is a spore-forming anaerobic Gram-positive bacillus. **Reservoirs and Mode of Transmission.** *C. difficile* is a member of the indigenous microflora in about 2%–3% of healthy, nonhospitalized adults. Hospitalized patients frequently become colonized with *C. difficile* as a result of its presence in the hospital environment. It is estimated that about 20%–30% of hospitalized patients are colonized with *C. difficile*. **Laboratory Diagnosis.** *C. difficile* is identified in the laboratory using a variety of phenotypic characteristics. However, diagnosis of *C. difficile*-associated diseases is most often accomplished using some type of commercial enzyme immunoassay or cytotoxin tissue culture assay.

resulting from the ingestion of preformed microbial toxins are called **microbial intoxications**. The distinction is based on where the toxin is actually produced—in the body (in vivo) or in the food (in vitro). The incubation time (the time that elapses between ingestion and onset of symptoms) is usually shorter in microbial intoxications. If toxin-producing bacteria are ingested, the incubation time will depend on the number of bacteria ingested, their generation time, and the amount of time it takes them to produce enough toxin to produce symptoms. According to the CDC, approximately 76 million cases of foodborne illness occur each year in the United States,

resulting in more than 5,000 deaths and 325,000 hospitalizations. CD-ROM Appendix 1 contains information pertaining to microbial intoxications.

BACTERIAL INFECTIONS OF THE GENITOURINARY SYSTEM

Urinary Tract Infections

Recall from Chapter 17 that UTIs can be divided into upper UTIs and lower UTIs. Upper UTIs include infections of the kidneys (nephritis or pyelonephritis) and ureters (ureteritis). Lower UTIs include infections of the

hemorrhagic *E. coli* (EHEC) Diarrhea. This disease consists of a hemorrhagic, watery diarrhea with abdominal cramping. Usually, patients have no fever or only a slight fever. About 5% of infected people (especially children younger than age 5 and the elderly) develop hemolytic-uremic syndrome (HUS), with anemia, low platelet count, and kidney failure. The first recognized outbreak of diarrhea caused by enterohemorrhagic *E. coli* (0157:H7) occurred in 1982, involving contaminated hamburger meat—hamburger meat contaminated with cattle feces. Since then, several well-publicized epidemics involving the same serotype have occurred. Not all of the outbreaks involved meat; some resulted from ingestion of unpasteurized milk or apple juice, lettuce, or other raw vegetables. It has been estimated that *E. coli* 0157:H7 infection accounts for as many as 73,000 cases of illness and 60 deaths in the United States per year.

Patient Care. Use Standard Precautions for hospitalized patients. Add Contact Precautions for diapered or incontinent patients.

Enterotoxigenic *E. coli* (ETEC) Diarrhea (Traveler's Diarrhea). This disease consists of a watery diarrhea with or without mucus or blood, vomiting, and abdominal cramping. Dehydration and low-grade fever may occur. Enterotoxigenic strains of *E. coli* are the most common cause of traveler's diarrhea worldwide and a common cause of diarrheal disease in children in developing countries.

Patient Care. Use Standard Precautions for hospitalized patients. Add Contact Precautions for diapered or incontinent patients.

ADDITIONAL INFORMATION

Pathogens. *E. coli* 0157:H7 (a serotype that possesses a cell wall antigen designated "0157" and a flagellar antigen designated "H7") is the most commonly involved EHEC serotype. Other EHEC serotypes include 026:H11, 0111:H8, and 0104:H21. These are all Gram-negative bacilli that produce potent cytotoxins called Shiga-like toxins—named for their close resemblance to Shiga toxin, produced by *Shigella dysenteriae*).

Reservoirs and Mode of Transmission. Reservoirs include cattle and infected humans. Transmission occurs via the fecal–oral route; inadequately cooked, fecally contaminated beef; unpasteurized milk; person-to-person contact; or fecally contaminated water.

Laboratory Diagnosis. *E. coli* 0157:H7 infection should be suspected in any patient with bloody diarrhea. Stool specimens should be inoculated onto sorbitol-MacConkey (SMAC) agar. Colorless, sorbitol-negative colonies should then be assayed for 0157 antigen using commercially available antiserum. Other immunodiagnostic procedures are available.

Pathogens. ETEC diarrhea is caused by many different serotypes of enterotoxigenic *E. coli* that produce a heat-labile toxin, a heat-stable toxin, or both.

Reservoirs and Mode of Transmission. Infected humans serve as reservoirs. Transmission occurs via the fecal–oral route; ingestion of fecally contaminated food or water.

Laboratory Diagnosis. ETEC diarrhea is diagnosed by isolation of the organism from stool specimens, followed by demonstration of enterotoxin production, molecular diagnostic procedures, or immunodiagnostic procedures.

urinary bladder (cystitis), the urethra (urethritis), and, in men, the prostate (prostatitis). Most UTIs are acquired via the ascending route, whereby the pathogen moves upward from the urethra. Far fewer UTIs occur via the descending route from the bloodstream to the kidneys.

A variety of indigenous microflora are found at and near the outer opening (meatus) of the urethra of both men and women. These microorganisms can ascend the urethra and gain access to the urinary bladder. UTIs may result from poor personal hygiene, sexual intercourse, the insertion of catheters, and other means. A patient with a UTI presents with dysuria (difficulty or pain on urination), lumbar pain, fever, and chills. The latter two symptoms are more common in pyelonephritis than in cystitis. The most common causes of UTIs are *E. coli* and other members of the family Enterobacteriaceae (especially *Proteus* and *Klebsiella* spp.) (Fig. 19-4). Other common causes of UTIs are *Enterococcus* spp., *Staphylococcus*

FIGURE 19-4. Many Gram-negative bacilli and many pink-staining polymorphonuclear neutrophils can be seen in this Gram-stained urine sediment from a patient with cystitis (urinary bladder infection). (From Winn WC Jr., et al. Koneman's Color Atlas and Textbook of Diagnostic Microbiology, 6th ed. Philadelphia: Lippincott Williams & Wilkins, 2006.)

TABLE 19-9   Bacterial Sexually Transmitted Diseases

DISEASE	ADDITIONAL INFORMATION
Genital Chlamydial Infections, Genital Chlamydiasis. *Chlamydia trachomatis* is considered to be the most common sexually transmitted pathogen. Different serovars of *C. trachomatis* cause different diseases. Serovars D through K are the major causes of nongonococcal urethritis (NGU) and epididymitis in men; and cervicitis, urethritis, endometritis, and salpingitis in women, causing mucopurulent urethral discharge, urethral itching, and burning on urination; may also cause infertility and proctitis in men. Most commonly causes endocervical and urethral infections, salpingitis, infertility, and chronic pelvic pain in women. Infection during pregnancy may result in premature rupture of membranes and preterm delivery as well as conjunctivitis and pneumonia in neonates. Genital chlamydial infection may be concurrent with gonorrhea. **Patient Care.** Use Standard Precautions for hospitalized patients.	**Pathogen.** Genital chlamydial infections are caused by certain serotypes of *C. trachomatis;* tiny, obligate intracellular, Gram-negative bacteria. (Less common causes of NGU are *Ureaplasma ureolyticum* [closely related to mycoplasmas], herpes simplex viruses, and *Trichomonas vaginalis*.) **Reservoirs and Mode of Transmission.** Infected humans serve as reservoirs. Transmission occurs via direct sexual contact or mother-to-neonate during birth. **Laboratory Diagnosis.** Identification of *C. trachomatis* by made by cell culture, staining, and immunodiagnostic procedures.
Gonorrhea. It is important to understand that not all clinical presentations of gonorrhea involve the genital tract. Gonorrhea may present as asymptomatic mucosal infection, ophthalmia neonatorum, urethritis, proctitis, pharyngitis, epididymitis, cervicitis, Bartholin gland infection, pelvic inflammatory disease, endometritis, salpingitis, peritonitis, and disseminated gonococcal infection. Patients with disseminated gonococcal infection have myalgia (muscular pain), arthralgia (joint pain), polyarthritis (inflammation of joints), and a characteristic dermatitis—skin lesions located primarily on the extremities. Urethral discharge and painful urination are common in infected men, usually starting 2–7 days after infection. Infected women may be asymptomatic for weeks or months, during which time severe damage to the reproductive system may occur. **Patient Care.** Use Standard Precautions for hospitalized patients.	**Pathogen.** Gonorrhea is caused by *Neisseria gonorrhoeae* (also known as gonococcus or GC), a Gram-negative diplococcus. Some strains (called penicillinase-producing *N. gonorrhoeae* or PPNG) possess plasmids containing the gene for penicillinase production; some strains are multidrug-resistant. **Reservoirs and Mode of Transmission.** Infected humans serve as reservoirs. Transmission occurs via direct mucous membrane-to-mucous membrane contact, usually sexual contact; adult-to-child (may indicate sexual abuse); and mother-to-neonate during birth. **Laboratory Diagnosis.** Gonorrhea in male patients can be diagnosed by the typical appearance of Gram-stained urethral discharge specimens, with numerous WBCs and numerous intracellular and extracellular Gram-negative diplococci (Fig. 19-5). Specimens are inoculated to chocolate agar or a modified chocolate agar (such as Thayer-Martin medium, Martin-Lewis medium, or Transgrow). β-Lactamase testing of isolates is performed, followed by antimicrobial susceptibility testing if the organism is β-lactamase positive. Isolates are usually identified using biochemical tests. Immunodiagnostic procedures are also available.
Syphilis. Syphilis is a treponemal disease that occurs in four stages: (a) primary syphilis—a painless lesion known as a chancre (refer back to Fig. 14-4 in Chapter 14), which develops at the site where *Treponema pallidum* entered the genital mucosa or skin through a break in the surface; (b) secondary syphilis—a skin rash (especially on the palms and soles) about 4–6 weeks later, with fever and mucous membrane lesions, followed by (c) a long latent period (as long as 5–20 years); and then (d) tertiary syphilis—with damage to the CNS, cardiovascular system, visceral organs, bones, sense organs, and other sites. Damage to the CNS or heart is usually not reversible.	**Pathogen.** Syphilis is caused by *T. pallidum*, a Gram-variable, tightly coiled spirochete that is too thin to be seen with brightfield microscopy (refer back to Fig. 4-18 in Chapter 4). **Reservoirs and Mode of Transmission.** Infected humans serve as reservoirs. Transmission occurs via direct contact with lesions, body secretions, mucous membranes, blood, semen, saliva, and vaginal discharges of infected people, usually during sexual contact; blood transfusions; or transplacentally from mother to fetus.

(continues)

TABLE 19-9	Bacterial Sexually Transmitted Diseases (continued)
DISEASE	**ADDITIONAL INFORMATION**
Patient Care. Use Standard Precautions for hospitalized patients.	**Laboratory Diagnosis.** Primary syphilis can be diagnosed by darkfield microscopy (refer back to Fig. 2-6 in Chapter 2) of material scraped from the margin of chancres. Many immunodiagnostic procedures are available, such as the rapid plasma reagin (RPR), Venereal Disease Research Laboratory (VDRL), and fluorescent treponemal antibody absorption (FTA-Abs) tests for detecting antibodies in serum or spinal fluid specimens and fluorescent antibody procedures for detecting antigen in material obtained from lesions or lymph nodes.

spp. (especially *S. aureus, Staphylococcus epidermidis,* and *Staphylococcus saprophyticus*), and *P. aeruginosa.*

UTIs may be acquired either within a healthcare setting (called healthcare-associated UTIs) or elsewhere (called community-acquired UTIs). UTIs are the most common type of healthcare-associated infection, often following urinary catheterization.

Infections of the Genital Tract

Common Bacterial Sexually Transmitted Diseases

Table 19-9 contains information pertaining to common bacterial STDs.

Less Common Bacterial Sexually Transmitted Diseases

Other bacterial pathogens may also be sexually transmitted. Three bacterial STDs, seen more often in parts of the world other than in the United States, are chancroid, granuloma inguinale, and lymphogranuloma venereum (LGV). Chancroid is caused by the Gram-negative bacterium *Haemophilus ducreyi.* Granuloma inguinale is a chronic infection caused by a Gram-negative bacterium named *Calymmatobacterium granulomatis (Donovania granulomatis).* LGV is a chlamydial infection involving the lymph nodes, rectum, and reproductive tract. It is caused by certain serotypes of *Chlamydia trachomatis.* It should be noted that many STDs are transmitted simultaneously; thus, when a patient is diagnosed with one STD, others should be sought.

BACTERIAL INFECTIONS OF THE CIRCULATORY SYSTEM

Rickettsial and Ehrlichial Infections of the Cardiovascular System

Recall that rickettsias and ehrlichias are obligate intracellular, Gram-negative bacteria. Table 19-10 contains information pertaining to rickettsial and ehrlichial diseases of the cardiovascular system.

Other Bacterial Infections of the Cardiovascular System

Infective Endocarditis

Infective (or infectious) endocarditis is usually caused by a bacterium or a fungus. It is characterized by the presence of vegetations (combinations of bacteria and blood clots) on or within the endocardium, most commonly involving a heart valve. Abnormal or damaged valves are most susceptible to infection, although valves can become contaminated during open heart surgery. The vegetations can break loose and be transported to vital organs, where they can block arterial blood flow. Obviously, such obstructions are very serious, possibly leading to strokes, heart attacks, and death.

The two most common types of infective endocarditis are acute bacterial endocarditis and subacute bacterial endocarditis (SBE). Acute bacterial endocarditis is usually caused by colonization of heart valves by virulent bacteria such as *S. aureus* (the most common cause), *S. pneumoniae, Neisseria gonorrhoeae, S. pyogenes,* and *Enterococcus faecalis.*

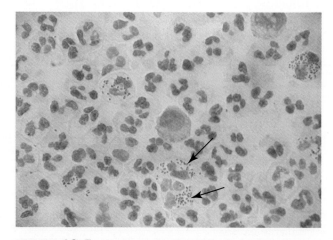

FIGURE 19-5. Gram-stained urethral exudate from a male patient with gonorrhea. Notice the numerous Gram-negative intracellular diplococci (arrows). (Courtesy of Joe Miller and the CDC.)

TABLE 19-10 Rickettsial and Ehrlichial Diseases of the Cardiovascular System

DISEASE	ADDITIONAL INFORMATION
Rocky Mountain Spotted Fever (Tickborne Typhus Fever). Rocky Mountain spotted fever (RMSF) is a tickborne rickettsial disease characterized by sudden onset of moderate-to-high fever, extreme exhaustion (prostration), muscle pain, severe headache, chills, conjunctival infection, and maculopapular rash on extremities on about the third day, which spreads to the palms, soles, and much of the body (Fig. 19-6). In about 4 days, small purplish areas (petechiae) develop as a result of bleeding in the skin. Although uncommon, death can result. RMSF occurs in all parts of the United States, especially the Atlantic seaboard. **Patient Care.** Use Standard Precautions for hospitalized patients.	**Pathogen.** The etiologic agent of RMSF is *Rickettsia rickettsii*, a Gram-negative bacterium. Like all rickettsias, *R. rickettsii* is an obligate intracellular pathogen; it invades endothelial cells (cells that line blood vessels). **Reservoirs and Mode of Transmission.** Reservoirs include infected ticks on dogs, rodents, and other animals. Transmission occurs via the bite of an infected tick. Person-to-person transmission rarely occurs—through blood transfusion. **Laboratory Diagnosis.** Immunodiagnostic procedures are used to diagnose RMSF.
Endemic Typhus Fever. Endemic typhus fever, also known as murine typhus fever and fleaborne typhus, is an acute febrile disease that is similar to, but milder than, epidemic typhus, which is described next. Symptoms include shaking chills, headache, fever, and a faint, pink rash. Endemic typhus has a worldwide occurrence, but is rare in the United States. **Patient Care.** Use Standard Precautions for hospitalized patients.	**Pathogen.** The etiologic agent of endemic typhus is *Rickettsia typhi*, a Gram-negative bacterium and obligate intracellular pathogen. **Reservoirs and Mode of Transmission.** Reservoirs include rats, mice, possibly other mammals, and infected rat fleas. Transmission occurs from rat to flea to human. Infected fleas defecate while feeding, and the rickettsiae in the feces are rubbed into the bite wound or other superficial abrasions. Person-to-person transmission does not occur. **Laboratory Diagnosis.** Immunodiagnostic procedures are used to diagnose endemic typhus.
Epidemic Typhus Fever. Epidemic typhus or louseborne typhus is an acute rickettsial disease, often with sudden onset of headache, chills, prostration, fever, and general pains. A rash appears on the fifth or sixth day, initially on the upper trunk, followed by spread to the entire body, but usually not to the face, palms, or soles. Epidemic typhus fever may be fatal if untreated. It occurs in cold climates in areas where people live under unhygienic conditions and are louse infested. In World War I, the body lice that transmitted epidemic typhus were referred to as "cooties" by soldiers. **Patient Care.** Use Standard Precautions for hospitalized patients.	**Pathogen.** The etiologic agent of epidemic typhus is *Rickettsia prowazekii*, a Gram-negative bacterium and obligate intracellular pathogen. **Reservoirs and Mode of Transmission.** Reservoirs include infected humans and body lice (*Pediculus humanus*; see Fig. 21–10 in Chapter 21). Transmission occurs from human to louse to human. Infected lice defecate while feeding, and the rickettsiae in the feces are rubbed into the bite wound or other superficial abrasions. **Laboratory Diagnosis.** Immunodiagnostic procedures are used to diagnose epidemic typhus.
Ehrlichiosis. Ehrlichiosis is an acute, febrile illness ranging from asymptomatic to mild to severe and life threatening. Patients usually present with acute influenza-like illness with fever, headache, and generalized malaise. Ehrlichiosis is reminiscent of RMSF, without the rash. The estimated fatality rate is about 5%. There are two types of ehrlichiosis: human monocytic ehrlichiosis (HME) and human granulocytic ehrlichiosis (HGE). Cases of HME are more common than HGE cases. Most HME cases have occurred in the southeast and mid-Atlantic states, whereas most HGE cases have occurred in states with high rates of Lyme disease (particularly Connecticut, Minnesota, New York, and Wisconsin). In these states, the tick that transmits the HGE agent is the same tick that transmits *Borrelia burgdorferi*, the etiologic agent of Lyme disease. **Patient Care.** Use Standard Precautions for hospitalized patients.	**Pathogens.** The etiologic agents of ehrlichiosis are Gram-negative coccobacilli that are closely related to rickettsias. They are obligate intraleukocytic pathogens. *Ehrlichia chaffeensis* invades human monocytes, causing HME. *Anaplasma phagocytophilum* invades human granulocytes, causing HGE. A canine species, *Ehrlichia ewingii*, has caused a small number of human cases. **Reservoirs and Mode of Transmission.** Reservoirs are unknown. Transmission occurs via tick bite. The two different types of ehrlichiosis seem to be transmitted by different species of ticks. **Laboratory Diagnosis.** Ehrlichiosis is diagnosed using immunodiagnostic procedures and nucleic acid assays.

FIGURE 19-6. Rocky Mountain spotted fever rash. (Courtesy of the CDC.)

FIGURE 19-8. *Yersinia pestis*, the etiologic agent of plague, in a Wright-stained blood smear. Note the safety-pin appearance that results from bipolar staining. (Courtesy of the CDC.)

In SBE, heart valves are infected by less virulent organisms such as alpha-hemolytic streptococci of oral origin (viridans streptococci), *S. epidermidis*, *Enterococcus* spp., and *Haemophilus* spp. Fungal endocarditis is rare, but cases of *Candida* and *Aspergillus* endocarditis do occur.

Oral streptococci can enter the bloodstream following minor or major dental procedures, oral surgery, and aggressive tooth brushing. Phlebotomy procedures and insertion of intravenous (IV) lines sometimes force organisms from the skin into the bloodstream. IV drug users are at high risk of developing infective endocarditis as a result of contaminated needles, syringes, and drug solutions.

Blood cultures are required for diagnosis of infective endocarditis. Treatment will depend on the specific pathogen involved and the antimicrobial susceptibility results.

Additional information pertaining to bacterial infections of the cardiovascular system is contained in Table 19-11.

FIGURE 19-7. Bull's eye rash of Lyme disease, technically known as erythema migrans. Recognition of this characteristic rash is a key component in the early diagnosis of Lyme disease. (Courtesy of James Gathany and the CDC.)

FIGURE 19-9. Lesion of tularemia caused by *Francisella tularensis*. (Courtesy of Dr. Brachman and the CDC.)

TABLE 19-11   Other Bacterial Infections of the Cardiovascular System

DISEASE	ADDITIONAL INFORMATION
Lyme Disease. Lyme disease or Lyme borreliosis is a tick-borne disease characterized by three stages: (a) an early, distinctive, targetlike, red skin lesion, usually at the site of the tick bite, expanding to a diameter of 15 cm, often with a central clearing (Fig. 19-7); (b) early systemic manifestations that may include fatigue, chills, fever, headache, stiff neck, muscle pain, joint aches, with or without lymphadenopathy; and (c) neurologic abnormalities (e.g., aseptic meningitis, facial paralysis, myelitis, and encephalitis) and cardiac abnormalities (e.g., arrhythmias, pericarditis) several weeks or months after the initial symptoms appear. The disease gets its name from the fact that the first U.S. cases occurred in Lyme, Connecticut. Since then, Lyme disease has been reported in 45 states (mainly the mid-Atlantic, Northeast and North Central states) and it occurs in many other areas of the world. Lyme disease is the most common arthropod-borne disease in the United States. **Patient Care.** Use Standard Precautions for hospitalized patients.	**Pathogen.** The etiologic agent of Lyme disease is *Borrelia burgdorferi*, a loosely coiled Gram-negative, spirochete (refer back to Fig. 4-28 in Chapter 4). **Reservoirs and Mode of Transmission.** Ticks, rodents (especially deer mice), and mammals (especially deer) serve as reservoirs. Transmission occurs via tick bite. Person-to-person transmission does not occur. **Laboratory Diagnosis.** Lyme disease is usually diagnosed by observation of the characteristic targetlike skin lesion, plus immunodiagnostic and molecular diagnostic procedures. *B. burgdorferi* can be grown in the laboratory on a special medium (Barbour-Stoenner-Kelley [BSK] medium at 33°C).
Plague. Plague is an acute, often severe zoonosis. Initial signs and symptoms may include fever, chills, malaise, myalgia, nausea, prostration, sore throat, and headache. **Bubonic plague** is named for the swollen, inflamed, and tender lymph nodes (buboes) that develop. Usually, the lymph nodes affected are those receiving drainage from the site of the bite of an infected flea. In about 90% of cases, the inguinal (groin area) lymph nodes are involved. **Pneumonic plague**, which is highly communicable, involves the lungs. It can result in localized outbreaks or devastating epidemics. **Septicemic plague** may lead to septic shock, meningitis, and death. **Patient Care.** Use Standard Precautions for hospitalized patients with bubonic and septicemic plague. Add Droplet Precautions for pneumonic plague patients, until 48 hours after initiation of effective therapy.	**Pathogen.** The etiologic agent of plague is *Yersinia pestis*, a nonmotile, bipolar-staining, Gram-negative coccobacillus, sometimes referred to as the plague bacillus. **Reservoirs and Mode of Transmission.** Reservoirs include wild rodents (especially ground squirrels in the United States) and their fleas, and, rarely, rabbits, wild carnivores, and domestic cats. Transmission is usually via flea bite (from rodent to flea to human). Transmission may also occur as a result of handling tissues of infected rodents, rabbits, and other animals, as well as droplet transmission from person to person (in pneumonic plague). **Laboratory Diagnosis.** Plague is diagnosed by observation of the typical appearance of *Y. pestis* (bipolar-staining bacilli that resemble safety pins) in Gram-stained or Wright-Giemsa–stained sputum, cerebrospinal fluid, or material aspirated from a bubo (Fig. 19-8). Diagnosis can also be made by culture, biochemical tests, and immunodiagnostic tests.
Tularemia. Tularemia, also known as rabbit fever, is an acute zoonosis with a variety of clinical manifestations, depending on the portal of entry of the pathogen into the body. Tularemia most often presents as a skin ulcer (Fig. 19-9) and regional lymphadenitis. Ingestion of the pathogen results in pharyngitis, abdominal pain, diarrhea, and vomiting. Inhalation of the pathogen results in pneumonia and septicemia, with a 30%–60% fatality rate. **Patient Care.** Use Standard Precautions for hospitalized patients.	**Pathogen.** The etiologic agent of tularemia is *Francisella tularensis*, a small, pleomorphic Gram-negative coccobacillus. Some strains are more virulent than others. **Reservoirs and Mode of Transmission.** Reservoirs include wild animals (especially rabbits, muskrats, and beavers), some domestic animals, and hard ticks. Transmission occurs via tick bite; ingestion of contaminated meat or drinking water, entry of organisms into a wound while skinning infected animals, inhalation of dust, or animal bites. Person-to-person transmission does not occur. **Laboratory Diagnosis.** Diagnosis of tularemia is by culture, biochemical tests, and immunodiagnostic procedures.

BACTERIAL INFECTIONS OF THE CENTRAL NERVOUS SYSTEM

Bacteria that can cause meningitis were discussed under "Infections of the CNS Having Multiple Causes" in Chapter 17. Additional information pertaining to bacterial infections of the central nervous system (CNS) is contained in Table 19-12.

DISEASES CAUSED BY ANAEROBIC BACTERIA

Some of the human diseases caused by anaerobic bacteria (usually referred to as "anaerobes") are shown in Table 19-13. Many infections that involve anaerobes are synergistic or polymicrobial infections.

DISEASES ASSOCIATED WITH BIOFILMS

Recall from Chapter 10 that biofilms are complex and persistent communities of assorted microbes. Biofilms exist in many environments, including certain anatomical sites within the human body. Listed here are some of the human diseases that are known to or thought to be associated with biofilms:

Bacterial endocarditis
Central venous catheter infection

TABLE 19-12	Bacterial Infections of the Central Nervous System
DISEASE	**ADDITIONAL INFORMATION**
Botulism (see CD-ROM Appendix 1, "Microbial Intoxications").	
Listeriosis. Generally, listeriosis is only a mild febrile illness in healthy, immunocompetent individuals. However, the disease can be manifested as meningoencephalitis and/or septicemia in newborns and elderly and/or immuno-suppressed adults, with fever, intense headache, nausea, vomiting, delirium, coma, occasionally collapse, shock, and death. Listeriosis causes fever and spontaneous abortion in pregnant women. **Patient Care.** Use Standard Precautions for hospitalized patients.	**Pathogen.** Listeriosis is caused by *Listeria monocytogenes*, a Gram-positive coccobacillus. **Reservoirs and Mode of Transmission.** Reservoirs include soil, water, mud, silage, infected mammals, humans, and soft cheeses (*Listeria* multiplies in contaminated refrigerated foods.) Transmission occurs via ingestion of raw or contaminated milk, soft cheeses, or vegetables. Listeriosis can also be transmitted from mother to fetus in utero or during passage through an infected birth canal. **Laboratory Diagnosis.** Listeriosis is diagnosed by isolation and identification of the pathogen from cerebrospinal fluid (CSF), blood, amniotic fluid, placenta, and other specimens. Gram-positive coccobacilli can be observed in Gram-stained smears of neonatal CSF.
Tetanus (Lockjaw). Tetanus is an acute neuromuscular disease induced by a bacterial exotoxin called tetanospasmin, with painful muscular contractions, primarily of the masseter (the muscle that closes the jaw) and neck muscles, spasms, and rigid paralysis (refer back to Fig. 14-9 in Chapter 14). Respiratory failure and death may result. **Patient Care.** Use Standard Precautions for hospitalized patients.	**Pathogen.** Tetanus is caused by *Clostridium tetani*, a motile, Gram-positive, anaerobic, spore-forming bacillus (refer back to Fig. 4-25 in Chapter 4) that produces a potent neurotoxin -called tetanospasmin. **Reservoirs and Mode of Transmission.** Reservoirs include soil contaminated with human, horse, or other animal feces (*C. tetani* is a member of the indigenous intestinal flora of humans and animals.) Spores of *C. tetani* are introduced into a puncture wound, burn, or needlestick by contamination with soil, dust, or feces. Under anaerobic conditions in the wound, spores germinate into vegetative *C. tetani* cells which produce the exotoxin in vivo. Person-to-person transmission does not occur. **Laboratory Diagnosis.** Diagnosis of tetanus is usually made on clinical and epidemiologic grounds. Attempts to isolate *C. tetani* from wounds or demonstrate antibody production are rarely successful.

TABLE 19-13   Some Human Diseases Caused by Anaerobic Bacteria

DISEASE	ANAEROBE(S) THAT CAUSE(S) THE DISEASE
Acne	*Propionibacterium acnes*
Actinomycosis	Various *Actinomyces* spp. and *Propionibacterium propionicus*
Acute necrotizing ulcerative gingivitis (also known as Vincent angina and trench mouth)	*Fusobacterium necrophorum* and anaerobic spirochetes
Antibiotic-associated diarrhea and pseudomembranous colitis	*Clostridium difficile*
Botulism	*Clostridium botulinum*
Brain abscess	Most often caused by *Bacteroides* and *Fusobacterium* spp. and anaerobic Gram-negative cocci; often polymicrobial
Gas gangrene (myonecrosis)	*Clostridium perfringens* (usually), *Clostridium novyi*, *Clostridium septicum*
Gynecologic and obstetric infectious processes	Many different types of anaerobes, including *Bacteroides* spp., clostridia, and anaerobic Gram-positive cocci
Intra-abdominal infectious processes	Many different types of anaerobes, including *Bacteroides* and *Fusobacterium* spp., *C. perfringens*, other clostridia, and anaerobic Gram-positive cocci; usually polymicrobial
Liver abscess	Many different types of anaerobes, including *Bacteroides*, *Fusobacterium*, *Clostridium*, and *Actinomyces* spp.
Oral/dental infectious processes (periodontitis)	Many different types of anaerobes, including *Porphyromonas*, *Wolinella*, and *Fusobacterium* spp. and anaerobic Gram-positive cocci
Perineal and perirectal infectious processes	Many different types of anaerobes, including *Bacteroides*, *Fusobacterium*, *Clostridium*, *Eubacterium*, and *Actinomyces* spp. and anaerobic Gram-positive cocci
Peritonitis	Many different types of anaerobes, including *Bacteroides* and *Clostridium* spp., *F. necrophorum*, and anaerobic Gram-positive cocci
Pleuropulmonary infectious processes	Many different types of anaerobes, including *Bacteroides*, *Porphyromonas*, *Actinomyces*, and *Eubacterium* spp., *Fusobacterium nucleatum*, and anaerobic Gram-positive cocci
Sinusitis	*Bacteroides* and *Fusobacterium* spp. and anaerobic Gram-positive cocci; often polymicrobial
Tetanus	*Clostridium tetani*

Chronic wounds
Cystic fibrosis lung infections
Gingivitis
Infection of prosthetic joints, heart valves, and intrauterine devices
Infectious kidney stones
Middle ear infections
Necrotizing fasciitis
Osteomyelitis
Periodontitis
Prostatitis

Sinusitis
Tooth decay
Urinary catheters
UTIs

RECAP OF MAJOR BACTERIAL INFECTIONS OF HUMANS

Table 19-14 provides a recap of some major bacterial infections of humans.

TABLE 19-14	Recap of Some Major Bacterial Infections of Humans
DISEASE	**BACTERIAL PATHOGEN**
Anthrax	*Bacillus anthracis* (a spore-forming, Gram-positive bacillus)
Cholera	*Vibrio cholerae* (comma-shaped Gram-negative bacilli)
Diphtheria	*Coynebacterium diphtheriae* (a Gram-positive bacillus)
Gas gangrene	*Clostridium perfringens* and some other *Clostridium* spp. (anaerobic, spore-forming, Gram-positive bacilli)
Gonorrhea	*Neisseria gonorrhoeae* (a Gram-negative diplococcus)
Legionellosis (Legionnaires' disease)	*Legionella pneumophila* and some other *Legionella* spp. (Gram-negative bacilli)
Leprosy (Hansen disease)	*Mycobacterium leprae* (an acid-fast bacillus)
Listeriosis	*Listeria monocytogenes* (a Gram-negative bacillus)
Lyme disease	*Borrelia burgdorferi* (a Gram-negative spirochete)
Plague	*Yersinia pestis* (a Gram-negative bacillus)
Rocky Mountain spotted fever	*Rickettsia rickettsii* (a Gram-negative bacillus; an obligate intracellular pathogen)
Salmonellosis	*Salmonella enteritidis* and *Salmonella typhimurium* (Gram-negative bacilli)
Shigellosis	*Shigella dysenteriae*, *Shigella flexneri*, *Shigella boydii*, and *Shigella sonnei* (Gram-negative bacilli)
Strep throat	*Streptococcus pyogenes* (a Gram-positive coccus)
Syphilis	*Treponema pallidum* (a tightly coiled spirochete)
Tetanus	*Clostridium tetani* (an anaerobic, spore-forming, Gram-positive bacillus)
Trachoma	Certain serotypes of *Chlamydia trachomatis* (a Gram-negative bacillus; an obligate intracellular pathogen)
Tuberculosis	Most cases are caused by *Mycobacterium tuberculosis* (an acid-fast bacillus)
Tularemia	*Francisella tularensis* (a Gram-negative bacillus)
Typhoid fever	*Salmonella typhi* (a Gram-negative bacillus)
Whooping cough (pertussis)	*Bordetella pertussis* (a Gram-negative coccobacillus)
Wound botulism	*Clostridium botulinum* (an anaerobic, spore-forming, Gram-positive bacillus)

APPROPRIATE THERAPY FOR BACTERIAL INFECTIONS

Recommendations for the treatment of infectious diseases change frequently. The bacterial infections described in this chapter must be treated using appropriate antibacterial drugs. Sources of updated information include *The Merck Manual* (http://www.merck.com/pubs) and WebMD (http://www.webmd.com). For certain bacterial diseases, antisera (e.g., for botulism and tetanus) are available for treatment. Additional information about antibacterial agents can be found in Chapter 9.

ON THE CD-ROM
- Terms Introduced in This Chapter
- Review of Key Points
- Insight:
  - A Closer Look at *Staphylococcus aureus*
  - A Closer Look at *Streptococcus pyogenes*
  - A Closer Look at *Streptococcus pneumoniae*
- Increase Your Knowledge
- Critical Thinking
- Case Studies
- Additional Self-Assessment Exercises

SELF-ASSESSMENT EXERCISES

After you have read this chapter, answer the following multiple-choice questions.

1. The most common STD in the United States is caused by:
   a. *Candida albicans.*
   b. *Chlamydia trachomatis.*
   c. *Neisseria gonorrhoeae.*
   d. *Trichomonas vaginalis.*
2. _____ is the most common cause of pneumonia in the world.
   a. *Chlamydophila pneumoniae*
   b. *Legionella pneumophila*
   c. *Mycoplasma pneumoniae*
   d. *Streptococcus pneumoniae*
3. Gas gangrene is always caused by:
   a. *Bacillus anthracis.*
   b. *Clostridium* spp.
   c. *Staphylococcus aureus.*
   d. *Streptococcus pyogenes.*
4. The bacterial species most frequently associated with necrotizing fasciitis is:
   a. *Francisella tularensis.*
   b. *S. aureus.*
   c. *S. pneumoniae.*
   d. *S. pyogenes.*
5. Which of the following diseases may be caused by *C. trachomatis*?
   a. inclusion conjunctivitis
   b. nongonococcal urethritis (NGU)
   c. trachoma
   d. all of the above
6. Which of the following organisms is the most common cause of urethritis?
   a. *C. albicans*
   b. *C. trachomatis*
   c. *N. gonorrhoeae*
   d. *T. vaginalis*
7. Which of the following organisms is the most common cause of cystitis?
   a. *C. trachomatis*
   b. *E. coli*
   c. *N. gonorrhoeae*
   d. *T. vaginalis*
8. Which of the following is the most common arthropod-borne disease in the United States?
   a. Lyme disease
   b. plague
   c. Rocky Mountain spotted fever
   d. tularemia
9. Which of the following diseases is *not* caused by a spirochete?
   a. Lyme disease
   b. plague
   c. relapsing fever
   d. syphilis
10. Which of the following associations is *incorrect*?
    a. Lyme disease . . . tick
    b. plague . . . rat flea
    c. Rocky Mountain spotted fever . . . tick
    d. typhoid fever . . . mosquito

20 FUNGAL INFECTIONS

CHAPTER OUTLINE

LEARNING OBJECTIVES

AFTER STUDYING THIS CHAPTER, YOU SHOULD BE ABLE TO:

- Categorize various fungal diseases by body system (e.g., respiratory system, circulatory system, etc.)
- Correlate a particular fungal disease with its major characteristics, etiologic agent, reservoir(s), mode(s) of transmission, and diagnostic laboratory procedures
- Briefly explain how fungi cause disease
- Classify a given fungal infection as being a superficial, cutaneous, subcutaneous, or systemic mycosis
- State several diseases caused by dimorphic fungi

INTRODUCTION

It would be impossible in a book this size to describe *all* of the human infectious diseases caused by fungi. Thus, only selected fungal diseases (mycoses) are described in this chapter. Readers should keep in mind that, although a certain fungal disease is described in one particular section of the chapter (e.g., under cardiovascular infections or respiratory infections), many fungal diseases have various clinical manifestations, affecting more than one anatomical site.

Fungal infections are also known as **mycoses** (sing., **mycosis**).

Mycoses are caused by fungi within three fungal categories: yeasts, moulds, and dimorphic fungi. Recall that dimorphic fungi are fungi that may grow as yeasts *or* moulds, depending on the temperature at which they are growing. Some fungi can also cause microbial intoxications, which are discussed in Appendix 1 of the CD-ROM.

Mycoses are caused by certain yeasts, moulds, and dimorphic fungi.

In 2007, only one fungal disease—coccidioidomycosis—was classified as a nationally notifiable infectious disease. Recall that cases of nationally notifiable infectious diseases must be reported to the Centers for Disease Control and Prevention (CDC). A total of 8,121 cases of coccidioidomycosis were reported to the CDC in 2007.

HOW DO FUNGI CAUSE DISEASE?

Unlike bacteria, fungi do not secrete toxins that cause damage to the host. Rather, the tissue damage associated with fungal infections results primarily from direct invasion of tissue, with subsequent displacement and destruction of vital structures, coupled with toxic effects of the inflammatory response.

Fungal pathogens cause disease by invasion and mechanical destruction of tissues and/or obstruction of the flow of bodily fluids.

Masses of fungal cells can cause obstruction of bronchi in the lungs and tubules and ureters in kidneys, leading to obstruction of the flow of bodily fluids. Certain fungi, such as *Aspergillus* and *Mucor* spp. can grow in the walls of arteries and veins, leading to occlusion and tissue necrosis resulting from a lack of oxygen.

CLASSIFICATION OF FUNGAL DISEASES

Fungal infections (mycoses) can be classified into the following four categories:

- **Superficial mycoses.** These are fungal infections of the outermost areas of the human body, including the outer surfaces of hair shafts and the outermost, nonliving layer of the skin (the epidermis). Superficial mycoses include otomycosis,[a] black piedra, white piedra, tinea (or pityriasis) versicolor, and tinea nigra. All are caused by moulds. Black piedra, caused by *Piedraia hortae*, is a fungal infection of scalp hair and, less commonly, eyebrows and eyelashes. White piedra, usually caused by *Trichosporon beigelii*, is a fungal infection of moustache, beard, pubic, and axilla hair. Tinea versicolor, caused by *Malassezia furfur*, is a ringworm infection that affects the skin of the chest or back and, less commonly, the arms, thighs, neck, and face. Tinea nigra, caused by *Hortaea werneckii*, is a ringworm infection of the palms of the hands, less commonly, the neck and feet.

  > Superficial mycoses are fungal infections of the outer surfaces of hair shafts and the outermost, nonliving layer of the skin (the epidermis).

- **Cutaneous, hair, and nail mycoses.** Fungal infections of the living layers of skin (the dermis), hair shafts, and nails—commonly called tinea infections or ringworm infections—are caused by a group of moulds collectively referred to as dermatophytes (Fig. 20-1).

[a] Otomycosis is a fungal infection of the outer ear canal, most often caused by a mould.

FIGURE 20-1. Various types of tinea infections.
(A) Tinea pedis (athlete's foot), **(B)** tinea corporis (ringworm of the trunk, shown here on the shoulder), **(C)** tinea capitis (ringworm of the head), **(D)** tinea cruris (ringworm of the groin area), and **(E)** tinea unguium (ringworm of the nails). (From Harvey RA, et al. Lippincott's Illustrated Reviews: Microbiology, 2nd ed. Philadelphia: Lippincott Williams & Wilkins, 2007.)

Tinea infections are named in accordance with the part of the anatomy infected. Examples include tinea barbae (infection of the beard and moustache), tinea capitis (scalp, eyebrows, eyelashes), tinea corporis (face, trunk, major limbs), tinea cruris (groin, perineal and perianal areas), tinea pedis (soles and between toes), and tinea unguium (nails).

> Fungal infections of the living layers of skin (the dermis), hair shafts, and nails are commonly called tinea or ringworm infections. They are caused by moulds collectively referred to as dermatophytes.

- **Subcutaneous mycoses.** These are fungal infections of the dermis and underlying tissues. They are more severe than superficial and cutaneous mycoses. Examples of subcutaneous mycoses are

> Subcutaneous mycoses, such as sporotrichosis, chromomycosis, and mycetomas, are fungal infections of the dermis and underlying tissues.

FIGURE 20-3. Mycetoma of the foot. (From Binford CH, Connor DH. Pathology of Tropical and Extraordinary Diseases, vol. 2. Washington, DC: Armed Forces Institute of Pathology, 1976.)

sporotrichosis, chromomycosis (chromoblastomycosis), and mycetomas (Fig. 20-2). Sporotrichosis is caused by *Sporothrix schenckii*, a dimorphic fungus, and typically affects the skin of an extremity. Chromomycosis, caused by various species of moulds, is a chronic, spreading infection of the skin and subcutaneous tissues, usually affecting a lower extremity. Mycetomas, caused by various moulds, are chronic granulomatous infections that involve the feet (usually), hands, or other areas of the body. Some of these subcutaneous mycoses can be quite grotesque in appearance (Fig. 20-3).

- **Systemic mycoses** (also known as generalized or deep-seated mycoses). These are the most serious types of fungal infections. They are fungal infections of internal organs of the body, sometimes affecting two or more organ systems

> Systemic mycoses—also known as generalized or deep-seated mycoses—are the most serious types of fungal infections.

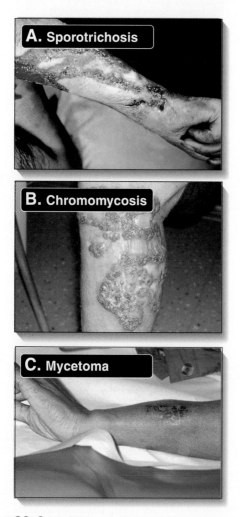

FIGURE 20-2. Subcutaneous mycoses. (A) The cutaneous–lymphatic form of sporotrichosis on a patient's arm, **(B)** chromomycosis on a patient's leg, **(C)** mycetoma on a patient's arm. (From Harvey RA, et al. Lippincott's Illustrated Reviews: Microbiology, 2nd ed. Philadelphia: Lippincott Williams & Wilkins, 2007.)

STUDY AID

Ringworm

The term *ringworm* is used in reference to some of the superficial and cutaneous mycoses, which more correctly are known as tinea infections. Be aware that diseases referred to as ringworm have absolutely *nothing* to do with worms. The term most likely arose long before fungi were known to be the cause of these lesions. Some of the lesions are circular and raised, prompting speculation that a worm lay coiled beneath the skin surface.

simultaneously—for example, simultaneous infection of the respiratory system and the bloodstream, or simultaneous infection of the respiratory tract and the central nervous system.

FUNGAL INFECTIONS OF THE SKIN

Dermatophytoses

Dermatophytoses are also known as *tinea* (ringworm) infections and *dermatomycoses.*

> Ringworm infections are fungal infections and have nothing to do with worms.

Diseases. (See preceding sections on superficial and cutaneous mycoses.) Some of the dermatomycoses cause only limited irritation, scaling, and redness. Others cause itching, swelling, blisters, and severe scaling.

Patient Care. Use Standard Precautions.

Pathogens. Dermatomycoses are caused by various filamentous fungi (moulds), collectively referred to as dermatophytes. Examples include species of *Microsporum, Epidermophyton,* and *Trichophyton.*

Reservoirs and Mode of Transmission. Infected humans and animals and soil serve as reservoirs. Transmission is by direct or indirect contact with lesions of humans or animals; or contact with contaminated floors, shower stalls, or locker room benches; barbers' clippers, combs, and hairbrushes; or clothing.

Laboratory Diagnosis. Microscopic examination of potassium hydroxide (KOH) preparations of skin scrapings or hair or nail clippings can reveal the presence of fungal hyphae (refer back to Fig. 13-14 [Chapter 13]). (The KOH preparation is described in CD-ROM Appendix 5.) Dermatophytes can be cultured on various media, including Sabouraud dextrose agar. Moulds are identified using a combination of macroscopic and microscopic observations (refer back to Chapter 13).

FUNGAL INFECTIONS OF THE RESPIRATORY SYSTEM

Infections of the Lower Respiratory Tract Having Multiple Causes

Information pertaining to infections of the lower respiratory tract having multiple causes is contained in Chapter 19.

Fungal Infections of the Lower Respiratory Tract

Table 20-1 contains information pertaining to fungal infections of the lower respiratory tract. Although they are not included in Table 20-1, moulds in the genera

FIGURE 20-4. *Aspergillus fumigatus* **hyphae in lung tissue from a patient with aspergillosis.** (From Schaechter M, et al. Mechanisms of Microbial Disease, 3rd ed. Philadelphia: Lippincott Williams & Wilkins, 1999.)

Aspergillus (Fig. 20-4) and *Penicillium* are also common causes of lower respiratory infections, especially in immunosuppressed patients. Infection is usually the result of inhalation of spores. In addition to the lungs, invasive aspergillosis can affect the sinuses, eyes, heart, kidneys, skin, and other organs. Infection with *Penicillium* spp.—penicilliosis—is usually a disseminated disease, involving lungs, liver, and skin.

FUNGAL INFECTIONS OF THE ORAL REGION

Thrush

Disease. Thrush is a yeast infection of the oral cavity. It is common in infants, elderly patients, and

TABLE 20-1 Fungal Infections of the Lower Respiratory Tract

DISEASE	ADDITIONAL INFORMATION
Coccidioidomycosis (Valley Fever). Coccidioidomycosis starts as a respiratory infection, with fever, chills, cough, and, rarely, pain. The primary infection may heal completely or may progress to the disseminated form of the disease, which is often fatal. Disseminated coccidioidomycosis may include lung lesions and abscesses throughout the body, especially in subcutaneous tissues, skin, bone, and the central nervous system. Other tissues and organs, such as inguinal lymph nodes, kidneys, thyroid gland, heart, pituitary gland, esophagus, and pancreas, may also be involved. **Patient Care.** Use Standard Precautions for hospitalized patients with draining lesions or pneumonia.	**Pathogen.** Coccidioidomycosis is caused by *Coccidioides immitis*, a dimorphic fungus. It exists as a mould in soil and on culture media (25°C), where it produces arthrospores (arthroconidia). In tissues, it appears as spherical yeast cells called spherules that reproduce by endospore formation. *C. immitis* arthrospores have potential use as a bioterrorist agent. **Reservoirs and Mode of Transmission.** Arthrospores are present in soil in arid and semiarid areas of the Western Hemisphere; in United States, from California to southern Texas; and in Mexico, Central America, and South America. Transmission occurs by inhalation of arthrospores, especially during wind and dust storms. It is not directly transmissible person to person or animal to person. **Laboratory Diagnosis.** Coccidioidomycosis is diagnosed by direct examination and culturing of sputum, pus, urine, cerebrospinal fluid, or biopsy materials. The mould form is highly infectious. All work must be performed in a biosafety level (BSL)-2 or BSL-3 facility (refer to CD-ROM Appendix 4). Skin tests, molecular diagnostic procedures, and immunodiagnostic procedures are also available.
Cryptococcosis. Cryptococcosis starts as a lung infection, but usually spreads via the bloodstream to the brain. The disease is described later in the chapter, in the section entitled "Fungal Infections of the Central Nervous System."	
Histoplasmosis. Histoplasmosis is a systemic mycosis of varying severity, ranging from asymptomatic to acute to chronic. The primary lesion is usually in the lungs. The acute disease involves malaise, fever, chills, headache, myalgia, chest pains, and a nonproductive cough (i.e., sputum is not produced). Histoplasmosis is the most common systemic fungal infection in AIDS patients. **Patient Care.** Use Standard Precautions for hospitalized patients.	**Pathogen.** Histoplasmosis is caused by *Histoplasma capsulatum* var. *capsulatum*, a dimorphic fungus that grows as a mould in soil and as a yeast in animal and human hosts (refer back to Fig. 5-13 in Chapter 5). **Reservoirs and Mode of Transmission.** Reservoirs include warm, moist soil containing a high organic content and bird droppings, especially chicken droppings, but also bat droppings in caves and around starling, blackbird, and pigeon roosts. Transmission occurs via inhalation of conidia (asexual spores) from soil. Bulldozing and excavation may produce aerosols of spores. Histoplasmosis is the most common systemic fungal disease in the United States, occurring primarily in the Ohio, Mississippi, and Missouri River valleys. Histoplasmosis is not transmitted from person to person. **Laboratory Diagnosis.** *H. capsulatum* yeasts may be observed in Giemsa- or Wright-stained smears of ulcer exudates, bone marrow, sputum, and blood. *H. capsulatum* produces mould colonies when incubated at room temperature and yeast colonies when incubated at body temperature. Conversion from the mould form to the yeast form can sometimes be accomplished in the laboratory. Skin tests and immunodiagnostic procedures are available.

TABLE 20-1	Fungal Infections of the Lower Respiratory Tract (continued)

DISEASE	ADDITIONAL INFORMATION
Pneumocystis Carinii Pneumonia (PCP, Interstitial Plasma-Cell Pneumonia). PCP is an acute-to-subacute pulmonary disease found in malnourished, chronically ill children; premature infants; and immunosuppressed patients, such as those with AIDS. Patients have fever, difficulty in breathing, rapid breathing, dry cough, cyanosis, and pulmonary infiltration of alveoli with frothy exudate. PCP is usually fatal in untreated immunosuppressed patients. It is a common contributory cause of death in AIDS patients. *Pneumocystis* causes an asymptomatic infection in immunocompetent people. **Patient Care.** Use Standard Precautions for hospitalized patients. Do not place PCP patients in the same room with an immunocompromised patient.	**Pathogen.** The etiologic agent of PCP is *Pneumocystis jiroveci* (formerly *P. carinii*). This organism has both protozoal and fungal properties. It was classified as a protozoan for many years, but is currently classified as a nonfilamentous fungus. **Reservoirs and Mode of Transmission.** Infected humans serve as reservoirs. The mode of transmission is unknown—perhaps direct contact, perhaps transfer of pulmonary secretions from infected to susceptible persons, perhaps airborne. **Laboratory Diagnosis.** Diagnosis of PCP is made by demonstration of *Pneumocystis* in material from bronchial brushings, open lung biopsy, lung aspirates, or smears of tracheobronchial mucus by various staining methods. *P. jiroveci* cannot be cultured.
Pulmonary Zygomycosis. The term *zygomycosis* (formerly mucormycosis or phycomycosis) refers to a disease caused by one of the many fungi in the class Zygomycetes. These fungi are widely distributed in soil and vegetative matter. Although being discussed in the section on lower respiratory diseases, these fungi cause diseases with a wide range of clinical manifestations. Other clinical syndromes caused by members of the Zygomycetes class include sinusitis, cerebral infection, cutaneous disease, gastrointestinal disease, and disseminated disease, which involve virtually every organ. **Patient Care.** Use Standard Precautions.	**Pathogens.** Many different fungi can cause zygomycosis, including some that are often referred to as bread moulds. These fungi, which include species of *Mucor*, *Rhizopus*, and *Absidia*, are responsible for the white or gray fuzzy growth seen on foods such as bread and cheese. The fuzziness is the result of aerial hyphae. **Reservoirs and Modes of Transmission.** Most commonly, humans become infected with zygomycetes by inhaling airborne spores, although ingestion and direct inoculation through traumatic breaks in the skin and mucous membranes can also lead to infection. Zygomycosis is not transmitted from person to person. **Laboratory Diagnosis.** Diagnosis of zygomycosis can be made by microscopic observation of distinctive, ribbon-like, broad, aseptate hyphae in tissue sections and by culture of biopsy tissue.

immunosuppressed individuals. White, creamy patches occur on the tongue, mucous membranes, and the corners of the mouth (Fig. 20-5). Thrush can be a manifestation of disseminated *Candida* infection (candidiasis). *Candida albicans* is the yeast and the fungus most commonly isolated from clinical specimens—sometimes isolated as a pathogen and sometimes isolated as a contaminant.

> *C. albicans* is the yeast and the fungus most commonly isolated from clinical specimens.

Pathogens. The yeast, *C. albicans* and related species.

Reservoir and Mode of Transmission. Infected humans serve as reservoirs. Transmission occurs by contact with secretions or excretions of mouth, skin, vagina, or feces of patients or carriers; also by passage from mother to neonate during childbirth and by endogenous spread (i.e., from one area of the body to another).

Laboratory Diagnosis. Thrush can be diagnosed by observation of yeast cells and pseudohyphae (strings of elongated buds) in microscopic examination of wet mounts, and by culture confirmation.

> Thrush is a yeast infection (most often a *Candida* infection) of the oral cavity.

FUNGAL INFECTIONS OF THE GENITOURINARY SYSTEM

Yeast Vaginitis

Disease. The three most common causes of vaginitis in the United States, each causing about one third of the cases, are *C. albicans* (a yeast), *Trichomonas vaginalis*

FIGURE 20-5. Oral candidiasis (thrush). (From Harvey RA, et al. Lippincott's Illustrated Reviews: Microbiology, 2nd ed. Philadelphia: Lippincott Williams & Wilkins, 2007.)

(a protozoan), and a mixture of bacteria (including bacteria in the genera *Mobiluncus* and *Gardnerella*). A saline wet mount preparation is usually used to diagnose vaginitis; this test procedure is described in CD-ROM Appendix 5. Typical symptoms of yeast vaginitis are vulvar pruritis (itching), a burning sensation, dysuria, and a white discharge. Vulvar erythema (redness) and rash sometimes occur. *C. albicans* causes approximately one third of the cases of vaginitis in the United States.

Pathogens. The yeast, *C. albicans*, causes about 85% to 90% of yeast vaginitis; other *Candida* spp. can also cause this disease.

Reservoir and Mode of Transmission. (See previous section on "Thrush.")

Laboratory Diagnosis. Yeast vaginitis can be diagnosed by microscopic examination of a saline wet mount of vaginal discharge material, in which yeasts and hyphae may be observed. The vaginal discharge material should also be cultured. *Candida* spp. grow well on blood agar and Sabouraud dextrose agar. *Candida* spp. can usually be identified using a commercial yeast identification minisystem. It is important to keep in mind that the vaginal microflora of up to 25% of healthy women can contain *Candida* spp.

FUNGAL INFECTIONS OF THE CIRCULATORY SYSTEM

Fungal endocarditis is rare, but cases of *Candida* and *Aspergillus* endocarditis do occur.

FUNGAL INFECTIONS OF THE CENTRAL NERVOUS SYSTEM

Cryptococcosis (Cryptococcal Meningitis)

Disease. Cryptococcosis starts as a lung infection, but spreads via the bloodstream to the brain. It usually presents as a subacute or chronic meningitis. Infection of the lungs, kidneys, prostate, skin, and bone may also occur. Cryptococcosis is a common infection in acquired immunodeficiency syndrome (AIDS) patients.

Patient Care. Use Standard Precautions for hospitalized patients.

Pathogens. Cryptococcosis can be caused by three subspecies of *C. neoformans*, an encapsulated yeast (refer back to Fig. 5-8 in Chapter 5). The capsule enables *C. neoformans* to adhere to mucosal surfaces and avoid phagocytosis by white blood cells.

Reservoirs and Modes of Transmission. Reservoirs include pigeon nests; pigeon, chicken, turkey, and bat droppings; and soil contaminated with bird droppings. Growth of *C. neoformans* is stimulated by the alkaline pH and high nitrogen content of bird droppings. Transmission occurs by inhalation of yeasts, often projected into the air by sweeping or excavation. Cryptococcus is not transmitted from person to person or animal to person.

Laboratory Diagnosis. Cryptococcal meningitis is often diagnosed by observing encapsulated, budding yeasts in cerebrospinal fluid specimens examined by an India ink preparation. (Details of the India ink preparation can be found in CD-ROM Appendix 5, Clinical Microbiology Laboratory Procedures.) Yeasts may also be observed in sputum, urine, and pus examined by an India ink preparation or Gram stain (refer back to Fig. 5-8 [Chapter 5]). *C. neoformans* can be cultured on routine media used in the Mycology Section. A sensitive cryptococcal antigen detection test is available.

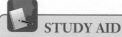
STUDY AID
Beware of Similar Sounding Names
Do not confuse *Cryptococcus neoformans* (a yeast) with *Cryptosporidium parvum* (a protozoan). Likewise, do not confuse **cryptococcosis** (a yeast infection) with **cryptosporidiosis** (a protozoan infection). *C. parvum* and cryptosporidiosis are described in Chapter 21.

TABLE 20-2	Recap of Some Major Fungal Infections of Humans
DISEASE	**FUNGAL PATHOGEN**
Aspergillosis	Various species of *Aspergillus* (moulds)
Black piedra	*Piedraia hortae* (a mould)
Coccidioidomycosis	*Coccidioides immitis* (a dimorphic fungus)
Cryptococcosis	*Cryptococcus neoformans* (an encapsulated yeast)
Dermatomycoses	Various filamentous fungi (moulds), collectively referred to as dermatophytes
Histoplasmosis	*Histoplasma capsulatum* (a dimorphic fungus)
Penicilliosis	Various species of *Penicillium* (moulds)
Pneumocystis pneumonia	*Pneumocystis jiroveci* (formerly *Pneumocystis carinii*) (a nonfilamentous fungus having both protozoal and fungal properties)
Sporotrichosis	*Sporothrix schenckii* (a dimorphic fungus)
Tinea nigra	*Hortaea werneckii* (a mould)
Tinea versicolor (pityriasis versicolor)	*Malassezia furfur* (a mould)
Thrush	*Candida albicans* (a yeast)
White piedra	Usually caused by *Trichosporon beigelii* (a mould)
Yeast vaginitis	*C. albicans* (a yeast)
Zygomycosis (mucormycosis, phycomycosis)	Various zygomycetes, including bread moulds

RECAP OF MAJOR FUNGAL INFECTIONS OF HUMANS

Table 20-2 provides a recap of some major fungal infections of humans.

APPROPRIATE THERAPY FOR FUNGAL INFECTIONS

Recommendations for the treatment of infectious diseases change frequently. The fungal diseases described in this chapter must be treated using appropriate antifungal drugs. Sources of updated information include *The Merck Manual* (http://www.merck.com/pubs) and WebMD (http://www.webmd.com). Additional information about antifungal agents can be found in Chapter 9.

ON THE CD-ROM
- Terms Introduced in This Chapter
- Review of Key Points
- Increase Your Knowledge
- Case Studies
- Additional Self-Assessment Exercises

SELF-ASSESSMENT EXERCISES

After you have read this chapter, answer the following multiple-choice questions.

1. Which of the following diseases is caused by an encapsulated yeast?
   a. Coccidioidomycosis
   b. Cryptococcosis
   c. Histoplasmosis
   d. Pneumocystis pneumonia
2. Which of the following diseases is *not* caused by a dimorphic fungus?
   a. Coccidioidomycosis
   b. Cryptococcosis
   c. Histoplasmosis
   d. Sporotrichosis
3. Which of the following diseases is a synonym for ringworm infection of the nails?
   a. tinea barbae
   b. tinea cruris
   c. tinea nigra
   d. tinea unguium
4. Which of the following is the most common systemic fungal disease in the United States?
   a. Cryptococcosis
   b. Coccidioidomycosis
   c. Histoplasmosis
   d. Pneumocystis pneumonia

5. One should associate the India ink preparation with diagnosis of which of the following?
   a. Cryptococcal meningitis
   b. thrush
   c. tinea pedis
   d. yeast vaginitis

6. Bread moulds are most commonly associated with which of the following diseases?
   a. thrush
   b. tinea versicolor
   c. vaginitis
   d. zygomycosis

7. Which of the following is the fungus most often isolated from human clinical specimens?
   a. *Candida albicans*
   b. *C. neoformans*
   c. *Histoplasma capsulatum*
   d. *Pneumocystis jiroveci*

8. Which of the following methods is the quickest and most common way to diagnose yeast vaginitis?
   a. culture
   b. India ink preparation
   c. KOH preparation
   d. saline wet mount

9. In the United States, *C. albicans* causes approximately _____ of the cases of vaginitis.
   a. 10%
   b. 25%
   c. 33%
   d. 50%

10. Tinea cruris is a ringworm infection of which of these body sites?
    a. feet
    b. groin area
    c. nails
    d. palms of the hands

PARASITIC INFECTIONS 21

LEARNING OBJECTIVES

AFTER STUDYING THIS CHAPTER, YOU SHOULD BE ABLE TO:

- Differentiate between the following: ectoparasites versus endoparasites; definitive hosts versus intermediate hosts; facultative parasites versus obligate parasites; and mechanical vectors versus biologic vectors
- Classify a particular parasitic infection as a protozoal or helminth disease
- Categorize various parasitic infections by body system (e.g., respiratory system, gastrointestinal tract, circulatory system)
- Correlate a particular parasitic infection (e.g., giardiasis) with its major characteristics, causative agent, reservoir(s), mode(s) of transmission, and diagnostic laboratory procedures

So, naturalists observe, a flea
Hath smaller fleas that on him prey
And these have smaller still to bite 'em;
And so proceed ad infinitum.

from Poetry, a Rhapsody, 1733
by Jonathan Swift (1667–1745)

INTRODUCTION

Although parasitology (the study of parasites) is considered a branch of microbiology, not all organisms studied in a parasitology course are microbes. In fact, of the three categories of organisms (parasitic protozoa, helminths, and arthropods) that are studied in a parasitology course, only one category—parasitic protozoa—contains microbes. Therefore, in this chapter, parasitic protozoa are discussed in greater detail than are helminths and arthropods.

It would be impossible in a book this size to describe *all* of the human infectious diseases caused by parasites. Thus, only selected parasitic diseases are described in this chapter. Although these diseases are described in one particular section of the chapter (e.g., under gastrointestinal infections), readers should keep in mind that some parasitic diseases have various clinical manifestations, affecting several body systems simultaneously, and that the pathogens may move from one body site to another.

Certain of the parasitic diseases described in this chapter are nationally notifiable infectious diseases, meaning that when a patient is diagnosed with one of these diseases in the United States, the information must be reported to the Centers for Disease Control and Prevention (CDC). As of 2007, there were four

TABLE 21-1	Nationally Notifiable Parasitic Diseases	
PARASITIC DISEASE	NO. OF NEW U.S. CASES REPORTED TO THE CDC IN 2007*
Cryptosporidiosis	11,170
Cyclosporiasis	93
Giardiasis	19,417
Malaria	1,408

Source: http://www.cdc.gov.
*These figures provide insight regarding how common or rare these diseases are in the United States. For updated information, go to the CDC web site; click on "Morbidity & Mortality Weekly Report"; then click on "Notifiable Diseases"; then click on the most recent year that is listed.

nationally notifiable parasitic diseases (see Table 21-1). These diseases are described in this chapter, as are some parasitic diseases that are not nationally notifiable.

DEFINITIONS

Parasitism is a symbiotic relationship that is of benefit to one party or symbiont (the parasite) at the expense of the other party (the **host**). Although many parasites cause disease, some do not. Even if a parasite is not causing disease, it is depriving the host of nutrients; therefore, parasitic relationships are always considered detrimental to the host.

Parasites are defined as organisms that live *on* or *in* other living organisms (hosts), at whose expense they gain some advantage. In addition to parasites of humans, there are

> Parasites are organisms that live on or in other living organisms, at whose expense they gain some advantage.

STUDY AID

What to Learn?

This chapter contains a large amount of information. Of primary importance will be your ability to later recall the name of the parasite that causes a particular parasitic disease and the manner in which the disease is transmitted. If applicable, you should be able to state the vector that is involved in the transmission of the disease. For example, if your teacher says "Chagas' disease," you should be able to state the name of the parasite that causes the disease (a flagellated protozoan named *Trypanosoma cruzi*), the manner in which Chagas' disease is transmitted (via the feces of infected reduviid bugs), and the vector involved in the transmission of Chagas' disease (reduviid bugs).

many types of plant parasites (i.e., parasites of plants) and many types of animal parasites (i.e., parasites of animals).

Parasites that live outside the host's body are referred to as **ectoparasites**, whereas those living inside the host are called **endoparasites**. Arthropods such as mites, ticks, and lice are examples of ectoparasites. Parasitic protozoa and helminths are examples of endoparasites.

> Parasites that live outside the host's body are ectoparasites; those that live inside the host are endoparasites.

The life cycle of a particular parasite may involve one or more hosts. If more than one host is involved, the **definitive host** is the one that harbors the adult or sexual stage of the parasite or the sexual phase of the life cycle. The **intermediate host** harbors the larval or asexual stage of the parasite or the asexual phase of the life cycle. Parasite life cycles range from simple to complex.

> The definitive host harbors the adult or sexual stage of the parasite or the sexual phase of the parasite's life cycle. The intermediate host harbors the larval or asexual stage of the parasite or the asexual phase of its life cycle.

There are one-, two-, and three-host parasites. Knowing the life cycle of a particular parasite enables epidemiologists and other healthcare professionals to control the parasitic infection through intervention at some point in the life cycle. In addition, parasitic infections are most often diagnosed by observing and recognizing a particular life cycle stage in a clinical specimen.

An **accidental host** is a living organism that can serve as a host in a particular parasite's life cycle, but is not a *usual* host in that life cycle. Some accidental hosts are **dead-end hosts**, from which the parasite cannot continue its life cycle.

A **facultative parasite** is an organism that can be parasitic but does not have to live as a parasite. It is capable of living an independent life, apart from a host. The free-living amebae that can cause keratoconjunctivitis and primary amebic meningoencephalitis (PAM) are examples of facultative parasites. An **obligate parasite**, on the other hand, has no choice; to survive, it must be a parasite. Most parasites that infect humans are obligate parasites.

> Facultative parasites are organisms that can be parasitic but are also capable of a free-living existence. Obligate parasites have no choice; to survive, they must be parasitic.

Parasitology is the study of parasites, and a **parasitologist** is someone who studies parasites. As previously stated, any upper-division or graduate-level parasitology course would be divided into three areas of study: the study of parasitic protozoa, of helminths, and of arthropods.

Medical parasitology is the study of parasites that cause human disease. The overall responsibility of the Parasitology Section of the Clinical Microbiology Laboratory is to assist clinicians in the diagnosis of parasitic diseases—primarily, parasitic diseases caused by endoparasites such as parasitic protozoa and helminths.

In general, parasitic infections are diagnosed by observing and recognizing various parasite life cycle stages in clinical specimens. Some life cycle stages (e.g., amebic cysts and *Cryptosporidium* oocysts) are extremely small. Finding them in specimens represents one of the greatest challenges faced by clinical microbiologists.

> In general, parasitic infections are diagnosed by observing and recognizing various parasite life cycle stages in clinical specimens.

HOW PARASITES CAUSE DISEASE

The manner in which parasites cause damage to their host varies from one species of parasite to another, and often depends on the number of parasites that are present. For helminths, the number that are present is often referred to as the "worm burden." Some parasites produce toxins, some produce harmful enzymes, some invasive and migratory parasites cause physical damage to tissues and organs, some cause the destruction of individual cells, and some cause occlusion of blood vessels and other tubular structures. Some parasites interfere with vital processes of the host, whereas others deprive their host of essential nutrients. In some cases, the host immune response to the presence of parasites or their products causes more injury than do the parasites themselves.

PARASITIC PROTOZOA

In the five-kingdom system of classification of living organisms, protozoa are in the kingdom Protista, together with algae. Some taxonomists prefer to place them in a kingdom by themselves—the kingdom Protozoa. Most protozoa are unicellular, but some are multicellular (colonial). Protozoa are classified taxonomically by their mode of locomotion. **Amebas** (amebae) move by means of pseudopodia (literally, "false feet"). **Flagellates** move by means of whiplike flagella. **Ciliates** move by means of hairlike cilia. Protozoa classified as *Sporozoa* (sporozoans) have no pseudopodia, flagella, or cilia, and therefore exhibit no motility.

> Protozoa are classified taxonomically by their mode of locomotion. Some move by pseudopodia, others by flagella, others by cilia, and some are nonmotile.

Not all protozoa are parasitic. For example, many of the pond water protozoa (e.g., *Paramecium* and *Stentor* spp.) studied in introductory biology and microbiology courses are not parasites. Although most protozoal parasites of humans are obligate parasites, some are facul-

tative parasites—capable of a free-living, nonparasitic existence, but also able to become parasites when they accidentally gain entrance to the body. *Acanthamoeba* spp. and *Naegleria fowleri* are examples of facultative parasites. These free-living amebas normally reside in soil or water, but can cause serious diseases when they gain entrance to the eyes or the nasal mucosa. From the nasal mucosa, they travel via the olfactory nerve into the brain and cause diseases affecting the central nervous system (CNS).

Because protozoa are tiny, protozoal infections are most often diagnosed by microscopic examination of body fluids, tissue specimens, or feces. Peripheral blood smears are usually stained with Giemsa stain, whereas fecal specimens are stained with trichrome, iron hematoxylin, or acid-fast stains. Most parasitic protozoal infections are diagnosed by observing trophozoites, cysts, oocysts, or spores in the specimen.

The *trophozoite* is the motile, feeding, dividing stage in a protozoan's life cycle, whereas cysts, oocysts, and spores are dormant stages (much like bacterial spores). Protozoal infections are primarily acquired by ingestion or inhalation of cysts, oocysts, or spores. Because of their fragile nature, only rarely do trophozoites serve as the infective stages.

> The trophozoite is the motile, feeding, dividing stage in the protozoal life cycle, and the cyst, oocyst, and spore are dormant stages. Protozoal infections are most often acquired by ingestion or inhalation of dormant stages.

PROTOZOAL INFECTIONS OF HUMANS

Protozoal Infections of the Skin

Leishmaniasis

Disease. There are three forms of leishmaniasis: cutaneous, mucocutaneous (or mucosal), and visceral. The cutaneous form starts with a papule that enlarges into a craterlike ulcer (Fig. 21-1). Individual ulcers may coalesce, causing severe tissue destruction and disfigurement. Visceral leishmaniasis, also known as kala-azar, is characterized by fever, enlarged liver and spleen, lymphadenopathy, anemia, leukopenia, and progressive emaciation and weakness. Death may result in untreated cases.

Patient Care. Use Standard Precautions for hospitalized patients.

Geographic Occurrence. Leishmaniasis occurs in many regions of the world, including Pakistan, India, China, the Middle East, Africa, South and Central America, and Mexico. Cases have also occurred in south central Texas. It is estimated that between 1.5 and 2 million people have leishmaniasis and that about 57,000 people die each year of the disease.

FIGURE 21-1. Patients with cutaneous leishmaniasis. ([A] From Binford CH, Connor DH. Pathology of Tropical and Extraordinary Diseases, vol. 1. Washington, DC: Armed Forces Institute of Pathology, 1976. [B] Courtesy of Dr. DS Martin and the CDC.)

Parasites. Leishmaniasis is caused by various species of flagellated protozoa in the genus *Leishmania*. The non-motile, intracellular form of the parasite is called an *amastigote*. The motile, extracellular form of the parasite is called a *promastigote*.

> Leishmaniasis is caused by various species of flagellated protozoa and is usually transmitted via the bite of an infected sand fly.

Reservoirs and Mode of Transmission. Reservoirs include infected humans, domestic dogs, and various wild animals. Leishmaniasis is principally a zoonosis and is usually transmitted via the bite of an infected sand fly. Transmission by blood transfusion and person-to-person contact have been reported.

Laboratory Diagnosis. Diagnosis of cutaneous and mucocutaneous leishmaniasis is made by microscopic identification of the amastigote form in stained preparations from lesions or by culture of the extracellular promastigote form on suitable media. Culture is rarely performed in clinical microbiology laboratories. In stained preparations, amastigotes are seen within macrophages and close to disrupted cells. An intradermal test, called the Montenegro test, and immunodiagnostic and molecular diagnostic procedures are also available. In the Montenegro test, an antigen derived from promastigotes is injected into the skin.

Protozoal Infections of the Eyes

Protozoal infections of the eyes include conjunctivitis and keratoconjunctivitis (inflammation of the cornea and conjunctiva), caused by amebas in the genus *Acanthamoeba*, and toxoplasmosis, caused by the sporozoan, *Toxoplasma gondii*. Although toxoplasmosis is described in this section of the chapter, there are many manifestations of toxoplasmosis in addition to ocular disease. Ocular manifestations of toxoplasmosis occur primarily in immunosuppressed patients, in whom the infection can lead to removal of the infected eyeball (enucleation). Amebic conjunctivitis and keratoconjunctivitis can also result in enucleation. Table 21-2 contains information about these diseases.

Protozoal Infections of the Gastrointestinal Tract

Of the many protozoal infections of the gastrointestinal tract, only amebiasis, balantidiasis, cryptosporidiosis, cyclosporiasis, and giardiasis are discussed here. As previously mentioned, the latter three diseases are nationally notifiable infectious diseases in the United States. Figure 21-2 and Table 21-3 contain information about protozoal infections of the gastrointestinal tract.

Protozoal Infections of the Genitourinary Tract

Trichomoniasis

Disease. Trichomoniasis is a sexually transmitted protozoal disease affecting both men and women. The disease is usually symptomatic in women, causing vaginitis with a profuse, thin, foamy, malodorous, greenish-yellowish discharge. It has been estimated that trichomoniasis accounts for approximately one third of the cases of vaginitis in the United States (another third is caused by *Candida albicans*, and another third by bacteria). In women, trichomoniasis may also present as urethritis

TABLE 21-2   Protozoal Infections of the Eyes

DISEASE	ADDITIONAL INFORMATION
Amebic Eye Infections. Amebic conjunctivitis and keratoconjunctivitis are amebic infections causing inflammation of the conjunctiva, corneal ulcers, pus formation, and severe pain. These infections can lead to loss of vision. The disease process is more rapid if corneal abrasions are present. **Patient Care.** Use Standard Precautions for hospitalized patients. **Geographic Occurrence.** Amebic eye infections occur in many countries on all continents.	**Parasites.** Amebic eye infections are caused by several species of amebas in the genus *Acanthamoeba*. Because these amebas are capable of either a free-living or a parasitic existence, they are referred to as facultative parasites. **Reservoirs and Mode of Transmission.** The amebas enter the eye from ameba-contaminated waters. Infections have occurred primarily in people who wear soft contact lenses and have used nonsterile, homemade cleaning or wetting solutions, or have become infected in ameba-contaminated spas or hot tubs. **Laboratory Diagnosis.** Amebic eye infections are diagnosed by microscopic examination of scrapings, swabs, or aspirates of the eye, or by culture on media seeded with *Escherichia coli* or another member of the family *Enterobacteriaceae*. The bacteria on the media serve as food for the amebas.
Toxoplasmosis. Toxoplasmosis is a systemic sporozoan infection that, in immunocompetent persons, may be asymptomatic or resemble infectious mononucleosis. However, serious disease, even death, may occur in immunodeficient persons. Disease typically involves the central nervous system, eyes (chorioretinitis), lungs, muscles, or heart. Cerebral toxoplasmosis is common in AIDS patients. Infection during early pregnancy may lead to fetal infection, causing death of the fetus or serious birth defects (e.g., brain damage). **Patient Care.** Use Standard Precautions for hospitalized patients. **Geographic Occurrence.** Toxoplasmosis occurs worldwide.	**Parasite.** Toxoplasmosis is caused by *Toxoplasma gondii*, an intracellular sporozoan. **Reservoirs and Mode of Transmission.** Definitive hosts include cats and other felines that usually acquire infection by eating infected rodents or birds. Intermediate hosts include rodents, birds, sheep, goats, swine, and cattle. Humans usually become infected by eating infected raw or undercooked meat (usually pork or mutton) containing the cyst form of the parasite or by ingesting oocysts that have been shed in the feces of infected cats. Oocysts may be present in food or water contaminated by feline feces. Children may ingest oocysts from sand boxes containing cat feces. Infection can also be acquired transplacentally, by blood transfusion, or by organ transplantation. **Laboratory Diagnosis.** Toxoplasmosis is typically diagnosed using immunodiagnostic procedures. Other diagnostic methods include demonstration of the parasite in stained body tissues or fluids obtained by biopsy or necropsy; and isolation of *T. gondii* using laboratory animals or cell culture.

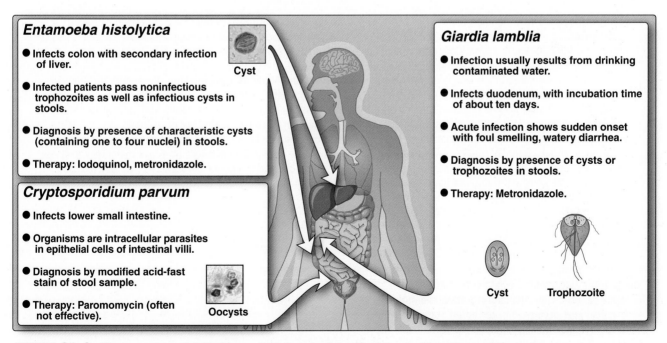

FIGURE 21-2. Three protozoal infections of the gastrointestinal tract. (From Harvey RA, et al. Lippincott's Illustrated Reviews: Microbiology, 2nd ed. Philadelphia: Lippincott Williams & Wilkins, 2007.)

TABLE 21-3   Protozoal Infections of the Gastrointestinal Tract

DISEASE	ADDITIONAL INFORMATION
Amebiasis. Amebiasis or amebic dysentery is a protozoal gastrointestinal infection that may be asymptomatic, mild, or severe and is often accompanied by dysentery, fever, chills, bloody or mucoid diarrhea or constipation, and colitis. The amebas may invade mucous membranes of the colon, forming abscesses and amebomas, which are granulomas that are sometimes mistaken for carcinoma. Amebas also may be disseminated via the bloodstream to extraintestinal sites, leading to abscesses of the liver, lung, brain, and other organs. Depending on their location, untreated extraintestinal amebic abscesses can be fatal. **Patient Care.** Use Standard Precautions for hospitalized patients. **Geographic Occurrence.** Amebiasis occurs worldwide.	**Parasite.** Amebiasis is caused by *Entamoeba histolytica*. Like all amebas, *E. histolytica* has two stages: the cyst stage, which is the dormant, infective stage, and the motile, metabolically active, reproducing trophozoite stage. **Reservoirs and Mode of Transmission.** Reservoirs include symptomatic and asymptomatic humans and fecally contaminated food or water. Transmission occurs in one of several ways: (a) via ingestion of fecally contaminated food or water containing cysts, (b) by flies transporting cysts from feces to food, (c) via the fecally soiled hands of infected food handlers, (d) by oral–anal sexual contact, or (e) by anal intercourse involving multiple sex partners. **Laboratory Diagnosis.** Amebic dysentery is diagnosed by microscopic observation of *E. histolytica* trophozoites and/or cysts in stained smears of fecal specimens. Amebic trophozoites and cysts are only 1 or 2 μm in diameter and thus are difficult to find in permanent stained smears of fecal material. It is also necessary for microbiology professionals to be able to differentiate *E. histolytica* from other pathogenic and nonpathogenic intestinal amebas. The presence of red blood cells within trophozoites indicates invasive amebiasis.
Balantidiasis. Balantidiasis is a protozoal gastrointestinal infection of the colon causing diarrhea or dysentery, colic, nausea, and vomiting. **Patient Care.** Use Standard Precautions for hospitalized patients. **Geographic Occurrence.** Although seen worldwide, balantidiasis is rare in the United States.	**Parasite.** Balantidiasis is caused by *Balantidium coli*, a ciliated protozoan (refer back to Fig. 5-3 in Chapter 5). *B. coli* is the only ciliate that causes disease in humans. Balantidiasis occurs more commonly in pigs than in humans. **Reservoirs and Mode of Transmission.** Reservoirs include pigs and anything that might be contaminated with pig feces (e.g., drinking water). Transmission most often occurs via ingestion of *B. coli* cysts in fecally contaminated food or water. **Laboratory Diagnosis.** Balantidiasis is diagnosed by observing and identifying *B. coli* trophozoites or cysts in fecal specimens, which may also contain blood and mucus. *B. coli* is the largest of the protozoa that infect humans.
Cryptosporidiosis. Cryptosporidiosis is a gastrointestinal infection caused by a coccidial protozoan. Coccidia are sporozoa. Cryptosporidiosis may be asymptomatic or may cause diarrhea, cramping, and abdominal pain. Less common symptoms include malaise, fever, anorexia, nausea, and vomiting. The disease may be prolonged, fulminant, and fatal in immunosuppressed patients. Children younger than 2 years of age, animal handlers, travelers, homosexuals, and day care center workers are particularly likely to be infected. Outbreaks in day care centers are common. Outbreaks have also been associated with drinking water, recreational use water, and drinking unpasteurized apple cider contaminated with cattle feces. **Patient Care.** Use Standard Precautions for hospitalized patients. Add Contact Precautions for diapered or incontinent patients. **Geographic Occurrence.** This disease has been reported worldwide. The largest waterborne outbreak that has ever occurred in the United States was the 1993 cryptosporidiosis outbreak in Milwaukee, WI, which affected more than 400,000 people.	**Parasite.** Cryptosporidiosis results from ingestion of oocysts of *Cryptosporidium parvum*, a coccidian (Other coccidial parasites of humans are in the genera *Cyclospora*, *Isospora*, and *Sarcocystis*.) **Reservoirs and Mode of Transmission.** Reservoirs include infected humans, cattle and other domestic animals. Fecal–oral transmission; from person to person, from animal to person, or via ingestion of contaminated water or food. **Laboratory Diagnosis.** Cryptosporidiosis can be diagnosed by microscopic observation of small (4–6 μm-diameter) acid-fast oocysts in stained smears of fecal specimens. Sensitive and specific immunodiagnostic procedures are also available.

TABLE 21-3   Protozoal Infections of the Gastrointestinal Tract (continued)

DISEASE	ADDITIONAL INFORMATION
Cyclosporiasis. Cyclosporiasis is a coccidial gastrointestinal infection, causing watery diarrhea (6 or more stools per day), nausea, anorexia, abdominal cramping, fatigue, and weight loss. The diarrhea lasts between 9 and 43 days in immunocompetent patients, and months in immunocompromised patients. **Patient Care.** Use Standard Precautions for hospitalized patients. **Geographic Occurrence.** Cyclosporiasis has been diagnosed in Asia, the Caribbean, Mexico, Peru, and the United States.	**Parasite.** Cyclosporiasis results from ingestion of oocysts of *Cyclospora cayetanensis*, a coccidian. **Reservoirs and Mode of Transmission.** Reservoirs include fecally contaminated water sources and produce that has been rinsed with fecally contaminated water. Transmission is primarily waterborne, but outbreaks have involved contaminated raspberries, basil, and lettuce. **Laboratory Diagnosis.** Diagnosis of cyclosporiasis is made by microscopic observation of the 8- to 9-μm-diameter acid-fast oocysts, which are about twice the size of *Cryptosporidium* oocysts. The oocysts autofluoresce a bright green to intense blue under ultraviolet fluorescence, when examined using appropriate filters.
Giardiasis. Giardiasis is a protozoal infection of the duodenum (the uppermost portion of the small intestine) and may be asymptomatic, mild, or severe. Patients experience diarrhea, steatorrhea (loose, pale, malodorous, fatty stools), abdominal cramps, bloating, abdominal gas, fatigue, and possibly weight loss. **Patient Care.** Use Standard Precautions for hospitalized patients. Add Contact Precautions for diapered or incontinent patients. **Geographic Occurrence.** This disease occurs worldwide.	**Pathogen.** Giardiasis is caused by *Giardia lamblia* (also called *Giardia intestinalis*), a flagellated protozoan (refer back to Fig. 5-4 in Chapter 5). Trophozoites attach by means of a ventral sucker to the mucosal lining of the duodenum. Trophozoites and/or cysts are expelled in feces. **Reservoirs and Mode of Transmission.** Reservoirs include infected humans, possibly beavers and other wild and domestic animals that have consumed water containing *Giardia* cysts; and fecally contaminated drinking water and recreational water. The disease commonly occurs in day care centers. Transmission occurs via the fecal–oral route, usually by ingestion of cysts in fecally contaminated water or foods, or from person to person by soiled hands to mouth (as occurs in day care centers). Large community outbreaks have resulted from drinking treated but unfiltered water. Filtration is necessary because the concentrations of chlorine used in routine water treatment do not kill *Giardia* cysts, especially in cold water. Smaller outbreaks have involved contaminated food, person-to-person transmission in day care centers, and fecally contaminated recreational water (e.g., swimming and wading pools). **Laboratory Diagnosis.** Giardiasis is usually diagnosed by microscopic observation of trophozoites and/or cysts in stained smears of fecal specimens or duodenal aspirates. The characteristic teardrop-shaped *Giardia* trophozoite contains two nuclei, giving it the appearance of a face (Fig. 21-3). It appears to be looking up at the person observing it microscopically. The *Giardia* trophozoite has been described as resembling an owl face, a clown face, or an old man with glasses. Immunodiagnostic procedures are also available.

or cystitis. Although rarely symptomatic in men, trichomoniasis may lead to prostatitis, urethritis, or infection of the seminal vesicles. Persons with trichomoniasis often also have other sexually transmitted diseases, especially gonorrhea.

Patient Care. Use Standard Precautions.

Geographic Occurrence. Trichomoniasis occurs worldwide.

Parasite. Trichomoniasis is caused by *Trichomonas vaginalis*, a flagellate.

Reservoirs and Mode of Transmission. Infected humans serve as reservoirs. Transmission occurs by direct contact with vaginal and urethral discharges of infected people during sexual

> Trichomoniasis is caused by a flagellated protozoan named *T. vaginalis* and is transmitted by direct contact with vaginal and urethral discharges of infected people.

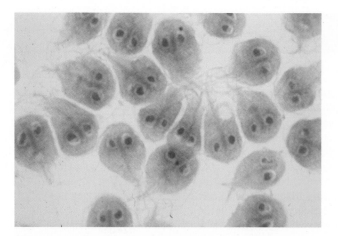

FIGURE 21-3. *Giardia lamblia* **trophozoites, which were cultured in a research laboratory.** *G. lamblia* trophozoites, 10 to 20 μm long by 5 to 15 μm wide, are easy to recognize in microscopically examined fecal specimens. Their two oval nuclei resemble eyes. As you observe a *Giardia* trophozoite through the microscope, it appears to be looking up at you.

FIGURE 21-4. *Trichomonas vaginalis* **and Gram-positive cocci, for size comparison.** *T. vaginalis* trophozoites (*arrows*) are easy to recognize in a saline wet mount preparation of a freshly collected specimen. Their flagella and undulating membrane cause them to be constantly in motion. When they die, however, they become spherical and cannot be distinguished from white blood cells. (From Harvey RA, et al. Lippincott's Illustrated Reviews: Microbiology, 2nd ed. Philadelphia: Lippincott Williams & Wilkins, 2007.)

intercourse. Because this organism exists only in the fragile trophozoite stage (there is no cyst stage), it cannot survive very long outside the human body.

Laboratory Diagnosis. Vaginitis caused by *T. vaginalis* can be diagnosed by performing a saline wet mount examination (described in CD-ROM Appendix 5) of freshly collected vaginal discharge material and observing the motile trophozoites (Fig. 21-4). Culture procedures are also available, but are rarely performed in clinical microbiology laboratories. *T. vaginalis* trophozoites are sometimes seen in urine and Papanicolaou (Pap) smears. Diagnosis of trichomoniasis in men can be accomplished by performing a saline wet mount of urethral discharge material or prostatic secretions.

Protozoal Infections of the Circulatory System

Table 21-4 contains information about protozoal infections of the circulatory system.

Protozoal Infections of the Central Nervous System

Protozoal infections of the CNS include African trypanosomiasis, amebic abscesses, PAM, and toxoplas-

STUDY AID

"Bugs"

Some people refer to all, or most, insects as bugs, but only one category of insects—class Insecta—actually contains bugs. Technically, true bugs are in the order Hemiptera. Included in this order are bed bugs, reduviid bugs, several types of water bugs, and many plant bugs.

mosis. Each of these diseases, except PAM, was discussed earlier in this chapter.

Primary Amebic Meningoencephalitis

Disease. PAM is an amebic disease causing inflammation of the brain and meninges, sore throat, severe frontal headache, hallucinations, nausea, vomiting, high fever, stiff neck. Unless diagnosed and treated promptly, death occurs within 10 days, usually on the fifth or sixth day.

Patient Care. Use Standard Precautions for hospitalized patients.

Geographic Occurrence. PAM has been reported worldwide.

Parasite. PAM is caused by *N. fowleri*, an ameboflagellate.[a] Amebas in the genera *Acanthamoeba* and *Balamuthia* can cause similar conditions.

> Primary amebic meningoencephalitis is caused by an ameboflagellate named *N. fowleri*.

Reservoirs and Mode of Transmission. Water and soil serve as reservoirs. The amebas usually enter the nasal passages of a person diving and/or swimming in ameba-contaminated water, such as ponds, lakes, "the old swimming hole," thermal springs, hot tubs, spas, and public swimming pools. After the amebas colonize the nasal tissues, they invade the brain and meninges by traveling along the olfactory nerves.

---

[a] *Naegleria fowleri* is classified as an ameboflagellate because its life cycle consists of three stages: trophozoite, a temporary flagellar stage known as ameboflagellate, and cyst.

TABLE 21-4   Protozoal Infections of the Circulatory System

DISEASE	ADDITIONAL INFORMATION
African Trypanosomiasis (African Sleeping Sickness). African trypanosomiasis is a systemic disease caused by flagellated protozoa in the bloodstream, known as hemoflagellates. Early stages of the disease include a painful chancre at the site of a tsetse fly bite, fever, intense headache, insomnia, lymphadenitis, anemia, local edema, and rash. Later stages of the disease include body wasting, falling asleep, coma, and death if untreated. The latter stages of the disease have given rise to the name African sleeping sickness or simply sleeping sickness. **Patient Care.** Use Standard Precautions for hospitalized patients. **Geographic Occurrence.** African trypanosomiasis is transmitted by the tsetse fly (Genus *Glossina*), so the disease only occurs in tropical Africa, where tsetse flies are found. It is estimated that more than 300,000 people have African trypanosomiasis and that about 66,000 people die each year of the disease.	**Pathogens.** Two subspecies of *Trypanosoma brucei* cause African trypanosomiasis. *T. brucei* ssp. *gambiense*, in western and central Africa, causes most cases of sleeping sickness; the disease may last several years. *T. brucei* ssp. *rhodesiense*, in eastern Africa, causes a more rapidly fatal form of African trypanosomiasis, usually lethal within weeks or a few months without treatment. **Reservoirs and Mode of Transmission.** Infected humans serve as reservoirs of *T. brucei* ssp. *gambiense*, whereas wild animals and domestic cattle are the primary reservoirs of *T. brucei* ssp. *rhodesiense*. Tsetse flies become infected when they ingest blood that contains the trypanosomes. The parasites then multiply and mature within the infected tsetse flies. Humans become infected when mature trypanosomes (trypomastigotes) are injected into the bloodstream as the infected tsetse flies take blood meals. **Laboratory Diagnosis.** African trypanosomiasis is diagnosed by observing and identifying trypomastigotes in blood, lymph node aspirates, or cerebrospinal fluid (Fig. 21-5). Immunodiagnostic procedures are also available.
American Trypanosomiasis (Chagas' Disease). American trypanosomiasis is also known as Chagas' disease, in honor of Carlos Chageas, who described the entire life cycle of *Trypanosoma cruzi* in 1909. In the acute stage of the disease, patients may present with an inflammatory response at the site of the reduviid bug bite, fever, malaise, lymphadenopathy, **hepatomegaly** (enlarged liver), and **splenomegaly** (enlarged spleen), although it may be asymptomatic. Chronic irreversible complications include heart damage, arrhythmias, enlarged esophagus (megaesophagus), and enlarged colon (megacolon). Life-threatening meningoencephalitis may occur. **Patient Care.** Use Standard Precautions for hospitalized patients. **Geographical Occurrence.** Chagas' disease occurs primarily in South America, Central America, and Mexico, although a few cases have been reported in the United States (by bug bite or blood transfusion). As increasing numbers of infected people enter the country from endemic areas, concern is growing in the United States about the safety of the blood supply. Currently, U.S. donor blood is not routinely screened for the presence of *T. cruzi*. It is estimated that between 16 million and 18 million people have Chagas' disease and that about 50,000 people die each year from the disease.	**Parasite.** The etiologic agent of American trypanosomiasis is *T. cruzi*, which occurs in two stages: a hemoflagellate (the trypomastigote form) and a nonmotile, intracellular parasite (the amastigote form). **Reservoirs and Mode of Transmission.** Reservoirs include infected humans and more than 150 species of domestic and wild animals, including dogs, cats, rodents, carnivores, and primates. The vectors of American trypanosomiasis are rather large bugs (see "Study Aid: Bugs" on page 364). They are known by many names, including reduviid bugs, triatome bugs, kissing bugs, and cone-nosed bugs. A bug becomes infected when it takes a blood meal from an infected animal. Later, when the bug takes a blood meal or feeds at the corner of a sleeping person's eye, the bug defecates. The person becomes infected by rubbing the insect feces—which contain the parasite—into the bite wound or eye. The characteristic unilateral swelling of the eyelid that occurs after *T. cruzi* is rubbed into the eye is called Romaña sign. Transmission by blood transfusion and organ transplantation also occurs. **Laboratory Diagnosis.** American trypanosomiasis is diagnosed by observation of trypomastigotes in blood (Fig. 21-6) or amastigotes in tissue (especially cardiac tissue) or lymph node biopsies. Immunodiagnostic procedures are also available. Xenodiagnosis is performed in endemic countries. In this procedure, sterile (uninfected), laboratory-raised reduviid bugs are allowed to take blood meals from persons suspected of having Chagas' disease. (The bite is painless.) The bugs are then taken to a laboratory, where their feces are periodically checked microscopically for the presence of the parasite.
Babesiosis. Babesiosis is a sporozoan disease that may include fever, chills, myalgia, fatigue, jaundice, and anemia. It is potentially severe and sometimes fatal, especially in splenectomized and elderly people. Patients may be simultaneously infected with *Borrelia burgdorferi*, the etiologic agent of Lyme disease, which is transmitted by the same species of tick.	**Parasites.** Babesiosis is caused by *Babesia microti* and other *Babesia* spp., including *Babesia divergens* in Europe. Like the malaria parasites, *Babesia* spp. are intraerythrocytic sporozoa (i.e., they live within erythrocytes). **Reservoirs and Mode of Transmission.** Reservoirs include rodents for *B. microti* and cattle for *B. divergens*. Transmission occurs by tick bite and rarely, by blood transfusion.

(continues)

TABLE 21-4   Protozoal Infections of the Circulatory System (continued)

DISEASE	ADDITIONAL INFORMATION
Patient Care. Use Standard Precautions for hospitalized patients. **Geographic Occurrence.** Babesiosis is an endemic disease in many parts of the world, including Europe, Mexico, and the United States. Most U.S. cases occur in New York and New England.	**Laboratory Diagnosis.** Babesiosis is diagnosed by observation and identification of intraerythrocytic *Babesia* parasites in Giemsa-stained blood smears. They resemble the early "ring forms" of malarial parasites—particularly *Plasmodium falciparum*—and thus must be differentiated from malarial parasites. Immunodiagnostic and molecular diagnostic procedures are also available.
Malaria. Malaria is a systemic sporozoan infection with malaise, fever, chills, sweating, headache, and nausea. The frequency with which the cycle of chills, fever, and sweating is repeated is referred to as periodicity, which depends on the particular species of malarial parasite that is causing the infection. The intermittent bouts of chills and fever are sometimes referred to as paroxysms. In addition to these symptoms, falciparum malaria may be accompanied by cough, diarrhea, respiratory distress, shock, renal and liver failure, pulmonary and cerebral edema, coma, and death. **Patient Care.** Use Standard Precautions for hospitalized patients. **Geographic Occurrence.** Malaria is one of the most important infectious diseases in the world. It is a major health problem in many tropical and subtropical countries, with an estimated 300–500 million cases and 1.5–2.7 million deaths annually. About 90% of all malaria cases occur in Africa, where approximately 1 million children die from malaria each year. Malaria is a nationally notifiable infectious disease in the United States. Most U.S. cases are imported, meaning that the disease was acquired outside of the country. A few nonimported, mosquito-transmitted cases of malaria occur in the United States each year.	**Parasites.** Human malaria is caused by four species in the genus *Plasmodium*: *Plasmodium vivax* (the most common species), *P. falciparum* (the most deadly), *Plasmodium malariae*, and *Plasmodium ovale*. These are intraerythrocytic sporozoan parasites. Infection with *P. vivax* and *P. ovale* results in chills and fever every 48 hours and is referred to as tertian malaria. *P. malariae* infection causes chills and fever every 72 hours and is referred to as quartan malaria. *P. falciparum* periodicity varies from 36–48 hours. Mixed infections—that is, infections involving more than one *Plasmodium* species—occur in certain geographic areas. Drug-resistant strains of *P. vivax* and *P. falciparum* are common. *Plasmodium* spp. have a complex life cycle involving a female *Anopheles* mosquito, the liver and erythrocytes of an infected human, and many life cycle stages (Fig. 21-7). **Reservoirs and Mode of Transmission.** Infected humans and infected mosquitoes serve as reservoirs. Most human infections occur as a result of injection of sporozoites into the bloodstream by an infected female *Anopheles* mosquito while taking a blood meal. Infection may also occur as a result of blood transfusion or the use of blood-contaminated needles and syringes. **Laboratory Diagnosis.** Malaria is diagnosed by observation and identification of intraerythrocytic *Plasmodium* parasites in Giemsa-stained blood smears (Fig. 21-8). Immunodiagnostic and molecular diagnostic procedures are being tested.

FIGURE 21-5. *Trypanosoma brucei* **trypomastigotes in a stained peripheral blood smear from a patient with African trypanosomiasis.** *T. brucei* trypomastigotes are 14 to 33 μm long by 1.5 to 3.5 μm wide. (From Winn WC Jr., et al. Koneman's Color Atlas and Textbook of Diagnostic Microbiology, 6th ed. Philadelphia: Lippincott Williams & Wilkins, 2006.)

FIGURE 21-6. *Trypanosoma cruzi* **trypomastigotes in a stained peripheral blood smear from a patient with American trypanosomiasis (Chagas' disease).** Several trypomastigotes of *T. cruzi*, with their typical "C" shape, can be seen among the red blood cells. (From Winn WC Jr., et al. Koneman's Color Atlas and Textbook of Diagnostic Microbiology, 6th ed. Philadelphia: Lippincott Williams & Wilkins, 2006.)

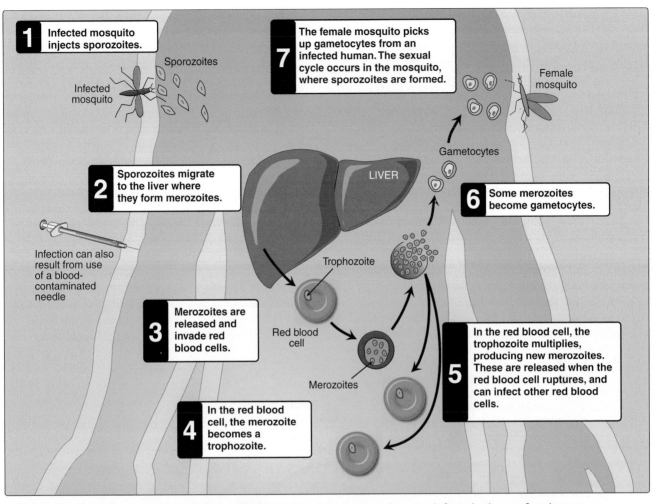

FIGURE 21-7. Life cycle of malarial parasites. Note that humans become infected when a female *Anopheles* mosquito injects sporozoites while taking a blood meal. Mosquitoes become infected when they ingest male and female gametocytes (at least one of each) while taking a blood meal. (From Harvey RA, et al. Lippincott's Illustrated Reviews: Microbiology, 2nd ed. Philadelphia: Lippincott Williams & Wilkins, 2007.)

FIGURE 21-8. Giemsa-stained peripheral blood smear showing *Plasmodium falciparum* trophozoites (*arrows*) within red blood cells. (From Binford CH, Connor DH. Pathology of Tropical and Extraordinary Diseases, vol. 1. Washington, DC: Armed Forces Institute of Pathology, 1976.)

Laboratory Diagnosis. Diagnosis of PAM can sometimes be made by microscopic examination of wet mount preparations of fresh cerebrospinal fluid (CSF). However, because they are colorless and transparent, amebas are difficult to see in wet mounts, unless the microscope light is turned very low. Phase-contrast microscopy is helpful. Smears of CSF sediment can be stained with Wright, Wright-Giemsa, Giemsa, or trichrome stain. Leukocytes and amebas are similar in appearance. Unfortunately, most cases of PAM are diagnosed after the patient's death through observation of amebas in stained sections of brain tissue.

HELMINTHS

The word **helminth** means parasitic worm. Although helminths are not microorganisms, the various procedures used to diagnose helminth infections are performed in the Parasitology Section of the Clinical Microbiology Laboratory. These procedures often involve the observation of microscopic stages—eggs and larvae—in the life cycles of these parasites. Helminths infect humans, other animals, and plants, but only helminth infections of humans are discussed here. The helminths that infect humans are always endoparasites.

Helminths are multicellular, eucaryotic organisms in the Kingdom Animalia. The two major divisions of helminths are roundworms (**nematodes**) and flatworms. The flatworms are further divided into tapeworms (**cestodes**) and flukes (**trematodes**).

Helminths (parasitic worms) are divided into roundworms (nematodes) and flatworms. Flatworms are further divided into tapeworms (cestodes) and flukes (trematodes).

The typical helminth life cycle includes three stages: the *egg*, the *larva*, and the *adult worm*. Adults produce eggs, from which larvae emerge, and the larvae mature into adult worms. Adult nematodes are either male or female. Cestodes and many trematodes are hermaphroditic,

The stages of the typical helminth life cycle are the egg, the larva, and the adult worm.

meaning that adult worms contain both male and female reproductive organs. Thus, it only takes one worm to produce fertile eggs.

The host that harbors the larval stage is called the *intermediate host*, whereas the host that harbors the adult worm is called the *definitive host*. Sometimes helminths have more than one intermediate host or more than one definitive host. The fish tapeworm, for example, is what is known as a three-host parasite, having one definitive host (human) and two intermediate hosts (a freshwater crustacean called a *Cyclops* and a freshwater fish) in its life cycle (Fig. 21-9). Fleas serve as intermediate hosts in the life cycle of the dog tapeworm, whereas dogs, cats, or humans can serve as definitive hosts.

Helminth infections are primarily acquired by ingesting the larval stage, although some larvae are injected into the

Helminth infections are usually diagnosed by observing (a) whole worms or segments of worms in clinical specimens—most often, fecal specimens, or (b) larvae or eggs in stained or unstained clinical specimens.

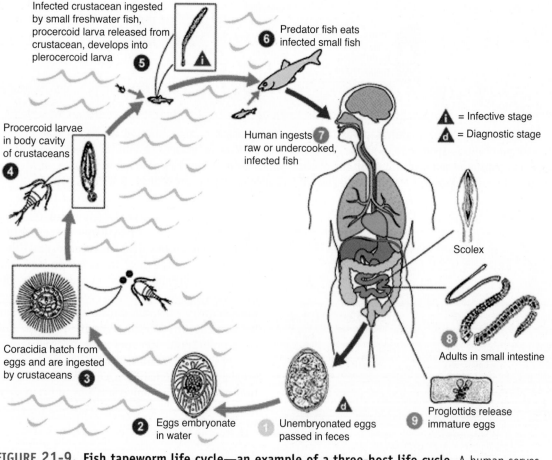

FIGURE 21-9. Fish tapeworm life cycle—an example of a three-host life cycle. A human serves as the definitive host, harboring the adult worm. A *Cyclops* species (a crustacean) serves as the first intermediate host, harboring the procercoid larva stage. A freshwater fish serves as the second intermediate host, harboring the plerocercoid larva (the infective stage). Humans become infected by ingesting the plerocercoid larva in raw or undercooked fish. (Courtesy of the CDC, Division of Parasitic Diseases.)

TABLE 21-5	Helminth Infections of Humans	
ANATOMIC LOCATION	**HELMINTH DISEASE**	**HELMINTH THAT CAUSES THE DISEASE**
Skin	Onchocerciasis (also known as "river blindness")	*Onchocerca volvulus* (N); microfilariae (tiny prelarval stages of these helminths are found in the skin
Muscle and Subcutaneous Tissues	Trichinosis Dracunculiasis	*Trichinella spiralis* (N) *Dracunculus medinensis* (N); also known as the guinea worm
Eyes	Onchocerciasis Loiasis	*Onchocerca volvulus* (N); microfilariae enter the eyes, causing an intense inflammatory reaction *Loa loa* (N); also known as the African eyeworm
Respiratory System	Paragonimiasis	*Paragonimus westermani* (T); the lung fluke
Gastrointestinal Tract	Ascariasis infection Hookworm infection Pinworm infection (enterobiasis) Whipworm infection (trichuriasis) Strongyloidiasis Beef tapeworm infection Dog tapeworm infection Dwarf tapeworm infection Fish tapeworm infection Pork tapeworm infection Rat tapeworm infection Fasciolopsiasis Fascioliasis Clonorchiasis	*Ascaris lumbricoides* (N); the large intestinal roundworm of humans *Ancylostoma duodenale* (N) or *Necator americanus* (N) *Enterobius vermicularis* (N) *Trichuris trichiura* (N) *Strongyloides stercoralis* (N) *Taenia saginata* (C) *Dipylidium caninum* (C) *Hymenolepis nana* (C) *Diphyllobothrium latum* (C) *Taenia solium* (C) *Hymenolepis diminuta* (C) *Fasciolopsis buski* (T); an intestinal fluke *Fasciola hepatica* (T); a liver fluke *Clonorchis sinensis* (T); also known as the Chinese or Oriental liver fluke
Circulatory System	Filariasis Schistosomiasis (also known as bilharzia)	*Wuchereria bancrofti* (N) and *Brugia malayi* (N); microfilariae of these helminths are found in the bloodstream Trematodes in the genus *Schistosoma*
Central Nervous System	Cysticercosis Hydatid cyst disease	Cysts (the larval stage) of the pork tapeworm (*Taenia solium*) are found in the brain *Echinococcus granulosis* (C) or *Echinococcus multilocularis* (C); in addition to the brain, hydatid cysts (the larval form of these helminths) can form in many other locations in the body

N, nematode; *C*, cestode; *T*, trematode.

body via the bite of infected insects, and others enter the body by penetrating skin. Helminth infections are usually diagnosed by observing whole worms or segments of worms in clinical specimens (usually, fecal specimens), or larvae or eggs in stained or unstained clinical specimens.

HELMINTH INFECTIONS OF HUMANS

The major helminth infections of humans are shown in Table 21-5. Additional information about helminth infections can be found on the CD-ROM.

APPROPRIATE THERAPY FOR PARASITIC INFECTIONS

Recommendations for the treatment of infectious diseases change frequently. The parasitic infections described in this chapter must be treated using appropriate antiprotozoal or antihelminth drugs.

Sources of updated information include *The Merck Manual* (http://www.merck.com/pubs) and WebMD (http://www.webmd.com). Additional information about antiprotozoal agents can be found in Chapter 9. Drugs used to treat helminth infections are also known as anthelmintics, anthelminthics, antihelmintics, and antihelminthics.

TABLE 21-6	Ways in which Arthropods May Be Involved in Human Diseases
TYPE OF INVOLVEMENT	**EXAMPLE(S)**
The arthropod may actually be the *cause* of the disease.	Scabies, a disease in which microscopic mites live in subcutaneous tunnels and cause intense itching.
The arthropod may serve as the *intermediate host* in the life cycle of a parasite.	Flea in the life cycle of the dog tapeworm. Beetle in the life cycle of the rat tapeworm. *Cyclops* sp. in the life cycle of the fish tapeworm. Tsetse fly in the life cycle of African trypanosomiasis. *Simulium* black fly in the life cycle of onchocerciasis. Mosquito in the life cycle of filariasis.
The arthropod may serve as the *definitive host* in the life cycle of a parasite.	Female *Anopheles* mosquito in the life cycle of malarial parasites.
The arthropod may serve as a *vector* in the transmission of an infectious disease.	Oriental rat flea in the transmission of plague. Tick in the transmission of Rocky Mountain spotted fever and Lyme disease. Louse in the transmission of epidemic typhus.

MEDICALLY IMPORTANT ARTHROPODS

There are many classes of arthropods, but only three are studied in a parasitology course: *insects* (class Insecta), *arachnids* (class Arachnida), and certain *crustaceans* (class Crustacea). The insects studied include lice, fleas, flies, mosquitoes, and reduviid bugs. Arachnids include mites and ticks. Crustaceans include crabs, crayfish, and certain *Cyclops* species. Arthropods may be involved in human diseases in any of four ways, as shown in Table 21-6.

FIGURE 21-10. Arthropod ectoparasites and vectors of human infectious diseases.
(A) *Dermacentor andersoni*, the wood tick; one of the tick vectors of Rocky Mountain spotted fever. **(B)** *Xenopsylla cheopis*, the oriental rat flea; the vector of plague and endemic typhus. **(C)** *Pediculus humanus*, the human body louse; a vector of epidemic typhus. **(D)** *Phthirus pubis*, the pubic louse; because of its appearance, it is also known as the crab louse. (From Winn WC Jr., et al. Koneman's Color Atlas and Textbook of Diagnostic Microbiology, 6th ed. Philadelphia: Lippincott Williams & Wilkins, 2006.)

Arthropods may serve as mechanical or biologic vectors in the transmission of certain infectious diseases. **Mechanical vectors** merely pick up the parasite at point A and drop it off at point B, similar to an overnight delivery service. For example, a housefly could pick up parasite cysts on the sticky hairs of its legs while walking around on animal feces in a meadow. The fly might then come through an open kitchen window and drop off the parasite cysts while walking on a pie cooling on the counter. A **biologic vector**, on the other hand, is an arthropod in whose body the pathogen multiplies or matures (or both). Many arthropod vectors of human diseases are biologic vectors. A particular arthropod may serve as both a host and a biologic vector. Refer back to Table 11-3 in Chapter 11 for a list of arthropods that serve as vectors of human infectious diseases. Several arthropods that serve as vectors of human diseases are shown in Figure 21-10.

ON THE CD-ROM
- Terms Introduced in This Chapter
- Review of Key Points
- Insight: A Closer Look at Helminths
- Increase Your Knowledge
- Critical Thinking
- Case Studies
- Additional Self-Assessment Exercises

SELF-ASSESSMENT EXERCISES

After studying this chapter, answer the following multiple-choice questions.

1. Humans develop malaria after the injection of *Plasmodium* _____ into the bloodstream by an infected female *Anopheles* mosquito when she takes a blood meal.
   a. male and female gametocytes
   b. schizonts
   c. sporozoites
   d. trophozoites

2. These *Plasmodium* life cycle stages must be ingested by a female *Anopheles* mosquito for the *Plasmodium* life cycle to continue in the mosquito.
   a. male and female gametocytes
   b. schizonts
   c. sporozoites
   d. trophozoites

3. Which of the following protozoal diseases is *not* transmitted via an arthropod vector?
   a. African trypanosomiasis
   b. American trypanosomiasis
   c. babesiosis
   d. giardiasis

4. Which of the following protozoal diseases is *least* likely to be transmitted via blood transfusion?
   a. American trypanosomiasis
   b. babesiosis
   c. malaria
   d. trichomoniasis

5. Which of the following protozoal diseases is *least* likely to be transmitted via an infected food handler who fails to wash his or her hands after using the bathroom?
   a. amebiasis
   b. cryptosporidiosis
   c. giardiasis
   d. toxoplasmosis

6. You are visiting a friend whose parents raise pigs. Which of the following diseases are you *most* likely to acquire by drinking well water at their farm?
   a. amebiasis
   b. balantidiasis
   c. cryptosporidiosis
   d. giardiasis

7. You are working on a cattle ranch. Which of the following diseases are you *most* apt to acquire as you perform your duties at the ranch?
   a. amebiasis
   b. balantidiasis
   c. cryptosporidiosis
   d. giardiasis

8. Which of the following protozoal diseases are you *most* likely to acquire by eating a rare hamburger?
   a. amebiasis
   b. balantidiasis
   c. giardiasis
   d. toxoplasmosis

9. Which of the following associations is incorrect?
   a. African trypanosomiasis . . . tsetse fly
   b. amebiasis . . . fecally contaminated water
   c. Chagas' disease . . . mosquito
   d. toxoplasmosis . . . cats

10. Which of the following is an example of an infectious disease that is caused by a facultative parasite?
   a. African trypanosomiasis
   b. giardiasis
   c. malaria
   d. PAM

ANSWERS TO SELF-ASSESSMENT EXERCISES

Chapter 1
1. a
2. b
3. d
4. d
5. b
6. b
7. d
8. b
9. b
10. b

Chapter 2
1. d
2. b
3. a
4. d
5. d
6. b
7. a
8. d
9. b
10. b

Chapter 3
1. c
2. c
3. b
4. c
5. c
6. c
7. b
8. c
9. a
10. c

Chapter 4
1. d
2. a
3. a
4. c
5. a
6. b
7. c
8. a
9. d
10. a

Chapter 5
1. d
2. d
3. b
4. c
5. d
6. c
7. d
8. a
9. d
10. d

Chapter 6
1. a
2. a
3. c
4. a
5. a
6. d
7. d
8. d
9. d
10. c

Chapter 7
1. c
2. a
3. d
4. a
5. c
6. d
7. d
8. b
9. c
10. a

Chapter 8
1. b
2. b
3. b
4. d
5. c
6. c
7. a
8. d
9. b
10. a

Chapter 9
1. c
2. d
3. b
4. d
5. b
6. c
7. a
8. b
9. b
10. c

Chapter 10
1. d
2. a
3. d
4. a
5. a
6. b
7. c
8. a
9. d
10. c

Chapter 11
1. b
2. d
3. a
4. d
5. a
6. b
7. a
8. c
9. c
10. d

Chapter 12
1. a
2. d
3. b
4. b
5. b
6. b
7. a
8. d
9. a
10. d

Chapter 13
1. d
2. c
3. c
4. d
5. c
6. c
7. c
8. d
9. d
10. d

Chapter 14
1. d
2. a
3. d
4. b
5. c
6. b
7. c
8. b
9. a
10. d

Chapter 15
1. b
2. a
3. d
4. d
5. d
6. a
7. d
8. d
9. a
10. c

Chapter 16
1. a
2. c
3. c
4. c
5. c
6. d
7. b
8. d
9. d
10. c

Chapter 17

1. a
2. b
3. d
4. c
5. a
6. b
7. a
8. a
9. a
10. a

Chapter 18

1. c
2. a
3. d
4. a
5. b
6. a
7. b
8. a
9. c
10. a

Chapter 19

1. b
2. d
3. b
4. d
5. d
6. b
7. b
8. a
9. b
10. d

Chapter 20

1. b
2. b
3. d
4. c
5. a
6. d
7. a
8. d
9. c
10. b

Chapter 21

1. c
2. a
3. d
4. d
5. d
6. b
7. c
8. d
9. c
10. d

Bacillus anthracis (buh-sil-us an-thray-sis). An aerobic, spore-forming, Gram-positive bacillus; the causative agent of anthrax in humans, cattle, swine, sheep, rabbits, guinea pigs, and mice; causes a cutaneous, respiratory, or gastrointestinal disease, depending on the portal of entry.

Bacteroides (bak-ter-oy-dez) species. Anaerobic, Gram-negative bacilli; common members of the indigenous microflora of the oral cavity, gastrointestinal tract, and vagina; opportunistic pathogens that cause various infections, including appendicitis, peritonitis, abscesses, and postsurgical wound infections.

Bordetella pertussis (bor-duh-tel-uh per-tus-sis). A fastidious, Gram-negative coccobacillus; the causative agent of whooping cough, which is also called pertussis.

Borrelia burgdorferi (boh-ree-lee-uh burg-door-fur-eye). A Gram-negative, loosely coiled spirochete; the causative agent of Lyme disease; transmitted from infected deer and mice to humans by tick bite.

Campylobacter jejuni (kam-pih-low-bak-ter juh-ju-nee). A curved, Gram-negative bacillus, having a characteristic corkscrew-like motility; often seen in pairs (described as a gull-wing morphology because a pair of curved bacilli resembles a bird); microaerophilic and capnophilic; a common cause of gastroenteritis with malaise, myalgia, arthralgia, headache, and cramping abdominal pain.

Chlamydia (kluh-mid-ee-uh) species. Pleomorphic, Gram-negative bacteria that are obligate intracellular pathogens; unable to grow on artificial media; etiologic agents of nongonococcal urethritis (NGU), trachoma, inclusion conjunctivitis, lymphogranuloma venereum, pneumonia, and psittacosis (ornithosis); different serotypes cause different diseases.

Clostridium botulinum (klos-trid-ee-um bot-yu-ly-num). An anaerobic, spore-forming, Gram-positive bacillus; common in soil; produces a neurotoxin called botulinum toxin, which causes botulism, a very serious and sometimes fatal type of food poisoning.

Clostridium difficile (klos-trid-ee-um dif-fuh-seal). An anaerobic, spore-forming, Gram-positive bacillus; it can colonize the intestinal tract, where overgrowth (superinfection) commonly occurs after ingestion of oral antibiotics; this organism produces two toxins—an enterotoxin that causes antibiotic-associated diarrhea (AAD) and a cytotoxin that causes pseudomembranous colitis (PMC); a common cause of healthcare-associated infections.

Clostridium perfringens (klos-trid-ee-um purr-frin-jens). An anaerobic, spore-forming, Gram-positive bacillus; common in feces and soil; the most common cause of gas gangrene (myonecrosis); produces an enterotoxin that produces a relatively mild type of food poisoning.

Clostridium tetani (klos-trid-ee-um tet-an-eye). An anaerobic, spore-forming, Gram-positive bacillus; common in soil; produces a neurotoxin called tetanospasmin, which causes tetanus.

Corynebacterium diphtheriae (kuh-ry-nee-bak-teer-ee-um dif-thee-ree-ee). A pleomorphic, Gram-positive bacillus; toxigenic (toxin-producing) strains cause diphtheria, whereas nontoxigenic strains do not.

Enterococcus (en-ter-oh-kok-us) species. Gram-positive cocci; common members of the indigenous microflora of the gastrointestinal tract; opportunistic pathogens; a fairly common cause of cystitis and healthcare-associated infections; some strains, called vancomycin-resistant enterococci (VRE), are multidrug resistant.

Escherichia coli (esh-er-ick-ee-uh koh-ly). A member of the family *Enterobacteriaceae*; a Gram-negative bacillus; a facultative anaerobe; a very common member of the indigenous microflora of the colon; an opportunistic pathogen; the most common cause of septicemia and urinary tract and healthcare-associated infections; some serotypes (called the enterovirulent *E. coli*) are always pathogens.

Francisella tularensis (fran-suh-sel-luh tool-uh-ren-sis). A Gram-negative bacillus; the causative agent of tularemia; may enter the body by inhalation, ingestion, tick bite, or penetration of broken or unbroken skin; tularemia frequently follows contact with infected animals (e.g., rabbits).

Fusobacterium (few-zoh-bak-teer-ee-um) species. Anaerobic, Gram-negative bacilli; common members of the indigenous microflora of the oral cavity, gastrointestinal tract, and vagina; opportunistic pathogens that cause various infections, including oral and respiratory infections.

Haemophilus influenzae (he-mof-uh-lus in-flu-en-zee). A fastidious, Gram-negative bacillus; a facultative anaerobe; encapsulated; found in low numbers as indigenous microflora of the upper respiratory tract; an opportunistic pathogen; a cause of bacterial meningitis, ear infections, and respiratory infections, but is *not* the cause of influenza (which is caused by influenza viruses); some strains are ampicillin resistant.

Helicobacter pylori (hee-luh-ko-bak-ter py-lor-ee). A curved, Gram-negative bacillus; capable of colonizing the stomach; a common cause of stomach and duodenal ulcers.

Klebsiella pneumoniae (kleb-see-el-uh new-moh-nee-ee). A member of the family *Enterobacteriaceae*; a Gram-negative bacillus; a facultative anaerobe; a common member of the indigenous microflora of the colon; an opportunistic pathogen; a fairly common cause of pneumonia and cystitis.

Lactobacillus (lak-toh-buh-sil-us) species. Gram-positive bacilli; some species are found in foods (e.g., yogurt, cheese); other species are common members of the indigenous microflora of the vagina and gastrointestinal tract; rarely pathogenic.

Legionella pneumophila (lee-juh-nel-luh new-mah-fill-uh). An aerobic, Gram-negative bacillus; common in soil and water; the causative agent of legionellosis (a type of pneumonia); can contaminate water tanks and pipes; has caused epidemics in hotels, hospitals, and cruise ships.

Listeria monocytogenes (lis-teer-ee-uh mon-oh-sigh-toj-uh-nees). A Gram-positive bacillus; the causative agent of listeriosis; can cause meningitis, encephalitis, septicemia, endocarditis, abortion, and abscesses; enters the body via ingestion of contaminated foods (e.g., cheese).

Mycobacterium leprae (my-koh-bak-teer-ee-um lep-ree). An aerobic, acid-fast, Gram-variable bacillus; referred to as the leprosy bacillus or Hansen's bacillus; the causative agent of leprosy (Hansen's disease); transmitted from person to person; has been found in wild armadillos, which are now used as laboratory animals to propagate this organism.

Mycobacterium tuberculosis (my-koh-bak-teer-ee-um tu-ber-kyu-loh-sis). An acid-fast, Gram-variable bacillus; causes tuberculosis; many strains are multidrug resistant.

Mycoplasma pneumoniae (my-koh-plaz-muh new-moh-nee-ee). A small, pleomorphic, Gram-negative bacterium; lacks a cell wall; the causative agent of atypical pneumonia.

Neisseria gonorrhoeae (ny-see-ree-uh gon-or-ree-ee). Also known as gonococcus or GC; a fastidious, Gram-negative diplococcus; microaerophilic and capnophilic; always a pathogen; causes gonorrhea; many strains are penicillin resistant.

Neisseria meningitidis (ny-see-ree-uh men-in-jih-tid-is). Also known as meningococcus; an aerobic, Gram-negative diplococcus; found as indigenous microflora of the upper respiratory tract of some people (referred to as carriers); a common cause of bacterial meningitis; also causes respiratory infections.

Nocardia (no-kar-dee-uh) species. Aerobic, acid-fast, Gram-positive bacilli; the causative agents of nocardiosis (a respiratory disease) and mycetoma (a tumorlike disease, most often involving the feet).

Peptostreptococcus (pep-toh-strep-toh-kok-us) species. Anaerobic, Gram-positive cocci; common members of the indigenous microflora of the gastrointestinal tract, vagina, and oral cavity; opportunistic pathogens that cause various infections, including abscesses, oral infections, and appendicitis.

Porphyromonas (porf-uh-row-mow-nus) species. Anaerobic, Gram-negative bacilli; common members of the indigenous microflora of the oral cavity and gastrointestinal tract; opportunistic pathogens that cause various infections, including abscesses, oral infections, and bite wound infections.

Prevotella (pree-voh-tel-luh) species. Anaerobic, Gram-negative bacilli; common members of the indigenous microflora of the vagina and gastrointestinal tract; opportunistic pathogens that cause various infections, including abscesses.

Proteus (pro-tee-us) species. Members of the family *Enterobacteriaceae*; Gram-negative bacilli; facultative anaerobes; common members of the indigenous microflora of the colon; opportunistic pathogens; a fairly common cause of cystitis.

Pseudomonas aeruginosa (su-doh-moh-nas air-uj-in-oh-suh). An aerobic, Gram-negative bacillus; produces a characteristic blue-green pigment (pyocyanin); has a characteristic fruity odor; causes burn wound, ear, urinary tract, and respiratory infections; one of the major causes of healthcare-associated infections; most strains are multidrug resistant and resistant to some disinfectants.

Rickettsia (rih-ket-see-uh) species. Gram-negative bacilli that are obligate intracellular pathogens; unable to grow on artificial media; the causative agents of typhus and typhuslike diseases (e.g., Rocky Mountain spotted fever); all rickettsial diseases are transmitted by arthropods (ticks, fleas, mites, lice).

Salmonella (sal-moh-nel-uh) species. Members of the family *Enterobacteriaceae*; Gram-negative bacilli; facultative anaerobes; a fairly common cause of food poisoning, especially cases caused by contaminated poultry; *Salmonella typhi* is the causative agent of typhoid fever.

Shigella (she-gel-uh) species. Members of the family *Enterobacteriaceae*; Gram-negative bacilli; facultative anaerobes; a major cause of gastroenteritis and childhood mortality in the developing nations of the world.

Staphylococcus aureus (staf-ih-low-kok-us aw-ree-us). (See "A Closer Look at *Staphylococcus aureus*" in the Chapter 19 section of the CD-ROM)

Streptococcus agalactiae (strep-toh-kok-us ay-guh-lak-tee-ee). Also known as group B streptococcus; a β-hemolytic, Gram-positive coccus; often colonizes the vagina; a frequent cause of neonatal meningitis.

Streptococcus pneumoniae (strep-toh-kok-us new-moh-nee-ee). (See "A Closer Look at *Streptococcus pneumoniae*" in the Chapter 19 section of the CD-ROM)

Streptococcus pyogenes (strep-toh-kok-us py-oj-uh-nees). (See "A Closer Look at *Streptococcus pyogenes*" in the Chapter 19 section of the CD-ROM)

Treponema pallidum (trep-oh-nee-muh pal-luh-dum). A very thin, tightly coiled spirochete; the causative agent of syphilis.

Vibrio cholerae (vib-ree-oh khol-er-ee). An aerobic, curved (comma-shaped), Gram-negative bacillus; halophilic; lives in salt water; the causative agent of cholera.

Yersinia pestis (yer-sin-ee-uh pes-tis). A Gram-negative bacillus; the causative agent of plague in humans, rodents, and other mammals; transmitted from rat to rat and rat to human by the rat flea.

C USEFUL CONVERSIONS

Length Conversions

To convert inches into centimeters, multiply by 2.54.
To convert centimeters into inches, multiply by 0.39.
To convert yards into meters, multiply by 0.91.
To convert meters into yards, multiply by 1.09.

1 mile (mi) = 1.609 kilometers
1 yard (yd) = 0.914 meter
1 foot (ft) = 30.48 centimeters
1 inch (in) = 2.54 centimeters
1 kilometer (km) = 0.62 mile
1 meter (m) = 39.37 inches
1 centimeter (cm) = 0.39 inch
1 millimeter (mm) = 0.039 inch

Note: Information about micrometers and nanometers can be found in Figure 2-1 in Chapter 2.

Volume Conversions

To convert gallons into liters, multiply by 3.78.
To convert liters into gallons, multiply by 0.26.
To convert fluid ounces into milliliters, multiply by 29.6.
To convert milliliters into fluid ounces, multiply by 0.034.

1 gallon (gal) = 3.785 liters
1 quart (qt) = 0.946 liter
1 pint (pt) = 0.473 liter
1 fluid ounce (fl oz) = 29.573 milliliters
1 liter (L) = 1.057 quarts
1 milliliter (mL) = 0.0338 fluid ounce

Weight Conversions

To convert ounces into grams, multiply by 28.4.
To convert grams into ounces, multiply by 0.035.
To convert pounds into kilograms, multiply by 0.45.
To convert kilograms into pounds, multiply by 2.2.

1 pound (lb) = 0.454 kilogram
1 ounce (oz) = 28.35 grams
1 kilogram (kg) = 2.2 pounds
1 gram (g) = 0.035 ounce
1 gram = 1,000 milligrams (mg)
1 gram = 1,000,000 micrograms (μg)

Temperature Conversions

To convert Celsius (°C) into Fahrenheit (°F), use
$°F = (°C \times 1.8) + 32$.
To convert Fahrenheit (°F) into Celsius (°C), use
$°C = (°F - 32) \times 0.556$.

GREEK LETTER			
Uppercase	**Lowercase**	**NAME**	**PRONUNCIATION**
A	α	Alpha	al-fah
B	β	Beta	bay-tah
Γ	γ	Gamma	gam-ah
Δ	δ	Delta	del-tah
E	ϵ	Epsilon	ep-si-lon
Z	ζ	Zeta	zay-tah
H	η	Eta	ay-tay
Θ	θ	Theta	thay-tah
I	ι	Iota	eye-o-tah
K	κ	Kappa	cap-ah
Λ	λ	Lambda	lamb-dah
M	μ	Mu	mew
N	ν	Nu	new
Ξ	ξ	Xi	zzEye
O	o	Omicron	om-ah-cron
Π	π	Pi	pie
P	ρ	Rho	row
Σ	σ	Sigma	sig-ma
T	τ	Tau	tawh
Υ	υ	Upsilon	oop-si-lon
Φ	ϕ	Phi	figh or fie
X	χ	Chi	kigh
Ψ	ψ	Psi	sigh
Ω	ω	Omega	o-may-gah

How to Get Started

1. Consult with your high school guidance counselor to learn how Dual Enrollment courses will apply to high school graduation and to ensure these courses will apply toward a degree program.

2. Visit **www.irsc.edu** to complete the IRSC Application for Admission. Click **Apply to IRSC.** Indicate "Dual Enrollment" as Enrollment Intention.

3. Complete the Dual Enrollment/Early Admission **Agreement** Form 508* (signed by you, your high school representative, and your parent/legal guardian) and submit <u>once</u> at any IRSC campus.

4. If required, take the P.E.R.T. (Postsecondary Education Readiness Test) at IRSC or request that official placement scores (enhanced ACT or SATI-Recentered) be sent to IRSC by ACT/SAT.

5. Register for IRSC classes at **www.irsc.edu** or any IRSC campus. (Must be at least 16 years of age to register online.)

6. <u>Each term</u>, complete and submit the Dual Enrollment Admission/**Registration** Form 68* (signed by you and your high school representative) at any IRSC campus before the Registration Deadline. Course and reference numbers must match your IRSC Schedule.

Note: Home Education students must also provide proof of enrollment in a home education program pursuant to S.232.02(4).

*IRSC forms are available at any IRSC campus or your high school guidance office.

A

Abiogenesis (ab'-ee-oh... ...can arise from nonliv[ing]... *neous generation* (Cha...

Acellular Microbe. ...cells (e.g., viruses, ...

Acid-Fast Stain. A... differentiates acid... teria; primarily ... tuberculosis (Ch...

Acidophile (uh-... acidic environ... *acidophilic* (Cha...

Acquired Imm... disease charac... tions and ma... ciency virus...

Acquired In... some poin...

Acquired ... to a drug...

Active Ac... quired a... (Chap....

Active ... fectio... the c...

Acute ... mor...

Acut... sho...

Ade... T... a...

A...

mycel... called *reproductive* ...

Aerotolerant Anaerobe (air-o...-...-air-obe). An organism that can live in the presence of oxygen but grows best in an anaerobic environment (an environment containing no oxygen) (Chap. 4).

Agammaglobulinemia (ay-gam'-uh-glob'-yu-luh-nee'-me-uh). Absence of, or extremely low levels of, the gamma fraction of serum globulin; the absence of immunoglobulins in the bloodstream (Chap. 16).

...uired *immunodeficiency syndrome*.

...ection Isolation Room (AIIR). A hospital ...acement for patients who require Airborne ...s; AIIRs are under negative pressure, and air ...uated from these rooms passes through high-...particulate air (HEPA) filters.

...**Precautions.** Standardized safety precautions ...practiced in a healthcare setting to prevent in-...transmitted by the airborne route (Chap. 12).

...'-gee), sing. *alga*. Eucaryotic, photosynthetic or-...s that range in size from unicellular to multicel-...includes many seaweeds (Chap. 5).

...**dal** (al'-juh-side-ul) **Agent.** A disinfectant or ...ical that specifically kills algae (Chap. 8).

...**iphile** (al'-kuh-luh-file). An organism that prefers ...line (basic) environments; such an organism is said ...be *alkaliphilic* (Chap. 8).

...**ergen** (al'-ur-jin). An antigen to which some people ...ecome allergic (Chap. 16).

...**meba** (uh-me'-bah), pl. *amebae*. A type of protozoan ...that moves by means of pseudopodia; in the phylum ...Sarcodina (which is a subphylum in some classification ...schemes) (Chap. 5).

Ames Test. A method of testing compounds to determine whether they are mutagenic (i.e., to see whether they cause mutations in bacteria); uses a mutant strain of *Salmonella* (Chap. 7).

Amino (uh-me'-no) **Acids.** The basic units or building blocks of proteins (Chap. 6).

Ammonification (uh-mon'-uh-fuh-kay'-shun). Conversion of nitrogenous compounds (e.g., proteins) into ammonia (Chap. 10).

Amphitrichous (am-fit'-ri-kus) **Bacterium.** A bacterium that possesses one flagellum or more than one flagellum at each end (pole) of the cell (Chap. 3).

Anabolic Reactions. Metabolic reactions that require energy for the creation of chemical bonds; also known as *biosynthetic reactions* (Chap. 7).

Anabolism (uh-nab'-oh-lizm). Term referring to all of the anabolic reactions that occur within a cell (Chap. 7).

Anaerobe (an'-air-obe). An organism that does not require oxygen for survival; can exist in the absence of oxygen (Chap. 4).

Anaphylactic (an-uh-fuh-lak'-tick) **Reactions.** Allergic reactions; may be localized or systemic; also known as *type I hypersensitivity reactions* (Chap. 16).

Anaphylactic (an-uh-fuh-lak'-tick) **Shock.** Shock after anaphylaxis; may lead to death (Chap. 16).

Anaphylaxis (an-uh-fuh-lak'-sis). An immediate, severe, sometimes fatal, systemic allergic reaction (Chap. 16).

Anoxygenic Photosynthesis (an'-ox-uh-gen'-ik foe-toe-sin'-thuh-sis). A type of photosynthesis in which oxygen is not produced (Chap. 4).

Antagonism (an-tag'-ohn-izm). As the term relates to the use of drugs, the use of two drugs that work against each other; also see *microbial antagonism* (Chap. 9).

Anthrax. A bacterial disease caused by *Bacillus anthracis*, a spore-forming Gram-positive bacillus (Chap. 19).

Antibacterial Agents. Technically, any physical or chemical agents that kill or inhibit the growth of bacteria; in this book, the term is reserved for drugs that are used to treat bacterial diseases (Chap. 9).

Antibiogram (an-tee-by'-oh-gram). The pattern of susceptible (S) and resistant (R) results obtained when antimicrobial susceptibility testing is performed on a particular microorganism (Chap. 12).

Antibiotic (an'-tee-by-ot'-tik). A substance produced by a microorganism that kills or inhibits the growth of other microorganisms (Chap. 1).

Antibiotic-Associated Diarrhea. A diarrheal disease that follows antibiotic therapy; usually caused by *Clostridium difficile*, a spore-forming, anaerobic, Gram-positive bacillus (Chap. 19).

Antibody (an'-tee-bod-ee). A glycoprotein produced by lymphocytes in response to an antigen; if it protects the host in some manner, it is referred to as a *protective antibody* (Chap. 15).

Anticodon (an-tee-ko'-don). A trinucleotide sequence that is complementary to a codon; found on a transfer RNA molecule (Chap. 6).

Antifungal Agents. Technically, any physical or chemical agents that kill or inhibit the growth of fungi; in this book, the term is reserved for drugs that are used to treat fungal diseases (Chap. 9).

Antigen (an'-tuh-jen). A substance, usually foreign, that stimulates the production of antibodies; an *anti*body *gen*erating substance; also known as an *immunogen* (Chap. 15).

Antigen–Antibody Complex. The structure produced as a result of the binding of an antibody to an antigen; also known as an *immune complex* (Chap. 16).

Antigen-Presenting Cell (APC). A macrophage that is displaying antigenic determinants on its surface (Chap. 16).

Antigenic (an-tuh-jen'-ick). If a molecule is antigenic, it stimulates the immune system to produce antibodies; such a molecule is also said to be *immunogenic* (Chap. 16).

Antigenic Determinant. The smallest part of an antigen capable of stimulating the production of antibodies; an antigenic molecule; also known as an *epitope* (Chap. 16).

Antigenic Variation. The ability of a microorganism to change its surface antigens (Chap. 16).

Antimicrobial (an'-tee-my-kro'-be-ul) **Agents.** Technically, any physical or chemical agents that kill or inhibit the growth of microorganisms; in this book, the term is reserved for drugs that are used to treat infectious diseases (Chap. 9).

Antiprotozoal Agents. Technically, any physical or chemical agents that kill or inhibit the growth of protozoa; in this book, the term is reserved for drugs that are used to treat protozoal diseases (Chap. 9).

Antisepsis (an-tee-sep'-sis). Prevention of infection by inhibiting the growth of pathogens (Chap. 8).

Antiseptic (an-tee-sep'-tick). An agent or substance capable of effecting antisepsis; usually refers to a chemical disinfectant that is safe to use on skin and other living tissues (Chap. 8).

Antiseptic Technique. Procedures followed to effect antisepsis; the use of antiseptics (Chap. 8).

Antiserum (an-tee-see'-rum). A serum containing specific antibodies; also known as an *immune serum* (Chap. 16).

Antitoxins (an-tee-tok'-sinz). Antibodies produced in response to a toxin; often capable of neutralizing the toxin that stimulated their production (Chap. 16).

Antiviral Agents. Technically, any physical or chemical agents that inactivate viruses; in this book, the term is reserved for drugs that are used to treat viral diseases (Chap. 9).

Apoenzyme. A protein that cannot function as an enzyme (i.e., cannot catalyze a chemical reaction) until it attaches to a cofactor (Chap. 6).

Arbovirus (are'-boh-vy'-rus). A virus that is transmitted by an arthropod; an arthropod-borne virus (Chap. 18).

Archaea (are-key'-uh). One of the three domains in the three-domain system of classification; members of this domain (archaeons) are procaryotes; the other two domains are *Bacteria* and *Eucarya* (Chap. 3).

Arthropod-borne Virus. See *arbovirus*.

Artificial Active Acquired Immunity. Active acquired immunity that is induced artificially (e.g., by injecting a vaccine into an individual) (Chap. 16).

Artificial Media. Culture media that are prepared in the laboratory; they do not occur naturally; also known as *synthetic media* (Chap. 8).

Artificial Passive Acquired Immunity. Passive acquired immunity that is induced artificially (e.g., by injecting antibodies into an individual) (Chap. 16).

Asepsis (a-sep'-sis). Literally, "without infection"; a condition in which living pathogens are absent (Chap. 8).

Aseptate Hyphae. Fungal hyphae that do not contain septa (cross-walls) (Chap. 5).

Aseptic Meningitis (ay-sep'-tick men-in-ji'-tis). A type of meningitis that is not caused by a pathogen or where the etiologic agent will not grow on standard bacteriological culture media; often used as a synonym for viral meningitis.

Aseptic (ay-sep'-tick) **Techniques.** Measures taken to ensure that living pathogens are absent (Chap. 8).

Asexual Reproduction. A type of reproduction in which a single organism is the sole parent; it passes copies of its entire genome to its offspring (Chap. 3).

Asymptomatic (ay'-simp-tow-mat'-ick) **Disease.** A disease having no symptoms; also referred to as a *subclinical disease* (Chap. 14).

Asymptomatic Infection. The presence of a pathogen in or on the body, without any clinical symptoms of disease; also referred to as a *subclinical infection* (Chap. 14).

Atopic (ay-tope'-ick) **Person.** Allergic person; one who suffers from allergies (Chap. 16).

Attenuated (uh-ten'-yu-ay-ted). An adjective meaning weakened, less pathogenic; used to describe certain microorganisms (Chap. 16).

Attenuated Vaccine. A vaccine prepared from an attenuated microorganism (Chap. 16).

Attenuation (uh-ten-yu-ay-'shun). The process by which microorganisms are attenuated (Chap. 16).

Autoclave (aw'-toe-klav). An apparatus used for sterilization by steam under pressure (Chap. 8).

Autogenous (aw-toj'-uh-nus) **Vaccine.** A vaccine prepared from microorganisms or cells obtained from the person's own body (Chap. 16).

Autoimmune (aw-toh-uh-myun') **Disease.** A disease in which the body produces antibodies directed against its own tissues (Chap. 16).

Autolysis (aw-tol'-uh-sis). Autodigestion; self-digestion (Chap. 3).

Autotroph (aw'-toe-trof). An organism that uses carbon dioxide as its sole carbon source (Chap. 7).

Avirulent (ay-veer'-yu-lent) **Strains.** Strains that are not virulent; not pathogenic; not capable of causing disease (Chap. 14).

Axial Filaments. Flagella-like fibrils that enable spirochetes to move in a spiral, helical, or inchworm manner.

B

B Cells (B Lymphocytes). The leukocytes that produce antibodies (Chap. 16).

Bacillus (bah-sil'-us), pl. *bacilli*. A rod-shaped bacterium; there is also a bacterial genus named *Bacillus*, made up of aerobic, Gram-positive, spore-forming bacilli (Chap. 2).

Bacteremia (bak-ter-ee'-me-uh). The presence of bacteria in the bloodstream (Chap. 13).

Bacteria (back-teer'-ee-uh). Microorganisms in the Domain *Bacteria* (Chap. 3).

Bacteria (back-teer'-ee-uh). One of the three domains in the three-domain system of classification; members of this domain (bacteria) are procaryotes; the other two domains are *Archaea* and *Eucarya* (Chap. 3).

Bacterial Vaginosis (BV). A vaginal infection caused by a variety of bacteria; an example of a *synergistic infection* (Chap. 17).

Bactericidal (bak-tear'-eh-sigh'-dull) **Agent.** A chemical agent or drug that kills bacteria; a *bactericide* (Chap. 8).

Bacteriocins (bak-teer'-ee-oh-sinz). Proteins produced by certain bacteria (those possessing bacteriocinogenic plasmids) that can kill other bacteria (Chap. 10).

Bacteriologist (back'-tier-ee-ol'-oh-jist). One who specializes in the science of bacteriology (Chap. 1).

Bacteriology (back'-tier-ee-ol'-oh-gee). The study of bacteria (Chap. 1).

Bacteriophage (back-tier'-ee-oh-faj). A virus that infects a bacterium; also known simply as a *phage* (Chap. 4).

Bacteriostatic (bak-tear'-ee-oh-stat'-ick) **Agent.** A chemical agent or drug that inhibits the growth of bacteria (Chap. 8).

Bacteriuria (bak-ter-ee'-yu'-ree-uh). The presence of bacteria in the urine (Chap. 13).

Bartholinitis (bar-toe-lin-eye'-tis). Inflammation of the Bartholin's gland in women (Chap. 17).

Basophil (bay'-so-fil). A type of granulocyte found in blood; its granules contain acidic substances (e.g., histamine) that attract basic dyes (Chap. 15).

Beneficial Mutation. A mutation that is of benefit to the mutant organism (Chap. 7).

β-Lactam Ring. One of the two double-ringed structures found in penicillin and cephalosporin molecules (Chap. 9).

β-Lactamases. Enzymes that destroy the β-lactam ring in antibiotics such as penicillin and cephalosporins (Chap. 9).

Binary (by'-nare-ee) **Fission.** A method of reproduction whereby one cell divides to become two cells; the method by which bacteria reproduce (Chap. 3).

Biochemistry (by-oh-kem'-is-tree). The chemistry of living organisms; the chemistry of life (Chap. 6).

Biocidal (by-o-sigh'-dull) **Agent.** A chemical agent that destroys living organisms, especially microorganisms (Chap. 8).

Biofilms. Complex and persistant communities of assorted microorganisms (Chap. 10).

Biogenesis (by-oh-gen'-uh-sis). The theory that life originates only from preexisting life and never from nonliving matter (Chap. 1).

Biologic Catalysts. Enzymes; biologic molecules that catalyze chemical reactions (Chap. 6).

Biologic Warfare (BW) Agents. Pathogens used as weapons in warfare (Chap. 11).

Biological Vector. An arthropod vector (such as a flea or tick) within which a pathogen multiplies or matures (Chap. 21).

Biology. The study of living organisms; the study of life (Chap. 1).

Bioremediation (by'-oh-ruh-meed'-ee-a-shun). The use of microorganisms to clean up industrial and toxic wastes (Chap. 1).

Biotechnology (by'-oh-tek-nol'-oh-gee). The use of living organisms or their derivatives to make or modify products or processes (Chap. 1).

Bioterrorist Agents. Pathogens used by terrorists (Chap. 11).

Biotherapeutic (by'-oh-ther-uh-pu'-tik) **Agents.** Microorganisms used for therapeutic purposes (to treat various diseases or conditions) (Chap. 10).

Biotype. The pattern of positive and negative biochemical test results obtained when a particular microorganism is tested; in some biochemical test systems (e.g., minisystems), biotype refers to the specific code number generated by the test results (Chap. 12).

Black Piedra (pee-a'-druh). A hair infection caused by the mould *Piedraia hortae* (Chap. 20).

Blocking Antibodies. Immunoglobulin G (IgG) antibodies produced by the body in response to allergy shots; they combine with allergens, thus preventing the allergens from attaching to IgE antibodies on the surface of basophils and mast cells (Chap. 16).

Botulinal (bot'-you-ly-nal) **Toxin.** The neurotoxin produced by *Clostridium botulinum*; causes botulism; known by various other names such as botulin and botulinum toxin (Chap. 14).

Botulism. A neurological disease caused by a neurotoxin (botulinal toxin) produced by *C. botulinum*, a spore-forming, anaerobic, Gram-positive bacillus (Chap. 19).

Brightfield Microscope. Alternate name for a compound light microscope; refers to the fact that objects are observed against a bright background (or bright field) (Chap. 2).

Broad-Spectrum Antibiotics. Antibiotics that are effective against a wide range of bacteria; they are effective against both Gram-positive and Gram-negative bacteria (Chap. 9).

Bronchitis (brong-ky'-tis). Inflammation of the mucous membrane lining of the bronchial tubes (Chap. 17).

Bronchopneumonia (brong'-ko-new-mow'-nee-uh). Combination of bronchitis and pneumonia (Chap. 17).

C

Calibrated Loop. A bacteriologic loop manufactured to contain a precise volume of liquid (usually 0.01 or 0.001 mL) (Chap. 13).

Candidiasis (kan-duh-dy'-uh-sis). Infection with, or disease caused by, a yeast in the genus *Candida*—usually *Candida albicans*; also known as *moniliasis* (Chap. 10).

Capnophile (cap'-no-file). An organism that grows best in the presence of increased concentrations of carbon dioxide; such an organism is said to be *capnophilic* (Chap. 4).

Capsid (kap'-syd). The external protein coat or covering of a virion (Chap. 4).

Capsomeres (kap'-so-meers). The individual protein subunits that make up the capsid of some virions (Chap. 4).

Capsule (kap'-sool). An organized layer of glycocalyx, firmly attached to the outer surface of a bacterial cell wall; some yeasts are also encapsulated (Chap. 3).

Carbohydrates (kar-boh-high'-drates). Organic compounds containing carbon, hydrogen, and oxygen in a ratio of 1:2:1; also known as *saccharides* (Chap. 6).

Carbuncle (kar'-bung-kul). A deep-seated pyogenic (pus-producing) infection of the skin, usually arising from a coalescence of furuncles (Chap. 17).

Carrier (keh'-ree-er). An individual having an asymptomatic infection that can be transmitted to other susceptible individuals (Chap. 10).

Catabolic (cat-uh-bohl'-ik) **Reactions.** Metabolic reactions that involve the breaking of chemical bonds and the release of energy; also known as *degradative reactions* (Chap. 7).

Catabolism (kuh-tab'-oh-lizm). Term referring to all the catabolic reactions that occur within a cell (Chap. 7).

Catalyst (kat'-uh-list). A substance (usually an enzyme) that speeds up a chemical reaction but is not itself consumed or permanently changed in the process (Chap. 6).

Catalyze (cat'-uh-lyz). To act as a catalyst; to speed up a reaction (Chap. 6).

Cell (sell). The smallest unit of living structure capable of independent existence (Chap. 3).

Cell-Mediated Immunity. A type of immunity involving many different cell types (e.g., macrophages, various types of lymphocytes), but where antibodies play only a minor role, if any; also known as *delayed hypersensitivity* (Chap. 16).

Cell Membrane (sell mem'-brain). The protoplasmic boundary of all cells; provides selective permeability and serves other important functions (Chap. 3).

Cell Theory. The theory stating that all living organisms are composed of cells (Chap. 3).

Cell Wall. The outermost layer of many types of cells (e.g., algal, bacterial, fungal, and plant cells); it serves to protect the cell (Chap. 3).

Cellular Microbe. A microbe that is composed of cells (e.g., bacteria, algae, protozoa) (Chap. 1).

Cellulose (sell'-you-los). A polysaccharide found in the cell walls of algae and plants (Chap. 3).

Centimeter (sen'-tuh-me-ter). One hundredth of a meter (Chap. 2).

Central Dogma. The flow of genetic information within a cell; from DNA to an mRNA molecule to a protein molecule (Chap. 6).

Cephalosporinase (sef'-uh-low-spore'-uh-nase). An enzyme that destroys the β-lactam ring in cephalosporin antibiotics; a type of β-lactamase (Chap. 9).

Cerebrospinal (sir-ee'-broh-spy'-nul) **Fluid (CSF).** The fluid within the spinal cord and the ventricles and cavities of the brain; also referred to simply as *spinal fluid* (Chap. 13).

Cervicitis (sir-vuh-sigh'-tis). Inflammation of the cervix (the part of the uterus that opens into the vagina) (Chap. 17).

Cestodes (sess'-toadz). A subcategory of flatworms; includes tapeworms (Chap. 21).

Chemically Defined Media. Types of culture media where the exact chemical composition is known (Chap. 8).

Chemoautotroph (keem'-oh-awe'-toe-trof). An organism that uses chemicals as an energy source and carbon dioxide as a carbon source; a type of autotroph (Chap. 7).

Chemoheterotroph (keem'-oh-het'-er-oh-trof). An organism that uses chemicals as an energy source and organic chemicals as a carbon source; a type of heterotroph (Chap. 7).

Chemokines. Chemotactic agents produced by various types of cells in the body (Chap. 15).

Chemolithotroph (keem'-oh-lith'-oh-trof). A type of chemotroph that uses inorganic compounds as a source of energy; also referred to as a *lithotroph* (Chap. 7).

Chemoorganotroph (keem'-oh-or-gan'-oh-trof). A type of chemotroph that uses organic compounds as a source of energy; also referred to as an *organotroph* (Chap. 7).

Chemosynthesis (keem'-oh-syn'-thuh-sis). The process of obtaining energy and synthesizing organic compounds from simple inorganic reactions; carried out by some chemoautotrophic bacteria (Chap. 7).

Chemotactic (keem'-oh-tack'-tick) **Agents.** Chemical substances that attract leukocytes; also referred to as *chemotactic factors*, *chemotactic substances*, and *chemoattractants* (Chap. 15).

Chemotaxis (keem'-oh-tack'-sis). The movement of cells in response to a chemical (e.g., the attraction of phagocytes to an area of injury) (Chap. 15).

Chemotherapeutic (keem'-oh-ther-uh-pyu'-tik) **Agent.** Any chemical used to treat any disease or medical condition (Chap. 9).

Chemotherapy (keem'-oh-ther'-uh-pee). The treatment of a disease (including an infectious disease) using chemical substances or drugs (Chap. 9).

Chemotroph (keem'-oh-trof). An organism that uses chemicals as an energy source (Chap. 7).

Chitin (ky'-tin). A polysaccharide found in fungal cell walls but not found in the cell walls of other microorganisms; also found in the exoskeleton of beetles and crabs (Chap. 3).

Chloroplast (klor'-oh-plast). A membrane-bound organelle found in the cytoplasm of algal and plant cells; a *plastid* that contains chlorophyll (Chap. 3).

Cholera. A diarrheal disease caused by *Vibrio cholerae*, a curved Gram-negative bacillus (Chap. 19).

Choleragin (kol'-er-uh-jen). The enterotoxin that causes cholera; produced by *V. cholerae* (Chap. 19).

Chromosomes (kro'-mow-soamz). Cellular structures where most (sometimes all) of the cell's genes are located; eucaryotic chromosomes consist of linear double-stranded DNA molecules and proteins (histones and nonhistone proteins); a procaryotic chromosome usually consists of a single, long, supercoiled, circular, double-stranded DNA molecule (Chap. 3).

Chronic Disease. A disease having an insidious (slow) onset and a long duration (Chap. 14).

Ciliates (sil'-ee-itz), sing. *ciliate*. Ciliated protozoa (Chap. 5).

Cilium (sil'-ee-um), pl. *cilia*. A thin, usually short, hair-like organelle of motility (Chap. 3).

Clean-Catch, Midstream Urine (CCMS urine). A urine specimen that has been collected in a manner that minimizes contamination with indigenous microflora; the proper type of specimen for a urine culture (Chap. 13).

Clinical Laboratory Scientists. Laboratory professionals possessing a baccalaureate degree in clinical laboratory science (medical technology); also known as *medical technologists* or *MTs* (Chap. 13).

Clinical Laboratory Technicians. Laboratory professionals possessing an associate degree in clinical laboratory technology (medical laboratory technology); also known as *medical laboratory technicians* or *MLTs* (Chap. 13).

Clinical Specimens. Various types of specimens (e.g., blood, urine, cerebrospinal fluid) collected from patients (Chap. 13).

Clinically Relevant Laboratory Results. Laboratory results that provide the physician with useful, accurate information about a patient's disease (Chap. 13).

Coagulase (ko-ag'-yu-lace). A bacterial enzyme that causes plasma to clot; converts fibrinogen (a plasma protein) to fibrin (Chap. 14).

Coccidioidomycosis (kok-sid-ee-oy'-doe-my-ko'-sis). A systemic mycosis caused by *Coccidioides immitis*, a dimorphic fungus (Chap. 20).

Coccobacillus (kok'-ko-buh-sil'-us), pl. *coccobacilli*. A very short bacillus (Chap. 4).

Coccus (kok'-us), pl. *cocci*. A spherical bacterium (Chap. 2).

Codon (koh'-don). A sequence of three consecutive nucleotides in a strand of mRNA that provides the genetic information (code) for a certain amino acid to be incorporated into a growing protein chain (Chap. 6).

Coenzyme (koh'-en-zym). A type of cofactor; several vitamins are coenzymes (Chap. 6).

Cofactor (koh'-fak'-tor). An ion or molecule essential for the enzymatic action of certain proteins (called apoenzymes) (Chap. 6).

Colicin (kol'-uh-sin). A type of bacteriocin produced by *Escherichia coli* and other closely related bacteria (Chap. 10).

Coliforms (ko'-lee-forms). *E. coli* and other lactose-fermenting members of the Family *Enterobacteriaceae* (Chap. 11).

Colitis (ko-ly'-tis). Inflammation of the colon (the large intestine) (Chap. 17).

Collagen (kol'-luh-jen). The major protein in the white fibers of connective tissue, cartilage, and bone (Chap. 14).

Collagenase (kol'-uh-juh-nace). A bacterial enzyme that causes the breakdown of collagen (Chap. 14).

Commensalism (ko-men'-sul-izm). A symbiotic relationship in which one party derives benefit and the other party is unaffected; many members of the indigenous microflora are commensals (Chap. 10).

Communicable (kuh-myun'-uh-kuh-bul) **Disease.** A disease capable of being transmitted from person to person (Chap. 11).

Community-Acquired Infection. Any infection acquired outside a healthcare setting (Chap. 12).

Competence (kom'-puh-tense). As used in this book, the ability of a bacterial cell to take up (absorb) free (naked) DNA from the environment; may lead to transformation (Chap. 7).

Competent Bacteria. Bacteria capable of taking up (absorbing) free (naked) DNA from the environment (Chap. 7).

Complement (kom'-pluh-ment). A protein complex of 25 to 30 components (including proteins designated C1 through C9) found in blood; involved in inflammation, chemotaxis, phagocytosis, and lysis of bacteria (Chap. 15).

Complement Cascade. The stepwise manner in which proteins of the complement system (complement components) interact with each other (Chap. 15).

Complex Media. Culture media, the exact chemical composition of which is unknown; often contain ground-up animal organs (e.g., brain, heart, liver) or yeast extract (Chap. 8).

Compound Light Microscope. A compound microscope that uses visible light as its source of illumination (Chap. 2).

Compound Microscope. A microscope containing more than one magnifying lens (Chap. 2).

Conidium (ko-nid'-ee-um), pl. *conidia*. An asexual fungal spore (Chap. 5).

Conjugate (kon'-ju-git) **Vaccine.** A vaccine prepared by linking a weakly antigenic molecule (e.g., bacterial capsule material) to a powerful antigen (Chap. 16).

Conjugation (kon-ju-gay'-shun). As used in this book, the union of two bacterial cells for the purpose of genetic transfer; *not* a reproductive process (Chap. 3).

Conjunctiva (kon-junk-ty'vuh). The mucous membrane that lines the eyelids and covers the anterior portion of the eyeball (Chap. 17).

Conjunctivitis (kon-junk'-tuh-vi'-tis). Inflammation of the conjunctiva (Chap. 17).

Constitutive Genes. Genes that are expressed at all times (Chap. 6).

Contact Precautions. Standardized safety precautions that are practiced in a healthcare setting to prevent infections transmitted by contact (Chap. 12).

Contagious Disease. A disease easily transmitted from one person to another; a type of communicable disease (Chap. 11).

Contamination (kon-tam-uh-nay'-shun). As used in this book, a condition indicating the presence of undesirable or accidentally introduced microorganisms (which would be referred to as *contaminants*) (Chap. 8).

Contractile Vacuole. An organelle that pumps water out of a protozoal cell (Chap. 5).

Convalescent (kon-vuh-less'-ent) **Carrier.** A person who no longer shows the signs or symptoms of a particular infectious disease but continues to harbor and transmit the causative agent during the convalescence period (Chap. 11).

Covalent (koh-vayl'-ent) **Bond.** A type of chemical bond in which two atoms share a pair of electrons (Chap. 6).

Crenated (kree'-nay-ted). Wrinkled, shriveled; (e.g., the appearance of erythrocytes placed into a hypertonic solution) (Chap. 8).

Crenation (kree-nay'-shun). The process of becoming, or state of being, crenated (Chap. 8).

Cryptococcosis (krip'-toe-kok-oh'-sis). A fungal infection caused by *Cryptococcus neoformans*, an encapsulated yeast (Chap. 20).

Cutaneous Anaphylaxis. Swelling and redness at the site where an antigen is injected intradermally or subcutaneously; also known as a *wheal-and-flare reaction* (Chap. 16).

Cyanobacteria (sigh'-an-oh-bak-tier'-ee-uh). A group of photosynthetic bacteria (Chap. 4).

Cyst. As the term applies to parasitology, the dormant, survival stage in a protozoan's life cycle; its tough wall enables the cyst to resist desiccation and temperature extremes (Chap. 5).

Cystitis (sis-ty'-tis). Inflammation or infection of the urinary bladder (Chap. 17).

Cytokines (sigh'-toe-kynz). Soluble chemical messages released by cells of the body; the manner in which different types of cells communicate with each other; examples include *lymphokines* (produced by lymphocytes) and *monokines* (produced by monocytes) (Chap. 16).

Cytokinesis (sigh'-toe-kuh-knee'-sis). Division of the cytoplasm, resulting in two daughter cells; follows mitosis (Chap. 3).

Cytology (sigh-tol'-oh-gee). The study of cells (Chap. 3).

Cytoplasm (sigh'-toe-plazm). A type of protoplasm; lies outside the nucleus of a eucaryotic cell (Chap. 3).

Cytoskeleton. A system of fibers (microtubules, microfilaments, and intermediate filaments) running throughout the cytoplasm of eucaryotic cells (Chap. 3).

Cytostome (sigh'-toe-stoam). A primitive mouth possessed by some protozoa (Chap. 5).

Cytotoxins (sigh'-tow-tok'-sinz). Toxic substances that inhibit or destroy cells (Chap. 14).

D

Darkfield Microscope. A compound light microscope that has been fitted with a darkfield condenser; refers to the fact that objects are observed against a dark background (or dark field) (Chap. 2).

Death Phase. The part of a bacterial growth curve during which no multiplication occurs and organisms are dying; the fourth and final phase in a bacterial growth curve (Chap. 8).

Decimeter (des'-uh-me-ter). One tenth of a meter (Chap. 2).

Decomposers. Microorganisms that decompose or break down substances (Chap. 1).

Definitive Host. In a parasitic relationship, the host that harbors the adult or sexual stage of a parasite, or the sexual phase of the parasite's life cycle (Chap. 21).

Dehydration Synthesis Reaction. An anabolic reaction in which two molecules are bonded together as a result of the loss of a water molecule; also called a *dehydrolysis reaction* (Chap. 6).

Dehydrogenation (dee-hy'-drah-jen-ay'-shun) **Reactions.** Chemical reactions in which a pair of hydrogen atoms is removed from a compound, usually by the action of enzymes called *dehydrogenases* (Chap. 7).

Delayed-Type Hypersensitivity (DTH) Reactions. Hypersensitivity reactions that usually take more than 24 hours to manifest themselves; also known as *cell-mediated immune reactions* and *type IV hypersensitivity reactions* (Chap. 16).

Denitrifying (dee'-ni-truh-fy-ing) **Bacteria.** Bacteria capable of converting nitrates into nitrogen gas; the process is known as *denitrification* (Chap. 10).

Dental Caries (kay'-reez). Tooth decay (Chap. 17).

Deoxyribonucleic (dee-ox'-ee-ry'-bow-new-clay'-ick) **Acid (DNA).** A macromolecule containing the genetic code in the form of genes (Chap. 3).

Dermatitis (der-muh-ty'-tis). Inflammation of the skin (Chap. 17).

Dermatophytes (der-mah'-toh-fytes). Fungi that cause superficial mycoses of the skin, hair, and nails; the cause of tinea infections (ringworm infections) (Chap. 20).

Dermis (der'-mis). The layer of skin containing blood and lymphatic vessels, nerves and nerve endings, glands, and hair follicles (Chap. 17).

Desiccation (des-uh-kay'-shun). The process of being desiccated (thoroughly dried) (Chap. 8).

Diarrhea (die-uh-ree'-uh). An abnormally frequent discharge of semisolid or fluid fecal matter (Chap. 17).

Differential (dif-er-en'-shul) **Media.** Culture media that enable microbiologists to readily differentiate one organism or group of organisms from another (Chap. 8).

Differential Staining Procedures. Bacterial staining procedures that enable differentiation of two groups of bacteria; (e.g., the Gram stain enables differentiation of Gram-positive bacteria from Gram-negative bacteria) (Chap. 4).

Dimorphic (dy-more'-fik) **Fungus.** A fungus that can exist either as a yeast or a mould (Chap. 5).

Dimorphism (dy-more'-fizm). A phenomenon whereby an organism can exist in two shapes or forms; (e.g., dimorphic fungi can exist either as yeasts or moulds) (Chap. 5).

Dipeptide (dy-pep'-tide). A protein consisting of two amino acids held together by a peptide bond (Chap. 6).

Diphtheria. A bacterial disease caused by toxigenic (diphtheria toxin-producing) strains of *Corynbebacterium diphtheriae*, Gram-positive bacilli (Chap. 19).

Diplobacilli (dip'-low-bah-sill'-eye). Bacilli arranged in pairs (Chap. 4).

Diplococci (dip'-low-kok'-sigh). Cocci arranged in pairs (Chap. 4).

Diploid (dip'-loyd) **Cells.** Eucaryotic cells containing two sets of chromosomes (Chap. 3).

Disaccharide (die-sack'-uh-ride). A carbohydrate consisting of two monosaccharides; examples include sucrose (table sugar), lactose (milk sugar), and maltose (malt sugar) (Chap. 6).

Disinfectant (dis-in-fek'-tent). A chemical agent used to destroy pathogens or inhibit their growth and vital activity; usually refers to a chemical agent used on nonliving materials (Chap. 8).

Disinfection (dis-in-fek'-shun). The process of destroying pathogens and their toxins (Chap. 8).

DNA Nucleotides. The building blocks of DNA; each DNA nucleotide consists of a nitrogenous base, deoxyribose, and a phosphate group (Chap. 6).

DNA Polymerase (poh-lim'-er-ace). The most important enzyme required in DNA replication (Chap. 6).

DNA Replication (rep-luh-kay'-shun). Production of two new DNA molecules (called *daughter molecules*) from one parent DNA molecule (Chap. 6).

DNA Vaccine. An experimental type of vaccine that stimulates host cells to produce numerous copies of a harmless microbial protein (antigen); the host's immune system then produces antibodies directed against the protein, and these antibodies protect the person from infection with the pathogen that possesses the protein; also known as a *gene vaccine* (Chap. 16).

Double Bond. A type of chemical bond, containing two pairs of shared electrons (Chap. 6).

Droplet Precautions. Standardized safety precautions that are practiced in a healthcare setting to prevent infections transmitted by droplets (Chap. 12).

Drug-Binding Site. A specific molecule on the surface of a cell that a particular drug attaches to (Chap. 9).

Dysentery (dis'-en-tay-ree). Frequent watery stools, accompanied by abdominal pain, fever, and dehydration; the stool specimens may contain blood or mucus (Chap. 17).

E

Ebola (ee-bow'-luh) **Virus.** An especially large virus that causes viral hemorrhaogic fever. (Chap. 18).

Ecology (ee-kol'-oh-jee). The branch of biology concerned with the total complex of interrelationships among living organisms; encompassing the relationships of organisms to each other, to the environment, and to the entire energy balance within a given ecosystem (Chap. 7).

Ecosystem (ee'-koh-sis-tem). An ecologic system that includes all the organisms and the environment within which they occur naturally (Chap. 7).

Ectoparasite (ek'-toh-par'-uh-site). A parasite that lives on the external surface of its host (Chap. 21).

Edema (uh-dee'-muh). Swelling caused by an accumulation of watery fluid in cells, tissues, or body cavities; swollen areas are described as being *edematous* (Chap. 15).

Ehrlichiosis. A bacterial disease caused by *Ehrlichia* spp., Gram-negative bacilli that are obligate intracellular pathogens (Chap. 19).

Electron (ee-lek'-tron) **Micrograph.** Photograph taken through the lens system of an electron microscope (Chap. 2).

Electron Microscope. A type of microscope that uses electrons as a source of illumination (Chap. 2).

Electron Transport Chain. A series of biochemical reactions by which energy is transferred in a step-wise manner; a major source of energy in some cells (Chap. 7).

Empiric (em-peer'-uh-kul) **Therapy.** Treatment or therapy that is initiated by a physician (or other healthcare professional) before receipt of test results (Chap. 9).

Empty Magnification. Microscopy term meaning an increase in magnification without any concurrent increase in resolving power (Chap. 2).

Encephalitis (en-sef-uh-ly'-tis). Inflammation or infection of the brain (Chap. 13).

Encephalomyelitis (en-sef-uh-low-my'-uh-ly'-tis). Inflammation or infection of the brain and spinal cord (Chap. 17).

Endemic (en-dem'-ick) **Disease.** A disease that is always present in a community or geographic area (Chap. 11).

Endemic Typhus. Synonym for fleaborne typhus fever; caused by *Rickettsia typhi*, a Gram-negative bacillus that is an obligate intracellular pathogen (Chap. 19).

Endocarditis (en'-doh-kar-dy'-tis). Inflammation of the endocardium (the innermost lining of the heart) (Chap. 17).

Endoenzyme (en'-doh-en'-zym). An enzyme produced by a cell that remains within the cell; an intracellular enzyme (Chap. 7).

Endometritis (en'-dough-me-try'-tis). Inflammation of the endometrium (the inner layer of the uterine wall) (Chap. 17).

Endoparasite (en-doh-par'-uh-site). A parasite that lives within the body of its host (Chap. 21).

Endoplasmic Reticulum (end-oh-plaz'-mick re-tick'-you-lum) **(ER).** A network of membranous tubules and flattened sacs in the cytoplasm of a eucaryotic cell; ER with attached ribosomes is called *rough ER* (*RER*) or *granular ER*; ER having no attached ribosomes is called *smooth ER* (*SER*) (Chap. 3).

Endospore (en'-dough-spore). Thick-walled, resistant body formed within a bacterial cell for the purpose of survival; a bacterial cell produces only one endospore, and from that endospore emerges (a process known as *germination*) one bacterial cell; also referred to as a *bacterial spore* (Chap. 3).

Endosymbiont (en'-doh-sym'-be-ont). The party in a symbiotic relationship that lives within the body of the other symbiont (Chap. 10).

Endotoxin (en-doh-tok'-sin). The lipid portion of the lipopolysaccharide found in the cell walls of Gram-negative bacteria; intracellular toxin (Chap. 14).

Enriched Media. Culture media that enable microbiologists to isolate fastidious organisms from samples or specimens and grow them in the laboratory (Chap. 8).

Enteric (en-tare'-ik) **Bacilli.** Gram-negative bacilli in the Family *Enterobacteriaceae* (Chap. 10).

Enteritis (en-ter-eye'-tis). Inflammation of the intestines, usually referring to the small intestine (Chap. 17).

Enterohemorrhagic *E. Coli.* Strains of *E. coli* that produce enterotoxins that cause bloody diarrhea and hemolytic uremic syndrome (Chap. 19).

Enterotoxigenic *E. Coli.* Strains of *E. coli* that produce toxins that cause diarrhea (Chap. 19).

Enterotoxin (en-ter-oh-tok'-sin). A bacterial exotoxin specific for cells of the intestinal mucosa (Chap. 14).

Enterovirulent *E. Coli.* Strains of *E. coli* that produce toxins that cause gastrointestinal diseases; examples include enterohemorrhagic *E. coli* and enterotoxigenic *E. coli* (Chap. 19).

Enzyme (en'-zyme). A protein molecule that catalyzes (causes or speeds up) a chemical reaction; remains unchanged in the process; a biologic catalyst (Chap. 6).

Eosinophil (ee-oh-sin'-oh-fil). A type of granulocyte found in blood; its granules contain basic substances (e.g., major basic protein) that attract acidic dyes (Chap. 15).

Eosinophilia (ee'-oh-sin-oh-fil'-ee-uh). An abnormally high number of eosinophils in the bloodstream (Chap. 15).

Epidemic (ep-uh-dem'-ick) **Disease.** A disease occurring in a higher than usual number of cases in a population during a given time interval (Chap. 11).

Epidemic Typhus. Synonym for louseborne typhus fever; caused by *Rickettsia prowazekii*, a Gram-negative bacillus that is an obligate intracellular pathogen (Chap. 19).

Epidemiology (ep-uh-dee-me-ol'-oh-jee). The study of relationships between the various factors that determine the frequency and distribution of diseases (Chap. 11).

Epidermis (ep-ee-derm'-is). The superficial epithelial portion of the skin (Chap. 17).

Epididymitis (ep-uh-did-uh-my'-tis). Inflammation of the epididymis (a tubular structure within the testis) (Chap. 17).

Epiglottitis (ep-ee-glot-eye-tis). Inflammation of the epiglottis (the mouth of the windpipe) (Chap. 17).

Episome (ep'-eh-som). An extrachromosomal element (plasmid) that may either integrate into the host bacterium's chromosome or replicate and function stably when physically separated from the chromosome (Chap. 7).

Epstein-Barr Virus. The virus that causes infectious mononucleosis; an oncogenic virus that causes several types of cancer. (Chap. 18).

Erysipelis (err-eh-sip'-uh-lis). An acute cutaneous cellulitis caused by *Streptococcus pyogenes* (Chap. 19).

Erythema (air-uh-thee'-muh). Redness of the skin; a reddened area of skin is described as being *erythematous* (Chap. 16).

Erythrocytes (ee-rith'-roh-sites). Red blood cells (Chap. 13).

Erythrogenic (ee-rith-roh-jen'-ick) **Toxin.** The exotoxin produced by *S. pyogenes* that causes scarlet fever; *erythrogenic* means "produces redness," referring to the red rash of scarlet fever (Chap. 14).

Essential Amino Acids. Amino acids that must be provided to an organism because the organism is unable to synthesize them (Chap. 6).

Essential Fatty Acids. Fatty acids that must be provided to an organism because the organism is unable to synthesize them (Chap. 6).

Essential Nutrients. Any nutrients that must be provided to an organism because the organism is unable to synthesize them (Chap. 7).

Etiologic (e'-tee-oh-loj'-ik) **Agent.** The causative agent of an infectious disease (i.e., the pathogen that causes the disease) (Chap. 1).

Etiology. Cause; as in the etiology of a disease (Chap. 1).

Eucarya (you-ker'-ee-uh). One of the three domains in the three-domain system of classification; alternate spelling = *Eukarya*; members of this domain are eucaryotes; the other two domains are *Archaea* and *Bacteria* (Chap. 3).

Eucaryotic (you'-kar-ee-ah'-tick) **Cells.** Cells containing a true nucleus; organisms possessing such cells are referred to as *eucaryotes*; can also be spelled eukaryotic (Chap. 3).

Exfoliative (eks-foh'-lee-uh-tiv) **Toxin.** The exotoxin produced by *Staphylococcus aureus* that causes staphylococcal scalded skin syndrome (SSSS); also known as *epidermolytic toxin* (Chap. 14).

Exoenzyme (ek-soh-en'-zyme). An enzyme produced by a cell that is released from the cell; an extracellular enzyme (Chap. 7).

Exotoxin (ek-soh-tok'-sin). A toxin that is released from the cell; an extracellular toxin (Chap. 14).

Exudate (eks'-yu-date). Any fluid (e.g., pus) that exudes (oozes) from tissue, often as a result of injury, infection, or inflammation (Chap. 17).

F

Facultative (fak'-ul-tay-tive) **Anaerobe.** An organism that can live either in the presence or absence of oxygen (Chap. 4).

Facultative Intracellular Pathogen. A pathogen that can live either intracellularly or extracellularly (Chap. 14).

Facultative Parasite. An organism that is capable of being a parasite, but is also capable of a free-living existence (Chap. 21).

Fascia (fash'-ee-uh). A sheet of fibrous tissue that envelops the body beneath the skin; also encloses muscles and groups of muscles (Chap. 19).

Fasciitis (fas-ee-eye'-tis). Inflammation in fascia (Chap. 19).

Fastidious (fas-tid'-ee-us) **Microorganisms.** Microorganisms that are difficult to isolate from specimens and grow in the laboratory, owing to their complex nutritional requirements (Chap. 1).

Fatty Acid. Any acid derived from fats by hydrolysis; fatty acids are the building blocks of lipids (Chap. 6).

Fermentation (fer-men-tay'-shun). An anaerobic biochemical pathway in which substances are broken down, and energy and reduced compounds are produced; oxygen does not participate in the process (Chap. 7).

Fermentative Pathways. Metabolic pathways in which oxygen does not participate (Chap. 7).

Fimbriae (fim'-bree-ee), sing. *fimbria* (fim'-bree-uh). See *pili* (Chap. 3).

Fixed Macrophages. Macrophages that remain localized within certain organs and tissues; also known as *histocytes* or *histiocytes* (Chap. 15).

Flagella (fluh-jel'-uh), sing. *flagellum*. Whiplike organelles of motility; procaryotic and eucaryotic flagella differ in structure; procaryotic flagella are composed of a protein called *flagellin*; eucaryotic flagella contain nine doublet microtubules arranged around two central microtubules (a 9 + 2 arrangement) (Chap. 3).

Flagellates (flaj'-eh-letz). Flagellated protozoa (Chap. 5).

Flagellin (flaj'-eh-lin). The protein of which bacterial flagella are composed (Chap. 3).

Fluorescence (floor'-es-ence) **Microscope.** A type of compound light microscope that uses an ultraviolet (UV) light source (Chap. 2).

Folliculitis (foh-lick-you-ly'-tis). Inflammation of a hair follicle, the sac that contains a hair shaft (Chap. 17).

Fomites (foh'-mitz). Inanimate objects or substances capable of absorbing and transmitting a pathogen (e.g., clothing, bed linens, towels, eating utensils) (Chap. 11).

Fungemia (fun-gee'-me-uh). The presence of fungi in the bloodstream (Chap. 13).

Fungi (fun'-ji), sing. *fungus*. Eucaryotic, nonphotosynthetic microorganisms that can be either saprophytic or parasitic (Chap. 5).

Fungicidal (fun-juh-sigh'-dull) **Agent.** A chemical agent or drug that kills fungi; a *fungicide* or *mycocide* (Chap. 8).

Furuncle (few'-rung-kul). A localized pyogenic (pusproducing) infection of the skin, usually resulting from folliculitis; often referred to as a *boil* (Chap. 17).

G

Gangrene (gang'-green). Necrosis (cell death) as a result of ischemia (lack of blood flow) (Chap. 19).

Gas Gangrene. Gangrene caused by *Clostridium* spp.; the gas that forms in the necrotic tissue is the result of bacterial fermentations; also known as *myonecrosis* (Chap. 19).

Gastritis (gas-try'-tis). Inflammation of the mucosal lining of the stomach (Chap. 17).

Gastroenteritis (gas'-tro-en-ter-eye'-tis). Inflammation of the mucosal linings of the stomach and intestines (Chap. 17).

Gene (jeen). A functional unit of heredity that occupies a specific space (locus) on a chromosome; contains the genetic information that will enable a cell to produce a protein (usually), an rRNA molecule, or a tRNA molecule (Chap. 3).

Gene Product. The molecule (usually a protein) that is coded for by a gene (Chap. 3).

Gene Therapy. The insertion of normally functioning genes into a cell to correct problems associated with abnormally functioning genes (Chap. 7).

Generation Time. The time required for a cell to split into two cells; also called the *doubling time* (Chap. 3).

Genetic (juh-net'-ick) **Code.** The sequence of nucleotide bases on a DNA molecule that provides the information necessary for cells to produce gene products (Chap. 6).

Genetic Engineering. The insertion of foreign genes into microorganisms to enable the microorganisms to produce specific gene products or to enable them to be used for other purposes (Chap. 1).

Genetics (juh-net'-iks). The branch of science concerned with heredity (Chap. 7).

Genotype (jeen'-oh-type). The complete genetic constitution of an individual (i.e., all of that individual's genes); also known as the *genome* (Chap. 3).

Genus (jee'-nus), pl. *genera*. The first name in binomial nomenclature; a genus contains closely related species (Chap. 3).

Germ. Slang term for pathogen (Chap. 1).

Germicidal (jer-muh-sigh'-dull) **Agent.** A chemical agent or drug that kills pathogens; a *germicide* (Chap. 8).

Gingivitis (jin-juh-vy'-tis). Inflammation or infection of the gingiva (gums) (Chap. 17).

Glucose (glue'-kohs). A biologically important, six-carbon monosaccharide; a hexose; $C_6H_{12}O_6$; also called *dextrose*; the product of complete hydrolysis of polysaccharides such as cellulose, starch, and glycogen (Chap. 6).

Glycocalyx (gly-ko-kay'-licks). Extracellular material that may or may not be firmly attached to the outer surface of a bacterial cell wall; capsules and slime layers are examples (Chap. 3).

Glycogen (gly'-koh-jen). A polysaccharide stored by animal cells as a food reserve; composed of numerous glucose molecules (Chap. 6).

Glycolysis (gly-kol'-eh-sis). The anaerobic, energy-producing breakdown of glucose into two molecules of pyruvic acid via a series of chemical reactions; an example of a biochemical pathway; also called *anaerobic glycolysis* (Chap. 7).

Glycosidic (gly-ko-sid'-ik) **Bond.** The covalent bond that holds monosaccharides together in carbohydrate molecules (Chap. 6).

Golgi (goal'-jee) **Complex.** A membranous system located within the cytoplasm of a eucaryotic cell; associated with the transport and packaging of secretory proteins; also known as *Golgi apparatus* or *Golgi body* (Chap. 3).

Gonococcal (gon-oh-kok'-ul) **Ophthalmia** (of-thal'-me-uh) **Neonatorum** (ne'-oh-nay-tor'-um). A bacterial eye disease of newborns caused by *Neisseria gonorrhoeae*, a Gram-negative diplococcus (Chap. 19).

Gonococcus (gon-oh-kok'-us), pl. *gonococci*. A slang term for *N. gonorrhoeae*; abbreviated GC (Chap. 13).

Gonorrhea (gon-oh-ree'-uh). A sexually transmitted bacterial disease caused by *N. gonorrhoeae*, a Gram-negative diplococcus (Chap. 19).

Gram Stain. A differential staining procedure named for its developer, Hans Christian Gram, a Danish bacteriologist; differentiates bacteria into those that stain blue to purple (called *Gram-positive bacteria*) and those that stain pink to red (called *Gram-negative bacteria*) (Chap. 4).

Granulocytes (gran'-yu-loh-sites). A category of leukocytes having prominent cytoplasmic granules; neutrophils, eosinophils, and basophils are examples (Chap. 15).

Growth Curve. As used in this book, a graphic representation of the change in size of a bacterial population over a period of time; includes a lag phase, a log phase, a stationary phase, and a death phase (Chap. 8).

H

Haloduric (hail-oh-dur'-ick) **Organisms.** Organisms capable of surviving in a salty environment (Chap. 8).

Halophiles (hail'-oh-file). Organisms whose growth is enhanced by a high salt concentration; such an organism is said to be *halophilic* (Chap. 8).

Hantavirus (hon'-tuh-vi-rus) **Pulmonary Syndrome (HPS).** A pulmonary disease caused by various hantaviruses. (Chap. 18).

Haploid (hap'-loyd) **Cells.** Eucaryotic cells containing only one set of chromosomes (Chap. 3).

Hapten (hap'-ten). A small, nonantigenic molecule that becomes antigenic when combined with a larger molecule (e.g., a carrier protein) (Chap. 16).

Harmful Mutation. A mutation that causes harm to the mutant organism (Chap. 7).

HBV. Hepatitis B virus; the causative agent of serum hepatitis (Chap. 18).

Helminth (hel'-minth). A parasitic worm (Chap. 21).

Hemolysin (he-moll'-uh-sin). A bacterial enzyme capable of lysing erythrocytes (Chap. 14).

Hemolysis (he-moll'-uh-sis). Destruction of erythrocytes in such a manner that hemoglobin is liberated into the surrounding environment (Chap. 8).

Hepatitis (hep-uh-ty'-tis). Inflammation of the liver (Chap. 17).

Heptose. A monosaccharide containing seven carbon atoms (Chap. 6).

Herpes Labialis (her'-peez lay-bee-al-us). A cold sore (fever blister) caused by herpes simplex viruses (Chap. 18).

Herpes Simplex Viruses. Viruses that cause a variety of infections, including cold sores (fever blisters), genital herpes, and shingles (Chap. 18).

Heterotroph (het'-er-oh-trof). An organism that uses organic chemicals as a source of carbon (Chap. 7).

Hexose. A monosaccharide containing six carbon atoms (Chap. 6).

Histamine (his'-tuh-meen). Potent chemical released from basophils and mast cells during allergic reactions; causes constriction of bronchial smooth muscles and vasodilation (Chap. 16).

HIV. Human immunodeficiency virus; the causative agent of AIDS (Chap. 4).

Holoenzyme. Apoenzyme plus cofactor; a whole (functional) enzyme (Chap. 6).

Healthcare-Associated Infection. Any infection acquired while one is hospitalized (or while a patient in some other healthcare facility) (Chap. 12).

Host. In a parasitic relationship, the organism on or in which a parasite lives (Chap. 10).

Host Defense Mechanisms. Mechanisms that serve to protect the body from pathogens and the infections they cause (Chap. 15).

Humoral Immunity. A type of immunity in which antibodies play a major role; also known as *antibody-mediated immunity* (*AMI*) (Chap. 16).

Hyaluronic (high'-uh-lu-ron'-ick) **Acid.** A gelatinous mucopolysaccharide that acts as an intracellular cement in body tissue (Chap. 14).

Hyaluronidase (high'-uh-lu-ron'-uh-dase). A bacterial enzyme that breaks down hyaluronic acid; sometimes called *diffusing* or *spreading factor*, because it enables bacteria to invade deeper into tissue (Chap. 14).

Hybridoma (high-brid-oh'-muh). A tumor produced in vitro by fusion of mouse tumor cells and specific antibody-producing cells; used in the production of monoclonal antibodies (Chap. 16).

Hydrocarbon (high-droh-kar'-bun). An organic compound consisting of only hydrogen and carbon atoms (Chap. 6).

Hydrolysis (hi-drol'-eh-sis) **Reaction.** A chemical process whereby a compound is cleaved into two or more simpler compounds with the uptake of the H and OH parts of a water molecule on either side of the chemical bond that is cleaved (Chap. 6).

Hypersensitivity (high'-per-sen-suh-tiv'-uh-tee) **Reactions.** Exaggerated immunologic reactions that result from an overly sensitive immune system (Chap. 16).

Hypertonic (hi-per-tahn'-ick) **Solution.** A solution having a greater osmotic pressure than cells placed into that solution; a higher concentration of solutes exists outside the cell (Chap. 8).

Hyphae (hy'-fee), sing. *hypha*. Long, thin, intertwined, cytoplasmic filaments that make up a mould colony (*mycelium*) (Chap. 5).

Hypogammaglobulinemia (high'-poh-gam'-uh-glob-yu-luh-nee'-me-uh). Decreased quantity of the gamma fraction of serum globulin, including a decreased quantity of immunoglobulins (Chap. 16).

Hypotonic (hi-poh-tahn'-ick) **Solution.** A solution having a lower osmotic pressure than cells placed into that solution; a lower concentration of solutes exists outside the cell (Chap. 8).

I

Iatrogenic (eye-at-roh-jen'-ick) **Infection.** An infection caused by medical treatment; literally, "physician induced," but could be caused by any healthcare professional (Chap. 12).

Immediate-Type Hypersensitivity Reactions. Hypersensitivity reactions that occur from within a few minutes to 24 hours after contact with a particular antigen (Chap. 16).

Immune (im-myun'). To be free from the possibility of acquiring a particular infectious disease; to be resistant to an infectious disease (Chap. 16).

Immunity (im-myu'-nuh-tee). The status of being immune or resistant to an infectious disease (Chap. 16).

Immunocompetent (im'-you-no-kom'-puh-tent) **Person.** A person who is able to mount a normal immune response; a person whose immune system is functioning properly (Chap. 16).

Immunodiagnostic (im'-yu-noh-dy-ag-nos'-tick) **Procedures.** Laboratory procedures used to diagnose infectious diseases by using the principles of immunology; used to detect either antigen or antibody in patients' specimens (Chap. 16).

Immunoglobulins (im-yu-noh-glob'-yu-lin). A class of glycoproteins, which contains antibodies (Chap. 16).

Immunohematology Laboratory. The laboratory where donor blood is collected, tested, and stored; often referred to as the *Blood Bank* (Chap. 13).

Immunologist (im-you-nol'-oh-jist). One who specializes in the science of immunology (Chap. 16).

Immunology (im-you-nol'-oh-je). The study of immunity and the immune system (Chap. 16).

Immunosuppressed (im'-you-no-sue-pressed) **Person.** A person whose immune system is not functioning properly; such persons are also said to be *immunodepressed* or *immunocompromised* (Chap. 16).

Impetigo (im-peh-ty'-go). A bacterial skin disease caused by *S. aureus* and/or *S. pyogenes* (Chap. 19).

In Vitro (in vee'-trow). In an artificial environment, as in a laboratory setting; used in reference to what occurs *outside* an organism (Chap. 1).

In Vivo (in vee'-voh). Used in reference to what occurs *within* a living organism (Chap. 1).

Inactivated Vaccine. A vaccine prepared from inactivated (killed) microorganisms (Chap. 16).

Incidence. The number of new cases of a particular disease in a defined population during a specific period of time (Chap. 11).

Inclusion Bodies. Distinctive clusters of virions, frequently formed in the nucleus or cytoplasm of cells infected with certain viruses (Chap. 4).

Incubation. In microbiology, refers to holding a culture at a particular temperature for a certain length of time (Chap. 8).

Incubator. In microbiology, the chamber within which cultures are held at a particular temperature for a certain length of time (Chap. 8).

Incubatory (in'-kyu-buh-tor'-ee) **Carrier.** A person capable of transmitting a pathogen during the incubation period of a particular infectious disease (Chap. 11).

India Ink Preparation. A laboratory procedure primarily used to presumptively diagnose cryptococcal meningitis (Chap. 20).

Indigenous Microflora (in-dij'-uh-nus my-crow-floor-uh). Microorganisms that live on and in the healthy body; also called *indigenous microbiota*; referred to in the past as normal flora (Chap. 1).

Inducible Genes. Genes that are not expressed all the time (Chap. 6).

Infection (in-fek'-shun). The presence and multiplication of a pathogen on or within the body; often used as a synonym for infectious disease (Chap. 14).

Infectious Disease (in-fek'-shus di-zeez'). Any disease caused by a microbe that follows colonization of the body by that microbe (Chap. 1).

Infestation (in-fes-tay'-shun). The presence of ectoparasites (e.g., lice) on the body (Chap. 21).

Inflammation (in-fluh-may'-shun). A nonspecific pathologic process consisting of a dynamic complex of cytologic and histologic reactions that occur in response to an injury or abnormal stimulation by a physical, chemical, or biologic agent (Chap. 15).

Inflammatory Exudate. An accumulation of fluid, cells, and cellular debris at a site of inflammation (Chap. 15).

Inoculation. In microbiology, refers to adding a specimen to some type of culture medium (Chap. 8).

Inorganic (in-or-gan'-ick) **Chemistry.** The science dealing with all types of chemicals except those classified as organic compounds (Chap. 6).

Inorganic Compounds. Chemical compounds in which the atoms or radicals consist of elements other than carbon. (Chap. 6).

Interferons (in-ter-fear'-onz). Small, antiviral glycoproteins produced by cells infected with an animal virus; interferons are cell-specific and species-specific, but not virus-specific (Chap. 15).

Interleukins (in-ter-lu'-kinz). Lymphokines and polypeptide hormones; interleukin 1 is produced by monocytes; interleukin 2 is produced by lymphocytes; a category of cytokines (Chap. 15).

Intermediate Host. In a parasitic relationship, the host that harbors the larval or asexual stage of a parasite, or the asexual phase of the parasite's life cycle (Chap. 21).

Intraerythrocytic Pathogen. A pathogen that lives within erythrocytes (Chap. 14).

Intraleukocytic Pathogen. A pathogen that lives within leukocytes (Chap. 14).

Intrinsic Resistance. Resistance to a particular drug that is the result of some naturally occurring property of a bacterial cell (Chap. 9).

Ischemia (is-key'-me-uh). Localized anemia as a result of mechanical obstruction of the blood supply (Chap. 19).

Isotonic (eye-soh-tahn'-ick) **Solution.** A solution having the same osmotic pressure as cells placed into that solution; when the concentration of solutes outside the cell equals the concentration of solutes inside the cell (Chap. 8).

K

Keratitis (ker-uh-ty'-tis). Inflammation of the cornea (Chap. 17).

Keratoconjunctivitis (ker'-at-oh-kon-junk'-tuh-vi'-tis). Inflammation of the cornea and conjunctiva (Chap. 17).

Killer Cell. A type of cytotoxic T cell involved in cell-mediated immune responses (Chap. 16).

Kinase (ky'-nace). A bacterial enzyme capable of dissolving clots; also known as *fibrinolysin* (Chap. 14).

Koch's Postulates. A series of scientific steps, proposed by Robert Koch, that must be fulfilled to prove that a specific microorganism is the cause of a particular disease (Chap. 1).

KOH Prep. See *potassium hydroxide preparation*.

Koplik Spots. Small red spots containing a minute bluish white speck; they appear on the buccal mucosa early in measles. (Chap. 18).

Krebs Cycle. A biochemical pathway that is part of aerobic respiration; also known as the *citric acid cycle*, *tricarboxylic acid*, and *TCA cycle* (Chap. 7).

L

L-Forms. Abnormal forms of bacteria that have lost part or all of their rigid cell walls; sometimes the result of exposure of an organism to an antimicrobial agent; also called *L-phase variants*; the "L" is derived from Lister Institute (Chap. 4).

Lag Phase. The part of a bacterial growth curve during which multiplication of the organisms is very slow or scarcely appreciable; the first phase in a bacterial growth curve (Chap. 8).

Laryngitis (lar-in-ji'-tis). Inflammation of the mucous membrane of the larynx (voice box) (Chap. 17).

Latent Infection. An asymptomatic infection capable of manifesting symptoms under particular circumstances or if activated (Chap. 14).

Lecithin (less'-uh-thin). A name given to several types of phospholipids that are essential constituents of animal and plant cells (Chap. 14).

Lecithinase (less'-uh-thuh-nace). A bacterial enzyme capable of breaking down lecithin (Chap. 14).

Legionellosis (lee-juh-nel-oh'-sis). A bacterial respiratory disease caused by Gram-negative bacilli in the genus *Legionella* (Chap. 19).

Leprosy (lep-roh-see). A bacterial disease of the skin, peripheral nerves, and testes caused by the acid-fast bacillus *Mycobacterium leprae*; Hansen disease is a synonym for leprosy (Chap. 19).

Lethal Mutation. A mutation that causes death of the organism possessing the mutation (Chap. 7).

Leukemia (lew-key'-me-uh). A type of cancer in which there is a proliferation of abnormal leukocytes in the blood (Chap. 13).

Leukocidin (lu-koh-sigh'-din). A bacterial exotoxin capable of destroying leukocytes (Chap. 14).

Leukocytes (lu'-koh-sites). White blood cells (Chap. 13).

Leukocytosis (lu'-koh-sigh-toe'-sis). An increased number of leukocytes in the blood (Chap. 15).

Leukopenia (lu-koh-pea'-nee-uh). A decreased number of leukocytes in the blood (Chap. 15).

Lichen (like'-in). An organism composed of a green alga (or a cyanobacterium) and a fungus; an example of a symbiotic relationship known as *mutualism* (Chap. 5).

Life Cycle. The generation-to-generation sequence of stages that occur in the history of an organism (Chap. 3).

Light Microscope. A type of microscope that uses visible light as a source of illumination; also called a *brightfield microscope* (Chap. 2).

Lipids (lip'-ids). Organic compounds containing carbon, hydrogen, and oxygen that are insoluble in water but soluble in so-called fat solvents such as diethyl ether and carbon tetrachloride (Chap. 6).

Lipopolysaccharide (lip'-oh-pol-ee-sack'-a-ride). A macromolecule of combined lipid and polysaccharide, found in the cell walls of Gram-negative bacteria (Chap. 4).

Listeriosis (lis-tear'-ee-oh'-sis). A bacterial disease caused by *Listeria monocytogenes*, a Gram-positive bacillus (Chap. 19).

Lithotroph (lith'-oh-trof). An organism that uses inorganic molecules as a source of energy; a type of chemotroph (Chap. 7).

Localized Infection. An infection that remains localized; that does not spread; also known as a *local infection* or *focal infection* (Chap. 14).

Logarithmic (log'-uh-rith-mik) **Growth Phase.** The part of a bacterial growth phase during which maximal multiplication is occurring by geometric progression; the second phase in a bacterial growth curve; also known as the *log phase* or *exponential growth phase* (Chap. 8).

Logarithmic (log'-uh-ryth-mik) **Scale.** A scale (as on graph paper) in which the values of a variable (e.g., number of organisms at a particular point in time) are expressed as logarithms (Chap. 8).

Lophotrichous (low-fot'-ri-kus) **Bacterium.** A bacterium that possesses two or more flagella at one end (pole) of the cell (Chap. 3).

Lyme Disease. A bacterial disease caused by *Borrelia burgdorferi*, a loosely coiled spirochete; transmitted by tick bite (Chap. 19).

Lymphadenitis (lim'-fad-uh-ny'-tis). Inflammation of a lymph node or lymph nodes (Chap. 17).

Lymphadenopathy (lim-fad-uh-nop'-uh-thee). A disease process affecting a lymph node or lymph nodes (Chap. 17).

Lymphangitis (lim-fan-ji'-tis). Inflammation of lymphatic vessels (Chap. 17).

Lymphokines (lim'-foh-kinz). Soluble proteins released by sensitized lymphocytes; examples include chemotactic factors and interleukins; lymphokines represent one category of *cytokines* (Chap. 16).

Lyophilization (ly-ahf'-eh-leh-zay'-shun). Freeze-drying; a method of preserving microorganisms and foods (Chap. 8).

Lysogenic (lye-so-jen'-ick) **Bacterium.** A bacterium in the state of lysogeny (Chap. 7).

Lysogenic Conversion. Alteration of the genetic constitution of a bacterial cell due to lysogeny (Chap. 7).

Lysogeny (lye-soj'-eh-nee). A situation in which viral genetic material is integrated into the genome of the host cell (Chap. 7).

Lysosome (lye'-so-som). A membrane-bound vesicle found in the cytoplasm of eucaryotic cells; contains a variety of digestive enzymes, including lysozyme (Chap. 3).

Lysozyme (lye'-so-zyme). A digestive enzyme found in lysosomes, tears, and other body fluids; especially destructive to bacterial cell walls (Chap. 15).

Lytic Cycle. When a virus takes over the metabolic machinery of the host cell, reproduces itself, and ruptures (lyses) the host cell so that the newly assembled virions can escape (Chap. 4).

M

Macrophage (mak'-roh-faj). A large phagocytic leukocyte that arises from a monocyte (Chap. 15).

Malaise (muh-laz'). A generalized feeling of discomfort or uneasiness (Chap. 17).

Mast Cell. A tissue cell that closely resembles a basophil (Chap. 16).

Mechanical Vector. An arthropod vector (e.g., a house fly) that merely transports a pathogen from "point A" to "point B," and within which the pathogen neither multiplies nor matures (Chap. 21).

Medical Asepsis (ay-sep'-sis). The absence of pathogens in a patient's environment (Chap. 12).

Medical Aseptic (ay-sep'-tick) **techniques.** Procedures followed and steps taken to ensure medical asepsis (Chap. 12).

Meiosis (my-oh'-sis). The type of cell division that results in the formation of haploid gametes; also known as *meiotic division* (Chap. 3).

Meninges (muh-nin'-jez), sing. *meninx.* As used in this book, the membranes that surround the brain and spinal cord (Chap. 17).

Meningitis (men-in-ji'-tis). Inflammation or infection of the meninges (Chap. 13).

Meningococcemia (meh-ninge'-oh-kok-see'-me-uh). The presence of *Neisseria meningitidis* in the blood (Chap. 13).

Meningococcus (meh-ninge'-oh-kok-us), pl. *meningococci.* A slang term for *N. meningitidis* (Chap. 13).

Meningoencephalitis (muh-ning'-go-en-sef-uh-ly'-tis). Inflammation or infection of the brain and its surrounding membranes (Chap. 13).

Mesophile (meez'-oh-file). A microorganism having an optimum growth temperature between 25°C and 40°C; such an organism is said to be *mesophilic* (Chap. 8).

Messenger RNA (mRNA). The type of RNA that contains the exact same genetic information as a single gene on a DNA molecule; also called *informational RNA* (Chap. 6).

Metabolic (met-uh-bol'-ik) **Reactions.** Chemical reactions that occur within cells; of two types—catabolic and anabolic reactions (Chap. 7).

Metabolism (muh-tab'-oh-lizm). The sum of all the chemical reactions occurring in a cell; consists of *anabolism* and *catabolism* (Chap. 3).

Metabolite (muh-tab'-oh-lite). Any chemical product of metabolism (Chap. 7).

Microaerophiles (my-krow-air'-oh-files). Organisms requiring oxygen, but in concentrations lower than the 20% to 21% found in air; they usually require around 5% oxygen (Chap. 4).

Microbial (my-krow'-be-ul). Pertaining to microorganisms (Chap. 1).

Microbial Antagonism (an-tag'-un-izm). The killing, injury, or inhibition of one microbe by substances produced by another (Chap. 10).

Microbial Ecology. Study of the interrelationships among microbes and the world around them (other microbes, other living organisms, and the nonliving environment) (Chap. 1).

Microbial Intoxication. A disease that results from ingestion of a toxin that was produced by a pathogen in vitro (outside the body) (Chap. 1).

Microbial Physiology. The study of the vital life processes of microbes (Chap. 7).

Microbicidal (my-krow'-buh-sigh'-dull) **Agent.** A chemical or drug that kills microorganisms; a *microbicide* (Chap. 8).

Microbiologist (my'-crow-by-ol'-oh-jist). One who specializes in the science of microbiology (Chap. 1).

Microbiology (my'-crow-by-ol'-oh-je). The study of microbes (Chap. 1).

Microbistatic (my-krow'-buh-stat'-ick) **Agent.** A chemical agent or drug that inhibits the growth of microorganisms (Chap. 8).

Microcolonies. Tiny clusters of bacteria within biofilms (Chap. 10).

Micrometer (my-crow'-me-ter). A unit of length, equal to one millionth of a meter and one thousandth of a millimeter (Chap. 2).

Microorganisms (my'-crow-or'-gan-izms). Very small organisms; usually microscopic; also called *cellular microbes*; includes bacteria, certain algae, protozoa, and certain fungi (Chap. 1).

Microscope (my'-crow-skope). An optical instrument that permits one to observe a small object by producing an enlarged image of the object (Chap. 1).

Microscopic (my-crow-skop'-ik). If an object is microscopic, it is so small that it can only be seen using a microscope (Chap. 2).

Microtubules (my-kro'-two-bules). Cylindrical, cytoplasmic tubules found in the cytoskeleton of eucaryotic cells; may be related to the movement of chromosomes during nuclear division (Chap. 3).

Millimeter (mill'-uh-me-ter). A unit of length equal to one thousandth of a meter (Chap. 2).

Mimivirus. An extremely large double-stranded DNA virus that has been recovered from amebas.

Minisystems. Miniaturized biochemical test systems; often used when attempting to speciate microorganisms that have been isolated from clinical specimens (Chap. 13).

Mitochondria (my-toe-kon'-dree-uh), sing. *mitochondrion*. Eucaryotic organelles involved in cellular respiration for the production of energy; energy factories of the cell (Chap. 3).

Mitosis (my-toe'-sis). The type of cell division that results in the formation of two daughter cells, each of which contains exactly the same number of chromosomes as the parent cell; also known as *mitotic division* (Chap. 3).

Molecular Epidemiology. Determining relatedness of two microbial isolates in a healthcare setting by genotypic methods (Chap. 12).

Monoclonal (mon-oh-klo'-nul) **Antibodies.** Antibodies produced by a clone of genetically identical hybrid cells (Chap. 16).

Monocyte (mon'-oh-site). A relatively large mononuclear leukocyte (Chap. 15).

Monosaccharides (mon-oh-sak'-uh-rides). Carbohydrates that cannot be broken down into any simpler sugar by simple hydrolysis; simple sugars containing three to nine carbon atoms (usually three to seven); the basic units or building blocks of polysaccharides (Chap. 6).

Monotrichous (mah-not'-ri-kus) **Bacterium.** A bacterium that possesses only one flagellum (Chap. 3).

Monounsaturated Fatty Acid. A fatty acid containing only one double bond (Chap. 6).

Morbidity Rate. The number of new cases of a particular disease that occurred during a specified time period per a specifically defined population (e.g., per 100,000) (Chap. 11).

Mortality Rate. The ratio of the number of people who died of a particular disease during a specified time period per a specified population (e.g., per 100,000); also known as the *death rate* (Chap. 11).

Mucormycosis (mew'-kor-my-koh'-sis). Infection caused by a bread mould; also known as *zygomycosis* (Chap. 20).

Mutagen (myu'-tah-jen). Any agent that can cause a mutation to occur; (e.g., radioactive substances, x-rays, or certain chemicals); such an agent is said to be *mutagenic* (Chap. 7).

Mutant (myu'-tant). A phenotype in which a mutation is manifested (Chap. 7).

Mutation (myu-tay'-shun). An inheritable change in the character of a gene; a change in the sequence of base pairs in a DNA molecule (Chap. 7).

Mutualism (myu'-chew-ul-izm). A symbiotic relationship in which both parties derive benefit (Chap. 10).

Mycelium (my-see'-lee-um), pl. *mycelia*. A fungal colony; composed of a mass of intertwined hyphae (Chap. 5).

Mycologist (my-kol'-oh-jist). One who specializes in the science of mycology (Chap. 1).

Mycology (my-kol'-oh-gee). The study of fungi (Chap. 1).

Mycosis (my-ko'-sis), pl. *mycoses*. A fungal disease (Chap. 5).

Mycotoxicosis (my'-ko-tox'-uh-ko-sis), pl. *mycotoxicoses*. A microbial intoxication caused by a mycotoxin (Chap. 5).

Mycotoxins (my'-ko-tox-inz). Toxins produced by fungi (Chap. 5).

Myelitis (my-uh-ly'-tis). Inflammation or infection of the spinal cord (Chap. 17).

Myocarditis (my'-oh-kar-dy'-tis). Inflammation of the myocardium (the muscular walls of the heart) (Chap. 17).

N

Nanobacteria (nah'-no-back-teer'-ee-uh). Especially small bacteria; less than 1 μm in diameter; the sizes of these bacteria are expressed in nanometers (Chap. 4).

Nanometer (nan'-oh-me'-ter). A unit of length, equal to one billionth of a meter and one thousandth of a micrometer (Chap. 2).

Narrow-Spectrum Antibiotics. Antibiotics that are only effective against a narrow range of bacteria (e.g., perhaps only effective against certain Gram-positive bacteria, or only effective against certain Gram-negative bacteria) (Chap. 9).

Natural Active Acquired Immunity. Active acquired immunity that is acquired naturally (e.g., by being infected with a particular pathogen) (Chap. 16).

Natural Killer (NK) Cell. A type of cytotoxic human blood lymphocyte (Chap. 16).

Natural Passive Acquired Immunity. Passive acquired immunity that is acquired in a natural manner (e.g., when a fetus receives the mother's antibodies in utero) (Chap. 16).

Necrosis (nuh-kro'-sis). Cell death (Chap. 19).

Negative Stain. A staining procedure in which unstained objects can be seen against a stained background (Chap. 3).

Nematodes (nem'-uh-toadz'). Roundworms (Chap. 21).

Nephritis (nef-ry'-tis). Inflammation of the kidneys (Chap. 17).

Neurotoxin (new'-roh-tok'-sin). A bacterial exotoxin that attacks the nervous system (Chap. 14).

Neutralism (new'-trul-izm). A symbiotic relationship in which organisms occupy the same niche but do not affect one another (Chap. 10).

Neutrophil (nu'-tro-fil). A type of granulocyte found in blood; its granules contain neutral substances that attract neither acidic nor basic dyes; also called a *polymorphonuclear cell*, *poly*, or *PMN* (Chap. 15).

Nitrifying Bacteria. Bacteria capable of converting ammonia to nitrites and nitrites to nitrates; the process is known as *nitrification* (Chap. 10).

Nitrogen Fixation. The process by which atmospheric nitrogen gas is converted into ammonia (Chap. 4).

Nitrogen-Fixing Bacteria. Bacteria capable of converting nitrogen gas into ammonia; the process is known as *nitrogen fixation* (Chap. 10).

Nonpathogen (non'-path'-oh-jen). A microorganism that does not cause disease; such an organism is said to be *nonpathogenic* (Chap. 1).

Nonspecific Host Defense Mechanisms. Host defense mechanisms directed against all types of invading pathogens and other foreign substances (Chap. 15).

Nuclear (new'-klee-er) **Membrane.** The membrane that surrounds the chromosomes and nucleoplasm of a eucaryotic cell (Chap. 3).

Nucleic (new-klay'-ick) **Acids.** Macromolecules consisting of linear chains of nucleotides; DNA, mRNA, tRNA, and rRNA are examples (Chap. 6).

Nucleolus (new-klee'-oh-lus). A dense portion of the nucleus of a eucaryotic cell; where ribosomal RNA (rRNA) is produced (Chap. 3).

Nucleoplasm (new'-klee-oh-plazm). That portion of a eucaryotic cell's protoplasm that lies within the nucleus (Chap. 3).

Nucleotides (new'-klee-oh-tides). The basic units or building blocks of nucleic acids, each consisting of a purine or pyrimidine combined with a pentose (either ribose or deoxyribose) and a phosphate group (Chap. 6).

Nucleus (new'-klee-us), pl. *nuclei*. That portion of a eucaryotic cell that contains the nucleoplasm and chromosomes (Chap. 3).

O

Obligate Aerobe (air'-obe). An organism that requires 20% to 21% oxygen (the amount found in the air we breathe) to survive (Chap. 4).

Obligate Anaerobe (an'-air-obe). An organism that cannot survive in oxygen (Chap. 4).

Obligate Intracellular Pathogen. A pathogen that must reside within another living cell; examples include viruses, chlamydias, and rickettsias (Chap. 1).

Obligate Parasite. An organism that can only exist as a parasite; incapable of a free-living existence (Chap. 21).

Octad. A packet of eight cocci (Chap. 4).

Oncogenic (ong-koh-jen'-ick). An adjective meaning cancer-causing (Chap. 17).

Oncogenic Viruses. Viruses capable of causing cancer; also known as *oncoviruses* (Chap. 4).

Oophoritis (oh-of-or-eye'-tis). Inflammation or infection on an ovary (Chap. 17).

Opportunistic Pathogen (op-poor-tune'-is-tick path'-oh-jen). A microbe with the potential to cause disease, but does not do so under ordinary circumstances; may cause disease in susceptible persons with lowered resistance; also called an *opportunist* (Chap. 1).

Opsonins (op'-soh-ninz). Substances (such as antibodies or complement fragments) that enhance phagocytosis (Chap. 15).

Opsonization (op'-suh-nuh-zay'-shun). The process by which bacteria (or other particles) are altered so that they may be more readily and more efficiently engulfed by phagocytes; often involves coating the bacteria with antibodies or complement fragments (Chap. 15).

Orchitis (or-ky'-tis). Inflammation or infection of the testes (Chap. 17).

Organelles (or'-guh-nelz). General term for the various and diverse structures contained within a eucaryotic cell (e.g., mitochondria, Golgi complex, nucleus, endoplasmic reticulum, and lysosomes) (Chap. 3).

Organic (or-gan'-ick) **Chemistry.** The study of organic compounds; the study of carbon and its covalent bonds (Chap. 6).

Organic Compounds. Chemical compounds composed of atoms (some of which are carbon) held together by covalent bonds (Chap. 6).

Osmosis (oz-moh'-sis). The process by which a solvent (e.g., water) moves through a semipermeable membrane from a solution having a lower concentration of solutes (dissolved substances) to a solution having a higher concentration of solutes (Chap. 8).

Osmotic (oz-maht'-ick) **Pressure.** A measure of the tendency for water to move into a solution by osmosis; always a positive value (Chap. 8).

Otitis (oh-ty'-tis) **Externa.** Inflammation or infection of the outer ear canal (Chap. 17).

Otitis Media. Inflammation or infection of the middle ear (Chap. 17).

Oxidation (ok-seh-day'-shun). As used in this book, the loss of one or more electrons, thus making the atom more electropositive (Chap. 7).

Oxidation–Reduction Reactions. Paired chemical reactions involving the transfer of one or more electrons from one compound to another; reactions which involve both oxidation and reduction; also known as *redox reactions* (Chap. 7).

Oxidative Pathways. Metabolic pathways requiring the participation of oxygen (Chap. 7).

Otomycosis. A fungal ear infection (Chap. 20).

Oxygenic Photosynthesis (ox'-uh-gen'-ik foe-toe-sin'-thuh-sis). A type of photosynthesis in which oxygen is produced (Chap. 4).

P

Paleomicrobiology (pay'-ee-oh-my'-crow-by-ol'-oh-je). The study of ancient microbes (Chap. 1).

Pandemic (pan-dem'-ick) **Disease.** A disease occurring in epidemic proportions in several to many countries; sometimes occurring worldwide (Chap. 11).

Papillomaviruses. Viruses that cause human warts and some types of carcinoma. (Chap. 18).

Parasite (par'-uh-sight). An organism that lives on or in another living organism (called the *host*) and derives benefit from the host (usually in the form of nutrients) (Chap. 1).

Parasitemia (par'-uh-suh-tee'-me-uh). The presence of parasites in the blood (Chap. 13).

Parasitism (par'-uh-suh-tizm). A symbiotic relationship that is beneficial to one party (the parasite) and detrimental to the other party (the host) (Chap. 10).

Parasitologist (par'-uh-suh-tol'-oh-jist). One who specializes in the science of parasitology (Chap. 1).

Parasitology (par'-uh-suh-tol'-oh-jee). The study of parasites (Chap. 1).

Parenteral (puh-ren'-ter-ul) **Injection.** Injection of substances directly into the bloodstream (Chap. 11).

Parotitis (par-oh-ty'-tis). Inflammation of the parotid gland (a salivary gland located near the ear); also known as *parotiditis*; epidemic parotitis is a synonym for mumps (Chap. 18).

Passive Acquired Immunity. Immunity or resistance acquired as a result of receipt of antibodies produced by another person or by an animal (Chap. 16).

Passive Carrier. A person who harbors a particular pathogen without ever having had the infectious disease it causes (Chap. 11).

Pasteurization (pas'-tour-i-zay'-shun). A heating process that kills pathogens in milk, wines, and other beverages (Chap. 1).

Pathogen (path'-oh-jen). Disease-causing microorganism; such an organism is said to be *pathogenic* (Chap. 1).

Pathogenesis (path-oh-jen-uh-sis). The steps or mechanisms involved in the development of a disease (Chap. 14).

Pathogenicity (path'-oh-juh-nis'-uh-tee). The ability to cause disease (Chap. 14).

Pathologist (pah-thol'-oh-jist). A physician who is a specialist in pathology (Chap. 13).

Pathology (pah-thol'-oh-gee). The study of disease, especially structural and functional changes that result from disease processes (Chap. 13).

Pellicle (pel'-uh-kul). As used in this book, a thickened outer membrane possessed by certain protozoa (Chap. 5).

Pelvic Inflammatory Disease (PID). Acute or chronic inflammation in the pelvic cavity, usually referring to infection of the female genital tract (Chap. 17).

Penicillinase. An enzyme that destroys the β-lactam ring in penicillin molecules; a type of β-lactamase (Chap. 9).

Pentose. A monosaccharide containing five carbon atoms (Chap. 6).

Peptide Bond. The name given to the covalent bond that holds amino acids together in protein molecules (Chap. 6).

Peptidoglycan (pep'-tuh-doh-gly'-kan). A complex structure found in the cell walls of bacteria, consisting of carbohydrates and proteins (Chap. 3).

Pericarditis (per'-ee-kar-dy'-tis). Inflammation of the pericardium (the membrane or sac around the heart) (Chap. 17).

Periodontal (purr'-ee-oh-don'-tul) **Disease.** Disease around the teeth (Chap. 17).

Periodontitis (purr'-ee-oh-don-ty'-tis). Inflammation or infection of the *periodontium* (tissues that surround and support the teeth) (Chap. 17).

Peritrichous (peh-rit'-ri-kus) **Bacterium.** A bacterium that possesses flagella over its entire surface (Chap. 3).

Peroxisome (per-ok'-suh-some). A membrane-bound organelle found in eucaryotic cells, within which hydrogen peroxide is both produced and degraded (Chap. 3).

Pertussis (purr-tus'-is). Synonym for whooping cough; a bacterial respiratory disease caused by *Bordetella pertussis*, a Gram-negative bacillus (Chap. 19).

Petri (pea'-tree) **Dish.** A shallow, circular container made of thin glass or clear plastic, with a loosely fitting, overlapping cover; used in microbiology laboratories for cultivation of microorganisms on solid media (Chap. 1).

Phagocyte (fag'-oh-site). A cell capable of ingesting bacteria, yeasts, and other particulate matter by phagocytosis; amebae and certain leukocytes are examples of phagocytic cells (Chap. 3).

Phagocytosis (fag'-oh-sigh-toe'-sis). Ingestion of particulate matter involving the use of pseudopodia to surround the particle (Chap. 3).

Phagolysosome (fag-oh-ly'-soh-sohm). A membrane-bound vesicle formed by the fusion of a phagosome and a lysosome (Chap. 15).

Phagosome (fag'-oh-sohm). A membrane-bound vesicle containing an ingested particle (e.g., a bacterial cell); found in phagocytic cells (Chap. 15).

Pharyngitis (far-in-ji'-tis). Inflammation or infection of the throat; sore throat (Chap. 17).

Phase-Contrast Microscope. A type of compound light microscope that can be used to observe unstained living microorganisms (Chap. 2).

Phenotype (fee'-no-type). Manifestation of a genotype; all the attributes or characteristics of an individual (Chap. 7).

Phospholipid (fos'-foh-lip'-id). A lipid containing glycerol, fatty acids, a phosphate group, and an alcohol; glycerophospholipids (also called *phosphoglycerides*) and sphingolipids are examples (Chap. 6).

Photoautotroph (foh'-toe-aw'-toe-trof). An organism that uses light as an energy source and carbon dioxide as a carbon source; a type of autotroph (Chap. 7).

Photoheterotroph (foh'-toe-het'-er-oh-trof). An organism that uses light as an energy source and organic compounds as a carbon source; a type of heterotroph (Chap. 7).

Photomicrograph. Photograph taken through the lens system of a compound light microscope (Chap. 2).

Photosynthesis (foe-toe-sin'-thuh-sis). Chemical process by which light energy is converted into chemical energy; an organism that produces organic substances in this manner is said to be *photosynthetic* (Chap. 3).

Phototroph (foh'-toe-trof). An organism that uses light as an energy source (Chap. 7).

Phycologist (fy-kol'-oh-jist). One who specializes in the science of phycology (Chap. 1).

Phycology (fy-kol'-oh-gee). The study of algae (Chap. 1).

Phycotoxicosis (fy'-koh-tox-uh-coh-sis), pl. *phycotoxicoses*. A microbial intoxication caused by a phycotoxin (Chap. 5).

Phycotoxins (fy'-ko-tox-inz). Toxins produced by algae (Chap. 5).

Phytoplankton (fy'-toh-plank'-ton). Microscopic marine plants and algae that are components of plankton (Chap. 1).

Pili (py'-ly), sing. *pilus*. Hairlike surface projections possessed by some bacteria (called *piliated bacteria*); most are organelles of attachment; also called *fimbriae*; certain specialized pili are called *sex pili*, (Chap. 3).

Pinocytosis (pin'-oh-sigh-toe'-sis). A process resembling phagocytosis but used to engulf and ingest liquids rather than solid matter (Chap. 5).

Piezophile (peez'-oh-file). An organism that thrives under high environmental pressure; such an organism is said to be *piezophilic* (Chap. 8).

Plague (playg). A bacterial disease caused by *Yersinia pestis*, a Gram-negative bacillus; transmitted by rodent fleas (Chap. 19).

Plankton (plank'-ton). Microscopic organisms in the ocean that serve as the starting point of many food chains (Chap. 1).

Plasma (plaz'-muh). The liquid portion of circulating blood (Chap. 13).

Plasma (plaz'-muh) **Cell.** An antibody-secreting cell produced by a stimulated B cell (Chap. 16).

Plasmid (plaz'-mid). An extrachromosomal genetic element; a molecule of DNA that can function and replicate while physically separate from the bacterial chromosome (Chap. 3).

Plasmolysis (plaz-moll'-uh-sis). Cell shrinkage as a result of a loss of water from the cell's cytoplasm (Chap. 8).

Plasmoptysis (plaz-mop'-tuh-sis). The escape of cytoplasm from a ruptured cell (Chap. 8).

Plastid. A membrane-bound organelle containing photosynthetic pigment; plastids are the sites of photosynthesis; a *chloroplast* is a plastid that contains chlorophyll (Chap. 3).

Pleomorphism (plee-oh-more'-fizm). Existing in more than one form; also known as *polymorphism*; an organism that exhibits pleomorphism is said to be *pleomorphic* (Chap. 4).

Pneumonia (new-mow'-nee-uh). Inflammation of one or both lungs (Chap. 17).

Polymer (pol'-uh-mer). A large molecule consisting of repeating subunits; nucleic acids, polypeptides, and polysaccharides are examples (Chap. 6).

Polypeptide (pol-ee-pep'-tide). A protein consisting of more than three amino acids held together by peptide bonds (Chap. 6).

Polyribosomes (pol-ee-ry'-boh-somz). Two or more ribosomes connected by a molecule of messenger RNA (mRNA) (Chap. 3).

Polysaccharide (pol-ee-sack'-uh-ride). Carbohydrate consisting of many sugar units; glycogen, cellulose, and starch are examples (Chap. 6).

Polyunsaturated Fatty Acid. A fatty acid containing more than one double bond (Chap. 6).

Population Growth Curve. A graph that represents changes in the number of viable bacteria in a population over time; constructed by plotting the logarithm ($\log_{10}$) of the number of viable bacteria (on the vertical or y axis) against the incubation time (on the horizontal or x axis) (Chap. 8).

Potassium Hydroxide Preparation. A laboratory procedure primarily used to observe fungal elements in skin scrapings, hair clippings, and nail clippings; usually referred to as the KOH prep (Chap. 20).

Preliminary Report. Any report furnished by the laboratory before publication of the final report (Chap. 13).

Prevalence. The number of cases of a particular disease existing in a given population during a specific period of time (period prevalence) or at a particular moment in time (point prevalence) (Chap. 11).

Primary Atypical Pneumonia. An older term for mycoplasmal pneumonia; caused by the bacterium, *Mycoplasma pneumoniae* (Chap. 19).

Primary Disease. The initial disease; often creates the conditions that lead to a secondary disease; if the primary disease is an infection, it is referred to as a *primary infection* (Chap. 14).

Primary Response. The immune response that occurs the first time an antigen enters a person's body (Chap. 16).

Prions (pree'-onz). Infectious protein molecules (i.e., proteins capable of causing certain diseases of animals and humans) (Chap. 4).

Procaryotic (pro'-kar-ee-ah'-tick) **Cells.** Cells lacking a true nucleus; organisms consisting of such cells are referred to as *procaryotes*; can also be spelled prokaryotic (Chap. 3).

Prophage (pro'-faj). During lysogeny, all that remains of the infecting bacteriophage is its DNA; in this form, the bacteriophage is referred to as a prophage (Chap. 7).

Prophylactic (pro'-fuh-lak'-tick) **Agent.** A drug used to prevent a disease (Chap. 17).

Prophylaxis (pro-fuh-lak'-sis). Prevention of a disease or a process that can lead to a disease (e.g., taking antimalarial medication in a malarious area) (Chap. 17).

Prostaglandins (pros-tuh-glan'-dinz). Physiologically active tissue substances that cause many effects, including vasodilation, vasoconstriction, and stimulation of smooth muscle (Chap. 15).

Prostatitis (pros-tuh-ty'-tis). Inflammation or infection of the prostate (Chap. 17).

Prostration (pros-tray'-shun). Significant loss of strength; the patient is prostrate (lying flat) (Chap. 13).

Protective Antibodies. Antibodies that protect an individual from infection or reinfection (Chap. 16).

Protective Environments. Hospital rooms for placement of patients who are especially vulnerable to infection; Protective Environments are under positive pressure, and vented air that enters these rooms passes through HEPA filters. (Chap. 12).

Proteins (pro'-teens). Macromolecules consisting of two, three, or more amino acids (Chap. 6).

Protists (pro'-tists). Members of the Kingdom Protista; includes algae and protozoa (Chap. 3).

Protoplasm (pro'-toe-plazm). The semifluid matter within living cells; *cytoplasm* and *nucleoplasm* are two types of protoplasm (Chap. 3).

Protozoa (pro-toe-zoe'-uh), sing. *protozoan*. Eucaryotic microorganisms frequently found in water and soil; some are pathogens; usually unicellular (Chap. 5).

Protozoologist (pro'-toe-zoe-ol'-oh-jist). One who specializes in protozoology (Chap. 1).

Protozoology (pro'-toe-zoe-ol'-oh-gee). The study of protozoa (Chap. 1).

Pseudohypha (su-doh-hy-fuh), pl. *pseudohyphae*. An elongated string of yeast buds (Chap. 5).

Pseudomembranous (soo-doe-mem'-bran-us) **Colitis** (koh-ly'-tis). Inflammation of the intestinal mucosa, with the formation and passage of pseudomembranous material in the stools; often a consequence of antibiotic therapy; most often caused by a cytotoxin produced by *C. difficile*, an anaerobic, spore-forming Gram-positive bacillus; also called *pseudomembranous* enterocolitis (Chap. 19).

Pseudomonicidal (su'-doh-moan-uh-side'-ul) **Agent.** A drug or disinfectant that kills *Pseudomonas* spp. (Chap. 8).

Pseudopodium (su-doe-poh'-dee-um), pl. *pseudopodia*. A temporary extension of protoplasm that is extended by an ameba or leukocyte for locomotion or the engulfment of particulate matter; also called a *pseudopod* (Chap. 5).

Psychroduric (sigh-krow-dur'-ick) **Organisms.** Organisms able to endure very cold temperatures (Chap. 8).

Psychrophile (sigh'-krow-file). An organism that grows best at a low temperature (0°C–32°C), with optimum growth occurring at 15°C to 20°C; such an organism is said to be *psychrophilic* (Chap. 8).

Psychrotroph (sigh'-krow-trof). A psychrophile that grows best at refrigerator temperature (4°C); such an organism is said to be *psychrotrophic* (Chap. 8).

Pure Culture. When only one type of organism is growing on or in a culture medium in the laboratory; no other types of organisms are present (Chap. 1).

Purine (pure'-een). A double-ringed nitrogenous base found in certain nucleotides and, therefore, in nucleic acids; adenine and guanine are purines found in both DNA and RNA (Chap. 6).

Purulent Exudate. A thick, greenish yellow exudate that contains many live and dead leukocytes; also known as *pus* (Chap. 15).

Pustule (pus'-chul). A small rounded elevation of the skin that contains purulent material (pus) (Chap. 17).

Pyelonephritis (py'-uh-low-nef-ry'-tis). Inflammation of certain areas of the kidneys, most often the result of bacterial infection (Chap. 17).

Pyogenic (py-oh-jen'-ick). Pus-producing; causing the production of pus (Chap. 15).

Pyogenic Microorganisms. Pathogens that cause pus-containing infectious processes (Chap. 15).

Pyrimidine (pi-rim'-uh-deen). A single-ringed nitrogenous base found in certain nucleotides and, therefore, in nucleic acids; thymine and cytosine are pyrimidines found in DNA; cytosine and uracil are pyrimidines found in RNA (Chap. 6).

Pyrogen (py'-roh-jen). A fever-producing substance; also referred to as a *pyrogenic substance* (Chap. 14).

R

R-Factor. A plasmid that contains multiple drug resistance genes; a bacterium that possesses an R-factor is multidrug-resistant (i.e., it is a "superbug"); the "R" stands for resistance (Chap. 7).

Receptors. Molecules on the surface of a host cell that a particular pathogen is able to recognize and attach to; also known as *integrins* (Chap. 14).

Reduction (ree-duk'-shun). As used in this book, the gain of one or more electrons, thus making the atom more electronegative (Chap. 7).

Regulatory T Cells. T cells that regulate various aspects of immune responses; helper T cells and suppressor T cells are examples (Chap. 16).

Reservoirs (rez'-ev-wars) **of Infection.** Places where pathogens are living and from which they can be transmitted to humans; reservoirs of infection may be living or nonliving; sometimes simply referred to as *reservoirs* (Chap. 11).

Resident Microflora. Members of the indigenous microflora that are more or less permanent residents (Chap. 10).

Resistance Factor. See *R-factor*.

Resolving Power. The ability of the eye or an optical instrument to distinguish detail, such as the separation of closely adjacent objects; also called *resolution* (Chap. 2).

Reticuloendothelial (ree-tick'-yu-loh-en-doh-thee'-lee-ul) **System (RES).** A collection of phagocytic cells that includes macrophages and cells that line the sinusoids of the spleen, lymph nodes, and bone marrow (Chap. 15).

Ribonucleic (ry-boe-new-klee'-ick) **Acid (RNA).** A macromolecule of which there are three main types: messenger RNA (mRNA), ribosomal RNA (rRNA), and transfer RNA (tRNA); found in all cells but only in certain viruses (called *RNA viruses*) (Chap. 3).

Ribosomal (rye-boh-so'-mul) **RNA (rRNA).** The type of RNA molecule found within ribosomes (Chap. 6).

Ribosomes (ry'-boh-soams). Organelles that are the sites of protein synthesis in both procaryotic and eucaryotic cells (Chap. 3).

Ringworm Infections. See *tinea infections*.

RNA Nucleotides. The building blocks of RNA; each RNA nucleotide consists of a nitrogenous base, ribose, and a phosphate group (Chap. 6).

RNA Polymerase (poh-lim'-er-ace). The enzyme required for transcription (Chap. 6).

Rocky Mountain Spotted Fever (RMSF). A bacterial disease caused by *Rickettsia rickettsii*, an obligate intracellular pathogen (Chap. 19).

Rough Endoplasmic Reticulum (RER). See *endoplasmic reticulum* (Chap. 3).

Rubella (roo-bell'-uh) **Virus.** The virus that causes rubella (German measles) (Chap.18).

Rubeola (roo-bee-oh'-luh) **Virus.** The virus that causes measles (Chap. 18).

S

Salmonellosis (sal'-moh-nel-oh'-sis). A diarrheal disease caused by Gram-negative bacilli in the genus *Salmonella* (Chap. 19).

Salpingitis (sal-pin-jy'-tis). As used in this book, inflammation of the fallopian tube (Chap. 17).

Sanitization (san'-uh-tuh-zay'-shun). The process of making something sanitary (healthful); usually involves reducing the number of microbes present to a safe level (Chap. 8).

Saprophyte (sap'-row-fight). An organism that lives on dead or decaying organic matter; such an organism is said to be *saprophytic* (Chap. 1).

Saturated Fatty Acid. A fatty acid containing no double bonds (Chap. 6).

Scanning Electron Micrograph. Photograph taken through the lens system of a scanning electron microscope (Chap. 2).

Scanning Electron Microscope. A type of electron microscope; enables the operator to observe the outer surfaces of specimens (i.e., to observe surface detail) (Chap. 2).

Sebaceous (seb-ay'-shous) **Gland.** An oil gland located in the dermis (Chap. 17).

Sebum (see'-bum). The oily secretion produced by sebaceous glands of the skin (Chap. 17).

Secondary Disease. A disease that follows an initial disease; if the secondary disease is an infection, it is referred to as a *secondary infection* (Chap. 14).

Secondary Response. The immune response that occurs the second time an antigen enters a person's body; also known as a *memory response* or an *anaphylactic response* (Chap. 16).

Selective Medium. A culture medium that allows a certain organism or group of organisms to grow while inhibiting growth of all other organisms (Chap. 8).

Selective Permeability. An attribute of membranes whereby only certain substances are able to cross the membranes (Chap. 3).

Semisynthetic Antibiotic. An antibiotic that has been chemically altered, usually to increase the drug's spectrum of activity (Chap. 9).

Sepsis. The presence of pathogens or their toxins in the bloodstream; often used as a synonym for *septicemia* (Chap. 8).

Septate Hyphae. Hyphae that contain septa (cross-walls) (Chap. 5).

Septic Shock. A type of shock resulting from sepsis or septicemia (Chap. 14).

Septicemia (sep-tuh-see'-me-uh). A serious disease consisting of chills, fever, prostration, and the presence of pathogens or their toxins in the blood (Chap. 13).

Serologic (ser-oh-loj'-ick) **Procedures.** Immunodiagnostic test procedures performed on serum (Chap. 16).

Serology (suh-rol'-oh-jee). That branch of science concerned with serum and serologic procedures (Chap. 13).

Serum (seer'-um), pl. *sera*. The liquid portion of blood that remains after coagulation (clotting) (Chap. 13).

Severe Acute Respiratory Syndrome (SARS). A pulmonary disease caused by SARS coronavirus (SARS-CoV) (Chap. 18).

Sex Pilus. A specialized pilus through which one bacterial cell (the donor cell) transfers genetic material to another bacterial cell (the recipient cell), in a process called *conjugation* (Chap. 3).

Sexual Reproduction. In this type of reproduction, two parents give rise to offspring that have unique combinations of genes inherited from both parents (Chap. 3).

Shigellosis (shig-uh-loh'-sis). A diarrheal disease caused by Gram-negative bacilli in the genus *Shigella* (Chap. 19).

Shingles. A painful nerve disease caused by reactivation of varicella virus (chickenpox virus) (Chap. 18).

Shock. A sudden, often severe, physical or mental disturbance, usually resulting from low blood pressure and a lack of oxygen in organs (Chap. 14).

Signs of a disease. Abnormalities indicative of disease that are discovered on examination of a patient; objective findings; examples include abnormal laboratory results; abnormal heart or breath sounds; lumps; abnormalities revealed by radiographs, computed tomographic scans, magnetic resonance imaging, electrocardiography, and ultrasound (Chap. 14).

Silent Mutation. A mutation that is neither beneficial nor harmful to the mutant organism; the organism is unaware of the mutation; also called a *neutral mutation* (Chap. 7).

Simple Microscope. A microscope containing only one magnifying lens (Chap. 2).

Simple Stain. A single dye that is used to stain objects (e.g., bacterial cells), enabling scientists to gain information about the objects (e.g., size, shape) (Chap. 4).

Single Bond. A type of chemical bond containing one pair of shared electrons (Chap. 6).

Sinusitis (sigh-neu-sigh'-tis). Inflammation of the lining of one or more of the paranasal sinuses (Chap. 17).

Slime Layer. An unorganized, loosely attached layer of glycocalyx surrounding a bacterial cell (Chap. 3).

Slime Mould. A eucaryotic organism having characteristics of protozoa and fungi; there are two types: cellular and acellular slime moulds (Chap. 5).

Smooth Endoplasmic Reticulum (SER). See *endoplasmic reticulum.*

Solute (sol'-yute). The dissolved substance in a solution; for example, sucrose (table sugar) when it is dissolved in water (Chap. 8).

Solution (soh-loo'-shun). A homogeneous molecular mixture; generally, a substance dissolved in water (referred to as an aqueous solution); solute plus solvent (Chap. 8).

Solvent (sol'-vent). A liquid in which another substance dissolves (Chap. 8).

Species (spe'-shez), pl. *species*. A specific member of a given genus; (e.g., *E. coli* is a species in the genus *Escherichia*); the name of a particular species consists of two parts—the generic name ("the first name") and the specific epithet ("the second name"); singular species is abbreviated sp., and plural species is abbreviated spp. (Chap. 3).

Specific Epithet. The second part ("second name") in the name of a species; the specific epithet cannot be used alone (Chap. 3).

Specific Host Defense Mechanisms. Host defense mechanisms directed against a specific invading pathogen; synonym for the immune system or the third line of defense (Chap. 15).

Spirochetes (spy'-roh-keets). Spiral-shaped bacteria; (e.g., *Treponema pallidum*, the causative agent of syphilis) (Chap. 3).

Splenomegaly (splen-oh-meg'-uh-lee). Enlargement of the spleen (Chap. 17).

Sporadic (spoh-rad'-ick) **Disease.** A disease that occurs occasionally, usually affecting only one person; neither endemic nor epidemic (Chap. 11).

Sporicidal (spor-uh-sigh'-dull) **Agent.** A chemical agent that kills spores; a *sporicide* (Chap. 8).

Sporulation (spor'-you-lay'-shun). Production of spores (Chap. 3).

Sputum. Pus that accumulates in the lungs of patients with lower respiratory tract infections such as pneumonia and tuberculosis (Chap. 13).

Standard Precautions. Safety precautions taken by healthcare workers to protect themselves and their patients from infection; these precautions are taken for *all* patients and *all* patient specimens (body substances); includes safety precautions previously referred to as universal precautions or universal body substance precautions (Chap. 12).

Staphylococci (staff"-eh-low-kok'-sigh). Cocci arranged in clusters, such as in the genus *Staphylococcus* (Chap. 4).

Staphylokinase (staf'-uh-low-ky'-nace). A kinase produced by *S. aureus* (Chap. 14).

Starch. A polysaccharide storage material found in plants (Chap. 6).

Stationary Phase. The part of a bacterial growth phase during which organisms are dying at the same rate at which new organisms are being produced; the third phase in a bacterial growth curve (Chap. 8).

STD. Sexually transmitted disease (Chap. 17).

Sterile (stir'-ill). Free of all living microorganisms, including spores (Chap. 8).

Sterile Techniques. Techniques used in an attempt to create an environment that is sterile (devoid of microbes) (Chap. 8).

Sterilization (stir'-uh-luh-zay'-shun). The destruction of *all* microbes in or on something (e.g., on surgical instruments) (Chap. 8).

Stigma. A photosensing (light sensing) organelle; also known as an *eyespot* (Chap. 5).

Streptobacilli (strep'-toh-bah-sill'-eye). Bacilli arranged in chains of varying lengths (Chap. 4).

Streptococci (strep'-toh-kok'-sigh). Cocci arranged in chains of varying lengths, such as in the genus *Streptococcus* (Chap. 4).

Streptokinase (strep'-toh-ky'-nace). A kinase produced by streptococci (Chap. 14).

Structural Staining Procedures. Staining procedures used to stain bacterial structures such as capsules, flagella, and endospores (Chap. 4).

Sty (Stye). Inflammation of a sebaceous gland that opens into a follicle of an eyelash (Chap. 17).

Syphilis (sif'-uh-lis). A sexually transmitted bacterial disease, caused by the spirochete *T. pallidum* (Chap. 19).

Subclinical Disease. See *asymptomatic disease*.

Substrate (sub'-strayt). The chemical substance that is acted upon or changed by an enzyme (Chap. 6).

Subunit Vaccine. A vaccine that uses antigenic (antibody-stimulating) portions of a pathogen, rather than using the whole pathogen; also known as an *acellular vaccine* (Chap. 16).

Superinfection (sue'-per-in-fek'-shun). An overgrowth or population explosion of one or more particular pathogens; often pathogens that are resistant to an antimicrobial agent that a patient is receiving (Chap. 9).

Surgical Asepsis. The absence of microorganisms in a surgical environment (e.g., an operating room) (Chap. 12).

Surgical Aseptic Techniques. Procedures followed and steps taken to ensure surgical asepsis (Chap. 12).

Symbionts (sim'-bee-ontz). The parties in a symbiotic relationship (Chap. 10).

Symbiosis (sim-bee-oh'-sis). The living together or close association of two dissimilar organisms (usually two different species) (Chap. 10).

Symptomatic Disease. A disease in which the patient experiences symptoms (Chap. 14).

Symptoms of a Disease. Indications of disease that are experienced by the patient; subjective; examples include aches and pains, chills, blurred vision, nausea (Chap. 14).

Synergism (sin'-er-jiz-um). When two or more drugs work together to accomplish a cure rate that is greater than either drug could accomplish by itself (Chap. 9).

Synergistic (sin-er-jis'-tik) **Infection.** An infection caused by the correlated action of two or more microorganisms; also known as a *polymicrobial infection*; examples include trench mouth and bacterial vaginosis (Chap. 10).

Synergistic Relationship. A symbiotic relationship in which two or more microorganisms work together to accomplish a task (e.g., to cause a synergistic infection) (Chap. 10).

Systemic Infection. An infection that has spread throughout the body; also known as a *generalized infection* (Chap. 14).

T

T Cells (T Lymphocytes). A category of leukocytes that play a variety of important roles in the immune system (Chap. 16).

T-Dependent Antigens. Antigens that require T-helper cells for their processing in the body (Chap. 16).

T-Independent Antigens. Antigens that do not require T-helper cells for their processing in the body (Chap. 16).

Taxa, sing. *taxon*. The names given to various groups in taxonomy; the usual taxa are kingdoms, phyla (or divisions), classes, orders, families, genera, species, and subspecies (Chap. 3).

Taxonomy (tak-sawn'-oh-me). The systematic classification of living things (Chap. 3).

Teichoic (tie-ko'-ick) **Acids.** Polymers found in the cell walls of Gram-positive bacteria (Chap. 4).

Temperate Bacteriophage. A bacteriophage whose genome incorporates into and replicates with the genome of the host bacterium; also known as a *lysogenic bacteriophage* (Chap. 4).

Tetanospasmin (tet'-uh-noh-spaz'-min). The neurotoxin produced by *Clostridium tetani* that causes tetanus (Chap. 14).

Tetanus (tet'-uh-nus). A bacterial disease of the central nervous system caused by a neurotoxin produced by *C. tetani*, an anaerobic, spore-forming Gram-positive bacillus (Chap. 19).

Tetrad. A packet of four cocci (Chap. 4).

Tetrose. A monosaccharide containing four carbon atoms (Chap. 6).

Thermal Death Point (TDP). The temperature required to kill all microorganisms in a liquid culture in 10 minutes at pH 7 (Chap. 8).

Thermal Death Time (TDT). The length of time required to kill all microorganisms in a liquid culture at a given temperature (Chap. 8).

Thermophile (ther'-mow-file). An organism that thrives at a temperature of 50°C or higher; such an organism is said to be *thermophilic* (Chap. 8).

Thrush. An oral infection caused by the yeast *C. albicans* (Chap. 20).

Tinea (tin'-ee-uh) **Barbae.** A fungal infection of the beard and moustache (Chap. 20).

Tinea Capitis. A fungal infection of the scalp, eyebrows, and eyelashes (Chap. 20).

Tinea Corporis. A fungal infection of the face, trunk, and major limbs (Chap. 20).

Tinea Cruris. A fungal infection of the groin and perineal and perianal areas (Chap. 20).

Tinea Infections. Fungal infections of the skin, hair, and nails; also called *ringworm infections*; named for the part of the body that is affected (Chap. 20).

Tinea Pedis. Also called *athlete's foot*; a fungal infection of the soles of the feet and between the toes (Chap. 20).

Tinea Unguium. A fungal infection of the nails; also called *onychomycosis* (Chap. 20).

Toxemia (tok-see'-me-uh). The presence of toxins in the blood (Chap. 13).

Toxigenicity (tok'-suh-juh-nis'-uh-tee) or **Toxinogenicity** (tok'-suh-no-juh-nisv-uh-tee). The ability to produce toxin; a microorganism capable of producing a toxin is said to be *toxigenic* (or *toxinogenic*) (Chap. 14).

Toxin (tok'-sin). As used in this book, a poisonous substance produced by a microorganism (Chap. 1).

Toxoid (tok'-soyd). A toxin that has been altered in such a way as to destroy its toxicity but retain its antigenicity; certain toxoids are used as vaccines (Chap. 16).

Toxoid Vaccine. A vaccine prepared from a toxoid (Chap. 16).

Trachoma (truh-koh'-muh). A bacterial eye disease caused by *Chlamydia trachomatis*, an obligate intracellular pathogen (Chap. 19).

Transcription (tran-skrip'-shun). Transfer of the genetic code from one type of nucleic acid to another; usually, the synthesis of an mRNA molecule using a DNA template (Chap. 6).

Transduction (trans-duk'-shun). Transfer of genetic material (and its phenotypic expression) from one bacterial cell to another via bacteriophages; in *generalized transduction*, the transducing bacteriophage is able to transfer any gene of the donor bacterium; in *specialized transduction*, the bacteriophage is able to transfer only one or some of the donor bacterium's genes (Chap. 7).

Transfer RNA (tRNA). The type of RNA molecule that is capable of combining with (and thus activating) a specific amino acid; involved in protein synthesis (translation); the anticodon on a tRNA molecule recognizes the codon on an mRNA molecule (Chap. 6).

Transferrin (trans-fer'-in). A glycoprotein, synthesized in the liver, used to store iron and deliver it to host cells (Chap. 15).

Transformation (trans-for-may'-shun). In microbial genetics, transfer of genetic information between bacteria via uptake or absorption of naked DNA; bacteria capable of absorbing naked DNA from their environment are said to be *competent* (Chap. 7).

Transient Bacteremia. A temporary bacteremia (Chap. 17).

Transient Microflora. Temporary members of the indigenous microflora (Chap. 10).

Translation (trans-lay'-shun). The process by which mRNA, tRNA, and ribosomes effect the production of proteins from amino acids; translation is also known as *protein synthesis* (Chap. 6).

Transmission-Based Precautions. Safety precautions taken by healthcare workers, in addition to standard precautions, to protect themselves and their patients from infection via airborne, contact, or droplet routes of transmission (Chap. 12).

Transmission Electron Micrograph. Photograph taken through the lens system of a transmission electron microscope (Chap. 2).

Transmission Electron Microscope. A type of electron microscope in which electrons are transmitted through very thin sections of specimens; enables the operator to observe internal detail (Chap. 2).

Trematodes (trem-uh-toadz). A category of flatworms; often referred to as *flukes* (Chap. 21).

Trench Mouth. Synonym for acute necrotizing ulcerative gingivitis (ANUG); also called *Vincent's angina*; involves painful, bleeding gums and tonsils, erosion of gum tissue, and swollen lymph nodes beneath the jaw; a synergistic infection involving two or more species of anaerobic bacteria of the indigenous oral microflora (Chap. 19).

Triglyceride (try-glis'-er-ide). A lipid that is composed of glycerol (a three-carbon alcohol) and three fatty acids; fats and oils are examples (Chap. 6).

Triose. A monosaccharide containing three carbon atoms (Chap. 6).

Tripeptide (try-pep'-tide). A protein consisting of three amino acids held together by peptide bonds (Chap. 6).

Triple Bond. A type of chemical bond containing three pairs of shared electrons (Chap. 6).

Trophozoite (trof-oh-zoe'-ite). The motile, feeding, dividing stage in a protozoan's life cycle (Chap. 5).

Tuberculocidal (too-bur'-kyu-low-sigh'-dull) **Agent.** A chemical or drug that kills the bacterium that causes tuberculosis (*Mycobacterium tuberculosis*); also known as a *tuberculocide* (Chap. 8).

Tularemia (too-luh-ree'-me-uh). A bacterial disease caused by *Francisella tularensis*, a Gram-negative bacillus (Chap. 19).

Tyndallization (tin-dull-uh-zay'-shun). A process of boiling and cooling in which spores are allowed to germinate and then the vegetative bacteria are killed by boiling again (Chap. 3).

Typhoid Fever. A bacterial disease caused by *Salmonella typhi*, a Gram-negative bacillus (Chap. 19).

U

Ubiquitous (you-bik'-wah-tus). Present everywhere (Chap. 1).

Ureteritis (you-ree-ter-eye'-tis). Inflammation or infection of a ureter (Chap. 17).

Urethritis (you-ree-thry'-tis). Inflammation or infection of the urethra (Chap. 17).

V

Vaccine (vak'-seen). Any preparation which, after injection (or ingestion, in some cases), produces active acquired immunity (Chap. 16).

Vaccinia (vak-sin'-ee-uh) **Virus.** The virus that causes cowpox (also known as *vaccinia*); used in a vaccine to convey resistance to smallpox (Chap. 18).

Vaginitis (vaj-uh-ny'-tis). Inflammation of the vagina (Chap. 10).

Vaginosis (vag-uh-no'-sis). Infection of the vagina, with no influx of leukocytes (Chap. 10).

Varicella (var-uh-sell'-uh) **Virus.** The virus that causes chickenpox (also known as *varicella*) and shingles (Chap. 18).

Variola (var-ee'-oh-luh) **Virus.** The virus that causes smallpox (also known as *variola*). (Chap. 18).

Vasoconstriction (vay'-so-kon-strik'-shun). A decrease in the diameter of blood vessels (Chap. 15).

Vasodilation (vay'-soh-die-lay'-shun). An increase in the diameter of blood vessels (Chap. 15).

Vectors (vek'-tour). As used in this book, invertebrate animals (e.g., ticks, mites, mosquitoes, fleas) capable of transmitting pathogens among vertebrates (Chap. 4).

Vegetative Hyphae. Hyphae that lie below the surface of whatever a fungal mycelium is growing on (Chap. 5).

Viable Plate Count. A laboratory technique used to determine the number of living bacteria in a milliliter of liquid; involves the use of plated media (Chap. 8).

Viral Rhinitis (rye-ny'-tis). A synonym for the common cold (Chap. 18).

Viremia (vy-ree'-me-uh). The presence of viruses in the blood (Chap. 13).

Viricidal (vy-ruh-sigh'-dull) **Agent.** A chemical or drug that inactivates a virus, rendering it noninfectious; can also be spelled *virucidal agent*; also known as a *viricide* or a *virucide* (Chap. 8).

Virion (veer'-ee-on). A complete, infectious viral particle (i.e., a virus that contains all of its parts) (Chap. 4).

Viroids (vi'-roydz). Infectious RNA molecules (i.e., RNA molecules capable of causing certain plant diseases) (Chap. 4).

Virologist (vi-rol'-oh-jist). One who studies or works with viruses (Chap. 1).

Virology (vi-rol'-oh-gee). That branch of science concerned with the study of viruses (Chap. 1).

Virulence (veer'-u-lenz). A measure of pathogenicity (i.e., some pathogens are more or less *virulent* than others) (Chap. 14).

Virulence Factors. Attributes or properties of a microorganism that contribute to its virulence or pathogenicity (e.g., certain exoenzymes and toxins produced by pathogenic bacteria) (Chap. 14).

Virulent (veer'-yu-lent) **Strains.** Strains that are pathogenic; capable of causing disease (Chap. 14).

Virulent Bacteriophage. A bacteriophage that regularly causes lysis of the bacteria it infects; causes the lytic cycle to occur (Chap. 4).

Viruses (vi'-rus-ez), sing. *virus*. Acellular microbes that are smaller than bacteria; obligate intracellular parasites; sometimes referred to as *infectious particles* rather than microbes (Chap. 4).

Vulvovaginitis (vul'-voh-vaj-uh-ny'-tis). Inflammation of the vulva (the external genitalia of women) and the vagina (Chap. 17).

W

Wandering Macrophages. Macrophages that migrate in the bloodstream and tissues; sometimes called *free macrophages* (Chap. 15).

Waxes. Lipids consisting of a saturated fatty acid and a long-chain alcohol (Chap. 6).

White Piedra. A fungal hair infection usually caused by the mould *Trichosporon beigelii* (Chap. 20).

Z

Zoonoses (zoh-oh-no'-seez), sing. *zoonosis*. Infectious diseases transmissible from animals to humans; also known as *zoonotic diseases* (Chap. 1).

Zooplankton (zoh'-oh-plank'-ton). Microscopic marine animals that are components of plankton (Chap. 1).

Page numbers in *italics* denote figures; those followed by an n or t indicate material in notes or tables, respectively.